PANCE PREP PEARLS

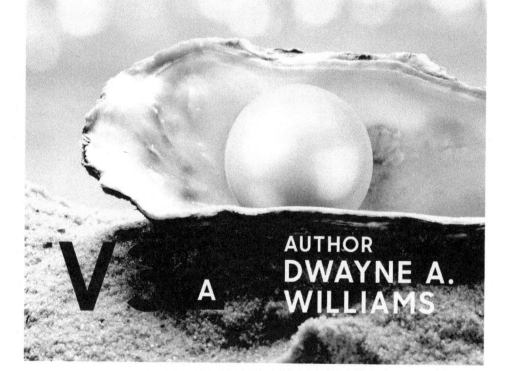

ISBN: 9781712861165
Imprint: Independently published
Kindle Direct Publishing Platform

Printed by Kindle direct publishing

DEDICATION

I would like to thank the Cornell and Long Island University Physician Assistant Programs for giving me the platform to teach. Thanks to my foundation teachers Marion Masterson, Medea Valdez, Gerard Marciano. A very special thanks to Stacey Hughes (words can't describe my gratitude to you), Sharon Verity and William Ameres for being my inspirational teachers as a student. To all those who contributed to making this profession great and to all my fellow educators who contribute to this field on so many levels.

Thanks to all of the owners of the photos. Your images helped to make this book a visual experience. Your contribution is invaluable. An extra special thanks to **Ian Baker**, the illustrator of most of the pictures in the book. You added a special touch to this project. Thanks Dr. Frank Gaillard and Jason Davis for your help during the process. Special thanks to **Kevin Young**, **Xiana Flowers & Kristen Risom** (the best illustrators I know!)

Special thanks to my parents Winifred & Robert Williams. Xiomara & Froylan Flowers (my second parents), Mercedes Avalon, Gilda Cain (the best nurse I know!) and my big brother Danilo Avalon.

To my gurus: Stacey Hughes, Tse-Hwa Yao, Ingrid Voigt, Dr. Antonio Dajer & Dr. Kenneth Rose.

Thanks to Isaak Yakubov (my Akim) for the Ultimate Mnemonic Comic Book and the amazing journey we have embarked on together. Thanks to Rachel Lehrer for allowing me to be a part of the FlipMed medical app project. I will make good on the promise I made to you.

Pamela Bodley, the world's best manager. You are the real boss lady!

Last but not least a very special thank you to my PPP warriors! I enjoy our interactions on social media and at conferences. This book would not have been the success it is without the support of each and every one you! YOU ARE A WARRIOR.....WARRIORS WIN!

PREFACE

STUDENTS

This book is designed for use in both didactic and clinical education. It is formatted to make you a rockstar on clinical rotations! It is a ***review book***, which means ***it is not meant to replace textbook-based education*** but as an additional study tool to enhance your knowledge base. Textbooks provide the foundation for understanding and learning medicine.

PRACTITIONERS

This book is purposed to increase your knowledge & retention of important clinical information and for use as a quick resource that is not time consuming.

THE STYLE OF PPP

Pance Prep Pearls is not written in the traditional style of a textbook but rather to feel like a collection of notes, drafts, charts, mnemonics and clinical pearls to make learning effective while entertaining. The use of bold and italics are to help you to organize the information and stress the importance of certain aspects of the disease states. The charts are designed for you to compare and contrast commonly grouped diseases and high-yield information. It is loaded with helpful algorithms to help you see the big picture on how to approach the disease.

I personally recommend that you use what I call the 5 P's of the ***Patient-Centered Learning Model*** as you study the different diseases:

1. **Pathophysiology:** imagine explaining the pathophysiology of a disease to your patient in 1 sentence (2 sentences maximum) in simple terms. Understanding the pathophysiology will often explain the clinical manifestations, physical examination findings, why certain tests are used and usually the treatment reverses the pathophysiology. This step is often skipped but is probably the most important (in terms of knowledge retention).
2. **Present** – based on the pathophysiology, how would this patient present? Know both the classic and the common findings and presentations (they aren't always the same).
3. **Pick it up**? – How would you diagnose the disease. Make sure to understand what is usually first line vs. gold standard (definitive diagnosis). Understand the indications and contraindications for each test.
4. **Palliate** – how do you treat (palliate) the disorder. Many people can list out the treatments but fail to remember first line treatments vs. alternative treatments. Make sure to understand the indications and contraindications of each treatment.
5. **Pharmacology** – understand the mechanism of action and understand why a medication is used for that disease. This helps to reinforce the pathophysiology as well as the presentation of the disease since the pharmacology often reverses the problem or treats the symptoms. A very important point is that if you see a medication that is used for different disorders, try to understand what connects the use of that drug to the different disorders.

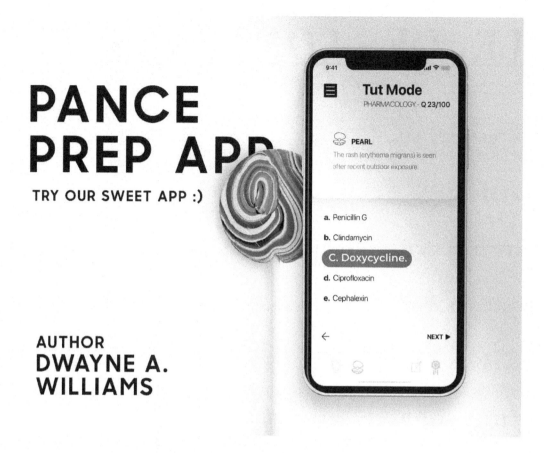

Over 8,600 clinically-based practice examination questions specifically formulated to enhance clinical skills and improve performance on examinations, such as the PANCE, PANRE, OSCES, USMLE, end of rotation examinations and comprehensive medical examinations.

This app will intuitively know your areas of weakness and give you a plan to improve your overall performance. Special clinical pearls, disease review, explanation of the answers, test taking strategies and much more.

3 modes,
Timed mode to simulate the exams
Tutor mode that allows you to review the disease states in addition to the questions and
improve mode to enhance your weak areas.

For every question in tutor mode, there is a feature for a hint to see if you are going in the right direction, answer explanation, a clinical pearl, and a bonus questions. Create your own examination based on organ systems or task areas. The ultimate study and exam preparation app!

TABLE OF CONTENTS

CHAPTER 1 - CARDIOVASCULAR DISORDERS

DILATED CARDIOMYOPATHY (DCMP)

- **Systolic dysfunction, leading to a dilated, weak heart.**

- Most common type of Cardiomyopathy (95%).

RISK FACTORS
- Most common 20-60 years of age, men.

ETIOLOGIES
- **Idiopathic most common cause** (may be familial).

- Infections: **viral most common** (especially the **enteroviruses - Coxsackievirus B**, Echovirus).

- Postviral myocarditis, HIV, Lyme disease, Parvovirus B19, Chagas disease.

- Toxic: **alcohol abuse, cocaine,** anthracyclines (eg, **Doxorubicin**), radiation.

- Pregnancy, autoimmune.
- Metabolic: eg, thyroid disorders, **vitamin B1 (thiamine) deficiency**.

CLINICAL MANIFESTATIONS
- **Systolic heart failure:**
  - Left-sided failure: L for Lung symptoms - dyspnea, fatigue.
  - Right-sided failure: peripheral edema, jugular venous distention, hepatomegaly, GI symptoms.
  - Embolic events, arrhythmias.

- Physical examination: **S3 gallop hallmark** (due to filling of a dilated ventricle). Mitral or tricuspid regurgitation.

DIAGNOSTIC STUDIES
- **Echocardiogram: diagnostic test of choice - left ventricular dilation** (large chamber), thin ventricular walls, **decreased ejection fraction**, ventricular hypokinesis. Similar findings to Systolic heart failure.

- Chest radiograph: **cardiomegaly**, pulmonary edema, pleural effusion.

- ECG: may show sinus tachycardia or arrhythmias.

MANAGEMENT
- **Standard systolic heart failure treatment:**
  Mortality reduction with ACE inhibitors, Beta blockers (eg, Metoprolol, Carvedilol), ARBs, Spironolactone. **Symptom control with diuretics**, Digoxin.

- Automated implantable cardioverter/defibrillator if ejection fraction < 35-30%.

STRESS (TAKOTSUBO) CARDIOMYOPATHY

- **Transient regional systolic dysfunction of the left ventricle** that can imitate Myocardial infarction, but is associated with the **absence of significant obstructive coronary artery disease or evidence of plaque rupture.**
- Risk factors: **postmenopausal women exposed to physical or emotional stress** (eg, death of relative, catastrophic medical diagnoses, acute medical illness).

PATHOPHYSIOLOGY

- Thought to be multifactorial, including **catecholamine surge** during physical or emotional stress, microvascular dysfunction, and coronary artery spasm.

CLINICAL MANIFESTATIONS

- Similar to Acute coronary syndrome (ACS) - eg, **substernal chest pain, dyspnea, syncope.**

DIAGNOSIS

- ECG: **ST elevations** (especially in the anterior leads similar to anterior MI). May have ST depressions.
- Cardiac enzymes: often positive.
- Coronary angiography: **absence of acute plaque rupture or obstructive coronary disease.** On examinations, this is an "*all the way question*", meaning the diagnosis is considered in patients with ACS with no evidence of obstructive coronary disease on coronary angiography.
- Echocardiogram: **transient** regional left ventricular systolic dysfunction, **especially apical left ventricular ballooning.** Usually performed after ACS has been ruled out.

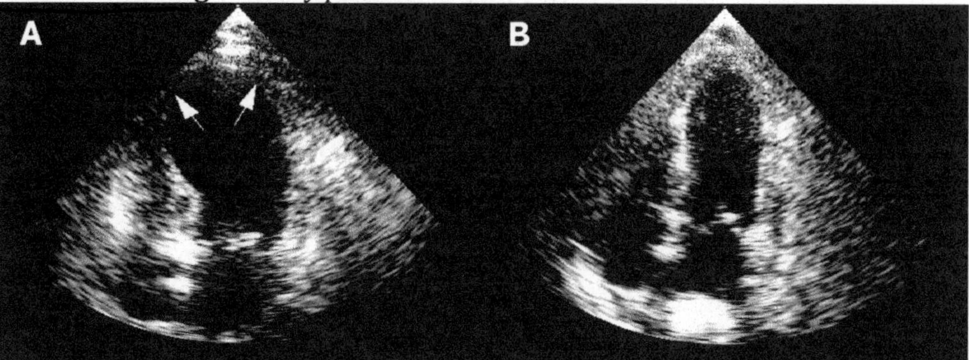

A) Echocardiograph showing dilatation of the left ventricle in the acute phase. (B) Resolution of left ventricular function on repeat echocardiograph 6 days later.

Photo credit: Tara C Gangadhar, Elisabeth Von der Lohe, Stephen G Sawada and Paul R Helft [CC BY 2.0 (https://creativecommons.org/licenses/by/2.0)]

INITIAL MANAGEMENT

- Because the initial presentation of Takotsubo cardiomyopathy presents similar to ACS, patients are treated as ACS with Aspirin, Nitroglycerin, Beta blockers, Heparin, and coronary angiography to rule out obstructive coronary artery disease.

SHORT-TERM MANAGEMENT

- Because Takotsubo cardiomyopathy is a transient condition, **conservative and supportive care is the mainstay of treatment** (eg, Beta blockers, ACE inhibitors for 3-6 months with serial imaging to assess for improvement).
- Anticoagulation in some with severe LV dysfunction (eg, EF <30%) or if thrombus is present.

RESTRICTIVE CARDIOMYOPATHY (RCMP)

- **Diastolic dysfunction in a non-dilated ventricle**, which **impedes ventricular filling** (decreased compliance). The stiff ventricle fills with great effort.

ETIOLOGIES

- **Infiltrative disease: Amyloidosis (most common), Sarcoidosis, Hemochromatosis**, Scleroderma, Metastatic disease, endomyocardial fibrosis.
- Chemotherapy, radiation therapy.

CLINICAL MANIFESTATIONS

- **Right-sided heart failure** > left-sided failure symptoms.
  - Right-sided failure: eg, peripheral edema, jugular venous distention, hepatomegaly, ascites, GI symptoms.
  - Left-sided failure: L for Lung symptoms (eg, **dyspnea most common complaint**, fatigue).
- **Kussmaul's sign**: the lack of an inspiratory decline or **increase in jugular venous pressure with inspiration.**
- Signs of heart failure. S3 may be heard. Pulmonary hypertension.

DIAGNOSIS

- **Echocardiogram: diagnostic test of choice – non-dilated ventricles with normal thickness** (may be slightly thick), **diastolic dysfunction, marked dilation of both atria.** Systolic function generally preserved in early disease. Bright speckled myocardium in Amyloidosis.
- Chest radiograph: normal ventricular chamber size, enlarged atria. Pulmonary congestion.
- ECG: low voltage QRS, arrhythmias.
- Increased BNP.
- **Endomyocardial biopsy: definitive diagnosis** (not used often).
  - Amyloidosis associated with apple-green birefringence with Congo-red staining.

MANAGEMENT

- No specific treatment.
- Treat the underlying disorder (eg, chelation for Hemochromatosis, Glucocorticoids for Sarcoidosis).
- Gentle diuresis for symptoms, vasodilators.

HYPERTROPHIC CARDIOMYOPATHY

- Autosomal dominant genetic disorder of inappropriate LV and/or RV hypertrophy with diastolic dysfunction.
- Subaortic outflow obstruction due to asymmetrical septal hypertrophy and systolic anterior motion of the mitral valve.

The obstruction worsens with

- Increased contractility (eg, exercise, Digoxin, beta agonists) and/or
- Decreased LV volume (eg, dehydration, decreased venous return, Valsalva maneuver).

CLINICAL MANIFESTATIONS

- **Dyspnea most common symptom,** fatigue, **angina** (chest pain), pre syncope, syncope, dizziness, **arrhythmias**. May be asymptomatic initially.
- **Sudden cardiac death,** especially in adolescent or preadolescent children **especially during times of extreme exertion** usually due to **Ventricular fibrillation.**

PHYSICAL EXAMINATION

- **Harsh systolic murmur** best heard at the **left sternal border**.
- **Increased murmur intensity** with **decreased venous return (eg, Valsalva, standing)** or decreased afterload (eg, Amyl nitrate).
- **Decreased murmur intensity** with **increased venous return (eg, squatting, supine, leg raise)** or increased afterload (eg, handgrip). Increased LV volume preserves outflow.
- May have **loud S4,** mitral regurgitation, S3, or pulsus bisferiens.

DIAGNOSIS

- **Echocardiography: asymmetric ventricular wall thickness (especially septal)** 15mm or greater, systolic anterior motion of the mitral valve, & small LV chamber size.
- ECG: **left ventricular hypertrophy,** anterolateral & inferior pseudo q waves, enlarged atria.

MANAGEMENT

- Focus on early detection, medical management, surgical management, and/or ICD placement.
- Medical: **Beta blockers first-line medical management.**
  Alternatives include **Calcium channel blockers** & Disopyramide.
- Surgical: Myomectomy usually performed in young patients refractory to medical therapy.
- Alcohol septal ablation: an alternative to surgical myomectomy.
- **Patients should avoid dehydration, extreme exertion, and exercise. Cautious use of Digoxin, Nitrates, and diuretics** (Digoxin increases contractility; Nitrates & diuretics decrease LV volume).

- **EXAM TIP**
- Aortic stenosis (AS) VS. Hypertrophic obstructive cardiomyopathy (HOCM)
- Both: angina, syncope, systolic murmur. Both murmurs go in the same direction with afterload maneuvers (eg, both increase with Amyl nitrate & both decrease with handgrip).
- **HOCM**: preload maneuvers that decrease LV volume **(eg, Valsalva, standing) will worsen the murmur of HOCM** whereas these maneuvers will decrease the intensity of most other murmurs (including AS). **Increased LV volume (eg, squatting, leg raise) will decrease the murmur of HOCM** whereas these maneuvers will increase the intensity AS. No carotid radiation.

Cardiomyopathy: disease of the heart muscle (myocardial tissue) with cardiac dysfunction NOT due to other heart diseases*

	DILATED CARDIOMYOPATHY (95%)	RESTRICTIVE CARDIOMYOPATHY (1%)	HYPERTROPHIC CARDIOMYOPATHY (4%)
DEFINITION	• **SYSTOLIC DYSFUNCTION ⇨ ventricular dilation** ⇨ "dilated, weak heart"	• **DIASTOLIC DYSFUNCTION** - Ventricular rigidity impedes ventricular filling (↓ ventricular compliance) • Preserved contractility early on in disease.	• **DIASTOLIC DYSFUNCTION** due to **impaired ventricular relaxation/filling.** • **SUBAORTIC OUTFLOW OBSTRUCTION:** - **hypertrophied septum** - **systolic anterior motion (SAM) of mitral valve** & SAM is **increased with: ❶ ↑contractility** (exertion) & **❷ ↓LV volume** (eg, ↓decreased venous return, dehydration).
ETIOLOGIES	•**Idiopathic MC cause,** autoimmune •**Viral myocarditis (eg, enteroviruses)** •**Toxic:** ETOH, cocaine, pregnancy • XRT, **doxorubicin,** daunorubicin	•**Infiltrative diseases** - **Amyloidosis most common (MC) cause** - Sarcoidosis, Hemochromatosis - Scleroderma, metastatic disease, Idiopathic	• **Inherited genetic disorder** of inappropriate LV and/or RV hypertrophy (especially septal).
CLINICAL MANIFESTATIONS	• Systolic heart failure symptoms - Dyspnea, edema, increased JVD • Embolic phenomena, Arrhythmias •**Viral Myocarditis: viral prodrome ⇨ signs of heart failure or chest pain, +cardiac enzymes, nonspecific ST-T changes.**	•RIGHT SIDED FAILURE more > left sided failure. •Dyspnea most common symptom. •Poorly tolerated tachyarrhythmias	• **Dyspnea most common initial complaint** (90%). • Angina pectoris • **Arrhythmias** AF; VT/VF (palpitations, syncope). • **Sudden cardiac death:** especially in adolescent/preadolescent children **(especially exertional)** due to **ventricular fibrillation.**
PHYSICAL	•L heart failure - Pulmonary congestion: rales, tachycardia, cough, pleural effusion •R heart failure - Peripheral edema, ↑JVP, hepatic congestion	•**Kussmaul's sign:** ↑JVP with inspiration •**R-sided heart failure** Peripheral edema, ↑JVP, hepatic congestion. •L-sided heart failure Crackles (rales).	•**Harsh systolic** crescendo-decrescendo murmur **@LLSB** - ↓**murmur intensity:** **↑venous return (eg, squatting, lying supine)** because ↑LV volume preserves outflow. Handgrip (increased afterload). - ↑**murmur intensity:** **↓venous return (Valsalva & standing) & exertion** - ↓LV volume & ↑contractility will ↓cardiac output. **Amyl nitrate** (decreases afterload). • Usually **no carotid radiation**. Normal pulse, **Loud S_4.** ± MR
DIAGNOSIS	•**Echocardiogram** most useful test: - ❶ **left ventricular dilation: thin ventricular walls** - ❷ **↓ejection fraction (EF)** - ❸ Regional or global LV hypokinesis. •***CXR:*** - Cardiomegaly, Pulmonary edema.	•**Echocardiogram:** - Ventricles nondilated with normal wall thickness. - **MARKED DILATION OF BOTH ATRIA** - **Diastolic dysfunction** with normal or near normal systolic function.	•**Echocardiogram:** - **Asymmetric wall thickness (septal),** SAM mitral valve. •ECG: - Left ventricular hypertrophy, septal q waves Avoid exertion, Implantable Defibrillator to prevent VF.
MANAGEMENT	•**Standard systolic heart failure treatment:** - **ACEI, Beta blockers,** Na restriction - Symptom control: **diuretics,** digoxin, - Implantable defibrillator if EF <35%	•No specific treatment Treat underlying cause	•**Medical: BETA BLOCKERS*** , Verapamil, Disopyramide. •Myomectomy, ETOH ablation •**Cautious use of digoxin, nitrates & diuretics** (digoxin ↑'es contractility while nitrates & diuretics ↓volume).

MYOCARDITIS

- Inflammation of the heart muscle. Most common in young adults.

PATHOPHYSIOLOGY

- Myocellular damage leads to myocardial necrosis & dysfunction, leading to Heart failure.

ETIOLOGIES

- Infectious: **viral most common (especially the enteroviruses - Coxsackievirus B)**, bacterial.
- Autoimmune eg, Systemic lupus erythematosus, Rheumatoid arthritis.
- Uremia, medications (eg, **Clozapine,** Methyldopa, antibiotics, Isoniazid, Cyclophosphamide, Indomethacin, Phenytoin, sulfonamides).

CLINICAL MANIFESTATIONS

- **Viral prodrome** – fever, myalgias, malaise for several days **followed by symptoms of systolic dysfunction (Dilated cardiomyopathy).**
- Heart failure symptoms: dyspnea, fatigue, exercise intolerance, **S3 gallop**.
- Other: **Megacolon, Pericarditis** (pericardial friction rub, effusion).

DIAGNOSTIC STUDIES

- Chest radiograph: **cardiomegaly** classic.
- ECG: nonspecific – sinus tachycardia most common, normal or may show Pericarditis (eg, diffuse ST elevations and PR depressions in the precordial leads).
- Labs: may have positive cardiac enzymes, increased ESR.
- Echocardiogram: **ventricular systolic dysfunction.** Also helpful to rule out other causes.
- **Endomyocardial biopsy: gold standard** – infiltration of lymphocytes with myocardial tissue necrosis. Usually reserved for severe or refractory cases.

MANAGEMENT

- **Supportive mainstay of treatment – standard Systolic heart failure treatment** (eg, ACE inhibitors, diuretics, Beta blockers).

BASH

BB ACE Spiro Hydral + Nitrates

ECG CHEAT SHEET

STEP 1: DETERMINE THE RHYTHM

Regular or Irregular?

☑ **Use Rhythm strip.** Check R-R intervals. If < 0.12 second difference, consider it a regular rhythm.

STEP 2: DETERMINE THE RATE

If ***Regular*** rhythm ⇨ 1500/# of small squares **OR** 300-150-100-75-60-50 method between an R-R interval.
If ***Irregular*** rhythm ⇨ count the number of R waves in a 6 second strip & multiply that number by 10.

STEP 3: DETERMINE THE QRS AXIS

	Normal	LAD	RAD
Lead I	+	+	-
aVF	+	-	+

***If Left Axis Deviation (LAD) based on I and aVF ⇨ check lead II.**
- **If QRS is predominantly positive in lead II ⇨ normal axis** (0° to -30°)
- **If QRS is predominantly negative in lead II ⇨ LAD** (< -30°)

STEP 4: EVALUATE THE P WAVES/PR INTERVAL

(Look in Lead II and V_1 for P wave morphology)

☑ **Sinus?** If positive/upright in I, II, avF & negative in avR. ***Each*** P wave followed by QRS complex.
☑ **PR interval normal?** Normal PRI = 0.12 - .20 sec (or 3-5 boxes). Prolonged (> .20); shortened (< .12)
☑ **Atrial enlargement?**

LEFT ATRIAL ENLARGEMENT

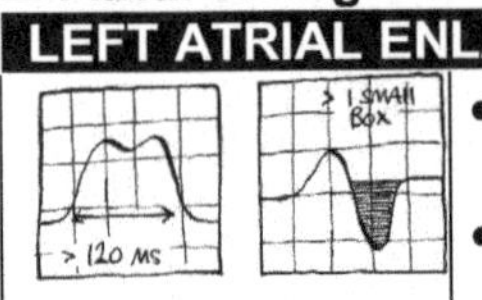

- ***m-shaped P wave in Lead II*** > .12 seconds (3 boxes)
- Biphasic P in V1 with larger terminal component

RIGHT ATRIAL ENLARGEMENT

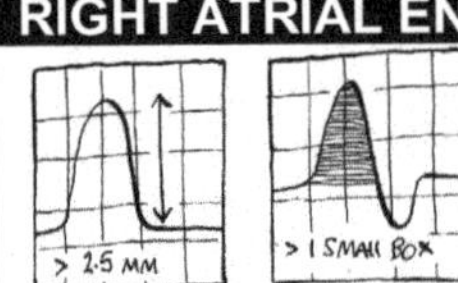

- ***tall P wave in Lead II ≥3 mm***
- Biphasic P in V1 with larger initial component

STEP 5: EVALUATE THE QRS COMPLEX

☑ **Narrow v. Wide** (normal < .12 seconds). If QRS is narrow, skip looking for bundle branch blocks.

☑ **Bundle Branch Blocks?**

Left BBB

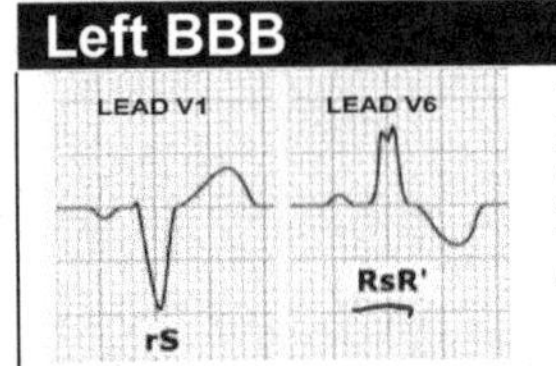

1. **Wide QRS** > 0.12 seconds
2. **Broad, slurred R in V5,6**
3. **Deep S** wave in **V1**
4. ST elevations V1-V3

Right BBB

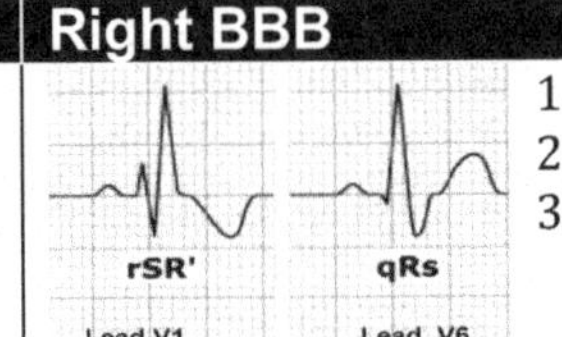

1. **Wide QRS** > 0.12 seconds
2. **RsR' in V1,2**
3. **Wide S** wave in **V6**

☑ **Ventricular Hypertrophy**

RIGHT VENTRICULAR HYPERTROPHY*:* look at V1: R>S in V1 or R >7 mm in height in V1

LEFT VENTRICULAR HYPERTROPHY*:*

Sokolow-Lyon criteria: S in V1 + R in V5 (or V6) >35 mm in men; >30 mm in women.

Cornell Criteria: R in aVL + S in V3 >28 mm in men; >20 mm in women.

☑ **Pathological Q waves?** Q wave >1 box (in depth or width).

STEP 6: EVALUATE ST SEGMENT

☑ ST depression or elevation >1 mm in depth/height?

STEP 7: EVALUATE T WAVES

☑ Any T wave inversions (TWI); T wave flattening? Is the QT interval prolonged?

SUMMARY OF THE 12 LEADS AND THEIR RELATION TO THE HEART

Coronary Artery Anatomy

The leads and their relation to the coronary arteries

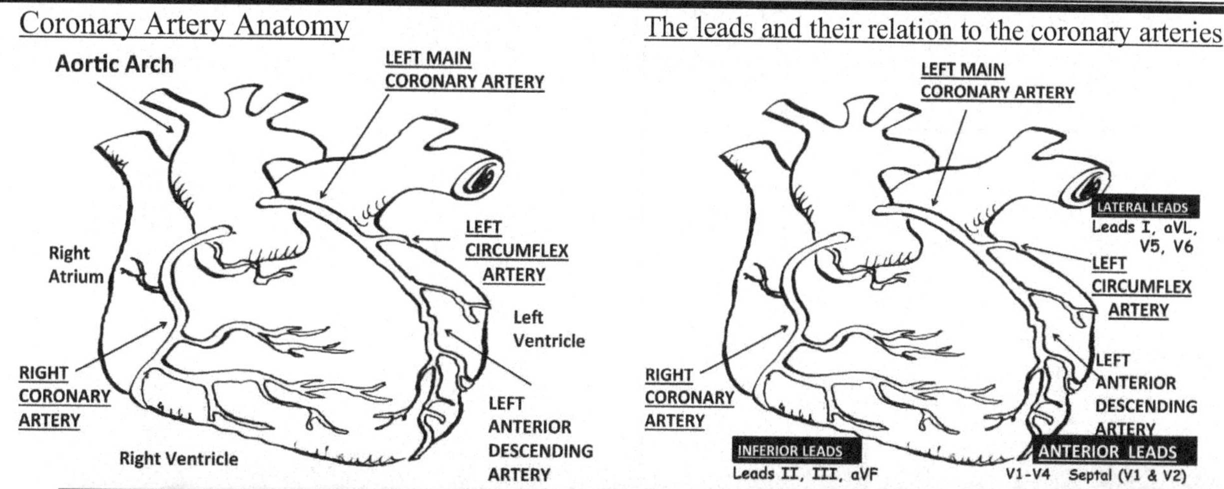

AREA OF INFARCTION	Q WAVES/ ST ELEVATIONS	ARTERY INVOLVED
ANTERIOR WALL	**V1 through V4**	**Left Anterior Descending** (LAD)
- SEPTAL	V1 & V2	Proximal LAD
LATERAL WALL	**I, aVL, V5, V6**	**Circumflex** (CFX)
ANTEROLATERAL	I, aVL, V4 + V5 + V6	Mid LAD +/- CFX
INFERIOR	**II, III, aVF**	**Right Coronary Artery** (RCA)
POSTERIOR WALL	**ST DEPRESSIONS V1-V2** (really the reciprocal changes since there are no "posterior" leads on a standard 12 lead ECG)	RCA, CFX

QRS AXIS DETERMINATION

Axis: the general direction of the impulses through the heart. It is the summation of all the vectors. Vectors move towards hypertrophy & away from infarction. **Normal QRS axis is -30° to +90°**

PERPENDICULAR	QUADRANT METHOD

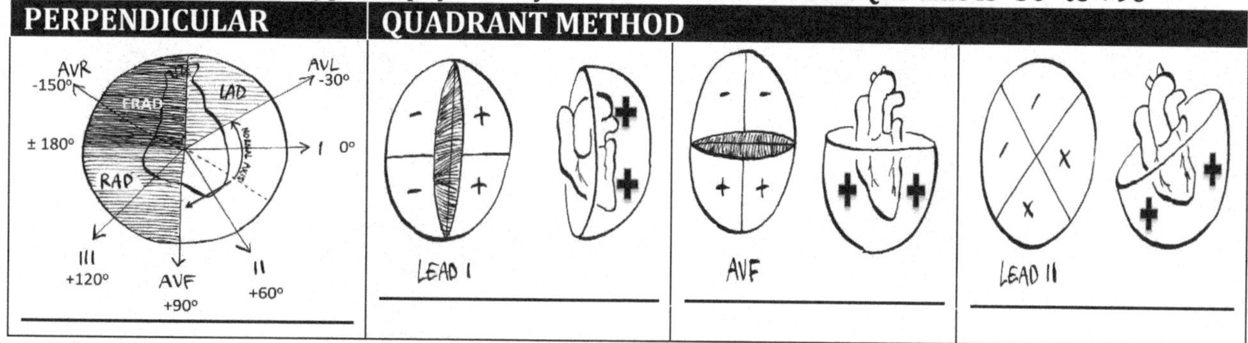

QUADRANT METHOD: If LAD (based on I and aVF) ⇨ check lead II. If QRS is predominantly negative in lead II ⇨ LAD

AXIS	Lead I	aVF	ETIOLOGIES OF LEFT & RIGHT AXIS DEVIATION
Normal	⊕	⊕	Normal
LAD	⊕	**-ve**	LBBB, LVH, inferior MI, elevated diaphragm, L anterior hemiblock, WPW
RAD	**-ve**	⊕	RVH, lateral MI, COPD, Left posterior hemiblock
ERAD	-ve	-ve	

LAD – vectors move towards hypertrophy (LVH) or away from infarction (inferior MI ± cause LAD).
RAD – vectors move towards hypertrophy (RVH) or away from infarction (lateral MI ± cause RAD).

BRADYCARDIA ALGORITHM

CHECK PULSE

↓ yes

UNSTABLE?
Hypotension
AMS
Refractory chest pain
Acute Heart Failure

Or Symptomatic?

no → **Monitor and Observe (No acute medical treatment needed)**

↓ yes

Atropine *1st line**
If Atropine not effective, options include:
- Epinephrine Infusion
- Dopamine Infusion
- Transcutaneous Pacing

EXCEPTION TO SYMPTOMATIC/UNSTABLE BRADYARRHYTHMIA RULE:
1. **3rd *Degree heart block*: transcutaneous pacing usually first line** followed by permanent pacemaker placement as definitive treatment.

ß-Blockers:
Metoprolol, Esmolol, Propranolol

Calcium Channel Blockers
Non-dihydropyridines*
Diltiazem, Verapamil

TACHYCARDIA ALGORITHM

CHECK PULSE

No → **Only 2 "shockable" rhythms using defibrillation (UNsynchronized cardioversion) are:**
❶ ventricular fibrillation &
❷ pulseless ventricular tachycardia*

↓ yes

UNSTABLE?
Hypotension
AMS
Refractory chest pain
Acute Heart Failure

yes → **UNSTABLE TACHYARRHYTHMIA**
- **SYNCHRONIZED Cardioversion***
- If regular, narrow QRS complex, may consider Adenosine

↓ no

Wide QRS?
≥ 0.12 seconds

yes → **Wide QRS Complex Tachycardia**
- **Antiarrhythmic: *Amiodarone****
  Lidocaine, Procainamide
- Cardiac Consult
- If regular, monomorpic, may consider Adenosine

↓ no

Narrow QRS Complex
- Vagal Maneuvers
- **Adenosine (if regular & narrow QRS)***
- **Beta Blocker or Calcium Channel Blocker**

Vagal Maneuvers: Hold breath & bear down or carotid massage (make sure no carotid bruits are present before performing)

STABLE NARROW-COMPLEX TACHYARRHYTHMIAS:
1. **ATRIAL FLUTTER OR A. FIB: Beta blocker or Calcium Channel Blocker 1st line.**
2. **WOLFF-PARKINSON-WHITE (WPW): Procainamide preferred.** Amiodarone. Avoid ABCD if wide complex (Adenosine, Beta blockers, CCBs, Digoxin).
3. **SVT:** Vagal maneuvers. **Adenosine first-line medical management.**
4. Sinus arrhythmia: treat the underlying cause.

SINUS RHYTHMS

Impulses originate at the SA (sinoatrial) node.

NORMAL SINUS RHYTHM (NSR)

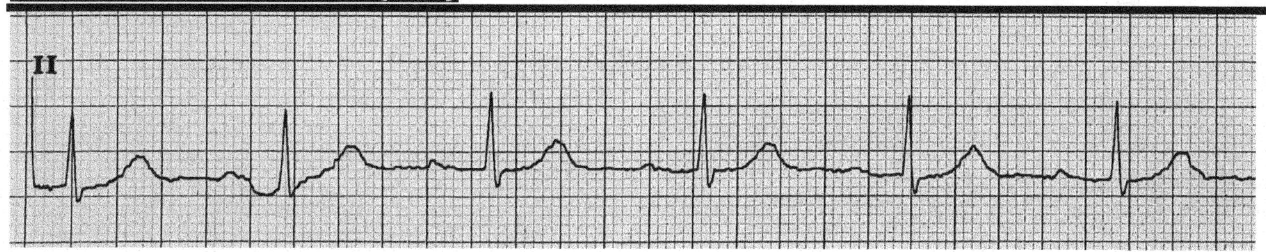

- Every P wave is followed by a QRS complex.
- P waves are positive/upright in leads I, II, aVF, & negative in aVR.
- Rate 60-100 bpm.

SINUS ARRHYTHMIA

- Irregular rhythm originating from the sinus node.
- **Normal variation of normal sinus rhythm** (meets the same criteria except that the **rhythm is irregular).**
- More commonly seen in children, young adults and patients with Sinus bradycardia.

PHYSIOLOGY

- Beat to beat variations with respiration - **rhythm increases with inspiration and decreases with expiration**, reflecting changes in stroke volume during respiration.

DIAGNOSIS

- ECG: normal-appearing P waves, beat to beat variation of the P-P interval (> .12 seconds), shorter intervals during inspiration (increased rate) and longer P-P intervals during expiration (decreased heart rate).

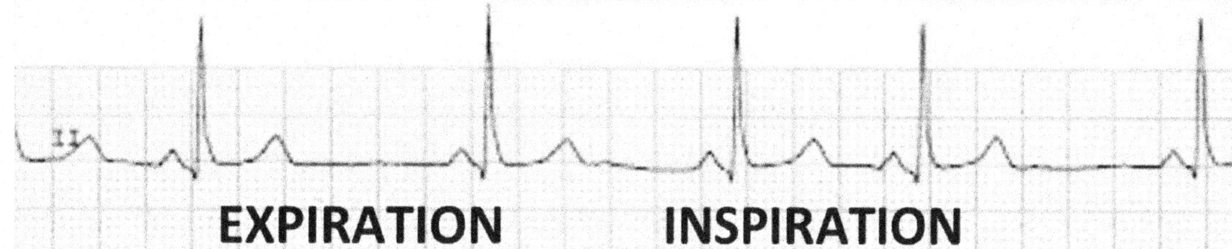

MANAGEMENT

- **None needed in most cases** (it is considered a normal variant).
- If symptomatic bradycardia occurs, Atropine is the first-line management.
- Transcutaneous pacing, Epinephrine, and Dopamine are second-line agents.

SINUS TACHYCARDIA

- Increased heart rate > 100 bpm originating from the sinus node.

ETIOLOGIES

- Physiologic: normal response to exercise, emotional stress. Normal in young children & infants.
- Pathologic: fever, hypovolemia, hypoxia, pain, infection, hemorrhage, hypoglycemia, anxiety, thyrotoxicosis, shock, sympathomimetics (eg, decongestants, cocaine).

DIAGNOSIS

- ECG: regular, rapid rhythm (> 100 bpm), normal-appearing P wave with every P followed by a QRS complex.

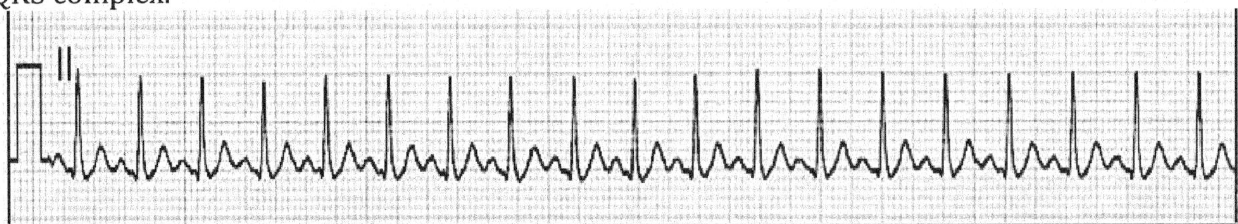

MANAGEMENT

- **Treat the underlying cause (first-line treatment).**
- Beta blockers (eg, Metoprolol) used in the management of persistent sinus tachycardia in the setting of Acute coronary artery syndrome.

SINUS BRADYCARDIA

- Decreased heart rate < 60 bpm originating from the sinus node.

ETIOLOGIES

- Physiologic: young athletes, vasovagal reaction, increased intracranial pressure, nausea, vomiting.
- Pathologic: Beta blockers, calcium channel blockers, digoxin, carotid massage, sinoatrial node ischemia, gram negative sepsis, & hypothyroidism.

DIAGNOSIS

- ECG: **regular, slow. rhythm (< 60 bpm), normal-appearing P wave** with every P followed by a QRS complex

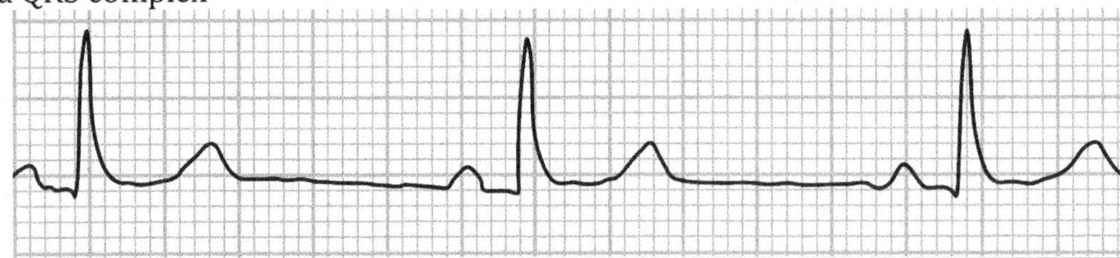

MANAGEMENT

- **Symptomatic or unstable: Atropine 1st-line treatment.**
  Epinephrine or transcutaneous pacing if not responsive to Atropine.
- **Asymptomatic: no treatment needed if physiologic.**
  Observation or cardiac consult may be needed if pathologic.

SICK SINUS SYNDROME (brady-tachy syndrome)

- Dysfunction of the sinus node that leads to a combination of **sinus arrest with alternating paroxysms of atrial tachyarrhythmias & bradyarrhythmias**.

ETIOLOGIES

- Sinus node fibrosis (most common), older age, corrective cardiac surgery, medications, systemic diseases that affect the heart.

CLINICAL MANIFESTATIONS

- Intermittent symptoms of bradycardia & or tachycardia: eg, palpitations, dizziness, lightheadedness, angina, dyspnea on exertion, presyncope, or syncope.

DIAGNOSIS

- ECG: alternating bradycardia (eg, sinus pause, SA exit block) and atrial tachyarrhythmias.

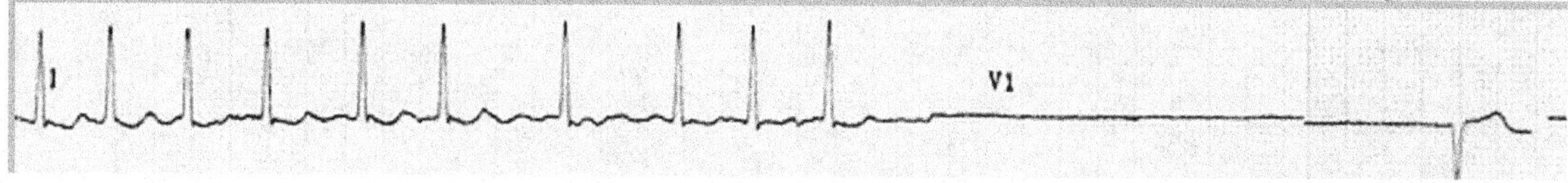

- Telemetry or ambulatory ECG monitoring may be needed to document episodes.

MANAGEMENT

- Stable: may not require urgent therapy as the symptoms are often transient.
- Hemodynamically unstable: Atropine first-line if medications are needed. Dopamine, epinephrine. Transcutaneous pacing.
- Long-term: permanent pacemaker definitive. Addition of an automatic implantable cardioverter defibrillator if alternating between tachycardia and bradycardia.

ATRIOVENTRICULAR CONDUCTION BLOCKS

AV BLOCK: interruption of the normal impulse from the SA node to the AV node (AV node dysfunction).

- **PR Interval (PRI) most helpful in determining the presence of AV conduction blocks.**

FIRST-DEGREE AV BLOCK

- AV node dysfunction leading to delayed but conducted impulses.

ETIOLOGIES

- Often a **normal variant** (individuals with high vagal tone without structural heart disease).
- Intrinsic AV node disease, acute myocardial infarction (eg, inferior wall MI), electrolyte disturbances (eg, hyperkalemia), AV nodal blocking drugs (eg, Digoxin, Beta-blockers & Calcium channel blockers), myocarditis due to Lyme, cardiac surgery.

CLINICAL MANIFESTATIONS

- Asymptomatic in most cases.
- If symptomatic, it is due to bradycardia-related decreased perfusion – fatigue, dizziness, dyspnea, chest pain, syncope, or in severe cases (hypotension or altered mental status).

DIAGNOSIS

- ECG: all atrial impulses are delayed but conducted to the ventricles = **prolonged PR interval** (> 0.20 seconds) + **all P waves are followed by QRS complexes.**

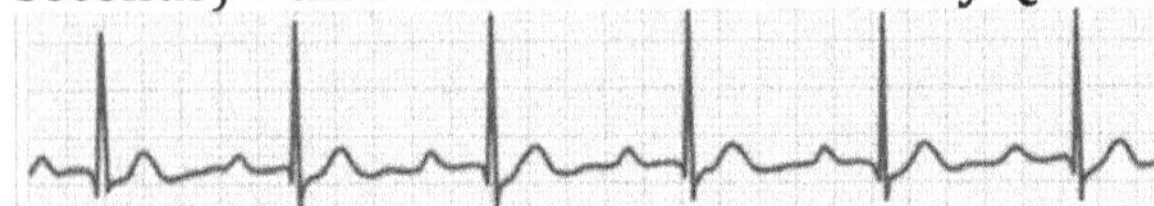

MANAGEMENT

- **Asymptomatic: no treatment**, observation. Cardiac consult in some cases.
- **Symptomatic: Atropine first-line**, epinephrine.
- Pacemaker definitive if persistently symptomatic & severe (PRI > 0.30 seconds).

SECOND DEGREE AV BLOCK

- 2nd = not all of the atrial impulses are conducted to the ventricles.
  This leads to some P waves that are not followed by QRS complexes ('dropped QRS').

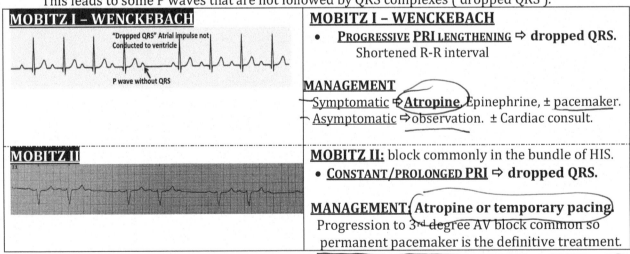

MOBITZ I – WENCKEBACH	MOBITZ I – WENCKEBACH
"Dropped QRS" Atrial impulse not Conducted to ventricle P wave without QRS	• **PROGRESSIVE PRI LENGTHENING ⇨ dropped QRS.** Shortened R-R interval **MANAGEMENT** Symptomatic ⇨ **Atropine**, Epinephrine, ± pacemaker. Asymptomatic ⇨ observation. ± Cardiac consult.
MOBITZ II	**MOBITZ II:** block commonly in the bundle of HIS. • **CONSTANT/PROLONGED PRI ⇨ dropped QRS.** **MANAGEMENT: Atropine or temporary pacing.** Progression to 3rd degree AV block common so permanent pacemaker is the definitive treatment.

MOBITZ I SECOND DEGREE AV BLOCK (Wenckebach)

- Interruption of electrical impulse at the AV node resulting in occasional non-conducted impulses.
- PATHOPHYSIOLOGY: AV node dysfunction (commonly above the bundle of HIS).

ETIOLOGIES

- Often a **normal variant** (individuals with high vagal tone without structural heart disease).
- **Inferior wall MI** (AV node ischemia), **AV nodal blocking agents** (eg, Beta blockers, Digoxin, Calcium channel blockers), myocarditis due to Lyme, hyperkalemia, cardiac surgery.

CLINICAL MANIFESTATIONS

- Asymptomatic in most cases.
- Bradycardia-related decreased perfusion – eg, fatigue, dizziness, dyspnea, chest pain, syncope, or in severe cases (hypotension or altered mental status).

DIAGNOSIS

- ECG: **progressive lengthening of the PR interval** until an **occasional non-conducted atrial impulse** (dropped QRS complex).

MANAGEMENT

- **Asymptomatic: no treatment**, observation. Cardiac consult in some cases.
- **Symptomatic: Atropine first-line**, Epinephrine.
- Pacemaker definitive if persistent.

MOBITZ II SECOND DEGREE AV BLOCK

- Interruption of electrical impulse at the AV node resulting in occasional non-conducted impulses.
- PATHOPHYSIOLOGY: AV node dysfunction (commonly at the bundle of HIS).

ETIOLOGIES

- **Rarely seen in patients without structural heart disease** - eg, myocardial ischemia, myocardial fibrosis, myocarditis (eg, Lyme disease), endocarditis.
- Iatrogenic – AV nodal blockers, post-catheter ablation, post-cardiac surgery.

CLINICAL MANIFESTATIONS

- Asymptomatic in most cases.
- Symptomatic: due to bradycardia-related decreased perfusion – fatigue, dizziness, dyspnea, chest pain, syncope, or in severe cases, hypotension or altered mental status.

DIAGNOSIS

- ECG: **constant PR interval** before & after the **non-conducted atrial beat** (dropped QRS complexes).
- If ischemia is suspected based on clinical picture, cardiac biomarkers, chest radiograph, and electrolytes should be ordered.

MANAGEMENT

- Initial: **transcutaneous pacing** or **Atropine for symptomatic bradycardia** with permanent pacemaker long-term management. These patients often do not respond to Atropine.
- Definitive: **permanent pacemaker required in many patients** because it often progresses to third degree AV block and is associated with complications of hypotension, and cardiac arrest.

THIRD DEGREE AV BLOCK

- **AV dissociation** = no atrial impulses reach the ventricles, so the atrial activity is independent of the ventricular activity.
- This leads to an escape rhythm from below the block.

ETIOLOGIES

- Myocardial ischemia **(inferior wall MI)**, **AV nodal blocking agents** (eg, Beta-blockers, Digoxin, Calcium channel blockers), endocarditis, myocarditis due to Lyme disease, cardiac surgery.
- Increased vagal tone, hypothyroidism, hyperkalemia, myocarditis.

CLINICAL MANIFESTATIONS

- May be asymptomatic.
- If symptomatic, it is due to **bradycardia**-related decreased perfusion especially during exertion (eg, fatigue, dyspnea, dizziness, chest pain, syncope) or in severe cases, hypotension or altered mental status.

DIAGNOSIS

- ECG: shows **regular P-P intervals & regular R-R intervals but they are not related to each other.** Patients are often bradycardic.

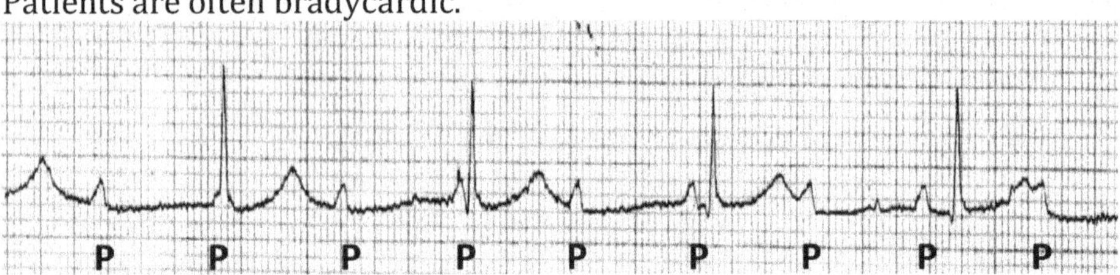

MANAGEMENT

- **Acute or symptomatic: transcutaneous pacing** often followed by permanent pacemaker placement.

- Definitive: permanent pacemaker placement.

HEART BLOCKS - REVIEW

1ST DEGREE:

- **Prolonged PRI, every P followed by QRS** (all conducted)

2nd degree = dropped QRS

(some NOT conducted)

- **MOBITZ 1: Progressive lengthening PRI – dropped QRS**

- **MOBITZ 2: Same length (may be prolonged) + Occasional dropped QRS**

3RD DEGREE

AV Dissociation (NONE are conducted)

ATRIAL DYSRHYTHMIAS

ATRIAL FLUTTER

- **1 irritable atrial focus** firing at a fast rate (atrial rate usually around 300 beats/min).
- Similar to Atrial fibrillation, there is an **increased risk of atrial thrombus formation that can lead to cerebral &/or systemic embolization** (eg, stroke).
- It may occur alone or be an interval rhythm between sinus tachycardia and atrial fibrillation.

CLINICAL MANIFESTATIONS

- Symptomatic: palpitations, dizziness, fatigue, dyspnea, & chest pain.
- **Unstable:** are due to hypoperfusion and can include **refractory chest pain, hypotension** (eg, systolic BP in double digits) or **altered mental status.**

DIAGNOSIS

- ECG: **flutter ("sawtooth") atrial waves** usually around 300 beats per minute (250-350 normal range) but **no discernable P waves**. The flutter waves are identical (1 ectopic atrial focus).

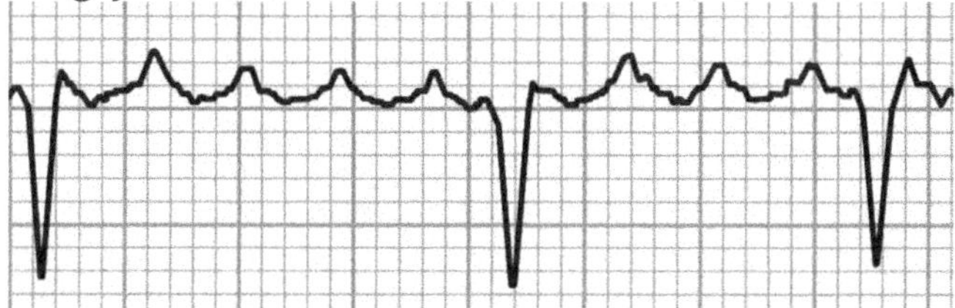

MANAGEMENT

- **Stable:** Vagal maneuvers. Rate control with **Beta blockers** (eg, Metoprolol, Atenolol, or Esmolol) OR non-dihydropyridine **Calcium channel blockers (eg, Diltiazem, Verapamil).**

- **Unstable: direct current (synchronized) cardioversion.**

- Anticoagulation: similar criteria (eg, CHA2DS2-VASc) for nonvalvular atrial fibrillation in patients at risk for embolization.

- Reversion to normal sinus rhythm:
  - **Radiofrequency catheter ablation (definitive management).**
  - Direct current cardioversion.
  - Class IA, IC, or III antiarrhythmics (eg, Ibutilide).

ATRIAL FIBRILLATION (AF)

- **Multiple irritable atrial foci** fire at fast rates.
- Similar to Atrial flutter, there is an **increased risk of atrial thrombus formation that can lead to cerebral &/or systemic embolization** (eg, stroke).
- Atrial fibrillation is the most common chronic arrhythmia. Most patients are asymptomatic.

ETIOLOGIES

Cardiac disease, ischemia, pulmonary disease, infection, cardiomyopathies, electrolyte imbalances, idiopathic, endocrine or neurologic disorders (eg, thyroid disorders), increasing age, genetics, hemodynamic stress, medications, drug or alcohol use. Men > women; Whites > blacks.

TYPES

- Paroxysmal: self-terminating within 7 days (usually <24 hours). ±Recurrent.
- Persistent: fails to self-terminate, lasts >7 days. Requires termination (medical or electrical).
- Permanent: persistent AF >1 year (refractory to cardioversion or cardioversion never tried).
- Lone: paroxysmal, persistent or permanent *without evidence of heart disease.*

CLINICAL MANIFESTATIONS

- Symptomatic: palpitations, dizziness, fatigue, & dyspnea.
- **Unstable:** are due to hypoperfusion and can include **hypotension** (eg, systolic BP in double digits), **altered mental status,** & **refractory** chest pain.

DIAGNOSIS

- ECG:

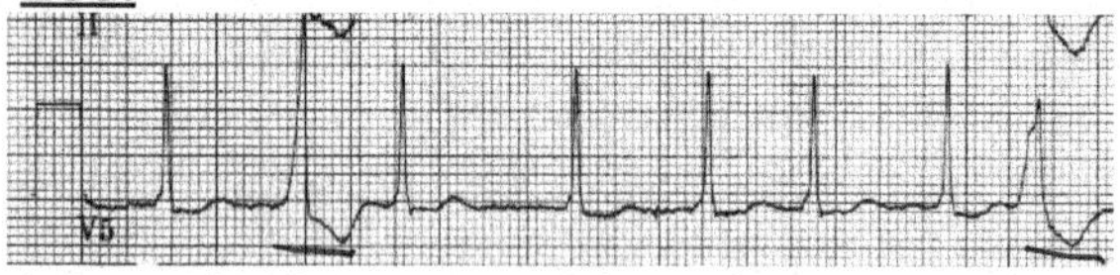

Ashman's phenomenon (seen here on 2nd & 8th beat)

- **Irregularly irregular rhythm with fibrillatory waves** (no discrete P waves).
- Often atrial rate >250 beats per minute.
- The AV nodal refractory period determines the ventricular rate.
- ± Ashman's phenomenon: occasional aberrantly conducted beats (wide QRS) after short R-R cycles.

- Cardiac monitoring: a Holter monitor or telemetry can be used if Atrial fibrillation is not seen on an ECG but is suspected.

MANAGEMENT

Stable:

- Rate control with **Beta blockers** (eg, Metoprolol, Atenolol, or Esmolol) OR non-dihydropyridine **Calcium channel blockers (eg, Diltiazem, Verapamil).**
- Digoxin may be used when Beta blockers or calcium channel blockers are contraindicated (eg, CHF or severe hypotension).

Unstable:

- **Direct current (synchronized) cardioversion.**

Long-term:

- Rate control usually preferred over rhythm control for long-term management.
- Direct current (synchronized cardioversion) or pharmacologic cardioversion.
- Radiofrequency catheter ablation or surgical "MAZE" procedure.
- Anticoagulation: similar criteria (eg, CHA2DS2-VASc) for nonvalvular atrial fibrillation in patients at risk for embolization.

CARDIOVERSION

- Direct current (synchronized cardioversion) or pharmacologic cardioversion. Cardioversion is most successful when performed within 7 days after the onset of Atrial fibrillation.
- **Echocardiogram is needed prior to cardioversion** to ensure there are no atrial clots.
- AF greater than 48 hours undergoing elective cardioversion, **anticoagulation for at least 3 weeks before cardioversion** or a transesophageal echocardiography-guided approach with abbreviated anticoagulation.
- AF < 48 hours undergoing elective cardioversion, anticoagulation prior is recommended.
- **Anticoagulation must be continued for 4 weeks after cardioversion.** With effective anticoagulation the stroke risk is decreased 3-fold after 4 weeks of anticoagulation.

CANDIDATES FOR ANTICOAGULATION WITH NONVALVULAR AF

- **CHA2DS2-VASc score** for nonvalvular Atrial fibrillation assess patients' risk for embolization. **Chronic oral anticoagulation** (eg, **Warfarin or Novel oral anticoagulants**) is **recommended for moderate to high risk (score of 2 or greater).**
- The use of anticoagulant therapy has been shown to reduce embolic risk by 70%.

ANTICOAGULATION RISK STRATIFICATION IN NONVALVULAR ATRIAL FIBRILLATION

CHA_2DS_2- VASc CRITERIA	POINTS	RECOMMENDED THERAPY
Congestive Heart Failure	1	≥ 2 **= Moderate to high risk:** **chronic oral anticoagulation recommended.**
Hypertension	1	
A_2ge ≥ 75y	2	
Diabetes Mellitus	1	1 = low risk: Based on clinical judgment, consideration of risk to benefit assessment & discussion with patient. Anticoagulation may be recommended in some cases.
S_2: Stroke, TIA, thrombus	2	
Vascular disease (prior MI, aortic plaque, peripheral arterial disease)	1	
Age 65 – 74y	1	0 = very low risk: No anticoagulation needed. May be recommended in some (based on clinical judgment & consideration of risk to benefit ratio).
Sex (female)	1	
MAXIMUM SCORE	**9**	

ANTICOAGULANT AGENTS:

1. **Non-vitamin K antagonist oral anticoagulants (NOAC):** *usually now preferred over Warfarin in most cases* due to similar or lower rates of major bleeding as well as lower risk of ischemic stroke, convenience of not having to check the INR, & less drug interactions.
   - **Dabigatran**: direct thrombin inhibitor (binds & inhibits thrombin).
   - **Rivaroxaban, Apixaban, Edoxaban**: factor Xa inhibitors.

2. **Warfarin:**
   Indications: may be preferred in some of the following patients – some with severe chronic kidney disease, contraindications to the NOAC (eg, HIV patients on protease inhibitor-based therapy, on CP450-inducing antiepileptic medications such as Carbamazepine, Phenytoin etc), patients already on Warfarin who prefer not to change, cost issues (Warfarin is less expensive). Warfarin usually bridged with heparin until Warfarin is therapeutic.
   Monitoring: International Normalized Ratio **(INR) goal of 2-3.** Prothrombin Time (PT).

3. Dual antiplatelet therapy: (eg, Aspirin + Clopidogrel). Anticoagulant monotherapy is superior to dual antiplatelet therapy. Dual antiplatelet therapy may be reserved for patients who cannot be treated with anticoagulation (for reasons OTHER than bleeding risk).

PAROXYSMAL SUPRAVENTRICULAR TACHYCARDIA (PSVT)

- Any **tachyarrhythmia originating above the ventricles** (either an atrial or atrioventricular nodal source).
- SVT is an umbrella term when a more specific term cannot be applied to a tachyarrhythmia originating above the ventricles.

PATHOPHYSIOLOGY: **reentry circuits**

- **AV node re-entrant tachycardia:** two pathways **(1 normal and 1 accessory pathway both within the AV node). Most common type.**
- AV reciprocating tachycardia: two pathways (1 normal and 1 accessory pathway outside of the AV node) – eg, Wolff-Parkinson-White (WPW) & Lown-Ganong-Levine syndrome (LGL).

CLINICAL MANIFESTATIONS

- Symptomatic: palpitations, dizziness, fatigue, dyspnea, & chest pain.
- **Unstable:** hypoperfusion can cause **hypotension** (eg, systolic BP in double digits), **altered mental status,** & refractory chest pain.

ECG

- **Orthodromic (95%): regular, narrow-complex tachycardia (no discernable P waves** due to the rapid rate) - "If you can't tell if the bump is a P or a T, then it must be SVT!"
- **Antidromic** (5%): **regular, wide-complex tachycardia** (mimics ventricular tachycardia).

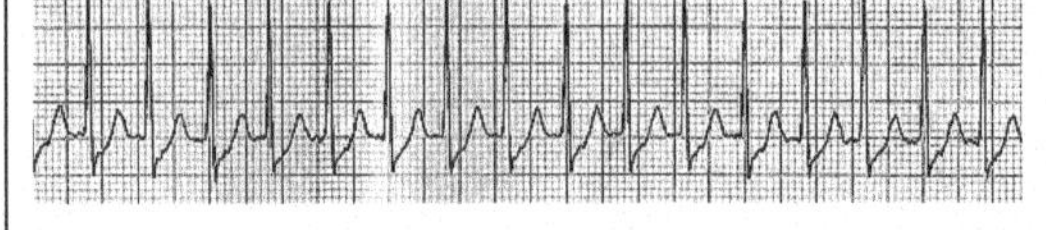	• Heart rate >100 bpm. • **Rhythm** usually **regular with narrow QRS complexes.** • P waves hard to discern due to the rapid rate.

MANAGEMENT

- **Stable (regular, narrow complex): Vagal maneuvers.**
  - AV nodal blockers – **Adenosine first-line medical management.**
  - Second-line: Calcium channel blockers (eg, Diltiazem); Beta blockers (eg, Metoprolol); Digoxin.
- **Stable (wide complex):** antiarrhythmics (eg, **Amiodarone**). **Procainamide if WPW suspected.**
- **Unstable: direct current (synchronized) cardioversion.**
- **Definitive: radiofrequency catheter ablation.**

WANDERING ATRIAL PACEMAKER (WAP) & MULTIFOCAL ATRIAL TACHYCARDIA (MAT)

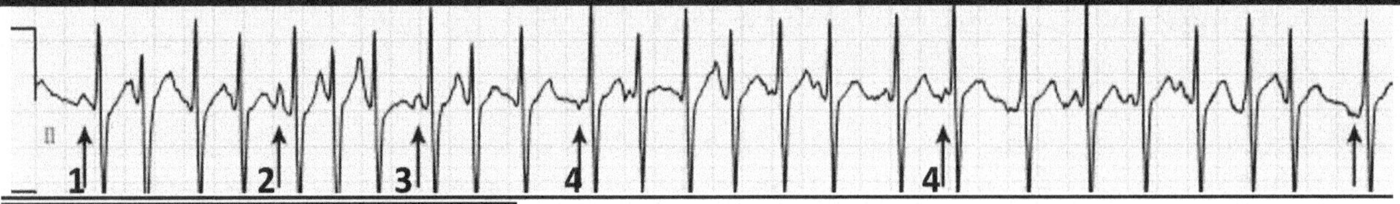

WANDERING ATRIAL PACEMAKER:

- Multiple ectopic atrial foci generate impulses that are conducted to the ventricles.
- **ECG: heart rate <100 bpm & ≥ 3 P wave morphologies.**

MULTIFOCAL ATRIAL TACHYCARDIA:

- Same as wandering atrial pacemaker except the heart rate is >100 bpm.
- **ECG: heart rate > 100 bpm & ≥3 P wave morphologies.**
- **MAT classically associated with severe COPD** (chronic obstructive pulmonary disease).

Difficult to treat: Calcium channel blocker (eg, **Verapamil)** or β-blocker used if LV function is preserved.

WOLFF-PARKINSON-WHITE (WPW)

- Preexcitation syndrome that is a type of AV reciprocating tachycardia (AVRT).

PATHOPHYSIOLOGY

- Accessory pathway (**Bundle of Kent**) outside of the AV node **"preexcites" the ventricles** (directly connects the atria & ventricles, bypassing the AV node), leading to a **delta wave** (slurred, wide QRS).

CLINICAL MANIFESTATIONS

- Most patients are asymptomatic but they are prone to the development of tachyarrhythmias.
- Symptomatic: palpitations, dizziness, fatigue, dyspnea, & chest pain.
- **Unstable:** are due to hypoperfusion and can include **hypotension** (eg, systolic BP in double digits), **altered mental status,** & refractory chest pain.

ECG: 3 components "WPW"

- **W**ave – **delta wave** (slurred QRS upstroke)
- **PR interval that is short**
- **Wide QRS** complexes (> 0.12 seconds)

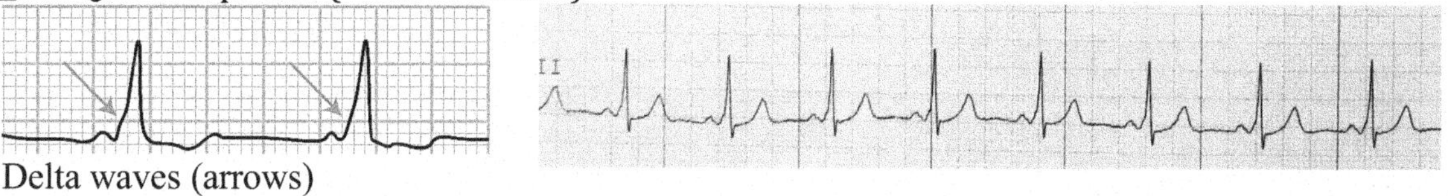

Delta waves (arrows)

MANAGEMENT

Stable (wide complex) tachycardia:

- Antiarrhythmics - **Procainamide preferred.** Amiodarone.
- **Avoid AV nodal blocking agents ABCD if wide QRS complexes** (Adenosine, Beta blockers, Calcium channel blockers, Digoxin) because they can lead to preferential conduction down the Bundle of Kent, worsening the tachycardia.

Unstable:

- **Direct current (synchronized) cardioversion.**

Definitive:

- **Radiofrequency catheter ablation definitive management -** electrically destroys the abnormal pathway. May be indicated if patients experience recurrent, symptomatic episodes.

AV JUNCTIONAL DYSRHYTHMIAS

- AV node/junction becomes the dominant pacemaker of the heart in AV junctional rhythms.
- Etiologies: sinus disease, coronary artery disease, most common rhythm seen with Digitalis toxicity, Myocarditis. May be seen in patients without structural heart disease.
- ECG: Regular rhythm. **P waves inverted (negative) if present** in leads where they are normally positive (I, II, aVF) **or are not seen**. Classically associated with a **narrow QRS** (± wide).
  - Junctional Rhythm: heart rate is usually 40-60 bpm (reflecting the intrinsic rate of the AV junction).
  - Accelerated Junctional: heart rate 60-100 bpm.
  - Junctional Tachycardia: heart rate >100 bpm.

Junctional rhythm with inverted P waves

Junctional rhythm with absent P waves

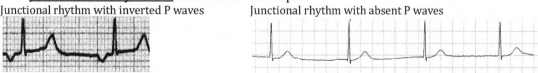

VENTRICULAR DYSRHYTHMIAS

PREMATURE VENTRICULAR COMPLEXES (PVC)

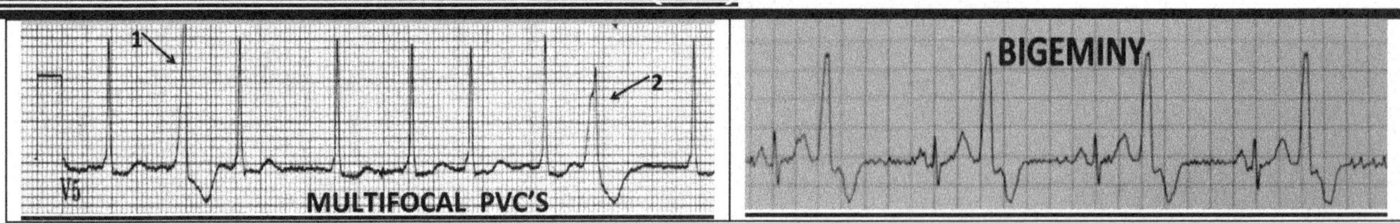

Unifocal (one morphology) **Multifocal** (>1 morphology) **Bigeminy** (every other beat is a PVC) **Couplet** (two PVCs in a row)

- **PVC:** premature beat originating from the ventricle ⇨ **wide, bizarre QRS occurring earlier than expected.** With a PVC, **the T wave is in the opposite direction of the QRS** usually. Associated with a **compensatory pause =** overall rhythm is unchanged (AV node prevents retrograde conduction).

MANAGEMENT
- **No treatment usually needed** (common finding on ECG).
- Most ventricular arrhythmias occur after a PVC.

VENTRICULAR TACHYCARDIA

- Defined as 3 or more consecutive PVCs at a rate >100 beats per minute (usually between 120-300).

CLASSIFICATION
- Sustained VT = duration at least 30 seconds. Non-sustained if < 30 seconds.
- Monomorphic (same QRS morphology) or Polymorphic.
- Torsades de pointes: a variant of polymorphic VT (waxing and waning QRS amplitude on ECG)

ETIOLOGIES:
- Underlying heart disease: **ischemic heart disease most common** (eg, post MI), structural heart defects, cardiomyopathies.
- **Prolonged QT interval**, electrolyte abnormalities (eg, **Hypomagnesemia,** hypokalemia, hypocalcemia), Digoxin toxicity.

CLINICAL MANIFESTATIONS
- Symptomatic: palpitations, dizziness, fatigue, dyspnea, & chest pain.
- **Unstable:** are due to hypoperfusion and can include **hypotension** (eg, systolic BP in double digits), **altered mental status,** & refractory chest pain.

ECG
- **Regular, wide complex tachycardia** with no discernable P waves.

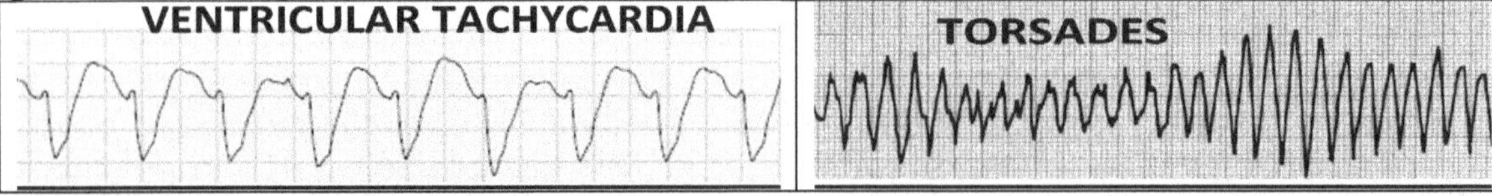

MANAGEMENT OF ACUTE TACHYARRHYTHMIAS

Stable sustained VT	**Antiarrhythmics (Amiodarone**, Lidocaine, Procainamide).
Unstable VT with a pulse	**Direct current (Synchronized) cardioversion.**
VT (no pulse)	- **Defibrillation (Unsynchronized cardioversion) + CPR** (treat similar to Ventricular Fibrillation).
Torsades de pointes	**IV Magnesium.** Correct electrolyte abnormalities.

TORSADES DE POINTES

- A **variant of polymorphic Ventricular tachycardia** (waxing and waning cyclic alterations of the QRS amplitude on ECG).

PATHOPHYSIOLOGY
- Prolonged repolarization and early afterdepolarization + triggered activity.

ETIOLOGIES
- **Prolonged QT interval**, electrolyte abnormalities (eg, **Hypomagnesemia, hypokalemia**, hypocalcemia), females > males. Congenital long QT syndrome.
- Medications: Digoxin, class IA antiarrhythmics (eg, Quinidine, Procainamide, Disopyramide), class III antiarrhythmics (Sotalol, Ibutilide), antibiotics (eg, **Macrolides**), antipsychotics, antidepressants, & antiemetics.

CLINICAL MANIFESTATIONS
- Symptomatic: palpitations, dizziness, fatigue, dyspnea, & chest pain.

DIAGNOSIS
- ECG: **polymorphic Ventricular tachycardia** (cyclic **alterations of the QRS amplitude on ECG around the isoelectric line**) aka sinusoidal waveform.
- Labs: rule out hypomagnesemia and hypokalemia.

MANAGEMENT
- **IV Magnesium sulfate first-line** (suppresses early afterdepolarizations, terminating the arrhythmia). Magnesium is effective in both terminating and preventing recurrent TdP. Correct electrolyte abnormalities.
- **Discontinue all QT prolonging drugs.**
- Isoproterenol and transvenous overdrive pacing may be used in refractory cases.

VENTRICULAR FIBRILLATION

- A type of cardiac death associated with ineffective ventricular contraction.

ETIOLOGIES
- Underlying heart disease: **ischemic heart disease most common** (eg, post MI), structural heart defects, cardiomyopathies, sustained Ventricular tachycardia.

CLINICAL MANIFESTATIONS
- **Unresponsive, pulseless patient, syncope.**

ECG
- Erratic pattern of electrical impulses, no P waves.

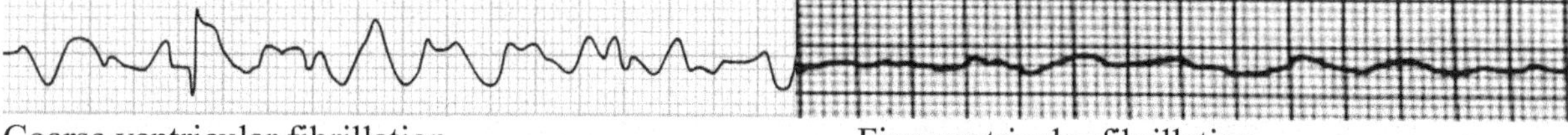

Coarse ventricular fibrillation — Fine ventricular fibrillation

MANAGEMENT
- **Unsynchronized cardioversion (Defibrillation) + CPR** (initiate ACLS)

PULSELESS ELECTRICAL ACTIVITY

- **Organized rhythm seen on a monitor but patient has no palpable pulse** (electrical activity is not coupled with mechanical contraction).

MANAGEMENT:

CPR + epinephrine + checks for "shockable" rhythm every 2 minutes.

ASYSTOLE (Ventricular standstill)

MANAGEMENT: treated the same as PEA

EARLY REPOLARIZATION ABNORMALITIES

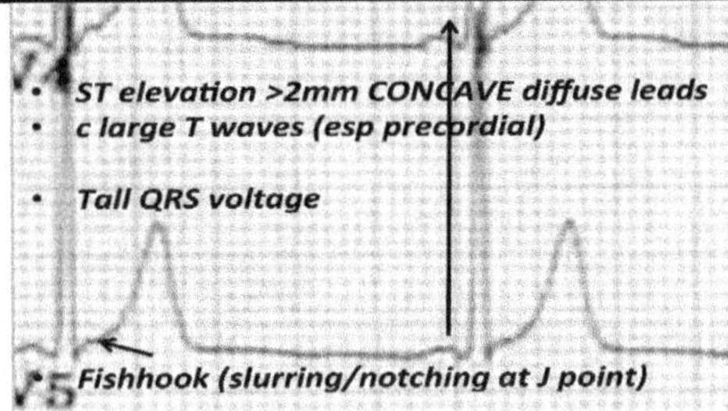

Usually a normal variant.
May be seen in thin, healthy males; African-American males.

EARLY REPOLARIZATION ABNORMALITIES

- **Diffuse CONCAVE ST elevations** >2 mm with **large T waves** (especially precordial).
- **Tall QRS voltage.**
- Fishhook (slurring/notching) at the J point.

LVH with Left Ventricular STRAIN

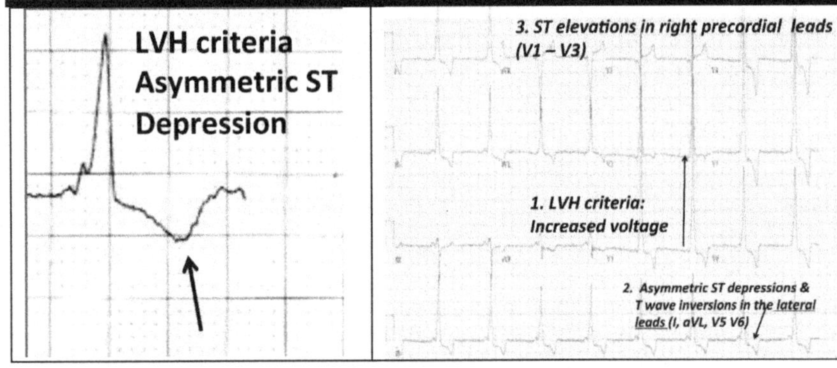

Often seen in patients with left ventricular hypertrophy (LVH) who also suffer from ischemic disease. The coronary artery supply is "strained" trying to supply the excess hypertrophic cardiac muscle.

BRUGADA SYNDROME

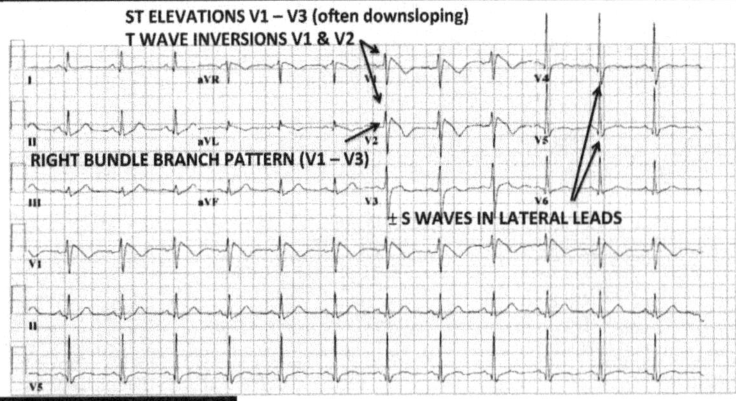

BRUGADA SYNDROME ECG PATTERNS

- **Right bundle branch block (RBB) pattern** (often incomplete).
- **ST elevation V_1-V_3** (often downsloping pattern).
- T wave inversions **V_1 & V_2, ±S wave in lateral leads.**

ANTI-ARRHYTHMIC AGENTS

CLASS I **NA+ CHANNEL BLOCKERS**	Decrease sodium conduction (especially depolarized cells). Affect phase 4 of depolarization (by blocking Na+ channel opening, they reduce SA node automaticity & cause membrane stabilization).
Class IA: **Procainamide** **Quinidine** Disopyramide	MOA: decrease conduction velocity, **prolong repolarization & refractory period. Prolong action potential** & increase excitation threshold. Ind: atrial AND ventricular arrhythmias (eg, SVT, reentrant tachycardias, VT especially if resistant to other meds). **Wolff-Parkinson White.** S/E: Torsades de pointes, hypotension, tachycardia, tinnitus. Caution if kidney dz. **Procainamide & Quinidine associated with drug-induced lupus-like syndrome.** Quinidine may enhance Digoxin toxicity.
Class IB: **Lidocaine** Tocainide	MOA: **decreases conduction velocity & shortens repolarization,** shortens action potential (affects ischemic as well as depolarized ventricular tissue – most useful in abnormal tissue as seen post MI) Indications: Stable VT (alternative). CI: narrow complex supraventricular tachycardia
Class IC: **Flecainide** Propafenone, Encainide	MOA: decreases conduction velocity significantly (↑QRS prolongation). Affects ventricular tissue in healthy cells. No effect on action potential duration. Ind: ventricular tachycardia (used as last line management).
CLASS II **BETA- BLOCKERS**	Antagonizes beta adrenergic receptors to different degrees by decreasing slope of phase 4 (decreased calcium currents – **decreased SA & AV node conduction**).
Cardio selective (β1): **Atenolol, Metoprolol, Esmolol** Nonselective (β1, β2): Propranolol, Sotalol Nonselective α & β1,2: Labetalol, Carvedilol	Ind: **rate control of atrial flutter, atrial fibrillation,** PSVT, ventricular tachycardias. Post MI. S/E: **Bradycardia, AV blocks,** hypotension, CNS (fatigue, depression, sexual dysfunction) **may mask the symptoms of hypoglycemia.** CI: sinus bradycardia, 2nd/3rd heart block, shock, CHF. Caution: Diabetes mellitus, peripheral vascular disease. **Nonselectives may cause bronchospasm in patients with asthma & COPD.** Glucagon is antidote for Beta-blocker toxicity.
CLASS III **K+ CHANNEL BLOCKERS**	Blocks K+ efflux during phase 3 ⇨ action potential prolongation & prolongation of effective refractory period, QT interval prolongation. **Amiodarone (Class III but possess characteristics of class I through IV)**
Amiodarone Ibutilide Dofetilide **Sotalol**	Ind: **atrial AND ventricular arrhythmias;** refractory SVT. S/E of Amiodarone: **pulmonary fibrosis, thyroid disorders** (contains iodine so can cause hyperthyroidism/hypothyroidism), corneal deposits (>6mos use), hepatotoxicity, blue-green skin discoloration, hypotension. Monitor TFTs, PFTs & LFTs in patients on long-term Amiodarone.
CLASS IV **Ca+2 CHANNEL BLOCKERS**	**Slows SA node & AV node conduction** (decreases L-type Ca+2 channels ⇨ decreased conduction speed, ↑PR interval, prolonged refractory period).
Verapamil **Diltiazem**	Ind: **atrial arrhythmias:** atrial flutter, atrial fibrillation, PSVT S/E: **peripheral edema,** bradycardia, AV blocks. Antimuscarinic S/E with **Verapamil (constipation,** dizziness, flushing).
Class V (Other)	Digoxin (cardiac glycoside). Ind: **A fib, heart failure** MOA: inhibit ATP-ase ⇨ positive inotrope, negative chronotrope/dromotrope

Nets play in **B K** for the **C**hampionship (Useful mnemonic to help remember the classes).
Also Note: Class I and III used primarily for rhythm control. Class II & IV primarily for rate control

ADENOSINE

INDICATIONS

- **Paroxysmal supraventricular tachycardia** (PSVT): **slows AV node conduction time and blocks AV nodal reentry pathways**. Short half-life (< 10 seconds) so followed by 5-10 cc IV saline flush.

- **Pharmacologic cardiac stress testing:** activates adenosine receptors (A1 & A2), producing **vasodilation of normal coronary arteries** (excluding diseased coronary arteries). This leads to a shunting effect to mimic increased demand. Adenosine is usually used with thallium-201 stress testing.

ADVERSE EFFECTS

- Common & short-lived: **chest discomfort, dyspnea, flushing**, lightheadedness, headache.
- Serious: **bronchospasm,** hypertension, arrhythmias, and myocardial infarction.

CAUTIONS/CONTRAINDICATIONS

- Use in patients with second and third degree heart block (without a pacemaker), WPW, wide complex tachycardias.
- Clinically active bronchospastic disorders (severe asthma/COPD), acute Myocardial ischemia.

AMIODARONE

MECHANISM OF ACTION

- **Class III antiarrhythmic** (K+ channel blocker) with class I through IV properties.
- Prolongs the action potential.

INDICATIONS

- **Most commonly used for stable wide-complex tachycardias** but useful for both atrial and ventricular arrhythmias, including refractory SVT.

ADVERSE EFFECTS

- IV use: **hypotension most common,** bradycardia, heart block, vasodilatation, polymorphic VT, phlebitis.
- Long-term use: corneal deposition with > 6 month use (most common side effect), **thyroid disorders:** hypo- or hyperthyroidism (contains iodine), **pulmonary fibrosis, increased LFTs**, blue-green discoloration of the skin. Monitor PFTs, TFTs, and LFTs for adverse effects.

CAUTION

- Procainamide and Amiodarone are not generally used together.
- Amiodarone is a cytochrome p450 inhibitor.

CONTRAINDICATIONS

- Second or third-degree heart block who do not have pacemakers, WPW with concurrent A fib.

NORMAL FETAL CIRCULATION

FETAL CARDIAC PHYSIOLOGY

- **FETAL CIRCULATION USES RIGHT TO LEFT SHUNTS.** The **fetus receives its nutrients & oxygen from the placenta** (not the fetal lungs). The oxygenated & nutrient-rich blood goes from the placenta to the right atrium. There are 2 right to left shunts that bypass the nonfunctioning fetal lungs:

1. **FORAMEN OVALE: which shunts** about 2/3 of the blood **from the right atrium directly into the left atrium.** The remaining 1/3 passes into the right ventricle. Most of the remaining 1/3 goes through the right ventricle and gets pumped into the pulmonary artery.

2. **DUCTUS ARTERIOSUS: shunts blood from the pulmonary artery directly into the aorta** (systemic circulation), bypassing the fetal lungs.

Note: as a baby takes its first breath, left side pressure becomes > right side pressure, promoting closure of these openings.

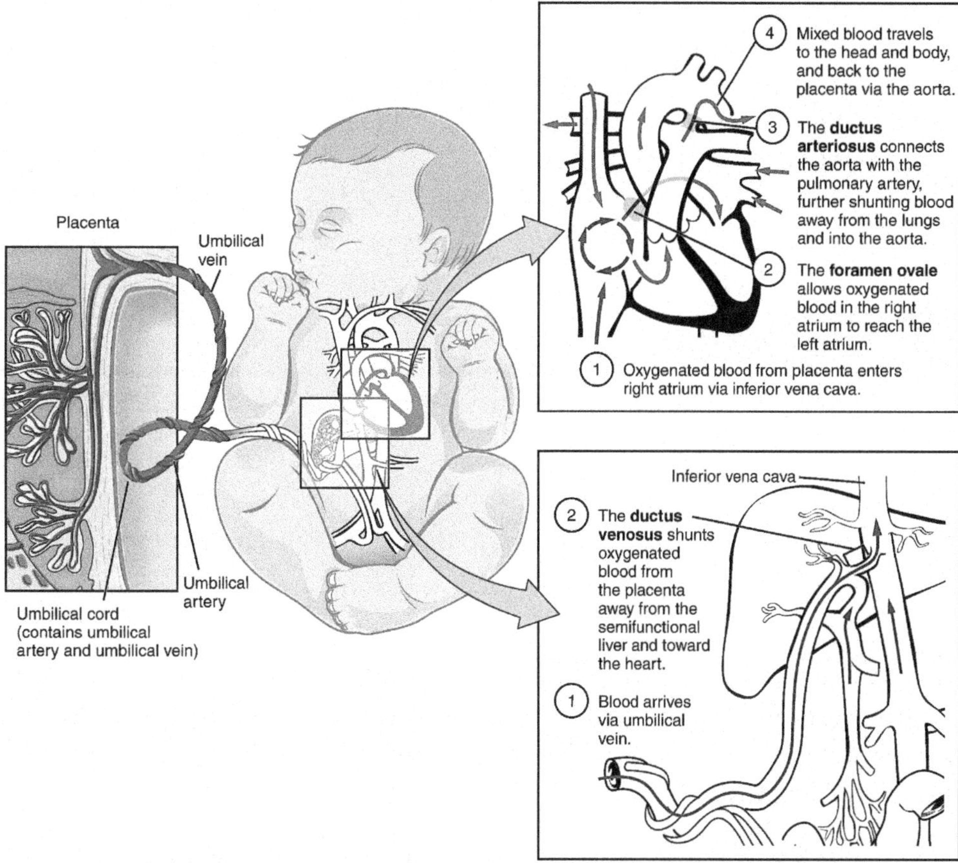

By OpenStax College [CC BY 3.0 (http://creativecommons.org/licenses/by/3.0)], via Wikimedia Commons

CLINICAL CORRELATION

Prostaglandins keep the ductus arteriosus patent (prostaglandins are vasodilators).

1. To **close a patent ductus arteriosus**, a **prostaglandin inhibitor** is given (eg, **IV indomethacin** or Ibuprofen). Most commonly used in preterm infants or within the 1st 10-14 days of life.
2. To **keep the ductus arteriosus open, administer prostaglandins.** In severe cyanotic diseases (eg, severe coarctation of the aorta, tetralogy of Fallot or transposition of the great vessels), a patent ductus arteriosus allows for mixing of the blood to improve cyanosis. **Prostaglandin E1 analogs** (eg, Alprostadil) maintains the ductus arteriosus open, reducing the cyanosis and improving circulation until surgical correction can be performed.

PEDIATRIC FUNCTIONAL MURMURS

Innocent (functional, physiologic) murmurs: non-pathologic, "functioning" murmurs caused by blood moving through the chambers.

Innocent murmurs tend to be soft, not associated with symptoms, position-dependent, often occurs during systole & seen in up to 40% of children at some point in their lives.

Systolic murmurs may be innocent or pathologic. *Diastolic murmurs are almost always pathological.*

STILL MURMURS

- **Most common innocent (physiologic) murmur.**
- Usually heard from 2 months of age until preadolescence.
- Pathophysiology: thought to be due to the vibration of the valve leaflets.

PHYSICAL EXAMINATION

- **Musical, vibratory, noisy, twanging,** low-pitched early to mid-systolic ejection murmur that is best heard in the inferior aspect of the **left lower sternal border & apex.**
- Minimal to no radiation (may radiate to the carotids).
- Diminishes with standing or Valsalva.
- Accentuated in the supine position and hyperdynamic states (eg, fever, anxiety).

CERVICAL VENOUS HUM

- 2nd most common innocent murmur (after Still's) & **most common continuous** benign murmur.
- Most commonly seen between 2-8 years of life.

PATHOPHYSIOLOGY

- Due to turbulent blood flow from blood returning to the heart at the junction between the jugular vein and the superior vena cava.

PHYSICAL EXAMINATION

- Soft, whirling, low-pitched **continuous murmur**, best heard in the right sternal border and right infraclavicular area in the upright position. The murmur does not radiate.
- Increased intensity: sitting or upright position with the head extended.
- **Decreased murmur intensity: supine, jugular compression, & rotation or flexion of the head,** Valsalva.

PULMONARY EJECTION MURMUR

- Usually heard in older children and adolescents.
- It is best heard in mid systole and in the left second intercostal space (or superior aspect of the left lower sternal border).
- Due to blood flowing across the pulmonary valve into the pulmonary artery. Commonly heard in older children & adolescents. Best heard in *mid-systole* in the **second left intercostal space** (or superior aspect of the left lower sternal border). Harsh in quality.

PATENT FORAMEN OVALE

- Covered but not sealed open communication between the right and left atria; however, a PFO is not considered an ASD because no septal tissue is missing (it is due to failed septal fusion).

CLINICAL MANIFESTATIONS
- Most are asymptomatic
- **Strokes from paradoxical embolism**, **cryptogenic stroke** (stroke with no other underlying cause), decompression sickness, migraine, and acute limb ischemia secondary to emboli.

DIAGNOSIS
- **Echocardiogram: best test to make the diagnosis.** Transthoracic echocardiogram is usually performed first but Transesophageal echocardiogram is more sensitive.

MANAGEMENT
- Percutaneous device closure, surgical PFO closure. Cryptogenic stroke: antiplatelet or anticoagulants.

ATRIAL SEPTAL DEFECT

- Abnormal opening in the atrial septum between the right and left atrium.
- Pathophysiology: allows for a left to right shunt (noncyanotic).
- Types: **ostium secundum most common type** (80%), ostium primum (associated with mitral valve abnormalities), sinus venosus, coronary sinus.

CLINICAL MANIFESTATIONS
- Most patients are asymptomatic or minimally symptomatic in childhood.
- Symptoms often initially occur in the third decade of life or later.
- Infants & young children: recurrent respiratory infection, failure to thrive, exertional dyspnea.
- Adolescents & young adults: exertional dyspnea, easy fatigability, palpitations, atrial arrhythmias, syncope, heart failure.
- May develop **paradoxical emboli** (stroke from venous clots) or dysrhythmias later in life.

PHYSICAL EXAMINATION
- **Systolic ejection** crescendo-decrescendo flow **murmur at the pulmonic area (left upper sternal border).**
- **Wide, fixed split S2 that does not vary with respirations**, loud S1, & hyperdynamic right ventricle.

DIAGNOSIS
- **Echocardiogram: best test to make the diagnosis.**
- ECG: incomplete RBBB. Crochetage sign (notching of the peak of the R wave in the inferior leads).
- CXR: cardiomegaly & increased cardiovascular markings.
- Cardiac catheterization: definitive but rarely needed.

MANAGEMENT
- **Small ASD < 5mm may be observed** (most small ASD spontaneously close in the first year if life).

- Surgical correction: if > 1cm or symptomatic (usually between 2-4 years of age).
  Percutaneous transcatheter closure vs. surgical intervention.

PATENT DUCTUS ARTERIOSUS

- Persistent communication between the descending thoracic aorta and main pulmonary artery after birth.

- Usually associated with a left to right shunt (noncyanotic).

- Risk factors: prematurity, female (2 times more common), fetal hypoxia.

PATHOPHYSIOLOGY
- **Continued prostaglandin E1 production** & low arterial oxygen content promotes patency.

CLINICAL MANIFESTATIONS
- Most are asymptomatic. Infants may develop poor feeding, weight loss, frequent lower respiratory tract infections, pulmonary congestion, infective endocarditis.

- Eisenmenger syndrome: pulmonary hypertension & cyanotic heart disease occurring when a left-to-right shunt switches and becomes a right-to-left shunt (cyanotic). Patients may develop cyanotic lower extremities (cyanosis and clubbing of the feet).

PHYSICAL EXAMINATION
- **Continuous machine-like** or "to and fro" **murmur loudest at the pulmonic area** (left upper sternal border).

- Wide pulse pressures **(bounding peripheral pulses)**, loud S2.

DIAGNOSIS
- **Echocardiogram: best initial test.**

- ECG: LVH, left atrial enlargement.

- CXR: normal or cardiomegaly.

- Cardiac catheterization: definitive but usually not necessary.

MANAGEMENT
- **NSAIDs first-line medical treatment** (eg, **IV Indomethacin,** Ibuprofen). NSAIDs inhibit prostaglandin synthesis.

- Surgical correction (eg, percutaneous catheter occlusion or surgical ligation) if no closure with Indomethacin. Best if done before 1-3 years of age.

COARCTATION OF THE AORTA

- Congenital **narrowing of the aortic lumen** at the distal arch or descending aorta. 2 times more common in males.

- Often associated with **bicuspid aortic valve** (70%), mitral valve defects, patent ductus arteriosus, and Turner syndrome.

PATHOPHYSIOLOGY

- Narrowing of the aorta most commonly at the insertion of the ductus arteriosus distal to the origin of the left subclavian vein results in hypertension in the arteries proximal to the lesion (eg, primary arteries supplying the upper extremities) with relative hypotension in the lower extremities.
- Over time, the body compensates by developing collaterals around the coarctation (eg, intercostal arteries).

TYPES

- Post-ductal (adult type) - narrowing occurs distal to the ductus arteriosum.

- Pre-ductal (infantile type) – narrowing occurs proximal to ductus arteriosum.

CLINICAL MANIFESTATIONS

- May range from asymptomatic to heart failure or shock after birth with closure of the patent ductus arteriosus.

- **Bilateral claudication,** dyspnea on exertion, syncope.

- Neonatal presentation: failure to thrive in infants, poor feeding 1-2 weeks after birth.

PHYSICAL EXAMINATION

- **Upper extremity systolic hypertension with lower extremity hypotension and/or diminished or delayed lower extremity pulses** (eg, femoral & dorsalis pedis pulses).

- Systolic murmur radiating to the back, scapula, or chest.

DIAGNOSIS

- **Echocardiography: confirmatory test** (narrowing of the aorta).

- CXR: **posterior rib notching** (due to increased intercostal artery collateral flow), **3 sign** (narrowed aorta looks like the notch of the number 3).

- ECG: left ventricular hypertrophy

- Angiography: gold standard

MANAGEMENT

- **Corrective surgery or transcatheter-based intervention** (eg, balloon angioplasty with or without stent placement), preferably in early childhood.

- **Prostaglandin E1 (eg, Alprostadil) preoperatively** to stabilize the condition - maintains a patent ductus arteriosus, reducing symptoms & improves lower extremity blood flow.

TETRALOGY OF FALLOT

- Constellation of 1) RV outflow obstruction 2) Right ventricular hypertrophy (RVH) 3) large unrestrictive VSD and 4) overriding aorta.

- **Most common cyanotic congenital heart disease** (associated with a **right-to-left shunt**).

- Risk factors: genetic & environmental factors. Associated with chromosome 22 deletion.

CLINICAL MANIFESTATIONS

- Infancy: **cyanosis most common presentation** (blue baby syndrome).

- Older children: exertional dyspnea, cyanosis that worsens with age. **Tet spells** – paroxysms of **cyanosis relieved with squatting** (squatting decreases right-to-left shunting, improving oxygenation). In infants, Tet spells are relieved with putting the knees to the chest.

PHYSICAL EXAMINATION

- **Harsh systolic murmur at left mid to upper sternal border** (VSD), **right ventricular heave** (RVH), digital clubbing, cyanosis.

DIAGNOSIS

- **Echocardiogram: test of choice.**

- CXR: **boot-shaped heart** (prominent right ventricle).

- ECG: RVH, right atrial enlargement.

MANAGEMENT

- **Surgical repair** performed ideally in the first 4-12 months of life.

- **Prostaglandin infusion prior to surgery to maintain a patent ductus arteriosus** (improves circulation).

- Prophylaxis for bacterial endocarditis

TRANSPOSITION OF THE GREAT ARTERIES (TOGA)

- Discordance between the aorta and pulmonary trunk (the aorta arises from the right ventricle and the pulmonary trunk arises from the left ventricle).

- Most common cyanotic heart disease presenting in the neonatal period (dextro).

TYPES

- **Dextro-TGA: most common. The aorta arises from the right ventricle & the pulmonary artery from the left ventricle,** leading to **two parallel circuits.** The systemic circuit sends systemic deoxygenated blood back to the systemic circulation. The pulmonary circuit sends oxygenated pulmonary venous blood back to the lungs. **Prior to surgical correction, survival is dependent upon the presence of shunts between the right and left circulations** (eg, patent ductus arteriosus, ASD, VSD).

- Levo-TGA: is **usually acyanotic**. The right atrium (RA) sends blood to the morphologic left ventricle (LV), which is on the right side physically. This morphologic LV sends blood to pulmonary system. The left atrium (LA) sends blood to morphologic right ventricle (RV) located on the left side; The morphologic right ventricle sends blood to the systemic circulation.

CLINICAL MANIFESTATIONS

- **Severe cyanosis & tachypnea within the first 30 days of life** not affected by exertion or the use of oxygen.

DIAGNOSIS

- **Echocardiogram: primary means of diagnosis.**

- Electrocardiography: may be normal or show right axis deviation or right ventricular hypertrophy.

- Chest radiography: **"egg on a string" appearance** - the heart appears as an egg on its side with the narrowed, atrophic thymus of the superior mediastinum appearing as the string. Mildly increased pulmonary vascular congestion, & mild cardiomegaly.

- Cardiac catheterization: gold standard but rarely used to make the diagnosis but may be used in therapeutic treatment (eg, balloon atrial septostomy).

MANAGEMENT

- **Arterial switch operation.**

- Prostaglandin E1 analog to maintain a patent ductus arteriosus & balloon atrial septostomy may be needed for temporary intercirculatory mixing prior to definitive surgical repair.

- Without treatment, 90% die by 1 year. 5 year survival rate after surgery >80%.

	ATRIAL SEPTAL DEFECT	PATENT DUCTUS ARTERIOSUS	COARCTATION OF AORTA	TETRALOGY OF FALLOT
DEFINITION	***Hole in atrial septum*** (opening between right & left atrium).	Communication between descending thoracic aorta & pulmonary artery	Congenital narrowing of descending thoracic aorta. Male:female 2:1	MC cyanotic congenital heart disease
SHUNT	Left to Right (Noncyanotic)	Left to Right (Noncyanotic)	Noncyanotic usually	***Right to Left (Cyanotic)****
ETIOLOGIES **PATHOPHYSIOLOGY**	• ***Ostium secundum MC**** (80%) • Ostium primum – associated with mitral regurgitation • Sinus venosus, coronary sinus • ASD 2nd MC cause of CHD (VSD MC)	Prematurity, perinatal distress & hypoxia delays closure, Rubella infection in the 1st trimester. Continued Prostaglandin E_2 production promotes patency	↑LV afterload with SNS activity & RAAS activation ⇨ HTN, LVH, CHF. ***<u>70% ALSO HAVE BICUSPID AORTIC VALVE*</u>***	❶ ***RV outflow obstruction*** – *pulmonary artery stenosis* ❷ ***RV Hypertrophy*** ❸ ***VSD (large unrestrictive)*** ❹ ***overriding aorta*** – between ventricles
CLINICAL MANIFESTATIONS	• ***Most patients asymptomatic or minimal in childhood until >30y.*** • <u>Infants/young children</u>: recurrent respiratory infections, failure to thrive, exertional dyspnea. • <u>Adolescents/Adults:</u> exertional dyspnea, easy fatigability, palpitations, atrial arrhythmias, syncope, heart failure. • Stroke (paroxysmal embolus)	• Most asymptomatic • Poor feeding, weight loss, frequent lower respiratory tract infections, pulmonary congestion • ***<u>Eisenmenger's syndrome:</u>*** pulmonary HTN ⇨ ***left to right shunt switches & becomes right to left shunt (cyanotic)***	• ***<u>Secondary HTN</u>**** • ***bilateral claudication,*** dyspnea on exertion, syncope. • <u>Infants:</u> failure to thrive, poor feeding, shock. <u>Types</u> • Infantile: preductal • Adult: postductal	• ***Blue Baby syndrome (cyanosis)*** • <u>Older:</u> exertional dyspnea, cyanosis worsens with age. • ***<u>"Tet-spells"*:</u>*** paroxysms of cyanosis – ***older children relieve spells by squatting*.*** • <u>Eisenmenger's syndrome:</u> seen with PDA, VSD, TOF (±ASD)
PHYSICAL EXAM FINDINGS	• ***Systolic ejection crescendo-decrescendo flow murmur @ <u>pulmonic area</u>**** (left upper sternal border). Sounds like PS (functional flow murmur). • ***<u>WIDELY SPLIT FIXED S_2:</u>* DOES NOT VARY WITH RESPIRATIONS.**** • *Loud S_1, hyperdynamic RV**	• *<u>CONTINUOUS MACHINERY MURMUR</u>** ***loudest @ pulmonic area.*** • ***Wide pulse pressure: <u>BOUNDING PERIPHERAL PULSES</u>**** LOUD S2 • Eisenmenger: normal hands (upper extremities) with cyanotic lower extremities (clubbed, blue toes)	• ***Systolic murmur that <u>radiates to the back/scapula/chest*</u>*** • ↑***<u>BP upper > lower extremities*</u>.*** • ***<u>Delayed/weak femoral pulses</u>**** ↓flow distal to obstruction in the lower extremities.	• ***Harsh holosystolic murmur @ <u>left upper sternal border</u>*** (sounds like PS). • ***Right ventricular heave.*** • Digital clubbing
DIAGNOSIS	• <u>CXR:</u> - cardiomegaly • <u>ECG:</u> - Incomplete RBB (rsR' in V_1 RAD) - <u>Crochetage sign</u>: notching of the peak of the R wave in inferior leads. • <u>Echocardiogram:</u> gold standard	• <u>CXR:</u> Normal or cardiomegaly • <u>ECG:</u> LVH, left atrial enlargement • <u>Echocardiogram:</u> gold standard	• <u>CXR:</u> - ***<u>Rib notching</u>*:*** ↑collateral circulation via intercostal arteries. - ***<u>"3 sign"</u>.**** Narrowed aorta looks like the notch of the number 3 • <u>ECG:</u> LVH • ***<u>Angiogram: gold standard.</u>**** CT scan	• <u>CXR:</u> - ***<u>Boot-shaped heart</u>**** Prominent right ventricle • <u>ECG:</u> ***Right ventricular hypertrophy**** Right atrial enlargement (RAE) • <u>Echocardiogram:</u> gold standard
MANAGEMENT	• Spontaneous closure likely in 1st year so may observe if small. • Surgical correction if symptomatic (usually between 2-4y)	• ***IV indomethacin 1st line tx**** (closes the PDA) • Surgical correction if indomethacin fails. Best if done before 1-3y of age.	• Surgical Correction • Balloon angioplasty ± stent • Prostaglandin E_1 (PGE_1) preoperatively (reduces symptoms, improves lower extremity blood flow)	Surgical repair performed in the first 4 – 12 months of life. PGE1 infusion: prevents ductal closure if patient in cyanotic patients prior to surgery.

ATRIAL SEPTAL DEFECT

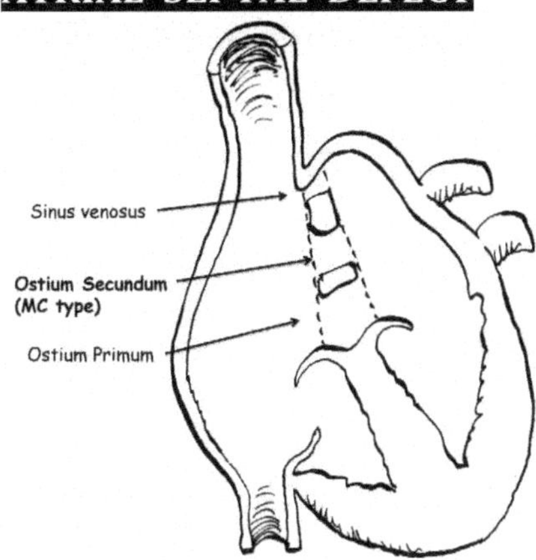

HALLMARKS

- Usually asymptomatic until >30y
- **Systolic ejection murmur** best heard at the pulmonic area.
- May develop stroke due to paradoxical emboli.
- **Widely fixed, split S2 (doesn't vary with respirations).**

PATENT DUCTUS ARTERIOSUS

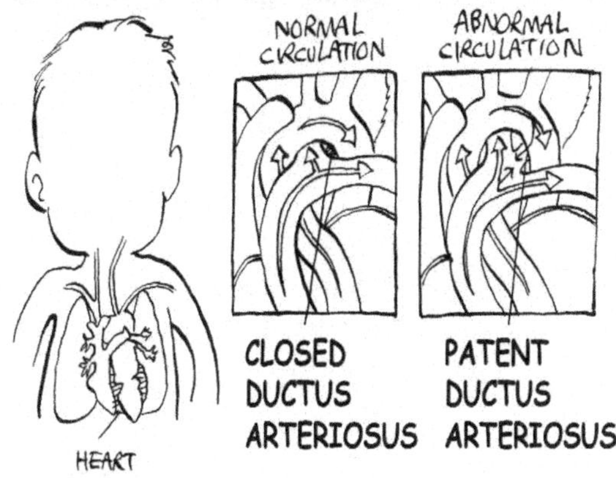

HALLMARKS

- **Continuous machinery murmur** loudest at the pulmonic area
- Wide pulse pressure - **bounding pulses**
- **IV Indomethacin 1st line to close a PDA in infants** (prostaglandin inhibition).

TETRALOGY OF FALLOT

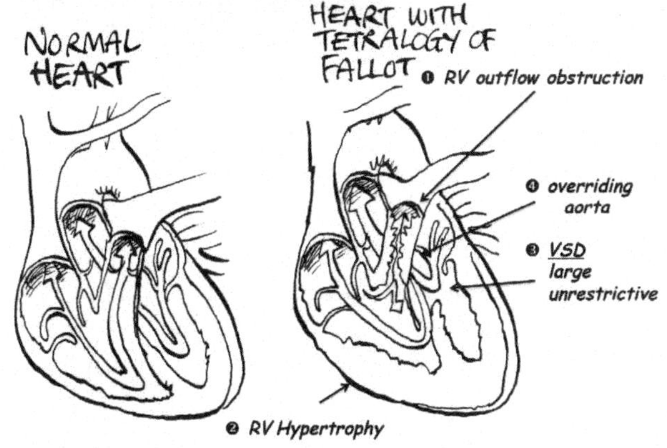

HALLMARKS

- MC cyanotic heart disease overall.
- Cyanosis in infants, **Tet spells** in older children (**periodic episodes of cyanosis relived with squatting** or putting an infant's knees to its chest).
- CXR: **boot-shaped heart**
- Management: surgical correction. Prostaglandin E1 prior to surgery to maintain patency of the ductus arteriosus.

COARCTATION OF THE AORTA

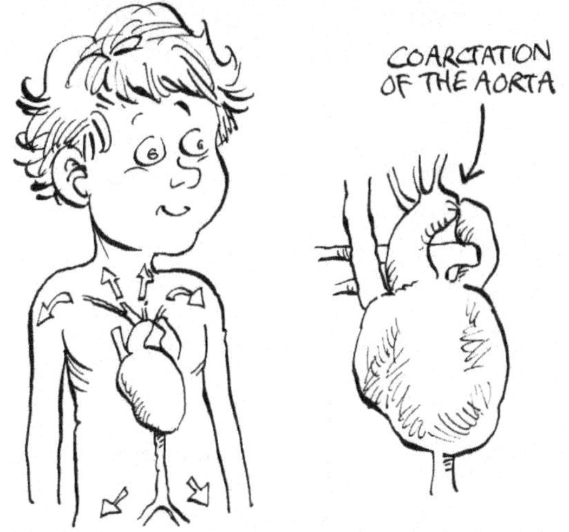

HALLMARKS

- 70% have a bicuspid aortic valve.
- Suspect in a child with 2ry **hypertension**, bilateral lower extremity claudication.
- Systolic murmur that radiates to the back, scapula or chest.
- **Systolic blood pressure in upper extremities > lower extremities.**
- Delayed or weak femoral pulses.
- CXR: **rib notching** (due to dilation of the intercostal arteries), **"3" sign** (shape of the coarctation).

VENTRICULAR SEPTAL DEFECT (VSD)

- Hole in the ventricular septum. Usually associated with a left to right shunt.
- **Most common type of congenital heart disease in childhood**.
- Small to moderate associated with a left to right shunt. Large (unrestricted) defects may eventually develop a right to left shunt (Eisenmenger syndrome).

TYPES

- Perimembranous: **most common type** (80%). Hole in the LV outflow tract near the tricuspid valve.
- Muscular: usually multiple holes in a **"swiss cheese"** pattern.
- Inlet (posterior): located posterior to the septal leaflet of the tricuspid valve.
- Supracristal (outlet): beneath the pulmonic valve. May have aortic valve insufficiency.

CLINICAL MANIFESTATIONS

- Small (restrictive): asymptomatic or mild symptoms. Normal pressure differences between the ventricles are maintained. Usually asymptomatic at birth and develop symptoms after a few weeks.
- Moderate: excessive sweating or fatigue, especially during feeds, lack of adequate growth, frequent respiratory infections.
- Large (unrestricted): severe symptoms. **No pressure differences between the ventricles.**
- Eisenmenger syndrome: right to left shunt occurring with large (unrestricted) VSDs.

PHYSICAL EXAMINATION

- **High-pitched harsh holosystolic murmur** best heard at the **lower left sternal border.**
- Smaller VSDs are usually louder and associated with more palpable thrills than larger ones.
- May be associated with a thrill or diastolic rumble at the mitral area.

DIAGNOSIS

- **Echocardiogram:** determines the size and location of VSD. **Echocardiogram usually preferred over catheterization.**

- ECG: LVH in mild to moderate disease. Combines RVH + LVH (Katz-Wachtel phenomenon).

- Chest radiograph: may be normal, show left atrial enlargement or right ventricular hypertrophy.

MANAGEMENT

- Observation: in small, asymptomatic VSDs (most close within 12 months).

- Patch closure: symptomatic infants or uncontrolled CHF, growth delay, recurrent respiratory infections. Large shunts repaired by 2 years of age to prevent pulmonary hypertension.

CONGENITAL CYANOTIC HEART DISEASES

5 Ts:

1. **TRUNCUS ARTERIOSUS** **1 vessel** instead of 2 normal vessels (aorta & pulmonary artery)

2. **TRANSPOSITION OF GREAT ARTERIES** **2 vessels switched** (aorta & pulmonary artery).

3. **TRICUSPID ATRESIA** (**3= tri**) absence of the **tri**cuspid valve leads to a hypoplastic right ventricle. An ASD & VSD must be present for blood to flow out of the right atrium.

4. **TETRALOGY OF FALLOT** (**4- tetra**): 4 problems: ❶ right ventricular outflow obstruction ex. pulmonary stenosis ❷ right ventricular hypertrophy ❸ overriding aorta & ❹ ventricular septal defect (large, unrestrictive).

5. **TOTAL ANOMALOUS PULMONARY VENOUS RETURN** (**5 vessels involved**): all 4 pulmonary veins connect to 1 vessel (superior vena cava) instead of the left atrium.

Hypoplastic left heart syndrome is often associated with mitral valve &/or aortic valve atresia.

PULMONARY ATRESIA

- Pulmonary atresia with intact intraventricular septum (PA/IVS) is characterized by **complete obstruction to right ventricular outflow** with varying degrees of right ventricular & tricuspid valve hypoplasia – **blood is unable to flow from the right ventricle into the pulmonary artery & the lungs.**

TYPES:

- Valvular (membranous): atretic pulmonary valve, small valve annulus with fused valve leaflets leading to a thin, intact membrane that causes right ventricular outflow tract obstruction.
- Muscular: obliteration of the muscular infundibulum. It is associated with severe right ventricular hypoplasia and increased coronary artery abnormalities.

CLINICAL MANIFESTATIONS

- Cyanosis due to right-to-left shunting at the atrial level. Improved survival if there is a patent ductus arteriosus.
- Single heart sound (due to a single semilunar valve – the aortic valve).
- Systolic murmur of tricuspid regurgitation

MANAGEMENT

- Maintain the patency of the ductus arteriosus (ex. prostaglandin E1 analog Alprostadil) to stabilize initially. Balloon atrial septostomy to improve the right to left atrial shunting.
- Surgical repair: definitive. If untreated, approximately 50% of these children die within 2 weeks of birth & 85% by six months.

TRICUSPID ATRESIA

- 2% of all congenital heart disease. Absence of the tricuspid valve leads to a hypoplastic right ventricle. A PDA or VSD is necessary for pulmonary blood flow and survival.

CLINICAL MANIFESTATIONS
- Cyanosis due to right-to-left shunting. Improved survival if there is a patent ductus arteriosus.
- Single heart sound (S_2).

DIAGNOSIS
- ECG: left ventricular hypertrophy.
- CXR: normal or enlarged cardiac silhouette with *decreased* pulmonary flow.

MANAGEMENT
- Maintain the patency of the ductus arteriosus (ex. prostaglandin E1 analog Alprostadil) to stabilize initially. Presence of VSD improves oxygenation of blood.
- Surgical repair: definitive. Subclavian artery to pulmonary shunt followed by a 2-staged surgical correction to direct systemic venous return directly to the pulmonary arteries.

HYPOPLASTIC LEFT HEART SYNDROME

- Failure of the development of the mitral valve, aortic valve, or the aortic arch ⇨ small ventricle unable to supply the normal systemic circulation requirements. 1% of all congenital heart disease.

CLINICAL MANIFESTATIONS
- Symptoms begin when the ductus arteriosus constricts, leading to cyanosis and heart failure.

DIAGNOSIS
- ECG: right ventricular hypertrophy.
- CXR: cardiomegaly.

MANAGEMENT
- Prostaglandin E1 to open the ductus arteriosus followed by surgical repair.

CORONARY ARTERY DISEASE (CAD)

- Pathologic process affecting the coronary artery disease, **usually due Atherosclerosis** (hardening and narrowing of the coronary arteries).
- **Inadequate tissue perfusion** due to imbalance between **increased demand & decreased coronary artery blood supply.**

MAJOR RISK FACTORS

- **Diabetes mellitus (worst risk factor, considered a CAD equivalent), smoking (most important modifiable risk factor),** hyperlipidemia, hypertension, men, age >45 in men or >55 in women & family history of coronary artery disease (eg, first-degree relative – father or brother before age 55 and in a mother or sister before the age of 65).

ANGINA PECTORIS

- A complication of Coronary artery disease leading to symptoms.

PATHOPHYSIOLOGY

- **Inadequate tissue perfusion** due to imbalance between **increased demand & decreased coronary artery blood supply.**
- Symptoms usually occur with occlusion 70% or greater.

CLINICAL MANIFESTATIONS

- **Chest pain: classic.** Although there is significant variation, the pain is classically **substernal, poorly localized, exertional, short in duration** (**< 30 minutes** but often resolves within 5 minutes of cessation of activity), exacerbated with activity or stress and **relieved with rest or Nitroglycerin,** may radiate to the arm, teeth, lower jaw, back, epigastrium, or shoulders.
- Associated symptoms: dyspnea, nausea, vomiting, diaphoresis, numbness, fatigue.
- Anginal equivalent: instead of chest pain, patients develop dyspnea, epigastric or shoulder pain. This is especially seen in women, elderly, diabetics, and obese patients.
- Physical examination is usually normal.

DIAGNOSIS

- Stable angina is usually a clinical diagnosis along with testing.
- **ECG: initial test if choice. ST depression classic finding,** T wave inversions, poor R wave progression, T wave pseudonormalization. **The resting ECG is normal in 50% of cases.**
- **Stress testing: most important noninvasive testing.** Options include stress ECG, myocardial perfusion imaging, or stress echocardiography.
- **Coronary angiography: definitive diagnostic test.** Defines location and extent of CAD.

MANAGEMENT

Medical:

- Typical outpatient regimen includes 4 drugs: **daily Aspirin + Beta blockers (both decrease mortality), sublingual Nitroglycerin as needed, and daily Statin.**
- Calcium channel blockers can be used in lieu of Beta blockers if Beta blockers are contraindicated or in Vasospastic disorders (eg, Prinzmetal).
- Reduction of risk factors: hypertension and DM control, exercise, diet, smoking cessation.

Revascularization: definitive management

- Percutaneous transluminal coronary angioplasty – 1 or 2 vessel disease in nondiabetics not involving the left main coronary artery, with normal or near-normal ejection fraction.
- Coronary artery bypass graft – **left main coronary artery stenosis, 3 vessel disease** (2 vessel disease in diabetics), or decreased left ventricular ejection fraction <40%

Class I: angina only with *unusually strenuous activity.* No limitations of activity.
Class II: angina with *more prolonged or rigorous activity.* Slight limitation of physical activity.
Class III: angina with usual daily activity. Marked limitation of physical activity.
Class IV: *angina at rest.* Often unable to carry out any physical activity.

STRESS TESTING IN CAD

- **Most useful noninvasive test** in the diagnosis of **Coronary artery disease.**

Stress ECG

- Indications: useful only **if baseline ECG is normal.**
- Positive findings include ECG changes (eg, ST depressions, T wave inversions, poor R wave progression) or reproduction of symptoms or signs.
- Limitations: does not locate the area of ischemia.

Myocardial perfusion imaging:

- Uses **Thallium or Technetium for imaging.**
- Indications: can be used if baseline ECG is abnormal. Gives information regarding the location & extent of ischemia.
- Can be performed either with exercise or a pharmacologic agent if the patient cannot exercise - vasodilators (eg, **Adenosine or Dipyridamole**).
- Contraindications to vasodilators: **bronchospastic disease,** hypotension, AV blocks.
- Theophylline and caffeine should be stopped 48 hours and 12 hours respectively.

Stress echocardiogram:

- Indications: can be used if baseline ECG is abnormal. Gives information regarding the location & extent of ischemia.
- Can be performed with exercise or pharmacologic if patient cannot exercise with **positive inotropes** (eg, **Dopamine or Dobutamine**).
- Contraindications to positive inotropes: severe LV outflow obstruction (eg, **Aortic stenosis**), ventricular arrhythmias, recent MI (1-3 days), or severe systemic hypertension.

Other considerations:

- During stress testing in patients without a history of coronary artery disease, antianginal medications (nitrates, beta blockers and calcium channel blockers) should be withheld 48 hours prior to stress testing.
- Patients with known history of coronary artery disease should continue their antianginal medications prior to stress testing. This allows for the evaluation of the efficacy of the patient's current treatment regimen and also to determine the appropriate level of exercise that is safe for the patient.

CORONARY ANGIOGRAPHY

- **Definitive diagnosis/gold standard.** "Cath" outlines the coronary artery anatomy. Angiography also defines location & extent of coronary artery disease (CAD).

Indications:

1. Confirm/exclude CAD in patients with symptoms consistent with CAD.
2. Confirm/exclude CAD in patients with negative noninvasive testing for CAD.
3. Patients who may possibly need revascularization (PTCA or CABG).

LONG-TERM MEDICAL MANAGEMENT OF STABLE ANGINA

Angina is chest pain brought on by exertion (due to ↓SUPPLY & ↑DEMAND) so the pharmacologic treatment is effective by increasing supply while simultaneously reducing demand.

PHARMACOLOGIC MANAGEMENT OF STABLE (CHRONIC) ANGINA	
β – BLOCKERS **Cardioselective (β_1):** **Metoprolol,** **Atenolol**	❶**↑myocardial blood supply: ↑O_2 by prolonging coronary artery filling times** (coronary arteries fill during diastole). Beta-blockers increase diastolic timing. ❷**↓Demand: reduces heart rate & myocardial O_2 requirements during exercise/stress** (negative chronotrope/inotrope). **Indications: 1st-line drug for Stable angina (reduces mortality**, decreases symptoms & prevents ischemic occurrences).
ASPIRIN	**Prevents platelet activation/aggregation** (by inhibiting cyclooxygenase ⇨ ↓**thromboxane A_2** & inhibiting prostaglandins). Does not directly address the supply & demand problem but prevents progression from chronic stable angina to acute coronary syndrome (the first step in ACS is thrombosis after plaque rupture). **Aspirin decreased mortality** & thrombosis risk. Cautious use in patients with active peptic ulcer disease or ↑bleeding risk.
NITROGLYCERIN **(Nitrates)** **Oral, spray, patch**	❶**↑myocardial blood supply:** ↑O_2 & ↑collateral blood flow to ischemic myocardium, **reduces coronary vasospasm** & ↑'es coronary artery dilation. ❷**↓demand:** ↓cardiac work: ↓**preload by venodilation.** ↓afterload. **Sublingual most effective.** Used when symptomatic or situations likely to induce angina. If no relief with 1st dose ⇨ give 2nd/3rd q5 minutes. No relief after 3rd dose, suspect ACS. Can be used prophylactically ~5 minutes before an activity likely to cause ischemia. Adverse effects: headache, flushing, tolerance, hypotension, peripheral edema, **tachyphylaxis** after 24h (allow nitrate-free period for 8h). Deteriorates with moisture, light, air. **Contraindications: SBP <90** mm Hg, **RV infarction, use of Sildenafil & other PDE-5 inhibitors.**
CA CHANNEL BLOCKERS **Nondihydropyridines:** **Diltiazem** **Verapamil (long acting)**	❶↑myocardial blood supply: prolongs diastolic filling times. Prevents/terminates ischemia induced by coronary vasospasm by increasing coronary vasodilation. ❷↓demand: ↓'es contractility, ↓'es heart rate (AV node blocker) ↓'es afterload. Indications: used in patients unable to use beta blockers; Prinzmetal angina.

Typical outpatient regimen includes 4 drugs:

- **Daily Aspirin + Beta blockers (both decrease mortality), sublingual Nitroglycerin as needed. Daily Statin.**

Reduction of risk factors: hypertension and DM control, exercise, diet, smoking cessation.

ASPIRIN FOR PRIMARY PREVENTION

- Low-dose Aspirin may be considered for primary prevention of atherosclerotic cardiovascular disease in select patients 40-70 years who are not at increased risk of bleeding.
- Low-dose Aspirin should not be administered on a routine basis for primary prevention in adults >70 years.
- Low-dose Aspirin should not be administered for primary prevention in any adult at any age with increased risk of bleeding.

ACUTE CORONARY SYNDROME (ACS)

- Symptoms of acute myocardial ischemia 2ry to **acute plaque rupture & varying degrees of coronary artery thrombosis (occlusion).**

SPECTRUM OF ACUTE CORONARY SYNDROMES			
	UA	NSTEMI	STEMI
HISTORY	Angina that is new in onset, crescendo, or at rest (usually >30 minutes). >90% occlusion can cause symptoms @ rest		
CORONARY THROMBOSIS	SUBTOTAL *occlusion*		TOTAL *occlusion*
ECG	ST DEPRESSIONS &/or T WAVE INVERSIONS		ST ELEVATIONS
CARDIAC ENZYMES	Negative	Positive (cell death) seen in both NSTEM & STEMI	

ETIOLOGIES

- **Atherosclerosis: (most common cause of MI)**. Plaque rupture ⇨ acute coronary artery thrombosis with platelet adhesion/activation/aggregation along with fibrin formation. Vasculitis, embolism.
- **Coronary artery vasospasm** (2%): **cocaine-induced, variant (Prinzmetal) angina.**

CLINICAL MANIFESTATIONS

- **Chest pain:** retrosternal pressure **not relieved with rest or nitroglycerin, pain at rest**, lasting **≥ 30 minutes**, may radiate to the lower jaw & teeth, left arm, epigastrium, back or shoulders or **change from typical pattern**. Pain at rest usually indicates >90% occlusion.
- Sympathetic stimulation - anxiety, diaphoresis, tachycardia, palpitations, nausea, vomiting, dizziness.
- Silent MI: ~25% are atypical/silent: eg, **women, elderly, diabetics & obese** patients. Atypical symptoms include: abdominal pain, jaw pain, or dyspnea without chest pain.

PHYSICAL EXAMINATION:

- Usually normal. Patients may be tachycardic.
- Inferior wall MI: may be associated with **bradycardia or heart blocks** (the RCA supplies the AV node in 90%). **May have S4** (especially with inferior MI). Triad of right ventricular infarction: **increased JVP + clear lungs + positive Kussmaul sign**.

DIAGNOSTIC STUDIES:

- 12 lead ECG
- Cardiac enzymes

- **STEMI: ST elevations >1mm in ≥ 2 anatomically contiguous leads with reciprocal changes in the opposite leads.**

ECG progression: **Hyperacute T waves first change ⇨ ST elevations ⇨** Q waves

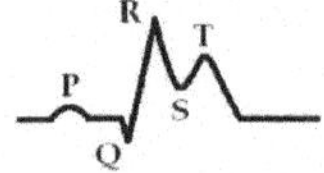

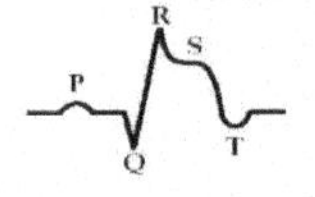

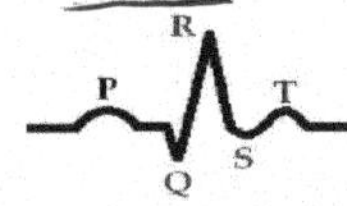

A new Left bundle branch considered an STEMI equivalent

AREA OF INFARCTION	Q WAVES/ST ELEVATIONS	ARTERY INVOLVED
ANTERIOR WALL	V1 through V4	Left Anterior Descending (LAD)
- SEPTAL	V1 & V2	Proximal LAD
LATERAL WALL	I, aVL, V5 & V6	Circumflex (CFX)
ANTEROLATERAL	I, avL, V4 through V6	Mid LAD or CFX
INFERIOR	II, III, avF	Right Coronary Artery (RCA)
POSTERIOR WALL	ST DEPRESSIONS V1-V2	RCA, CFX

Cardiac Markers 3 sets 8 hours apart - **CK-MB & Troponin most commonly ordered**

	Appears	Peaks	Returns to baseline
CK/CK-MB	4-6h	12-24h	3-4d
Troponin I & T	4-8h	12-24h	**7-10 days (most sensitive & specific)**
Myoglobin	2-4h (fastest)	4-6h	1d

^Troponin may be falsely elevated in patients with renal failure, advanced heart failure, acute PE, CVA.

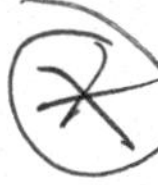

MANAGEMENT OF ACUTE CORONARY SYNDROME OVERVIEW

- **AMI PROTOCOL: ECG within 10 minutes; Door to thrombolytics within 30 minutes; Door to PCI within 90 minutes (± 30 minutes).**
  - **"MONA regimen" – M**orphine, **O**xygen, **N**itrates, **A**spirin (Morphine if no pain relief with nitrates)

STEMI:	ß blockers, NTG, Aspirin, Heparin, **ACEI, REPERFUSION (MOST IMPORTANT).**
UA or NSTEMI:	ß blockers, NTG, Aspirin, Heparin. NO emergent reperfusion!
COCAINE-INDUCED MI	ASA, NTG, heparin, anxiolytics **(avoid β blockers because of vasospasm).**

ACUTE CORONARY SYNDROMES

Symptoms associated with ischemia or infarction

Perform brief history/exam
Obtain cardiac markers
Oxygen @4L/min (especially if O2 sat <94% on room air)
Aspirin (160mg to 325mg) ***chewed for fast absorption***
Nitroglycerin (sublingual/spray)
Morphine (consider if pain not relieved by Nitroglycerin)
Obtain ECG: within first 10 minutes of entering the ER
EKG INTERPRETATION

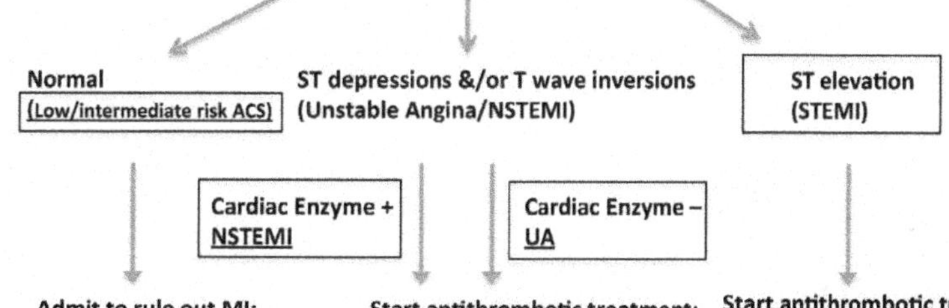

Admit to rule out MI:
◆**Serial ECG's**
◆**Serial cardiac markers**

Start antithrombotic treatment:
- **Heparin (UFH or LMWH)**
- Consider: Clopidogrel
- Consider: GPIIb/IIIa

Consider adjunctive treatment:
- ***β-Blockers***
- Nitroglycerin

Assess TIMI risk score

Start antithrombotic treatment:
- **Heparin (UFH or LMWH)**
- Consider: Clopidogrel
- Consider: GPIIb/IIIa

Consider adjunctive treatment:
- ***β-Blockers***
- Nitroglycerin

Symptoms <12 hours

REPERFUSION!!**
◆**Door to PCI (90 min) OR**
◆**Door to Fibrinolysis (30 min)**

ACS MANAGEMENT

Normal ECG:
MONA + Serial enzymes & ECGs

UA or NSTEMI:
MONA, Heparin, beta blockers
TIMI or HEART risk assessment.

STEMI:
MONA, Heparin, beta blockers, REPERFUSION.*
ACE inhibitors for long term.

Inferior or Posterior wall STEMI:
Oxygen, aspirin, heparin, IV fluids, reperfusion
(no IV Morphine or IV Nitroglycerin)

Cocaine-induced MI & Prinzmetals:
Calcium channel blockers treatment of choice. MONA, Heparin
Avoid selective beta blockers (unopposed alpha constriction)

Use of Phosphodiesterase-5 inhibitors:
NO nitroglycerin*

ANTERIOR AND LATERAL WALL MI

- **Complete occlusion** of the **left anterior descending artery (anterior) or left circumflex (lateral).**

ECG
- **Anterior MI: ST elevations in leads V1 through V4** with reciprocal changes (ST depressions) in the inferior leads (II, III, aVF).
- **Lateral MI: ST elevations in leads I, aVL, V5, V6** with reciprocal changes (ST depressions) in the inferior leads (II, III, aVF).
- Cardiac enzymes: **positive.**

MANAGEMENT
- Initial: **Aspirin (chewed), Nitroglycerin**, Oxygen (if hypoxic), Morphine (if nitro fails to relieve pain).
- Adjunctive: **Heparin, Beta blockers** if no contraindications (eg, hypotension, cardiogenic shock, bradycardia), **Clopidogrel.**
- In STEMI, long-term management with ACE inhibitors slow progression to Heart failure.

Reperfusion:
- **Percutaneous coronary intervention (PCI) ideally within 90 minutes of ER presentation of PCI-capable hospital and within 12 hours of chest pain onset.**
- Thrombolytics within 30 minutes of ER presentation is an alternative to catheterization if PCI is not possible (including transfer to a PCI capable hospital within the first 120 minutes).

INFERIOR or POSTERIOR WALL MI

- **Complete occlusion of the right coronary artery (RCA)** in 80%.
- In 20% the posterior descending artery is a branch of the left circumflex artery.

PHYSICAL EXAMINATION
- **Bradycardia or heart blocks** (the RCA supplies the AV node in 90%).
- **May have S4** (especially with inferior MI).
- Triad of right ventricular infarction: **increased JVP + clear lungs + positive Kussmaul sign**.

DIAGNOSIS
- ECG: **ST elevations in inferior leads (II, III, & aVF)** with reciprocal changes (ST depressions) in leads I & aVL. Right-sided ECGs may increase diagnosis (lead V4R). Posterior: ST depressions in V1 - V4.
- Cardiac enzymes: **positive.**

MANAGEMENT
- Initial: antithrombotic therapy (**Aspirin, Heparin**), IV fluids, oxygen. Clopidogrel.
- **Avoid Nitroglycerin and Morphine in inferior and posterior wall MIs** (right-sided MIs are preload dependent to maintain cardiac output).
- Adjunctive: Beta blockers if no contraindications (eg, hypotension, cardiogenic shock, bradycardia).

Reperfusion:
- **Catheterization lab preferred (ideally within 90 minutes of ER presentation and within 12 hours of chest pain onset).**
- Thrombolytics within 30 minutes alternative to catheterization if access to cath lab is not timely.

CONSERVATIVE MANAGEMENT

- Used in patients whose chest pain began >12 hours (without current/active chest pain) or low TIMI:
  - **Aspirin** (± **Clopidogrel** x 9 months), **statin, beta blocker, ACE Inhibitor. Nitroglycerin** as needed.

COMPLICATIONS OF MYOCARDIAL INFARCTION

- **Arrhythmias (eg, ventricular fibrillation), ventricular aneurysm/rupture,** cardiogenic shock, papillary muscle dysfunction, heart failure, left ventricular wall rupture.
- **Dressler syndrome: post-MI pericarditis** + fever + pulmonary infiltrates.

ADJUNCTIVE THERAPY	
Drug	**Comment**
ß-blockers Cardioselective: • **Metoprolol** • **Atenolol**	Mechanism of action: • Beta-receptor blockade leads to decrease in cardiac output, myocardial oxygen demand, blood pressure, heart rate, & contractility (except those with intrinsic sympathetic activity); decreased renin secretion, decreased post myocardial infarction-induced ventricular remodeling. Often titrated to pulse <70. Indications: • Stable angina • Acute coronary syndrome (Unstable angina, non-ST elevation MI, ST elevation MI) • STEMI: 15% ↓**in mortality in STEMI** (decrease wall tension, prevents MI complications). Adverse effects: • Fatigue, depression, erectile dysfunction, bronchospasm. Contraindications: **Congestive heart failure, bradycardia** (HR <50), **heart block** (2nd/3rd), **hypotension** (SBP <100), **severe reactive airway disease** (severe asthma/COPD), **shock, cocaine-induced MI** (causes unopposed ↑alpha 1-mediated vasoconstriction).
Nitrates	Mechanism of action: • **Increased myocardial blood supply** – increases coronary artery blood flow & collateral circulation as well as reduces coronary artery vasospasm. Vasodilatation occurs due to stimulation of guanylate cyclase, which increases cGMP. • Decreases cardiac demand – **decreased preload & afterload.** Routes: • Sublingual, translingual, transdermal, transmucosal, ointment, IV, oral sustained-release. Indications: • **Stable angina, Acute coronary syndrome, Pulmonary edema, Heart failure, CHF**, hypertensive emergencies, vasospastic disorders (eg, Prinzmetal angina), Esophageal varices (prophylaxis). • Administration: administered sublingual if chest pain occurs. Given up to 3 doses 5 minutes apart. Can be used prophylactically 5 minutes before an activity likely to cause ischemia. Adverse effects: • Headache, flushing, tolerance, hypotension, peripheral edema, **tachyphylaxis** after 24 hours (allow for nitrate-free period for 8 hours), reflex tachycardia. Deteriorates with light, moisture, air. Contraindications for IV: • **Systolic blood pressure < 90 mmHg, RV infarction** (inferior or posterior wall MI), **use of phosphodiesterase-5 inhibitors (eg, Sildenafil).**
ACE Inhibitors	Indications: • **STEMI: slows the progression of CHF** during & after STEMI by ↓**ventricular remodeling,** (↓mortality) especially in patients with CHF, STEMI, LBBB, ejection fraction <40%. • Given within the first12-24 hours (after the patient is stable). • Adverse effects: **angioedema & cough (due to ↑bradykinin – a potent vasodilator),** renal failure, **hyperkalemia.** • Contraindications: severe hypotension (SBP <100 mm Hg), renal failure, pregnancy.
Morphine	Relieves pain, ↓anxiety, venodilation ⇨ ↓preload.

ANTITHROMBOTIC & ANTIPLATET TREATMENT	
ANTI-PLATELET DRUGS	
Aspirin	**Prevents platelet activation/aggregation**. Inhibits COX ⇨ ↓thromboxane A_2 **Chewed for faster absorption.** 20% reduction in death from MI.
ADP INHIBITORS **Clopidogrel** Prasugrel Ticlopidine	Ind: **Good in patients with Aspirin allergy.** Give if conservative strategy or if PCI planned. 20% ↓in death/MI/stroke. MOA: **inhibits ADP-mediated platelet aggregation**. Caution if CABG planned within 7 days, hepatic/renal impairment, bleeding.
GP IIb/IIIa Inhibitors Eptifibatide, Tirofiban Abciximab	MOA: inhibits the final pathway for platelet aggregation. Indication: good for UA, NSTEMI, patients undergoing PCI. CI: internal bleeding within 30 days; major trauma/surgery, thrombocytopenia.
ANTICOAGULANTS	
UNFRACTIONATED HEPARIN	MOA: **binds to & potentiates antithrombin III's ability to inactivate Factor Xa, inactivates thrombin (Factor IIa),** inhibiting fibrin formation. Prevents new clot formation (however, does not dissolve existing clots). Ind: **ACS patients with ECG changes or ⊕ cardiac markers** (↓ in death/MI).
LOW MOLECULAR WEIGHT HEPARIN **Enoxaparin** Dalteparin	MOA: **binds to & potentiates antithrombin III's ability to inactivate Factor Xa.** LMWH more specific to Factor Xa than UFH. Ind: **Same as UFH.** LMWH superior to UFH: longer ½ life (~12 hours) no need for IV infusion or PTT monitoring, ↓incidence of Heparin-induced thrombocytopenia, more reliable dosing. Long ½ life may be an issue for CABG. S/E: **thrombocytopenia** (obtain CBC prior to use). Obtain serum creatinine level (must be renally dosed if renal impairment to prevent complications).
Fondaparinux	Direct factor Xa inhibitor (binds to & enhances antithrombin). No direct effect on thrombin.

To form a clot, Factor Xa convers prothrombin (II) ⇨ thrombin (Factor IIa). Thrombin activates fibrinogen⇨ fibrin clot.

REPERFUSION IN ST ELEVATION MI (STEMI)

- **Mainstay of treatment –** done **within 12 hours of symptom onset.**
- **Either PCI** (percutaneous transluminal coronary angioplasty) **or thrombolytics**

PCI (Percutaneous Coronary Intervention):

- **Best within 3 hours of symptom onset (especially within 90 minutes). PCI superior to thrombolytics**.
- Good especially for cardiogenic shock, large anterior MI, prior CABG and if thrombolytics are contraindicated.
- Coronary Artery Bypass Graft: 3-vessel disease, L main coronary artery, ↓left ventricle EF <40%.

THROMBOLYTIC (FIBRINOLYTIC) THERAPY: Used if PCI is not an option/unable to get PCI early

THROMBOLYTIC (FIBRINOLYTIC) THERAPY	
Drug	**Comments**
Tissue Plasminogen Activators:	MOA: **dissolves clot by activating tissue plasminogen ⇨ plasmin.** Plasmin is a proteolytic enzyme that degrades fibrin.
• **Alteplase (rTPA)**	Ind: **STEMI (earlier patency of coronary artery, shorter half-life),** thrombotic strokes, pulmonary embolism. S/E: **higher rebleed risk.** Expensive.
• Reteplase (RPA)	↑ potency. Used in STEMI, pulmonary embolism.
• Tenecteplase (TNK)	Long ½ life. Used in STEMI.
Streptokinase	MOA: binds to plasminogen, activating it into plasmin. Derived from streptococcus. Ind: Less effective than TPA so only used in patients in whom PCI is contraindicated & patient has a high risk of intracerebral hemorrhage (**least chance of intracranial bleeding with streptokinase), cheap.** S/E: derived from streptococcus so usually only given once (tolerance develops).

Unlike antithrombotic drugs that prevents new clots, thrombolytics (fibrinolytics) dissolve existing clots.

CORONARY VASOSPASM DISORDERS

VASOSPASTIC (VARIANT, PRINZMETAL) ANGINA

- Symptoms and signs (such as **rest angina**) due to **coronary artery vasospasm.**

TRIGGERS

- Cold weather, exercise, alpha-agonists (eg, Pseudoephedrine, cocaine), hyperventilation.

RISK FACTORS

- females, > 50 years, smokers, history of other vasospastic disorders (eg, Raynaud phenomenon, Migraine).

CLINICAL MANIFESTATIONS

- **Chest pain: at rest (especially midnight to early morning),** usually **not exertional** and not relieved with rest.

DIAGNOSIS

- ECG: **transient ST elevations** in the affected artery **that resolve with symptom resolution (ST elevations may resolve with Calcium channel blockers or Nitroglycerin)**. May have ST depressions.
- Angiography: rules out coronary artery disease and may show evidence of coronary **vasospasm during angiography, especially with the use of Ergonovine,** hyperventilation, or Acetylcholine. Like Takotsubo cardiomyopathy, this is an "all the way" question. The diagnosis is made after coronary angiography is performed to rule out obstructive CAD.

MANAGEMENT

- **Calcium channel blockers first-line** (eg, Diltiazem, Verapamil, Amlodipine, Nicardipine) given at night.
- Nitroglycerin second-line.
- During an acute chest pain episode prior to the diagnosis, Aspirin and heparin may be given until atherosclerotic disease is ruled out.
- **Beta blockers are avoided** as they may lead to unopposed vasospasm.

COCAINE-INDUCED MYOCARDIAL INFARCTION

PATHOPHYSIOLOGY:

- **Coronary artery vasospasm** due to cocaine's activation of the sympathetic nervous system & alpha-1 receptors ⇨ vasoconstriction of the coronary arteries. MI may occur if vasoconstriction is prolonged (due to decreased blood flow).

DIAGNOSIS

- ECG: **transient ST elevations classic.** May induce myocardial infarction if prolonged constriction.

MANAGEMENT

- **Calcium channel blockers & nitrates drugs of choice to reverse the vasospasm.**
- Often treated with Aspirin, Heparin & benzodiazepines until atherosclerotic disease is ruled out.
- **Avoid nonselective β-blockers in cocaine-induced MI - ↑risk of vasospasm (unopposed α_1 constriction).**

HEART FAILURE (HF)

Heart failure: inability of the heart to pump sufficient blood to meet the metabolic demands of the body at normal filling pressures. **Coronary artery disease (CAD) most common cause (eg, post MI).**

FORMS OF HEART FAILURE

These terms are not mutually exclusive: eg, left-sided systolic failure or left-sided diastolic failure etc.

1. **LEFT-SIDED vs. RIGHT-SIDED**

   L-SIDED: **most common causes are coronary artery disease & hypertension.**
   Others include: valvular disease & Cardiomyopathies.

   R-SIDED: **most common cause of R-sided failure is L-sided failure.**
   Pulmonary disease (COPD, Pulmonary hypertension), Mitral stenosis.

2. **SYSTOLIC vs. DIASTOLIC**

   SYSTOLIC: **↓ ejection fraction, ± S_3 gallop. Systolic most common form of heart failure.**
   - Etiologies: **post Myocardial infarction, Dilated cardiomyopathy,** Myocarditis.

   DIASTOLIC: **preserved ejection fraction (normal/↑EF), ± S_4 gallop = forced atrial contraction into a stiff ventricle.** Associated with normal cardiac size.
   - Etiologies: **Hypertension, Left ventricular Hypertrophy, elderly,** valvular heart disease, Cardiomyopathies (hypertrophic, restrictive), Constrictive pericarditis.

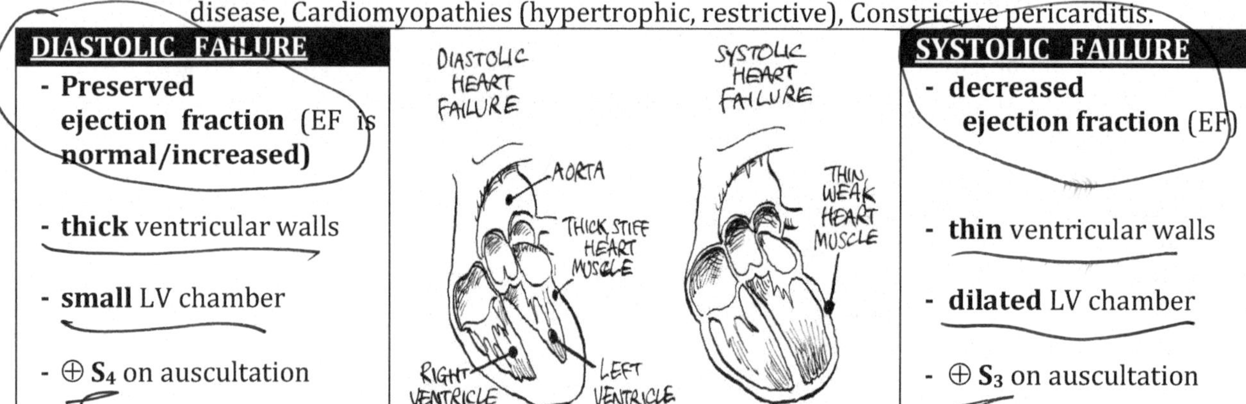

DIASTOLIC FAILURE	SYSTOLIC FAILURE
- **Preserved ejection fraction** (EF is **normal/increased)**	- **decreased ejection fraction** (EF)
- **thick** ventricular walls	- **thin** ventricular walls
- **small** LV chamber	- **dilated** LV chamber
- ⊕ **S_4** on auscultation	- ⊕ **S_3** on auscultation

3. **HIGH OUTPUT v. LOW OUTPUT**

   High output: the metabolic demands of the body exceeds normal cardiac function.
   – thyrotoxicosis, wet beriberi, severe anemia, AV shunting, Paget's disease of the bone.

   Low output: inherent problem of myocardial contraction, ischemia, chronic hypertension.

4. **ACUTE V. CHRONIC**

   Acute: largely systolic (eg, hypertensive crisis, acute MI, papillary muscle rupture).

   Chronic: typically seen in patients with dilated cardiomyopathy or valvular disease.

PATHOPHYSIOLOGY OF HEART FAILURE

Initial insult leads to ↑**afterload,** ↑**preload** &/or ↓**contractility**. The injured heart tries makes short-term compensations that, over time, promote cardiovascular deterioration. Compensations include:

❶ Sympathetic nervous system activation
❷ Myocyte hypertrophy/remodeling
❸ RAAS activation: fluid overload, **ventricular remodeling**/hypertrophy ⇨ CHF

CLINICAL MANIFESTATIONS

Left-sided Heart failure

- Increased pulmonary venous pressure from **fluid backing up into the lungs (L for Lungs and L-sided).**
- **Dyspnea most common symptom.** Includes exertional, orthopnea, paroxysmal nocturnal dyspnea. **Fatigue.** Chronic, nonproductive cough or productive with pink, frothy sputum.

Physical examination:

- **Pulmonary edema & congestion: rales** (fluid in the alveoli), **rhonchi**, wheezing. Tachypnea (rapid, shallow breathing).
- **Cheyne-Stokes breathing** - deeper, faster breathing with gradual decrease & periods of apnea, cyanosis.
- **S3 gallop with Systolic heart failure. S4 gallop with Diastolic heart failure.**
- Dusky pale skin, diaphoresis, **cool extremities**

NEW YORK HEART ASSOCIATION FUNCTIONAL CLASS

Class I - No symptoms, no limitation during ordinary physical activity.
Class II – Mild symptoms (dyspnea &/or angina), slight limitation during ordinary activity.
Class III – Symptoms cause marked limitation in activity (even with minimal exertion) comfortable only at rest.
Class IV – Symptoms even while at rest, severe limitations, & inability to carry out physical activity.

Right-sided Heart failure

- Increased systemic venous pressure from **fluid backing up into the roads (R for R-sided and 3 Roads** = inferior vena cava, superior vena cava, & hepatic circulation).
- IVC: **peripheral edema:** pitting edema of the legs, cyanosis.
- SVC: **jugular venous distention** due to increased jugular venous pressure.
- **GI & hepatic congestion:** anorexia, nausea, vomiting, hepatojugular reflux (increased JVP with liver palpation), hepatosplenomegaly.

DIAGNOSIS

Heart failure

Echocardiogram: diagnostic test of choice in the outpatient setting to make the diagnosis of Heart failure. It measures ejection fraction, assesses ventricular function, & may reveal the cause. **Ejection fraction most important determinant of prognosis** (EF <35% associated with increased mortality).

- **Systolic Heart failure: decreased ejection fraction, thin ventricular walls, & dilated LV chamber.**
- **Diastolic Heart failure: preserved ejection fraction** (normal or increased), thick ventricular walls, & small LV chamber.

Congestive (Decompensated) Heart failure (CHF):

- **Chest radiograph and BNP are the initial tests of choice for suspected CHF.**

- Chest radiograph: cephalization of flow followed by Kerley B lines (linear lucencies in the peripheral lung fields), butterfly (bat wing) appearance followed by cardiomegaly, pleural effusions, and **pulmonary edema**. **CHF most common cause of pleural effusions** (90% of all transudates).

- B-type natriuretic peptide: helpful to identify CHF as the cause for dyspnea. Indicates severity & prognosis. Ventricles release B-type natriuretic peptides during volume overload (congestive heart failure) in attempt to reverse the process (causing ↓renin-angiotensin-aldosterone activation, ↓total body fluid volume, ↑sodium excretion).
    - **BNP >100 = CHF is likely**. N-terminal pro-BNP may also be used. Cardiac enzymes to r/o MI.

LONG -TERM MANAGEMENT OF HEART FAILURE

Initial management: ACEI (& diuretic for symptoms). ACEI > beta blockers best 2 drugs for ↓mortality.

	DRUG/INTERVENTION	COMMENTS
	Diet/exercise	Na restriction <2g/d; fluid restriction <2L/d, exercise, smoking cessation
VASODILATORS (↓ AFTERLOAD)	**ACE INHIBITORS** **"PRILS"** Captopril Enalapril Ramipril Benazepril Lisinopril Quinapril Trandolapril	Mechanism of action (MOA): • Decreased preload, decreased afterload, **decreased aldosterone production,** (decreased synthesis of angiotensin II). Potentiates other **vasodilators** (eg, bradykinin, prostaglandins, nitric oxide). Increases exercise tolerance, **decreases ventricular remodeling.** Indications: • **First-line therapy for Heart failure** with reduced ejection fraction (**most effective singular medication for mortality benefit**), decreased rehospitalization. A diuretic may be added for symptom control. Adverse effects: • **Hyperkalemia. Nonproductive cough & angioedema (due to increased bradykinin)**, first-dose hypotension, azotemia, renal insufficiency. Contraindications: • **Pregnancy** (teratogenic), hypotension, severe renal insufficiency, bilateral renal artery stenosis. • Although there has been some concern about their effectiveness in African-Americans, the available evidence is **not** sufficient to support a difference in ACE inhibitor use based on race.
	BETA-BLOCKERS **Carvedilol** nonselective ($\beta_{1,2}$,α_1) **Metoprolol & Bisoprolol** (cardioselective: β_1 only)	Mechanism of action: • Decreases harmful effects of sustained sympathetic & renin activation, **reduces ventricular size & remodeling**, increases ejection fraction (EF) long-term (after initial transient decrease in EF for the first 1- 10 weeks), & prevents arrhythmias. Start at low doses and titrate every 2 weeks. Indications: • Heart failure with reduced ejection fraction **with no or minimal current evidence of fluid retention** (especially class II –III). • 35% **decrease mortality.** • **Usually added after ACEI** or ARB if additional treatment is needed. Adverse effects: • **Discontinue or reduce beta-blocker dose in decompensated CHF.** Carvedilol not selective (so may cause dizziness, hypotension 2ry to alpha-1 receptor blockade).
	ANGIOTENSIN II RECEPTOR BLOCKERS (ARB) Losartan Valsartan Candesartan Irbesartan	Mechanism of action • **Blocks effects of angiotensin II** (not its production, so there is no increase in bradykinin ⇨ no cough/angioedema). Indications: • **Patients unable to tolerate ACEI.** Adverse effects: Hyperkalemia, pregnancy (teratogenic).
	HYDRALAZINE + NITRATES COMBINED	Mechanism of action: • Nitroglycerin decreased preload & afterload, Hydralazine decreases afterload. Indications: • **African-Americans with NYHA class III to IV HF with LVEF < 40% despite optimal therapy** with BB, ACEI (or ARB), aldosterone agonist (if indicated) and diuretics or if they are unable to tolerate those therapies. May be used in non-African-Americans with hypertension & mitral regurgitation refractory to conventional treatment. • **The combination is associated with decreased mortality.** Adverse effects: • Dizziness, headache, tachyphylaxis (8 hour nitrate-free period to prevent it).

↓PRELOAD		
	DIURETICS **LOOP DIURETICS** **Furosemide** (Lasix) **Bumetanide** **Torsemide**	Mechanism of action: • Inhibits water transport across Loop of Henle ⇨ ↑excretion of H_2O, Cl^-, Na^+, K^+. Indications: • **Most effective treatment for symptoms for mild-moderate CHF.** Adverse effects: • Volume depletion, decreased electrolytes (Cl^-, Na^+, K^+), **hyperglycemia, hyperuricemia**, sulfa allergies, hypochloremic metabolic alkalosis.
	POTASSIUM SPARING DIURETICS **Spironolactone** **Eplerenone**	Mechanism of action: • **Aldosterone antagonist.** Weak diuretic, most useful in combo with loop diuretics to minimize potassium loss & inhibit RAAS. • **Decreased mortality** (due to aldosterone antagonism). Indications: • Added to ACEI, ARB in patients with class II HF with EF of 30% or class III to IV with LVEF < 35%. Adverse effects: • **Hyperkalemia, gynecomastia, metabolic acidosis.** • Eplerenone less likely to cause gynecomastia. Contraindications: • Renal failure, hyponatremia.
	Hydrochlorothiazide **Metolazone**	Adverse effects: • Hyponatremia, hypokalemia, metabolic alkalosis, hyperuricemia, hyperglycemia.

POSITIVE INOTROPES		
	SYMPATHOMIMETICS **(Positive Inotropes)** **DIGOXIN**	Mechanism of action: • Cardiac glycoside that is a **positive inotrope** (increased contraction), negative chronotrope (decreases heart rate by increasing vagal tone), and **negative dromotrope** (slows conduction velocity). Its positive inotropic effects are due to Na/K pump inhibition, increasing calcium-mediated contraction. Indications: • **Systolic heart failure** (decreases rate of hospitalization **but does not decrease mortality)** • **Atrial fibrillation** (eg, patients in whom Beta blockers and/or Calcium channel blockers are contraindicated, such as hypotension or CHF). Adverse effects: • CNS: seizures, dizziness. GI: anorexia common early finding, nausea, vomiting, diarrhea. Gynecomastia. • Digitalis effect on ECG: PVCs most common, **downsloping of the ST segment**. Digitalis toxicity • **Digitalis toxicity directly causes Hyperkalemia but Hypokalemia predisposes to Digoxin toxicity.** • Clinical manifestations: **GI symptoms most common** (nausea, vomiting, abdominal pain), **visual changes (yellow/green color changes**, double vision, halos around lights), Arrhythmias (eg, **bradycardia** > tachycardia, atrial fibrillation with a slow ventricular response), headache, confusion. • Management: Digoxin-specific antibody (DSFab), Magnesium.
	Dobutamine	↑contractility (β_1 agonist), produces peripheral vasodilation.
	Dopamine	High doses acts as β/α agonist. at low doses, acts as a diuretic by ↑renal blood flow.

Nesiritide	MOA: **synthetic BNP (↓'es** RAAS activity, ↑'es Na^+ excretion). Only used in ER or inpatient settings.

IVABRADINE

Mechanism of action:

- Selective sinus node inhibitor (slows the sinus rate).

Indications:

- Associated with ↓hospitalization & ↓mortality.
- Used in symptomatic chronic stable heart failure with LVEF ≤35%, in sinus rhythm with a resting pulse of ≥70 bpm & already maxed out on the beta-blocker dose or are unable to take beta-blockers.

SACUBITRIL-VALSARTAN

Mechanism of action:

- Sacubitril is an angiotensin receptor neprilysin inhibitor ⇨ increased levels of natriuretic peptides. Valsartan is an angiotensin II receptor blocker.

Indications:

- Reduces mortality & ↓hospitalization for chronic heart failure (Class II-IV) with reduced EF.

IMPORTANT PRINCIPLES IN THE MANAGEMENT OF SYSTOLIC HEART FAILURE

- **ACE inhibitors are the single most effective medications for mortality benefit in Heart failure with reduced ejection fraction (systolic heart failure).**
- Beta-blockers (Carvedilol, Metoprolol, Bisoprolol) are often added to ACE inhibitors for additional mortality benefit.
- **Medications that decrease mortality:** ACE inhibitors, Beta blockers, Angiotensin receptor blockers, angiotensin receptor-neprilysin inhibitors, Hydralazine plus Nitrate, and aldosterone antagonists.
- Automated Implantable Cardioverter Defibrillator in patients with EF <35% (because these patients tolerate arrhythmias poorly).

Medications with no mortality benefit

- **There is no mortality benefit of non-Dihydropyridine Calcium channel blockers** (Verapamil, Diltiazem) **in the management of Heart failure with reduced ejection fraction and there may be a possible deleterious effect** (they have a greater depressive effect on cardiac conduction and contractility and are somewhat less potent dilators in comparison to the Dihydropyridines).
- Digoxin is associated with decreased hospitalization but no mortality benefit.

CONGESTIVE (DECOMPENSATED) HEART FAILURE (CHF)

CLINICAL MANIFESTATIONS

- Left-sided: pulmonary symptoms (dyspnea, cough, rales). Think **L for L-sided and Lungs.**
- Right-sided: systemic symptoms (eg, increased JVP, lower extremity edema, hepatojugular reflux, GI symptoms). Think **R for R-sided and roads to the heart** (IVC, SVC).

DIAGNOSIS

- **Chest radiograph:** cephalization of flow, Kerley B lines (linear lucencies in the peripheral lung fields), butterfly (bat wing) appearance, cardiomegaly, pleural effusions, and **pulmonary edema**.
- **BNP:** levels > 100 make CHF likely

MANAGEMENT: LMNOP

- **Lasix (furosemide):** decreases dyspnea & peripheral edema (removes fluid off of the lungs).
- **Morphine:** decreases dyspnea, venodilator (decreased preload), and decreased anxiety. Not used often.
- **Nitrates (venodilators):** venodilation & some arterial dilation, anxiolytic, analgesic
- **Oxygen:** relieves the sensation of dyspnea.
- **Position:** sit patient up, have legs dangle over bed to decrease preload/venous return. **Positive pressure (ventilation).**

CXR FINDINGS IN CONGESTIVE HEART FAILURE

Cephalization of flow ⇨ Kerley B lines ⇨ batwing appearance ⇨ pulmonary edema.

Cephalization: ↑vascular flow to the apices as a result of increased pulmonary venous pressure. Occurs with pulmonary capillary wedge pressures of 12-18mm Hg (normal PCWP is 6 – 12 mm Hg).

Kerley B Lines (PCWP 18-25 mmHg)

Short linear markings @ lung periphery

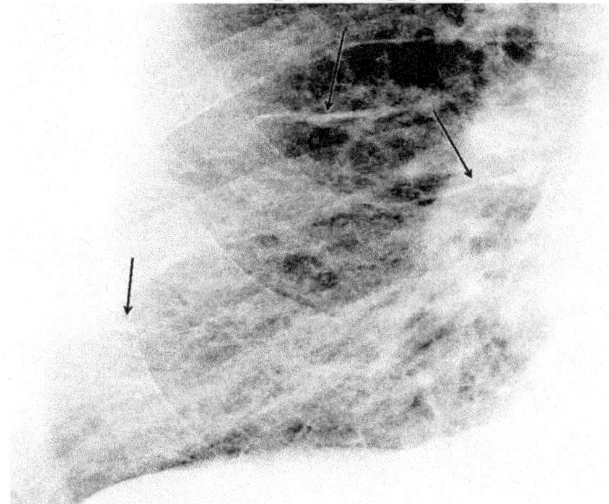

Butterfly (Batwing) Pattern (PCWP >25mmHg)

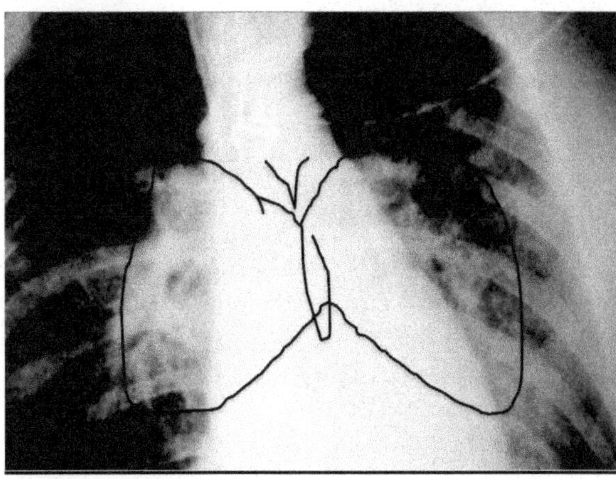

CONGESTIVE HEART FAILURE SIGNS

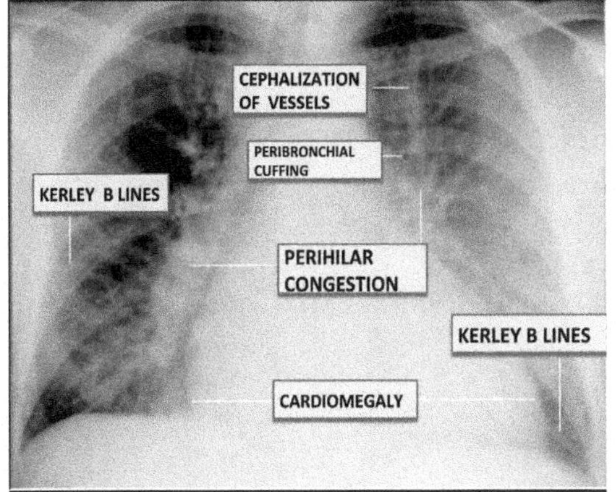

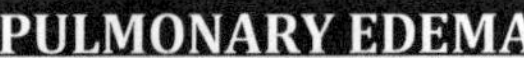

PULMONARY EDEMA

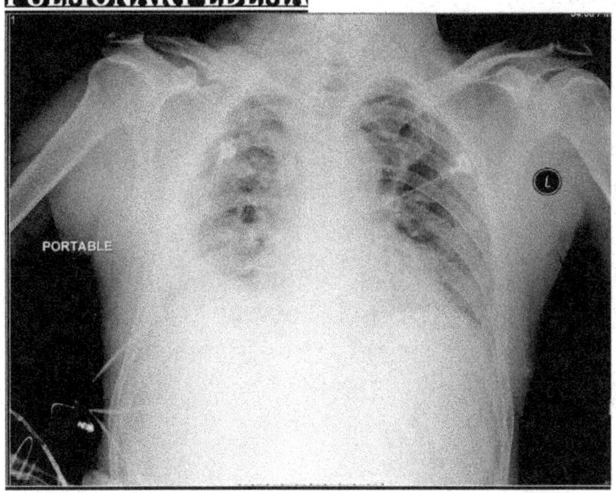

DIASTOLIC HEART FAILURE

MANAGEMENT

- Heart rate control, blood pressure control, relief of ischemia (eg, Beta blockers, ACE inhibitors), Calcium channel blockers. Diuretics for volume overload.
- Note that although Calcium channel blockers may be used in Diastolic heart failure, they can worsen Systolic heart failure.

HYPERTENSION

2017 ACC/AHA GUIDELINES			
Classification	Systolic Blood pressure		Diastolic blood pressure
Normal BP	**<120**	and	**<80**
Elevated BP	**120 – 129**	and	**<80**
Stage I Hypertension	**130 – 139**	or	**80-89**
Stage II Hypertension	**≥ 140**	or	**≥ 90**

DEFINITION

- **Systolic blood pressure of 130 mmHg or more and/or diastolic blood pressure 80 mmHg or more.**
- The elevations must be **at least 2 different readings on at least 2 different visits.**

ETIOLOGIES

Primary (essential):

- **Most common cause (95%) – due to idiopathic etiology.**
- Associated with increased salt sensitivity, increases sympathetic activity, and increased mineralocorticoid activity.

Secondary: 5%

- Due to an underlying, often correctable cause.
- **Renovascular most common cause of secondary** (4%) – eg, renal artery stenosis.
- Endocrine (0.5%): Cushing syndrome, Hyperaldosteronism.
- Pheochromocytoma, Coarctation of the aorta, sleep apnea, alcohol use, oral contraceptives, COX-2 inhibitors.

COMPLICATIONS

- **Cardiovascular:** coronary artery disease, heart failure, myocardial infarction, left ventricular hypertrophy, aortic dissection, aortic aneurysm, peripheral vascular disease.
- **Neurologic:** TIA, stroke (CVA), ruptured aneurysms, encephalopathy.
- **Nephropathy:** renal stenosis & sclerosis. **HTN second most common cause of end stage renal disease in the US** (after Diabetes mellitus).
- **Optic:** retinal hemorrhage, blindness, retinopathy.

WORKUP

- Initial workup includes 12 lead ECG (document LVH), funduscopy (retinopathy), creatinine, cholesterol, urine albumin to creatinine ratio.

MANAGEMENT

- Lifestyle management: **initial management of choice of a newly diagnosed hypertensive –** salt restriction, smoking cessation, exercise, diet, weight reduction.
  - Weight loss: achieve BMI 18.5-24.9. Smoking cessation, sodium restriction: ≤2.4 g/day.
  - Dash Diet: ↑ fruits & vegetables with ↓saturated/total fats & low sodium.
  - Exercise: ≥30 minutes of exercise/day for most of the week.
  - Limited alcohol consumption: ≤2 drinks/d in men; ≤1 drink/d in women (& patients with low BMI).

- **Medical management in patients who fail a trial of diet and exercise.**

- **Blood pressure target is less than 140/90 mmHg** (< 150/90 mmHg in adults 60 years of age or older).

- Treatment results in 50% ↓ of heart failure; 40% ↓of strokes, 20-25% ↓of myocardial infarctions.

PHARMACOLOGIC MANAGEMENT OF HYPERTENSION

INITIAL HYPERTENSIVE THERAPY IN UNCOMPLICATED HTN (NON AFRICAN-AMERICANS)

Any 1 of the 4 classes:

1. **Thiazide-type diuretics**
2. **ACE inhibitors**
3. **Angiotensin II receptor blockers**
4. **Calcium channel blockers**

HYPERTENSIVE THERAPY WITH COEXISTING CONDITIONS

COMORBID DISEASE	OPTIMUM THERAPY
Angina	**β-blockers, Calcium channel blockers (CCB)**
Post Myocardial Infarction	**ACE Inhibitors, β-blockers,**
Systolic Heart Failure	**ACEI, ARB, β blockers,** diuretics
Diabetes mellitus, Chronic kidney disease	**ACEI, ARB**
Isolated systolic HTN in elderly	Diuretics, CCB
Osteoporosis	Thiazides
BPH	**α_1 blockers**
African- Americans	**Thiazides, calcium channel blockers**
Young, Caucasian males	Thiazides, ACEI, ARBs
Gout	**Calcium Channel Blockers** Losartan is the only ARB that doesn't cause hyperuricemia.

COMORBID DISEASE	LIKELY TO HELP
Atrial flutter or fibrillation	**β-blockers, Calcium channel blockers (CCB)**
Raynaud phenomenon	Dihydropyridine calcium channel blockers
Hyperthyroidism	Beta blockers (eg, Propranolol)
Essential tremors	Beta blockers (eg, Propranolol)
Migraine	β-blockers, Calcium channel blockers

DISEASE	ADVERSE EFFECT ON COMORBID CONDITIONS
Depression	**β-blockers,** Central-acting alpha-2 agonists
Gout	Thiazides and Loop diuretics
Hyperkalemia	ACEI, ARBs, renin inhibitors, aldosterone antagonists
Hyponatremia	Thiazides
SEVERE renal disease	ACEI, ARBs, renin inhibitors

DISEASE	CONTRAINDICATED
Angioedema	ACEI
SEVERE renovascular disease	ACEI, ARBs, renin inhibitors
2nd or 3rd degree heart block	Beta blockers, Non-dihydropyridine CCBs (Verapamil, Diltiazem)

PHARMACOLOGIC MANAGEMENT OF HYPERTENSION

	DRUG/INTERVENTION	COMMENTS
DIURETICS	**DIURETICS** **Hydrochlorothiazide** **Chlorthalidone** Metolazone	Mechanism of action: • Affect blood pressure by reducing blood volume, prevent kidney Na^+/water reabsorption at **distal diluting tubule**. Lower urinary calcium excretion. Adverse effects: • **Hyponatremia, hypokalemia,** mild cholesterol elevations, **hyperuricemia, & hyperglycemia** (therefore caution in patients with Diabetes or Gout). **Hypercalcemia.**
	Loop diuretics **Furosemide, Bumetanide**	Mechanism of action: • Inhibit water transport across Loop of Henle ⇨ ↑excretion of water, Cl, Na, K. Strongest class of diuretics. Adverse effects: • Volume depletion, **hypokalemia/**natremia/calcemia, hyperuricemia, hypochloremic metabolic alkalosis, ototoxicity; **hyperlipidemia, hyperglycemia.** • Contraindicated if **sulfa allergy.**
	Potassium sparing diuretics **Spironolactone** **Amiloride** **Eplerenone**	Mechanism of action: • **Inhibit aldosterone-mediated Na/H_2O absorption** (spares potassium). Weak diuretic, most useful in combo with loop diuretics to minimize potassium loss. Adverse effects: • **Hyperkalemia,** metabolic acidosis, **Gynecomastia with Spironolactone.** • Contraindications: renal failure, hyponatremia
VASODILATORS	**ACE INHIBITORS** **Captopril** **Enalapril** **Ramipril** **Benazepril**	Mechanism of action: • **Cardioprotective, synergistic effect when used with thiazides**; ↓preload/afterload, (↓synthesis of AG II/aldosterone production), potentiates other vasodilators (bradykinin, prostaglandins, nitric oxide); ↑'es exercise tolerance. Improves insulin's action. Indications: • **HTN** (especially if **history of diabetes mellitus, nephropathy, CHF, old MI)** Adverse effects • **1st-dose hypotension, azotemia/renal insufficiency**, **hyperkalemia** (can be ameliorated with low salt, diuretics), **cough & angioedema (due to ↑bradykinin), hyperuricemia.** • Contraindications: pregnancy.
	ANGIOTENSIN II RECEPTOR BLOCKERS (ARB) Lo**sartan** Val**sartan** Irbe**sartan** Cande**sartan**	Mechanism of action: • Similar actions as ACE inhibitors but binds and blocks the angiotensin II receptor. Does not increase bradykinin production. Indications: • **Consider in patients not able to tolerate Beta-blockers/ACEI or in addition to ACEI.** Adverse effects: • **Hyperkalemia. Contraindicated in pregnancy.**

CALCIUM CHANNEL BLOCKERS **Dihydropyridines** **Nifedipine** **Amlodipine** **Non-dihydropyridines** **Verapamil** **Diltiazem**	Mechanism of action: • **Dihydropyridines: potent vasodilators (little or no effect on cardiac contractility or conduction)** neutral or increased vascular permeability. Dihydropyridines most commonly used in HTN. • **Non-dihydropyridines affect cardiac contractility & conduction** as well as potent vasodilators, reduces vascular permeability. Adverse effects • Vasodilation: **headache, dizziness, lightheadedness, flushing, peripheral edema. Constipation with verapamil.** Contraindications: • CHF (especially nondihydropyridines). • **2nd/3rd heart block.** Patients taking beta blockers (non-dihydropyridines)
β – BLOCKERS **Cardioselective (β1):** **Atenolol, Metoprolol, Esmolol** **Nonselective (β1, β2):** **Propranolol** **Both α & β1,2:** **Labetalol, Carvedilol**	Mechanism of action: • Catecholamine inhibitor. **Blocks "adrenergic" renin release.** • Not usually used as first line therapy in general unless there is a comorbid condition in which beta blockade is helpful. Adverse effects: • **Fatigue, depression, impotence;** may mask tachycardic symptoms of hypoglycemia in DM **(so use with caution in diabetic patients).** • Caution if **hypotensive or HR <50 bpm** Contraindications: • **2nd/3rd heart block, decompensated heart failure.** • **Nonselective agents CI in asthma/COPD** and may worsen peripheral vascular disease/Raynaud's phenomenon.
α1 BLOCKERS **Prazosin** **Terazosin** **Doxazosin**	Mechanism of action: • Alpha blockade leads to peripheral arterial dilation. • Generally not used as first-line therapy generally but may be helpful in patients with hypertension + benign prostatic hypertrophy. Adverse effects: • **1st-dose syncope, dizziness, headache,** weakness.

HYPERTENSIVE URGENCY

- **SBP > 180 mmHg and/or DBP >120 mmHg without evidence of end organ damage**.

CLINICAL MANIFESTATIONS

- General: headache (most common), dyspnea, chest pain, focal neurologic deficits, altered mental status, delirium, seizures, nausea, vomiting.

MANAGEMENT

- Gradual **reduction of mean arterial pressure by no more than 25% over 24-48 hours with oral medications** (eg, Clonidine, Captopril, Labetalol, Nicardipine, Furosemide).
- Treatment goals are blood pressure ≤160/100 mmHg.

ORAL DRUGS USED FOR HYPERTENSIVE URGENCIES		
Drug	**Mechanism of Action**	**Adverse Effects**
Clonidine	**Centrally acting α-2 adrenergic agonist (short-term use only)**	Headache, tachycardia, nausea, vomiting, sedation, fatigue dry mouth, **rebound hypertension if discontinued abruptly - (mimics Pheochromocytoma).**
Captopril	ACE Inhibitor	Angioedema, Acute kidney injury.
Furosemide	Loop diuretic	Electrolyte abnormalities, alkalosis.
Labetalol	$\alpha_1 \beta_1 \beta_2$ blocker	CI in severe asthma/COPD, AV heart block, congestive heart failure.
Nicardipine	Calcium channel blocker	Reflex tachycardia, headache, nausea

HYPERTENSIVE EMERGENCY

- **SBP > 180 mmHg and/or DBP >120 mmHg** with **evidence of end organ damage**.

CLINICAL MANIFESTATIONS

- General: headache (most common), dyspnea, chest pain, focal neurologic deficits, altered mental status, delirium, seizures, nausea, vomiting.
- Neurologic: encephalopathy, stroke (hemorrhagic or ischemic), seizure.
- Cardiac: Acute coronary syndrome, Aortic dissection, Acute heart failure (pulmonary edema). Workup includes CXR, ECG, cardiac enzymes, BNP.
- Renal: Acute kidney injury, proteinuria, hematuria (glomerulonephritis).
- Retinal: malignant Hypertension, severe (Grade IV) retinopathy.

MANAGEMENT

- **IV blood pressure reduction agents.** For most hypertensive emergencies, **mean arterial pressure should be reduced gradually by about 10-20% in the first hour and by an additional 5-15% over the next 23 hours**.

The 3 main exceptions are as follows:

- Acute phase of an ischemic stroke: blood pressure is usually not lowered unless it is ≥ 185/110 mmHg in patients who are candidates for reperfusion treatment OR ≥ 220/120 mmHg in patients who are not candidates for reperfusion.
- Acute aortic dissection: systolic blood pressure is rapidly lowered to a goal of 100-120 mmHg within 20 minutes.
- Intracerebral hypertension: treatment depends on different factors.

EMERGENCY	FIRST LINE	NOTES
NEUROLOGIC HTN ENCEPHALOPATHY	**Nicardipine or Clevidipine** **Labetalol,** Fenoldopam Sodium Nitroprusside	Must r/o stroke. **HTN encephalopathy often presents with confusion, headache, nausea & vomiting.** Symptoms improve with lowering of BP. Nitroprusside, Nitroglycerin & Hydralazine may increase intracranial pressure.
HEMORRHAGIC STROKE	Nicardipine or Labetalol	Benefits vs. risks of lowering blood pressure must be weighed in hemorrhagic strokes.
ISCHEMIC STROKE	Nicardipine or Labetalol	*Avoid cerebral hypoperfusion if ischemic.* Reduce blood pressure ONLY if BP is: ≥220/120 (not a thrombolytic candidate). ≥185/110 (if a thrombolytic candidate).
CARDIOVASCULAR AORTIC DISSECTION	***β-blocker*: *Esmolol, Labetalol*** Sodium Nitroprusside (± add to beta blocker) Nicardipine, Clevidipine	Decreases shearing forces. Beta blocker tx target: systolic BP 100-120mmHg & pulse <60 bpm achieved within 20 minutes.
ACUTE CORONARY SYNDROME	**Nitroglycerin** **Beta blockers** (eg, Esmolol, Metoprolol) Nitroprusside	*Nitroglycerin not used if suspected right ventricular infarction or phosphodiesterase - 5 inhibitor use within 24-48h (eg, Sildenafil).*
ACUTE HEART FAILURE	**Nitroglycerin, Furosemide** Nitroprusside	Avoid Hydralazine & Beta blockers in CHF. Only if no evidence of cardiac ischemia.

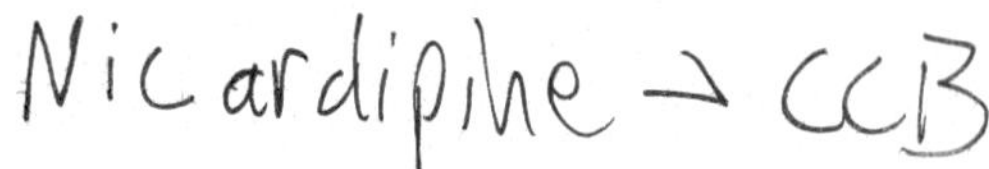

POSTURAL (ORTHOSTATIC) HYPOTENSION

- Hypotension within 2-5 minutes of quiet standing (or after a 5 minute period of supine rest) defined by **at least 20 mmHg fall in systolic pressure and/or at least 10 mmHg fall in diastolic pressure.**
- Common in older patients > 65 years.

ETIOLOGIES
- Impaired autonomic function and/or decreased intravascular volume.
- Medications: includes antihypertensives (eg, Alpha blockers, Nitroglycerin, ACE inhibitors), diuretics, narcotics, antipsychotics, antidepressants, and alcohol consumption
- Neurologic: include diabetic neuropathy, Parkinson disease, polyneuropathies etc.
- Hypovolemia (eg, Loop diuretics, hemorrhage or vomiting).

CLINICAL MANIFESTATIONS
- Due to cerebral hypoperfusion – dizziness, lightheadedness, palpitations, blurred vision, darkening of visual fields, and/or syncope.

WORKUP
- Blood pressure measurement
- **Tilt table test:** blood pressure reduction at a 60-degree angle.
- Labs (eg, hematocrit, electrolytes, BUN, creatine, glucose) to evaluate for anemia or dehydration.

MANAGEMENT
- Initial management: **conservative initial management of choice - increasing salt and fluid intake,** gradual positional changes, compression stockings or abdominal binder, exercise, and discontinuation of offending medications. Caffeine may be helpful.
- **Fludrocortisone is the first-line medical management** if persistent symptoms despite nonpharmacologic measures.
- Midodrine (alpha-1 agonist) or Droxidopa (pressor agent) may be used in patients if additional therapy is needed or if the patient is unable to take Fludrocortisone.
- Avoiding the flat position, sleeping with the head of the bed raised 30-45 degrees if refractory to medical therapy.

REFLEX-MEDIATED SYNCOPE

- Neurally-mediated syncope.

VASOVAGAL SYNCOPE
- Due to vasovagal hypotension (self-limited systemic hypotension associated with bradycardia and/or peripheral venodilation/vasodilation).
- **Most common cause of syncope**, especially without apparent neurologic or cardiovascular disease.
- Triggers: blood phobia, emotional stress/fear, pain, trauma.
- Manifestations: **prodromal phase** (eg, dizziness, lightheadedness, epigastric pain, palpitations, blurred vision, darkening of visual fields) followed by syncope followed by a postdromal phase.

CAROTID SINUS SYNCOPE
- Syncope with minor stimulation of the carotid sinus (eg, shaving, putting on neckties, wearing a tight collar, head turning, or applying minor pressure to the carotids).

SITUATIONAL SYNCOPE
- Triggers include defecation, micturition, coughing/sneezing, post-prandial, or trigger points.

CIRCULATORY SHOCK

- **Inadequate organ perfusion & tissue oxygenation** to meet the body's oxygenation requirements. **Often associated with hypotension (but not always). Shock is determined by EITHER:**
  1. **Low cardiac output** – **OR**
  2. **Low systemic vascular resistance** (SVR). SVR = the resistance to blood flow through the circulatory system (determined by peripheral blood vessels). Peripheral vasoconstriction increases SVR. Vasodilation decreases SVR.

4 MAIN TYPES OF SHOCK	
1. HYPOVOLEMIC	**loss of blood or fluid volume** (eg, hemorrhage).
2. CARDIOGENIC	**primary myocardial dysfunction** ⇨reduced cardiac output (eg, MI).
3. OBSTRUCTIVE	**extrinsic or intrinsic obstruction to circulation** (eg, pericardial tamponade).
4. DISTRIBUTIVE	**maldistribution of blood flow** from essential organs to nonessential organs (eg, septic or neurogenic shock).

PATHOPHYSIOLOGY OF SHOCK

1. **Inadequate tissue perfusion:** inability to meet the body's metabolic oxygen requirements ⇨ metabolic acidosis & organ dysfunction.
2. **Autonomic nervous system activation:** in an attempt to improve systemic O_2 delivery.
   - Sympathetic nervous system activation: causes vasoconstriction (↑SVR) & ↑contractility (to ↑CO). ↑Norepinephrine, dopamine & cortisol release. The ↑SVR helps to maintain cerebral & cardiac perfusion by causing vasoconstriction of splanchnic, musculoskeletal & renal blood flow.
   - RAAS activation: water & sodium retention (↓urine output to minimize renal water & salt loss). Also causes vasoconstriction to help maintain cardiac output.
3. **Systemic effects of shock:**
   - ATP depletion ⇨ ion pump dysfunction leading to cellular dysfunction, cell swelling, & death.
   - **Metabolic acidosis**: due to lack of oxygen ⇨ cells resort to anaerobic metabolism, producing **lactic acid** as a byproduct. Order lactate levels as part of workup.
   - Multiorgan Dysfunction Syndrome (MODS): physiologic consequences of shock on organ systems. Includes lung, kidney, heart, & brain dysfunction as well as DIC (disseminated intravascular coagulation).
   - Multisystemic Organ Failure (MSOF): organ failure if the conditions persist.

CLINICAL MANIFESTATIONS OF SHOCK

1. Generally acutely ill, altered mental status, decreased peripheral pulses, tachycardia, skin usually cool and mottled (may be warm and flushed in distributive shock), systolic blood pressure <110 mmHg (some patients in shock may be normotensive initially).
2. Laboratory tests: include CBC, BMP (Chem-7), lactate, coagulation studies, cultures (to look for potential infectious sources), ABG and other studies depending on the likely etiology.

GENERAL MANAGEMENT OF SHOCK ABCDE's

1. **Airway:** may need intubation.
2. **Breathing:** mechanical ventilation & sedation decreases the work of breathing (reducing the oxygen demand associated with tachypnea).
3. **Circulation:** isotonic crystalloids (Normal Saline, Lactated Ringer's). Often given multiple liters & titrated to central venous pressure (CVP) of 8-12mmHg OR urine output of 0.5ml/kg/hr (30ml/hr) OR an improved heart rate.
4. **Delivery of Oxygen:** monitor lactate levels.
5. **Endpoint of Resuscitation:** urine output (UOP): 0.5ml/kg/hr, CVP 8-12mmHg, mean arterial pressure (MAP) 65-90mmHg, central venous oxygen concentration >70%.

HYPOVOLEMIC SHOCK

- **LOSS OF BLOOD OR FLUID VOLUME** due to hemorrhage or fluid loss.

ETIOLOGIES

- **Hemorrhagic:** eg, GI bleed, AAA rupture, massive hemoptysis, trauma, ectopic pregnancy, postpartum hemorrhage.

- **Non-blood fluid loss:** GI: vomiting, bowel obstruction, pancreatitis; severe burns, diabetic ketoacidosis (causes osmotic diuresis in response to hyperglycemia).

PATHOPHYSIOLOGY

Loss of blood or fluid volume ⇨ ↑heart rate, vasoconstriction (↑SVR), hypotension, ↓cardiac output.

Body's response to hypovolemia:

- rapid: peripheral vasoconstriction, ↑cardiac activity.

- sustained: arterial vasoconstriction, Na^+/water retention, ↑cortisol.

CLINICAL MANIFESTATIONS

Loss of volume ⇨ ↑heart rate (tachycardia), hypotension, ↓CO (oliguria or anuria), vasoconstriction (↑SVR) ⇨ **pale cool dry skin/extremities, slow capillary refill >2 seconds, ↓skin turgor, dry mucous membranes,** AMS.

Usually does not cause profound respiratory distress.

CLASSES OF HEMORRHAGIC SHOCK		
I	< 15% blood loss	Pulse usually normal, systolic blood pressure (SBP) usually normal.
II	15 – 30% blood loss	**Tachycardia** (pulse >100). SBP usually >100mmHg.
III	30 – 40% blood loss	Tachycardia, **decreased systolic blood pressure** (<100mmHg), confusion, decreased urine output.
IV	>40% blood loss	Tachycardia, decreased SBP, **lethargy, no urine output.**

DIAGNOSIS

Hallmark:

Vasoconstriction (↑SVR), hypotension, ↓CO & decreased pulmonary capillary pressure.

- CBC: ↑Hgb/Hct = dehydration (hemoconcentration). ↓Hgb/Hct is late sign in hemorrhagic shock.

- Decreased CVP (central venous pressure)/PCWP (pulmonary capillary wedge pressure).

MANAGEMENT

1. ABCDE's, Insert 2 large bore IV lines or a central line.
2. **Volume resuscitation: crystalloids (Normal Saline or Lactated Ringer's)** often given 3-4 liters to restore blood volume. Monitor urine output to assess success of resuscitation.
3. Control the source of hemorrhage to prevent further sequelae. ± Packed RBC blood transfusion if severe hemorrhage: (O-negative or cross-matched).
4. Prevention of hypothermia, treat any coagulopathies.

CARDIOGENIC SHOCK

- **PRIMARY CARDIAC/MYOCARDIAL DYSFUNCTION** ⇨ inadequate tissue perfusion ⇨ ↓CO (cardiac output) with ↑systemic vascular resistance (SVR). Often systolic in nature.
- Cardiogenic often produces increased respiratory effort/distress whereas hypovolemic does not.

ETIOLOGIES

Cardiac disease: myocardial infarction, myocarditis, valve dysfunction, congenital heart disease, cardiomyopathy, arrhythmias.

PATHOPHYSIOLOGY

↓CO & evidence of tissue hypoxia in the presence of adequate intravascular volume. Sustained hypotension in the presence of **↑pulmonary capillary wedge pressure** (>15mmHg).

Vasoconstriction (↑SVR), hypotension, ↓CO ,& ↑ pulmonary capillary wedge pressure.

MANAGEMENT

1. Oxygen, isotonic fluids (**avoid aggressive IV fluid treatment - use smaller amounts of fluid**).
   NOTE CARDIOGENIC SHOCK IS THE ONLY SHOCK IN WHICH LARGE AMOUNTS OF FLUIDS AREN'T GIVEN.
2. **Inotropic support:** drugs to increase myocardial contractility & cardiac output:
   - Dobutamine (positive inotrope), Epinephrine (positive inotrope & vasoconstrictor).
   - Amrinone may be used if refractory (Amrinone is a phosphodiesterase-3 inhibitor that is a positive inotrope).
   - Intraaortic balloon pump support.
3. **Treat the underlying cause:** eg, MI: early angioplasty or thrombolytics.

OBSTRUCTIVE SHOCK

- **OBSTRUCTION OF BLOOD FLOW DUE TO PHYSICAL OBSTRUCTION OF HEART OR GREAT VESSELS.**
- Intrinsic or extrinsic (↑external pressure on the heart decreases the heart's ability to pump blood).

ETIOLOGIES:

1. **Massive pulmonary embolism**: obstruction to pulmonary artery blood flow. Cyanosis, tachycardia, hypotension, VQ mismatch, hemoptysis. ECG: $S_1Q_3T_3$, sinus tachycardia. ABG: PaO_2 <80mmHg, ↑A-a gradient. Low CO, ↑peripheral resistance, ↑CVP.
2. **Pericardial Tamponade:** blood in the pericardial space prevents venous return to the heart, causing obstruction. **Beck's triad**: muffled heart sounds, systemic hypotension & ↑JVP.
3. **Tension pneumothorax**: positive air pressure causes external pressure on the heart. **Hyperresonance to percussion & decreased breath sounds on the affected side. Mediastinal & tracheal shift to the contralateral side**, SQ emphysema, ↑JVP.
4. **Aortic dissection:** proximal dissections. May also cause hypovolemic shock.

MANAGEMENT

Oxygen, isotonic fluids, inotropic support: dobutamine, epinephrine, intra-aortic balloon pump.

Treat the underlying cause:

Pulmonary Embolism: heparin, thrombolytics. ± Embolectomy.

Pericardial tamponade ⇨ pericardiocentesis.

Tension pneumothorax ⇨ needle decompression.

Proximal dissections usually require surgical intervention.

DISTRIBUTIVE SHOCK

- **EXCESS VASODILATION & ALTERED DISTRIBUTION OF BLOOD FLOW** (increased venous capacity) with shunting of blood flow from vital organs (ex. heart, kidney) to non-vital tissues (eg, skin, skeletal muscle). **Hallmark: ↓CO, ↓SVR, ↓PCWP.**
- **An important EXCEPTION IS EARLY SEPTIC SHOCK - ASSOCIATED WITH ↑CO & ↓SVR so warm extremities often noted in these patients.** Septic shock is the most common type of distributive shock.

1. SEPTIC SHOCK:

PATHOPHYSIOLOGY: infective organisms activate the immune system ⇨ **host produces systemic inflammatory response** ⇨ cytokines cause prompt peripheral vasodilation ⇨ **↓SVR**), increased capillary permeability (initiating shock) & end organ thrombosis. These (normally local) responses to infection occur in a systemic fashion, affecting multiple organs.

CLINICAL MANIFESTATIONS: warm shock: hypotension with **WIDE PULSE PRESSURE**, bounding arterial peripheral pulses. **Only major type of shock associated with ↑CO (fast capillary refill time; warm, flushed extremities).**

SIRS (Systemic Inflammatory Response Syndrome): at least 2 of the 4 following:

1. Temperature: fever >38°C (100.4° F) or hypothermia <36°C (96.8°F)
2. Pulse: > 90 bpm
3. Respiratory rate: >20 or $PaCO_2$ <32mmHg
4. WBC count: >12,000 cells/hpf or <4,000 cells/hpf

Sepsis = **SIRS + focus of infection. Often associated with ↑LACTATE (>4mmol/L).**

Severe sepsis = **SIRS + MSOF (multi system organ failure).**

Septic shock = **Sepsis + refractory hypotension** despite fluid administration (SBP <90mmHg, MAP <65mmHg or drop in SBP 40mmHg from baseline).

MANAGEMENT:

1. **Broad spectrum IV antibiotics:** (pan culture before initiating). Zosyn + Ceftriaxone or Imipenem. Choose depending on suspected organisms (Gentamicin for Pseudomonas, Vancomycin for MRSA, Clindamycin or Metronidazole for intrabdominal infections, Ceftriaxone in asplenic patients to cover *N. meningitidis* & *H. influenzae*).
2. **IV fluid Resuscitation: isotonic crystalloids** (Normal saline, Lactated Ringer's)
3. **Vasopressors:** if no response to 2-3L of IV fluids with goal of MAP >60mmHg. ± IV hydrocortisone.

2. ANAPHYLACTIC SHOCK:

IgE-mediated severe systemic hypersensitivity reaction. History of incest bite/stings, food or drug allergy, recent IV contrast. Symptoms usually begin within 60 minutes of exposure.

PHYSICAL EXAM: pruritus, hives, angioedema ⇨ respiratory distress, stridor, sensation of "lump in throat", hoarseness (life threatening laryngeal edema).

MANAGEMENT: Epinephrine 1st line (0.3mg IM of 1:1000 repeat q5-10min as needed). If cardiovascular collapse, give Epinephrine 1mg IV (1:10,000). **Airway management, antihistamines** (Diphenhydramine 25-50mg IV blocks H_1, Ranitidine IV blocks H_2), IV fluids. **Observe patient for 4-6 hours** because up to 20% of patients have a biphasic phenomenon (return of symptoms 3-4 hours after the initial reaction).

3. NEUROGENIC SHOCK:

due to **acute spinal cord injury**, regional anesthesia.

PATHOPHYSIOLOGY: autonomic sympathetic blockade ⇨ unopposed ↑vagal tone. ⇨ **bradycardia & hypotension.** Loss of sympathetic tone ⇨warm, dry skin.

CLINICAL: warm skin, normal or ↓HR, ↓SVR, hypovolemia, **WIDE pulse pressure.**

Management: fluids, pressors +/- corticosteroids.

4. ENDOCRINE SHOCK:

eg, **Adrenal insufficiency (Addisonian crisis).**

Management: Hydrocortisone 100mg IV (often unresponsive to fluids & pressors).

	PATHOPHYSIOLOGY	ETIOLOGIES	CO	PCWP	SVR	CLINICAL MANIFESTATIONS
HYPOVOLEMIC	***LOSS OF BLOOD OR FLUID VOLUME*** ⇨ ↑PVR & ↑HR to maintain CO.	**Hemorrhage:** GI bleed, AAA rupture etc. **Fluid loss**: GI: vomiting, diarrhea, pancreatitis, severe burns etc.	Decreased	***Decreased***	Increased	•***Pale, cool, mottled skin*** •***Prolonged capillary refill*** •***Decreased skin turgor, dry mucous membranes*** •*Usually no severe respiratory distress*
CARDIOGENIC	***PRIMARY MYOCARDIAL ABNORMALITY*** ⇨ heart unable to maintain CO	•Myocardial Infarction •Myocarditis •Valvular disease •Cardiomyopathies •Arrhythmias	Decreased	***Increased***	Increased	•***Severe respiratory distress*** •***Cool clammy skin***
OBSTRUCTIVE	***EXTRINSIC OR INTRINSIC OBSTRUCTION of heart or great vessels***	•Pericardial tamponade •Massive Pulmonary Embolism •Tension Pneumothorax •Aortic dissection	Decreased	***Increased***	Increased	•***Severe respiratory distress*** •***Cool clammy skin***
DISTRIBUTIVE 4 types (below)	***MALDISTRIBUTION OF BLOOD & VASODILATION*** with shunting of blood away from vital to non vital organs	•Septic •Neurogenic •Anaphylactic •Hypoadrenal			***Decreased***	
1. SEPTIC	Severe host immune response	Bacteria				
Early (warm)	Vasodilation		***Increased****	↑ or ↓	***Decreased***	•***↑CO*: WARM, FLUSHED EXTREMITIES & skin, brisk capillary refill, bounding pulses, WIDE pulse pressure*** • ***ONLY SHOCK ASSOC WITH ↑CO****
Late (cool)			Decreased	Decreased	Increased	Cool clammy skin
2. NEUROGENIC	Sympathetic blockade ⇨ unopposed vagal tone on vessels ⇨ vasodilation	Acute spine injury	Decreased	Decreased	Decreased	•***HYPOTENSION without tachycardia**** •± ***BRADYCARDIA****
3. ANAPHYLACTIC	***IgE mediated*** systemic HSN reaction with histamine release ⇨ vasodilation leading to ↑capillary permeability	•Insect bites/stings •Food allergies •Drug allergies •Recent IV contrast	Decreased	Decreased	Decreased	•***Pruritus, hives, ± angioedema*** •± throat fullness, hoarseness, wheezing •Recent h/o of insect bite/sting, food, drug or IV contrast
4. HYPOADRENAL	Decreased corticosteroid & mineralocorticoid activity	Adrenal insufficiency (Addisonian crisis)	Decreased	Decreased	Decreased	• ***Low serum glucose.*** •***Hypotension refractory to fluids & pressors***

SVR = Systemic Vascular Resistance CO = Cardiac Output PCWP = Pulmonary Capillary Wedge Pressure

HYPERLIPIDEMIA

ETIOLOGIES

1. Hypercholesterolemia: hypothyroidism, pregnancy, kidney failure.
2. Hypertriglyceridemia: Diabetes Mellitus, ETOH, obesity, steroids, estrogen.

CLINICAL MANIFESTATIONS OF HYPERLIPIDEMIA

1. Most patients are asymptomatic. Hypertriglyceridemia may cause pancreatitis.
2. May develop Xanthomas (eg, Achilles tendon) or Xanthelasma (lipid plaques on the eyelids).

GOALS

- Weight reduction, increased exercise.
- Dietary restriction of cholesterol & carbohydrates, decreased trans fatty acids.
- Goal of lipid-lowering agents: plaque stabilization, reversal of endothelial dysfunction, thrombogenicity reduction & atherosclerosis regression.

SCREENING FOR HYPERLIPIDEMIA

Based on risks: sex, age, cardiac risk factors such as smoking, hypertension, family history of coronary heart disease (first-degree male relative with CHD before age 55; first-degree female relative with CHD before age 65).

1. American College of Cardiology/American Heart Association: (2019): in adults between the ages 20 to 39 who are free of cardiovascular disease (CVD) it is "reasonable" to assess risk factors every 4 – 6 years to calculate their 10-year CVD risk.

There is considerable controversy regarding the optimal age for initiating screening.

- Higher risk = >1 risk factor (hypertension, smoking, family hx) or 1 severe risk factor. initiate screening at age 20 to 25 for males; 30 - 35 for females.

- Lower risk: initiate screening at age 35 for males; 45 for females.

LIPID GUIDELINES FOR THE INITIATION OF STATIN THERAPY

Determined by a 10-year and lifetime risk calculator instead of strict numbers only. The risk factors include: gender, age, race, smoking, blood pressure, blood cholesterol levels & Diabetes mellitus. It recommends treatment in the following patients:

1. Patients with type 1 or 2 Diabetes Mellitus between the ages 40-75 years of age.

2. Patients without cardiovascular disease ages 40-75 years of age & ≥7.5% risk for having a heart attack or stroke within 10 years.

3. People ≥21 years of age with LDL levels ≥190 mg/dL.

4. Any patient with any form of clinical atherosclerotic cardiovascular disease.

5. Patients <19 years of age with familial hypercholesterolemia.

BENEFIT OF LIPID LOWERING MEDICATIONS

- **Best meds to lower elevated LDL ⇨ Statins,** Bile acid sequestrants.
- **Best meds to lower elevated triglycerides ⇨ Fibrates,** Niacin.
- **Best meds to increase HDL ⇨ Niacin,** Fibrates.
- Type II DM ⇨ Statins, Fibrates

HMG-COA REDUCTASE INHIBITORS (STATINS) **Simvastatin** **Pravastatin** **Lovastatin** **Atorvastatin** **Rosuvastatin**	Mechanism of action: • **Inhibit the rate-limiting step in hepatic cholesterol synthesis** via inhibition of the enzyme HMG-CoA reductase. • Increase LDL receptors, promoting LDL clearance. Reduce triglycerides. Indications: • **Best drug to decrease LDL levels.** • Statins have been shown to decrease cardiovascular complications. Adverse effects: • Muscle damage (eg, myalgias, **myositis, Rhabdomyolysis**). • Statins may also cause increased liver function tests, hepatitis (most common), gastrointestinal symptoms, Diabetes mellitus. Considerations: • Atorvastatin, Rosuvastatin can be taken any time of the day, most of the others are taken in the evening. LFTs order prior to the initiation of statin therapy. Drug interactions: • Drugs that inhibit the CP450 system (eg, Erythromycin, Diltiazem, -azoles) may increase drug levels. Contraindications: • Active hepatic disease, persistent elevated LFTs, pregnancy, & breastfeeding.
NICOTINIC ACID (Niacin)	Mechanism of action: • increases HDL (delays HDL clearance). Decreases hepatic production of LDL & its precursor VLDL. Decreases triglycerides. Indications: • **Best drug to increase HDL levels.** Adverse effects: • Increased prostaglandins (eg, **flushing, warm sensation, pruritus**, headache). **Pretreatment of 30 minutes with NSAIDs or Aspirin can be given to counter flushing.** • Dry skin, hyperuricemia (may precipitate gout), **hyperglycemia**, hepatotoxicity. GI symptoms (nausea, vomiting, dyspepsia) – **GI symptoms reduced if taken with meals.** Contraindications: • Active Peptic ulcer disease, active liver disease, arterial bleeding.
FIBRATES • **Fenofibrate** • **Gemfibrozil**	Mechanism of action: • **Inhibit triglyceride synthesis, increase the activity of lipoprotein lipase** (stimulating catabolism of triglyceride-rich lipoproteins), increase HDL synthesis & decrease LDL synthesis. • Indications: **best drugs to decrease triglycerides.** Adverse effects: • headache, dizziness, GI symptoms, increased liver function tests, **increased gallstones**. They are also associated with myalgias & myositis (especially with concomitant statin use). • The only fibrate FDA approved to be used in combination with a Statin is Fenofibric acid. Contraindications: • Active hepatobiliary disease, severe renal disease, breastfeeding, Gemfibrozil + Repaglinide.

BILE ACID SEQUESTRANTS • Cholestyramine • Colestipol • Colesevelam	Mechanism of action: • **Bile acid sequestrant** (binds bile acids in the intestine, blocking enterohepatic reabsorption of bile acids), reduces cholesterol pool, lowers intrahepatic cholesterol. Because the liver has to make new bile acids, it increases its LDL receptors, **decreasing LDL levels.** Indications: • Often used in combination with a Statin to reduce LDL levels, mild to moderate increases in HDL. **Safe in pregnancy** (not systemically absorbed). Cholestyramine used to treat **pruritus associated with biliary obstruction.** Adverse effects: • GI side effects (nausea, vomiting, bloating, crampy abdominal pain), increased LFTs. • **Increased triglyceride levels.** • Osteoporosis with long-term use. Interactions: • **May impair absorption other medications** (eg, **antibiotics, Digoxin, Warfarin**, fat-soluble vitamins) so these medications should be taken 1 hour before or 4 hours after BAS. Contraindications: • Severe hypertriglyceridemia, complete biliary obstruction.
EZETIMIBE	Mechanism of action: • Inhibits intestinal cholesterol absorption. Indications: • Often used in combination with a Statin to reduce LDL levels. Adverse effects: • Headache, diarrhea, increased LFTs (especially with Statin use).

INFECTIVE ENDOCARDITIS

- Infection of the endothelium/valves 2ry to colonization (eg, during transient/persistent bacteremia).
- **Mitral valve most common valve involved** (M>A>T>P).
  Exception is IV drug use - tricuspid valve most common in IV drug users.
- Risk factors: increased age, rheumatic heart disease, IV drug use, immunosuppression, prosthetic heart valves, congenital heart disease.

TYPES

Acute bacterial endocarditis:
- Infection of **normal valves** with a virulent organism (eg, ***S. aureus***).

Subacute bacterial endocarditis:
- Indolent infection of **abnormal valves** with less virulent organism (eg, ***S. viridans***).

IV drug-related endocarditis:
- **Most commonly due to *S. aureus* (especially MRSA).** Pseudomonas, Candida.

Prosthetic valve endocarditis:
- **Early (within 60 days): *Staphylococcus epidermis* most common.**
- Late (after 60 days) resembles native valve endocarditis.

ORGANISMS

***Staphylococcus aureus*:**
- Most common cause of **ACUTE** infective endocarditis (rapidly progressive). **Affects normal valves.**
- Also common in patients with **IV drug use** (especially **MRSA**).

Streptococcus viridans
- Most common cause of **SUBACUTE** infective endocarditis.
- **Affects damaged valves.**
- Part of the oral flora (associated with **poor dentition or dental procedures**).

Staphylococcus epidermis:
- Most common organism in early **prosthetic valve endocarditis** (especially within 60 days of the procedure).

Enterococcus:
- Seen especially in men >50 years with a recent history of **gastrointestinal or genitourinary procedure**.

HACEK organisms
- (Haemophilus aphrophilus, Actinobacillus, Cardiobacterium hominis, Eikenella corrodens, Kingella kingae) are gram- negative organisms that are hard to culture. Suspect these organisms in patients with endocarditis & **negative blood cultures**.

Streptococcus bovis:
- Especially in patients with colon cancer or ulcerative colitis.

CLINICAL MANIFESTATIONS
- Generalized constitutional symptoms: **persistent fever most common**, malaise, fatigue, anorexia etc.
- **New onset of a murmur** or worsening of an existing murmur.
- **Osler nodes**: painful or tender raised violaceous nodules on the pads of the digits and the palms (may be seen on the thenar or hypothenar eminence).
- **Janeway lesions**: **painless** erythematous **macules** on the palms & soles.
- **Splinter hemorrhages** (linear reddish-brown lesions under the nail bed), petechiae (skin or mucous membranes).
- **Roth spots:** retinal hemorrhages with central clearing.
- Splenomegaly, septic arterial or pulmonary emboli, glomerulonephritis

DIAGNOSTIC STUDIES

- **Blood cultures:** (before antibiotic initiation). **3 sets** at **least 1 hour apart** if the patient is stable.
- ECG: at regular intervals to assess for new conduction abnormalities (prone to arrhythmias).
- Echocardiogram: obtain TTE first; consider TEE if TTE is nondiagnostic or increased suspicion. **Transesophageal echocardiogram (TEE) much more sensitive than TTE** (>90% v 50% in NVE) (82%v 36% in PVE) so may be used in patients with suspected Prosthetic valve endocarditis.
- **Labs:** CBC: leukocytosis, anemia (normochromic, normocytic); ↑ESR/Rheumatoid Factor.

MODIFIED DUKE CRITERIA	
MAJOR	MINOR
• **SUSTAINED BACTEREMIA** 2 ⊕ **blood cultures** by organism known to cause endocarditis. • **ENDOCARDIAL INVOLVEMENT**: documented by either: - **⊕ echocardiogram**: (vegetation, abscess, valve perforation, prosthetic dehiscence) - clearly established **new valvular regurgitation** (aortic or mitral regurgitation)	• Predisposing condition abnormal valves, IVDA, indwelling catheters, etc. • **Fever** (>38° C /100.4°F). • **Vascular & embolic phenomena:** Janeway lesions, septic arterial or pulmonary emboli, ICH. • **Immunologic phenomena:** - Osler's nodes, Roth spots, ⊕ Rheumatoid factor - Acute glomerulonephritis • ⊕ Blood culture not meeting major criteria. • ⊕ echocardiogram not meeting major criteria (eg, worsening of existing murmur).
Clinical criteria for infective endocarditis: 2 major OR 1 major + 3 minor OR 5 minor (80% accuracy)	

major = 3 minor

INDICATIONS FOR SURGERY

- Refractory CHF; persistent or refractory infection, invasive infection, prosthetic valve, recurrent systemic emboli, fungal infections.

MANAGEMENT OF INFECTIVE ENDOCARDITIS: suggested **Empiric therapy:**

NATIVE VALVE	• **Anti-staphylococcal penicillin** (eg, **Nafcillin, Oxacillin) plus either Ceftriaxone or Gentamicin**. • Vancomycin substituted if Penicillin allergy or MRSA suspected.
PROSTHETIC VALVE	• **Vancomycin + Gentamicin + Rifampin**
FUNGAL	• Amphotericin B (treat 6-8 weeks). • Patients often need surgical intervention for fungal cases

Penicillin & Vancomycin have great gram-positive coverage.
Gentamicin & Ceftriaxone have great gram-negative coverage.

- In acute Endocarditis, antibiotics are started promptly after culture data is obtained.
- In subacute Endocarditis, if the patient is hemodynamically stable, antibiotics may be delayed in order to properly obtain blood culture data, especially if prior treatment with antibiotics.
- Adjust the antibiotic regimen based on organism, culture & sensitivities. Fever may persist up to 1 week after appropriate antibiotic therapy has been initiated.
- **Duration of therapy usually 4-6 weeks** (with aminoglycosides used only for the first 2 weeks).

Gentamicin

	ENDOCARDITIS PROPHYLAXIS INDICATIONS
Cardiac conditions	1. **Prosthetic (artificial) heart valves.** 2. **Heart repairs using prosthetic material (not including stents).** 3. **Prior history of endocarditis.** 4. **Congenital heart disease.** 5. Cardiac valvulopathy in a transplanted heart.
Procedures	1. **Dental:** involving manipulation of gums, roots of the teeth, oral mucosa perforation. 2. **Respiratory:** surgery on respiratory mucosa, rigid bronchoscopy. 3. **Procedures involving infected skin/musculoskeletal tissues** (including abscess incision & drainage).
Regimens	• **Amoxicillin 2g 30-60 minutes before** the procedures listed above. • **Clindamycin 600mg** if penicillin allergic. • Macrolides or Cephalexin are other options.

NOTE prophylaxis is no longer routinely recommended for gastrointestinal or genitourinary procedures.

NOTE prophylaxis no longer routinely recommended for most types of valvular heart disease (including mitral valve prolapse, bicuspid aortic valve, acquired mitral or aortic valve disease, hypertrophic cardiomyopathy).

Good oral hygiene recommended to reduce temporary episodes of bacteremia.

LIBMAN-SACKS ENDOCARDITIS

- **Nonbacterial thrombotic endocarditis** (marantic endocarditis) is a noninfectious endocarditis due to sterile platelet thrombi deposition on the affected valve. It most commonly affects the mitral and aortic valves.

ETIOLOGIES

- Can be seen with malignancy, **systemic lupus erythematosus**, antiphospholipid antibody syndrome, rheumatic fever, and other inflammatory conditions.

CLINICAL MANIFESTATIONS

- Most patients are asymptomatic and are usually afebrile.
- Symptoms are usually due to emboli to the skin, kidney, extremities, and spleen.

MANAGEMENT

- Manage the SLE.
- May need anticoagulation.

ACUTE PERICARDITIS

- Inflammation of the pericardium, the outer layer of the heart.
- Fibrinous or serofibrinous: eg, post MI, infectious.
- Serous: autoimmunity (eg, SLE, RA).

ETIOLOGIES

- **2 most common causes are idiopathic & viral (especially Coxsackievirus & Echovirus)**, neoplastic.
- **Dressler syndrome** (post MI pericarditis + fever + pleural effusion)
- Autoimmune, uremia, bacterial, radiation, medications.

CLINICAL MANIFESTATIONS

- **Chest pain:** sudden onset of **pleuritic** (sharp, worse with inspiration), **persistent, postural (worse when supine & improved with sitting forward)**. Pain may radiate to the shoulder, back, neck, arm, or epigastric area.
- **Pericardial friction rub:** best heard at end expiration while upright and leaning forward. 3 components.

DIAGNOSTIC STUDIES

- **ECG:** diagnostic test of choice – **diffuse ST elevations in the precordial leads with associated PR depressions** in those leads (aVR associated with the opposite – PR elevations and ST depressions). May have cardiac enzyme positivity.
- Echocardiogram: useful to evaluate for an associated pericardial effusion and/or signs of cardiac tamponade.

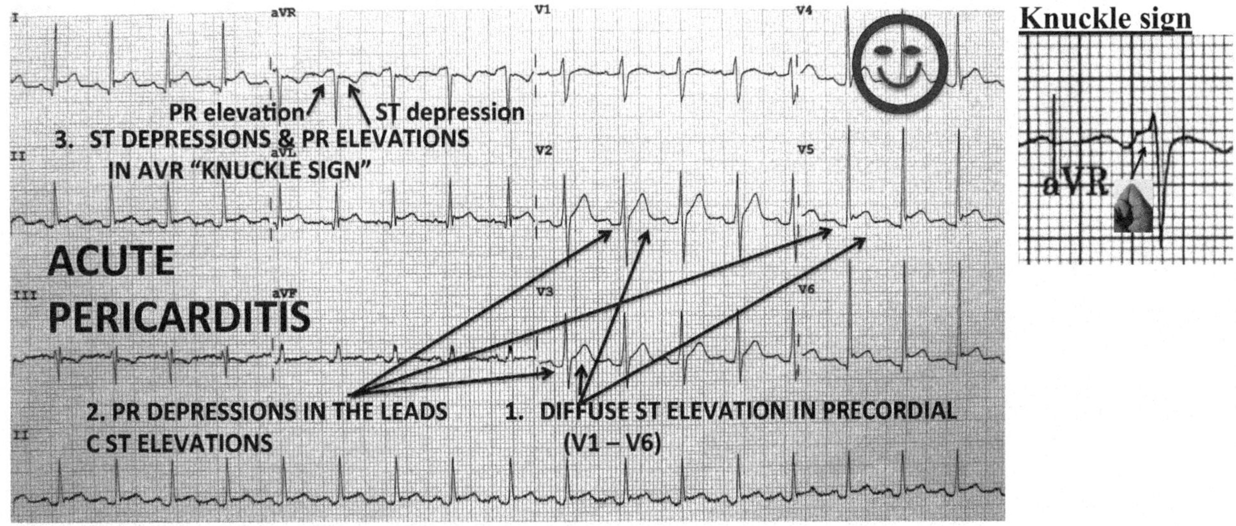

MANAGEMENT

- Anti-inflammatory meds: **NSAIDs or Aspirin first-line** x 7-14 days (symptoms usually subside in 1-2 days).
- Colchicine second-line.
- Dressler syndrome: **Aspirin or Colchicine** (avoid NSAIDS because they can interfere with myocardial scar formation).

PERICARDIAL EFFUSION

- Accumulation of fluid in the pericardial space.
- Normally, about 5-15 ml of fluid is in the pericardial space.

ETIOLOGIES

- Same causes of acute Pericarditis (eg, viral, idiopathic, immune, malignancy – lung cancer most common, breast second most common, aortic dissection, uremia).

CLINICAL MANIFESTATIONS

- Chest pain (if associated with acute Pericarditis), dyspnea, fatigue.
- Physical examination: **decreased (muffled) heart sounds** (due to fluid).

DIAGNOSIS

- **Echocardiogram: test of choice** increased fluid in the pericardial space.
- ECG: **electrical alternans** (alternating amplitudes of the QRS complexes) in large effusions. **Low QRS voltage.**

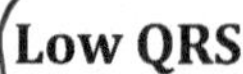

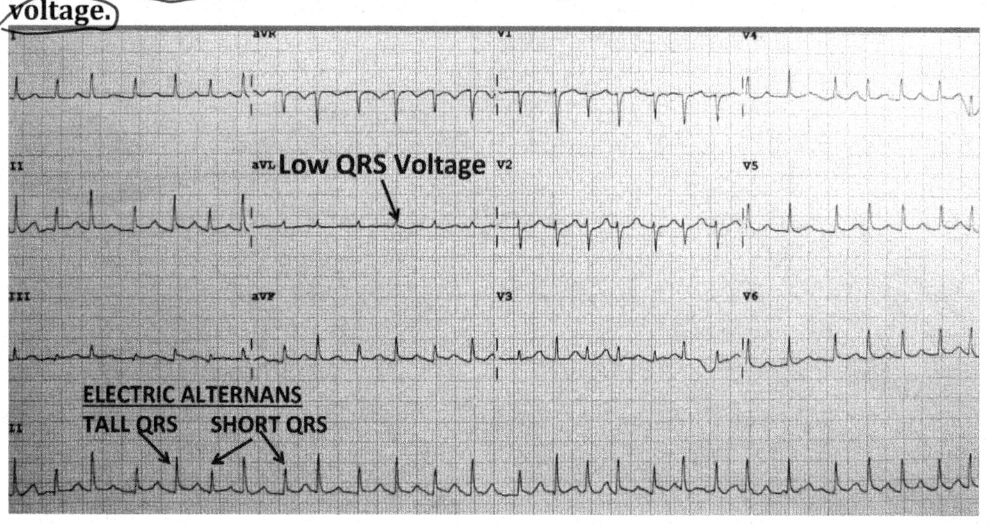

- Chest radiograph: not used in the diagnosis. Findings may include appearance of the heart as a "water bottle" (not sensitive or specific).

MANAGEMENT

- Treat the underlying cause (eg, acute Pericarditis). Serial echocardiography if necessary.
- Large effusions may need pericardiocentesis for symptomatic relief.

CARDIAC TAMPONADE

- **Pericardial effusion causing significant pressure on the heart, impeding cardiac filling, leading to decreased cardiac output and shock** (medical emergency).
- **The rate of accumulation of fluid is more critical than the volume.** A rapid accumulation of as little as 150ml of fluid can cause tamponade, while as much as 1 liter can slowly accumulate if the pericardium is compliant. Usually starts on the right side because the right walls are thinner.
- Etiologies: complication of acute Pericarditis or trauma. Malignancy is the most common nontraumatic cause of Tamponade.

CLINICAL MANIFESTATIONS
- **Beck's triad: distant (muffled) heart sounds, increased JVP, and systemic hypotension.**
- Pulsus paradoxus: exaggerated (>10 mmHg) decrease in systolic blood pressure with inspiration.
- Dyspnea, fatigue, peripheral edema, shock, reflex tachycardia, cool extremities.

DIAGNOSTIC STUDIES
- **Echocardiogram: pericardial effusion + diastolic collapse of cardiac chambers.**
- ECG: signs of pericardial effusion (low voltage QRS complexes, electrical alternans).
- Chest radiograph: may show an enlarged cardiac silhouette.
- Right heart catheterization: equalization of pressures in diastole.

MANAGEMENT
- **Pericardiocentesis (immediate)** to remove the pressure.
- Volume resuscitation and pressor support if needed. Pericardial window drainage if recurrent.

CONSTRICTIVE PERICARDITIS

- Loss of pericardial elasticity (thickening, fibrosis & calcification) leading to **restriction of ventricular diastolic filling.**
- Pathophysiology: fibrosis limits ventricular filling, decreasing stroke volume and cardiac output.
- Etiologies: any cause of acute Pericarditis. In the US, idiopathic and viral are the most common causes. Worldwide, Tuberculosis is the leading cause.

CLINICAL MANIFESTATIONS
- Dyspnea most common symptom, fatigue, orthopnea.
- Right-sided heart failure signs: **increased jugular venous distention**, peripheral edema, nausea, vomiting, increased hepatojugular reflex, **Kussmaul's sign** (the lack of an inspiratory decline or an increase in jugular vein pressure with inspiration).
- **Pericardial knock**: high pitched diastolic sound similar to S3 (sudden cessation of ventricular filling).

DIAGNOSTIC STUDIES
- Chest radiograph: pericardial calcification may be seen especially on lateral view, clear lung fields. Normal or slightly increased heart size, Square root sign on cardiac catheterization.
- **Echocardiography: pericardial thickening and/or calcification**. Also used to rule out Restrictive cardiomyopathy. **"Square root" sign** – early diastolic dip followed by a plateau of diastasis.
- **CT scan or MRI:** more sensitive than echocardiography – **pericardial thickening or calcification.**

MANAGEMENT
- Diuretics for symptom relief as well as reduction of edema and venous pressure.
- Pericardiectomy definitive management.

PERICARDIAL DISEASES

	ACUTE PERICARDITIS	PERICARDIAL EFFUSION	PERICARDIAL TAMPONADE	CONSTRICTIVE PERICARDITIS
DEFINITION	***Inflammation of the pericardium.***	↑ fluid in pericardial space.	***Pericardial effusion ⇨ pressure on the heart* ⇨ limits ventricular diastolic filling & ↓cardiac output.***	***Fibrotic, calcified pericardium limits ventricular diastolic filling***
ETIOLOGIES	•***2 most common causes are idiopathic*** (probably postviral) & ***viral (esp Enteroviruses: Coxsackievirus & Echoviruses).*** •Neoplastic, autoimmune (SLE, RA) •Inflammatory, vascular etc. •***Dressler's syndrome: post MI***	Same as acute pericarditis.	Same as pericarditis. May be traumatic.	Same as pericarditis Chronic inflammation
CLINICAL MANIFESTATIONS	**5 P's of pericarditis:** •**Chest Pain** -***Pleuritic*** (sharp pain worse with inspiration)* -***Postural (pain worse supine, relieved with sitting forward).**** -***Persistent*** chest Pain • ***Pericardial Friction Rub***	•***Distant (muffled) heart sounds.**** •± sx of pericarditis.	•***BECK'S TRIAD**** ❶***Distant heart sounds (effusion)*** ❷↑***JVP*** (jugular venous pressure) ❸ ***Systemic HYPOtension*** •***Pulsus paradoxus*** – drop >10mmHg of systolic BP with inspiration (pulses disappear with inspiration). -***Kussmaul's sign: ↑JVP c inspiration.***	•***Dyspnea MC sx**** •***R-SIDED FAILURE SX*:*** -***Peripheral edema*** -***↑JVP*** - ***Hepatic congestion, N/V*** • ***PERICARDIAL KNOCK* 3rd heart*** sound from sudden cessation of ventricular filling •***Pulsus paradoxus*** •***Kussmaul's sign***
DIAGNOSIS	•ECG: -***Diffuse ST elevations**** (concave up) ***in precordial leads with PR depressions in same leads**** ⇨ T wave inversions ⇨ resolution. -aVR: ST depression & PR elevation. •ECHOCARDIOGRAM: -Normal (± pericardial effusion). Used mainly to r/o tamponade.	•ECG: -***Low voltage QRS complex**** -***Electric Alternans*** •ECHOCARDIOGRAM: -↑***pericardial fluid.*** -No hemodynamic compromise.	•ECG: -***Low voltage QRS complexes**** -Electric Alternans •ECHOCARDIOGRAM: -↑pericardial fluid + ***diastolic collapse of cardiac chambers* hemodynamic compromise.***	 •**ECHOCARDIOGRAM:** -***PERICARDIAL THICKENING* & calcification****
MANAGEMENT	•***ASPIRIN OR NSAIDs tx of choice**** •***Colchicine 2nd line*** •***Steroids if refractory (sx > 48h)*** •***Dressler's syndrome: Aspirin or Colchicine***	•***Treat underlying cause*** •*Pericardial window if recurrent*	•***PERICARDIOCENTESIS****	•***PERICARDIECTOMY****

THE 5 GOLDEN RULES TO CONQUER MURMURS

RULE 1 - QUALITY OF THE MURMUR

- **HARSH/RUMBLE SOUNDS = think STENOSIS: AS, MS:** abnormal forward flow of blood through (stenotic) valve that should be open. Stenotic lesions lead to pressure overload. Regurgitation leads to volume overload.

- **BLOWING sound – think REGURGITATION: AR, MR:** abnormal backflow of blood (regurgitation) through an incompletely closed valve. Regurgitation leads to volume overload.

RULE 2

- **Increase in venous return increases the intensity of ALL murmurs EXCEPT hypertrophic cardiomyopathy & the click of mitral valve prolapse** (murmur of hypertrophic is decreased & ejection click is delayed/occurs later).

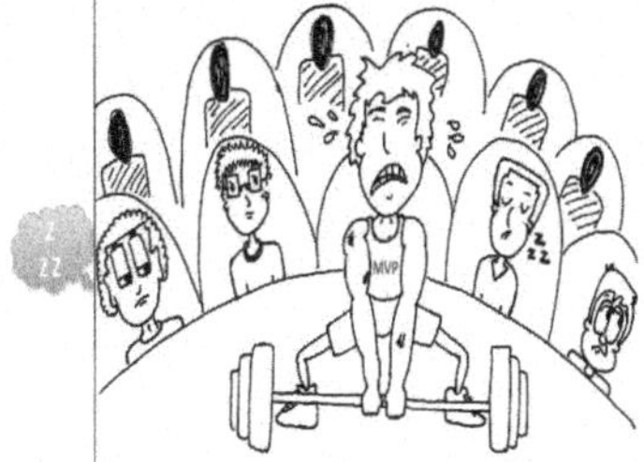

Increase venous return
- **Supine position**
- **Squatting**
- **Leg elevation**

When the **MVP** with **hypertrophied arms squatted**, the **sound** of the crowd **got lower** in anticipation

RULE 2 Continued

- **Decrease in venous return decreased the intensity of ALL murmurs EXCEPT hypertrophic cardiomyopathy & the click of mitral valve prolapse** (murmur of hypertrophic is intensified & ejection click occurs earlier/increased prolapse).

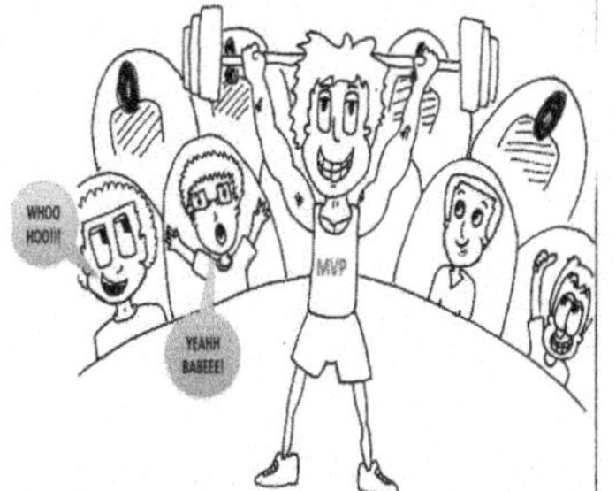

decrease venous return
- **Standing**
- **Valsalva maneuver**

When the **MVP with hypertrophied** arms stood up, the **sound** of the crowd got **louder**

RULE 3

- The right-sided murmurs sound like the left-sided versions (eg, TR sounds like MR, AS sounds like PS, AR sounds like TR)

The 2 things that distinguish them are

- ❶ the location of intensity &
- ❷**inspiration increases the intensity of Right-sided murmurs** (inspiration decreases the intensity of left-sided murmurs)

AORTIC: RIGHT UPPER STERNAL BORDER
PULMONIC: LEFT UPPER STERNAL BORDER
AORTIC
PULMONIC
MITRAL
TRICUSPID: LEFT LOWER STERNAL BORDER
TRICUSPID
MITRAL: APEX

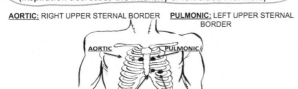

RULE 4

•RADIATION

Axilla – Mitral Regurgitation

Carotid – Aortic Stenosis

RULE 5 TIMING:

"AR MS rest" DIASTOLIC murmurs

Aortic Regurgitation & Mitral stenosis - diastolic murmurs

Aortic stenosis & Mitral regurgitation - systolic murmurs

MURMUR ACCENTUATION MANEUVERS

POSITION

- **AORTIC:** **SITTING UP & LEANING FORWARD ACCENTUATES AORTIC MURMURS** (AS, AR).
- **MITRAL:** **LYING ON LEFT SIDE ACCENTUATES MITRAL MURMURS** (MS, MR).

INCREASED VENOUS RETURN

- ↑venous return INCREASES ALL MURMURS/opening Snap (left & right side)
  - squatting, leg raise, lying down
- Exceptions: ↓ murmur of hypertrophic cardiomyopathy & delayed ejection click (decreased prolapse/shorter murmur duration) of mitral valve prolapse (MVP)

DECREASED VENOUS RETURN

- ↓venous return (Valsalva/standing) DECREASES ALL MURMURS/Opening Snap (left & right side).
- Exceptions: ↑murmur of hypertrophic cardiomyopathy & earlier ejection click (increased prolapse & longer murmur duration) of MVP

INSPIRATION

- Inspiration ↑'es venous return on right side:
  ↑ALL murmurs/opening snap on the R side (↓ejection click R side)
    - **Right-sided murmurs best heard with inspiration.**
- Inspiration ↓'es venous return on left side:
  ↓ALL murmurs/opening snap on the L side (earlier ejection click on the L side)

EXPIRATION

- Expiration ↑'es venous return on left side:
  ↑ALL murmurs/opening snap on the L side (delayed ejection click on the L side)
    - **Left-sided murmurs best heard after maximal expiration.**
- Expiration ↓'es venous return on right side:
  ↓ALL murmurs/opening snap on the R side (earlier ejection click R side).

HANDGRIP

- **↑'es afterload** (by compressing the arteries of the upper extremity) leading to ↓LV emptying (decreased forward flow & **increased backward flow**).
    - **Outflow murmurs (eg. AS, hypertrophic cardiomyopathy)** and MVP ↓ **with handgrip** (note that *handgrip & amyl nitrate are the only maneuvers that affect hypertrophic cardiomyopathy & AS in the same direction* – because both maneuvers affect AFTERLOAD & FORWARD FLOW). Because handgrip increases afterload, the increased afterload prevents blood from being ejected from the ventricles, lessening the blood flowing through the stenotic aortic valve and less blood ejected in hypertrophic cardiomyopathy.
    - **Regurgitant murmurs (AR, MR) ↑ with handgrip** (due to ↑backward flow); MS ↑'es due to ↑afterload.

AMYL NITRATE

- **↓'es afterload** (direct arteriolar vasodilator) leading to ↑LV emptying (increases forward flow & decreases backward flow of blood).
    - AS, MVP, hypertrophic cardiomyopathy murmur ↑ with amyl nitrate
    - **Regurgitant murmurs (AR, MR) ↓ with amyl nitrate**
      This is why afterload reducers like ACEI are used in the management of AR, MR.

AORTIC STENOSIS (AS)

- Pathophysiology: LV outflow obstruction leads to a fixed cardiac output, increased afterload, Left ventricular hypertrophy (LVH), and eventually LV failure.
- Most common valvular disease. Symptoms usually occur when Aov orifice <1 cm^2 (Normal 3-4 cm^2).

ETIOLOGIES
- **Degenerative: calcifications,** wear and tear, especially > 70 years of age.
- **Congenital & Bicuspid valve** common in patients < 70 years of age.
- Rheumatic heart disease: may be isolated or accompanied with Aortic regurgitation.

CLINICAL MANIFESTATIONS
- Once symptomatic, lifespan is dramatically reduced. Dyspnea is the most common symptom.
- **Angina: most common symptom** (5 year mean survival), **syncope** (3 years), **CHF** (2 years).

PHYSICAL EXAMINATION
- **Systolic crescendo-decrescendo murmur best heard at the right upper sternal border, radiating to the carotid artery.**
- **Increased murmur intensity: sitting while leaning forward,** increased venous return (eg, **squatting, supine, and leg raise**), expiration.
- Decreased murmur intensity: decreased venous return (eg, **Valsalva, standing**), inspiration, **handgrip** (due to decreased ejection of blood)
- **Weak, delayed carotid pulse** (pulsus parvus et tardus), narrow pulse pressure.

DIAGNOSTIC STUDIES
- Echocardiogram: best test - small aortic orifice, LVH, thickened or calcified aortic valve.
- ECG: **left ventricular hypertrophy**. Left atrial enlargement, atrial fibrillation.
- Chest radiograph: nonspecific – postaortic dilatation, aortic valve calcification, pulmonary congestion.
- Cardiac catheterization: definitive diagnosis (may be used prior to surgery).

MANAGEMENT
- **Surgical therapy: aortic valve replacement only effective treatment (treatment of choice)**
  Indications for AoV replacement (AVR): symptomatic AS, asymptomatic severe AS (↓EF or area <0.6cm^2).
  - -Mechanical: prolonged durability but thrombogenic (eg, stroke), bleeding. Must be placed on long-term anticoagulant therapy.
  - - Bioprosthetic: less durable but minimally thrombogenic (usually used in patients that that are not candidates for anticoagulant). Heterograft (porcine valve); pericardial.

- Percutaneous aortic valvuloplasty (PAV): results in 50% ↑AoV area, but 50% restenosis at 6-12 months so used as a bridge to AVR, if not a surgical candidate, or in pediatric patients.

- Intraaortic balloon pump: used for temporary stabilization as a bridge to valve replacement.

- Medical therapy: no medical treatment truly effective.
  - No exercise restrictions in patients with mild AS.

Severe AS prior to surgery:
- Because patients are dependent on preload to maintain cardiac output ⇨ **avoid physical exertion/venodilators** (eg, nitrates)/**negative inotropes** (Ca^{+2} channel blockers, β-blockers).

AORTIC REGURGITATION (AR) or AORTIC INSUFFICIENCY (AI)

- Incomplete aortic valve closure lead to LV volume overload with eventual LV dilation and heart failure.

ETIOLOGIES

- Acute: acute MI, aortic dissection, endocarditis. Can lead to pulmonary edema.
- Chronic: aortic dilation - Marfan syndrome, inflammatory disorders, rheumatic fever, Syphilis, HTN.

PHYSICAL EXAMINATION

- **Diastolic blowing decrescendo murmur best heard at the left upper sternal border** (high-pitched).
- **Increased murmur intensity: sitting while leaning forward,** increased venous return (eg, **squatting, supine and leg raise**), expiration, **handgrip**.
- **Decreased murmur intensity:** decreased venous return (eg, **Valsalva, standing**), inspiration, **amyl nitrate.**
- Austin-Flint murmur: mid-late diastolic rumble at the apex secondary to retrograde regurgitant jet competing with antegrade flow from the left atrium into the left ventricle.
- **Bounding pulses** due to increased stroke volume. Pulsus bisferiens can be seen (especially with combined AS + AR or severe AR).
- **Wide pulse pressure:**

Classic Signs of WIDENED PULSE PRESSURE in AR/AI (seen ONLY with chronic AR/AI)	
SIGN	**DESCRIPTION**
Water Hammer pulse	**Swift upstroke & rapid fall of radial pulse accentuated with wrist elevation.**
Corrigan's pulse	Similar to water hammer pulse but referring specifically to the carotid artery.
Hill's sign	Popliteal artery systolic pressure > brachial artery by 60mmHg **(most sensitive).**
Duroziez's sign	Gradual pressure over femoral artery ⇨ systolic and diastolic bruits.
Traube's sound (pistol shot)	Double sound heard @ femoral artery c partial compression of femoral artery.
De Musset's sign	**Head-bobbing** with each heartbeat (low sensitivity).
Müller's sign	Visible systolic pulsations of the uvula.
Quincke's pulses	Visible **fingernail bed pulsations** with light compression of fingernail bed.

DIAGNOSTIC STUDIES

- Echocardiogram: regurgitant jet.
- Cardiac catheterization: definitive diagnosis (may be used prior to surgery).

MANAGEMENT

- Medical therapy: **afterload reduction** improves forward flow (eg, ACE inhibitors, ARBs, Nifedipine, Hydralazine).

- Surgical therapy: definitive management. Indicated in acute or symptomatic AR, asymptomatic AR with LV decompensation (EF < 55% - patients with AR normally have higher than normal ejection fraction).

MITRAL STENOSIS (MS)

PATHOPHYSIOLOGY
- Obstruction of flow from LA to LV 2ry to narrowed mitral orifice ⇨ blood backs up into the left atrium.
- ↑**L-atrial pressure/volume overload** ⇨ pulmonary congestion ⇨ **pulmonary HTN** ⇨ CHF.

ETIOLOGIES
- **Rheumatic heart disease is almost always the cause.** Most common in the 3rd/4th decade.
- Congenital, left atrial myxoma, thrombus, valvulitis (SLE, amyloid, carcinoid).

CLINICAL MANIFESTATIONS
- Slow progression until symptoms occur (then progression becomes rapid).
- Pulmonary symptoms: **dyspnea** (most common symptom), pulmonary edema, **hemoptysis,** cough, frequent bronchitis, **pulmonary HTN** (if rheumatic in origin, symptoms usually begins in 20s – 30s).
- **Atrial fibrillation:** secondary to atrial enlargement ⇨ thromboembolic events (ex. CVA).
- Right-sided heart failure: due to prolonged pulmonary hypertension.
- **Mitral facies = ruddy (flushed) cheeks with facial pallor** (chronic hypoxia).
- Signs of left atrial enlargement: dysphagia (esophageal compression), Ortner's syndrome: recurrent laryngeal nerve palsy due to compression by the dilated left atrium ⇨ hoarseness.

PHYSICAL EXAMINATION
- **Prominent S1** (forceful closure of mitral valve), **opening snap** (forceful opening of mitral valve), loud P2.
- Low-pitched, **mid-diastolic rumbling murmur** best heard at the apex.
- **Increased murmur intensity: left lateral decubitus position,** expiration, isometric exercise, increased venous return (eg, **squatting, leg raise, lying supine**).
- Decreased murmur intensity: decreased venous return (eg, **Valsalva, standing**), inspiration.
- Increased severity of MS: shorter A2-OS duration, prolonged murmur duration.

DIAGNOSIS
- ECG: **left atrial enlargement** (P wave > 3 mm, biphasic P wave in V1 and V2), **atrial fibrillation, pulmonary hypertension** (RVH, right axis deviation).
- **Echocardiography: most useful noninvasive tool.**
- Chest radiograph: left atrial enlargement (eg, straightening of the left border, prominent pulmonary arteries, posterior displacement of the esophagus, elevation of left mainstem bronchus).
- Cardiac catheterization: most accurate but rarely done.

MANAGEMENT
- **Percutaneous balloon valvuloplasty: best treatment for symptomatic MS in younger patients** with noncalcified valves or if refractory to medical therapy.
- Mitral valve replacement: reserved if mitral valvuloplasty is contraindicated or with unfavorable valve morphology.
- Medical: diuretics and sodium restriction for edema & volume overload. Rate control of Atrial fibrillation with Beta blockers, Calcium channel blockers, or Digoxin.
- Anticoagulation in patients with Atrial fibrillation (eg, Warfarin).

MITRAL REGURGITATION

PATHOPHYSIOLOGY

- Abnormal, retrograde blood flow from the left ventricle into the left atrium, leading to **left atrial dilation & increased pulmonary pressure.**

ETIOLOGIES

- Leaflet abnormalities: **mitral valve prolapse most common cause in US**. Rheumatic fever most common cause in developing countries. Endocarditis, valvulitis, annulus dilation **(LV dilation),** Marfan syndrome.
- Papillary muscle dysfunction: myocardial ischemia or infarction, cardiomyopathy.
- Ruptured chordae tendinae: collagen vascular disease, dilated cardiomyopathy.

CLINICAL MANIFESTATIONS

- Chronic: heart failure symptoms (eg, **dyspnea most common**, fatigue), **atrial fibrillation**, hemoptysis, hypertension.
- Acute: pulmonary edema, hypotension.

PHYSICAL EXAMINATION

- **Blowing holosystolic murmur** best heard at the **apex with radiation to the axilla** (high-pitched).
- **Increased murmur intensity: left lateral decubitus position,** expiration, isometric exercise, increased venous return (eg, squatting, leg raise, lying supine), **handgrip**.
- **Decreased murmur intensity:** decreased venous return (eg, Valsalva, standing), inspiration, **amyl nitrate.**
- Widely split S2, laterally displaced PMI, S3, soft S1 (if severe).

DIAGNOSIS

- **Echocardiogram: most useful noninvasive test –** hyperdynamic LV, regurgitant jet.
- ECG: nonspecific – left atrial enlargement, LVH, atrial fibrillation.
- Chest radiograph: nonspecific – left atrial enlargement, LVH, pulmonary edema.

MANAGEMENT

- Medical: **symptom control with afterload reducers** (eg, **ACE inhibitors, ARBs**, Hydralazine, Nitrates), or diuretics (do not reduce progression of the disease.
- Surgical: **repair preferred over replacement –** indicated if EF 60% or less or refractory to medical therapy.

MITRAL VALVE PROLAPSE (MVP)

- The leaflets of the mitral valve bulge (prolapse) into the left atrium during systole.
- **MVP most common cause of Mitral regurgitation (MR) in the US.**
- **Most common in young women** (15 – 35 years of age). Seen in 2-5% of the population.

ETIOLOGIES:
- **Myxomatous degeneration of the mitral valve.**
- Connective tissue diseases eg, Marfan or Ehlers-Danlos syndromes, Osteogenesis imperfecta.

CLINICAL MANIFESTATIONS:
- **Most are asymptomatic.**
- **Autonomic dysfunction** - anxiety, **atypical chest pain, panic attacks, palpitations** from arrhythmias, syncope, dizziness, fatigue.
- Symptoms associated with MR progression (not common) – dyspnea, fatigue, CHF.
- Stroke (rare)

PHYSICAL EXAMINATION:
- May have narrow AP diameter, low body weight, hypotension, scoliosis, pectus excavatum.
- **Mid-late systolic ejection click** best heard at the apex. May be associated with mid-late systolic murmur (MR).
  - **Any maneuver that makes the LV smaller (decreases preload) results in an earlier click** & longer murmur duration (eg, Valsalva, standing) due to increased prolapse.
  - **Maneuvers that make the LV bigger (increases preload) results in a delayed click** & shorter murmur duration (eg, squatting, leg raise, supine) due to decreased prolapse. Handgrip.

DIAGNOSIS
- **Echocardiography** – posterior bulging leaflets with tissue redundancy.

MANAGEMENT
- **Reassurance in most patients** (MVP is associated with a good prognosis).
- **Beta blockers only used in patients with autonomic dysfunction.**
- Mitral valve repair or replacement is reserved for MVP with severe MR to prevent CHF.
- Endocarditis prophylaxis is not needed.

PULMONIC STENOSIS (PS)

- Right ventricular outflow obstruction of blood across the pulmonic valve.
- **Almost always congenital** & a **disease of the young** (eg, Congenital rubella syndrome).

PHYSICAL EXAMINATION
- Harsh mid-systolic ejection crescendo-decrescendo murmur (maximal at the left upper sternal border) radiates to the neck.
  - **Murmur increases with inspiration.** The longer the murmur duration = ↑stenosis.
  - Systolic ejection click (often "buried" in S1), Wide split S_2 (delayed P_2), ± S_4

MANAGEMENT
- Balloon valvuloplasty is the preferred treatment.

PULMONIC REGURGITATION (PR)

ETIOLOGIES

- **Almost always congenital.** Pulmonary hypertension, tetralogy of Fallot, endocarditis, rheumatic heart disease.

PATHOPHYSIOLOGY

- Retrograde blood flow from pulmonary artery into RV ⇨ R-sided volume overload.

CLINICAL MANIFESTATIONS:

- Most clinically insignificant. If symptomatic ⇨R-sided failure symptoms.

PHYSICAL EXAMINATION

- **Graham-Steell murmur: brief decrescendo early diastolic murmur @ LUSB** (2nd L ICS) **with full inspiration.** Severe pulmonary HTN ↑'es the velocity of the regurgitation.
    - **↑(augmented) murmur:↑venous return** (squatting, supine, **inspiration).**
    - ↓ (diminished) murmur: ↓ venous return (Valsalva, standing, expiration).

MANAGEMENT

- No treatment needed in most (most well tolerated).

TRICUSPID STENOSIS (TS)

- Blood backs up into the right atrium ⇨↑ right atrial enlargement ⇨ right-sided heart failure.

PHYSICAL EXAMINATION

- Mid-diastolic murmur at the left lower sternal border (Xyphoid, 4th intercostal space). Low frequency.
    - **↑ intensity**: ↑venous return: (squatting, laying down, leg raising, **inspiration).**
    - Opening snap (OS): usually occurs later than the opening snap of mitral stenosis.

MANAGEMENT

- Medical: decrease right atrial volume overload with diuretics & Na^+ restriction.
- Surgical: commissurotomy or replacement if right heart failure or ↓cardiac output.

TRICUSPID REGURGITATION

PHYSICAL EXAMINATION

- Holosystolic, blowing, high-pitched murmur at the subxyphoid area (left mid sternal border).
- Little to no murmur radiation.
- ↑murmur intensity: ↑venous return: (ex. squatting, inspiration).
- **Carvallo's sign: increased murmur intensity with inspiration** (due to increased right sided blood flow during inspiration). Helps to distinguish TR from MR. ±Pulsatile liver.

MANAGEMENT

- Medical: diuretics (for volume overload & congestion). If LV dysfunction - standard HF therapy.
- Surgical: suggested for patients with severe TR despite medical therapy. Repair >replacement.

	AORTIC STENOSIS (AS)	MITRAL STENOSIS (MS)	AORTIC REGURGITATION	MITRAL REGURGITATION	MITRAL VALVE PROLAPSE
PATHO PHYSIOLOGY	• ***LV outflow obstruction ⇨ fixed CO*.*** • ***↑afterload ⇨ LVH****	• ***Obstruction of flow from LA to LV ⇨ ↑L-atrial enlargement & ↑LA pressure ⇨ pulm HTN***	• ***Backflow from Aorta to LV ⇨ LV volume overload****	• ***Backflow from LV into LA ⇨ LV volume overload* ⇨ ↓CO***	*Myxomatous degeneration of mitral valve* (floppy, redundant valve)
ETIOLOGIES	• ***Degeneration (>70y)**** • ***Congenital (<70y)**** • Rheumatic disease	• ***Rheumatic Heart disease (RHD) MC cause by far****	• Rheumatic disease, HTN • Endocarditis, Marfan • Syphilis • Ankylosing spondylitis	• ***MVP MC cause**** • Rheumatic, Endocarditis • Ischemia (ruptured papillary muscle/chordae tendinae post MI)	• ***MC in young women*** • Connective tissue disease (ex Marfan, Ehrlos Danlos)
CLINICAL	• ***Angina*** (5y survival s AVR) • ***Syncope*** (3y s AVR) • ***CHF*** (2y s AVR)	• ***R-SIDED heart failure**** • ***Pulmonary HTN - Hemoptysis*** • ***ATRIAL FIBRILLATION**** • ***Mitral Facies**** (flushed cheeks)	• ***L-SIDED heart failure****	• Acute: pulmonary edema, ***dyspnea*** • Chronic: A fib, CHF. May have Pulmonary HTN (not as often as MS)	• ***Most asymptomatic*** • ❶***Autonomic dysfunction:*** chest pain, panic attacks; arrhythmias causing palpitations, syncope, dizziness, fatigue • ❷ ***Sx associated with MR progression:*** fatigue, dyspnea, CHF. • ❸ Stroke, endocarditis, PVC's
MURMUR	• ***SYSTOLIC "EJECTION" CRESCENDO-DECRESCENDO @ RUSB**** • ***Later peaking murmur = ↑severity***	• ***DIASTOLIC RUMBLE @ APEX (LOW) IN LLD**** *May be preceded by* ***OPENING SNAP**** • Shorter S_2-OS duration = ↑severity	• ***DIASTOLIC DECRESCENDO BLOWING @ LUSB.*** ***↑'es with handgrip**** ***↓ with amyl nitrate*** • ***±Austin Flint Murmur:*** mid-late diastolic rumble @ apex	• ***BLOWING HOLOSYSTOLIC MURMUR @ APEX*** ***↑'es with handgrip, LLD**** ***↓'es with amyl nitrate***	• ***MID TO LATE SYSTOLIC EJECTION CLICK* @ apex. ↓venous return (Valsalva, standing, inspiration) ⇨ earlier click (↑prolapse) & longer murmur duration*** • ***±mid-late systolic murmur (MR)***
RADIATION	• ***CAROTID ARTERIES****	• ***NO RADIATION***	• ***Along L-sternal border***	• ***AXILLA****	
PULSE	• ***PULSUS PARVUS ET TARDUS**** (weak, delayed pulse) • ***Narrow pulse pressure****	• Usually reduced intensity (due to decreased cardiac output)	• ***BOUNDING PULSES* (↑SV)*** • ***WIDE pulse pressure**** • Pulse Bisferiens (if combined AS +AR)*	May have a brisk upstroke (due to hyperdynamic ventricle) from ↑preload & ↓afterload	
PHYSICAL EXAM	• LV heave due to LV hypertrophy	Left atrial enlargement	• Hill- popliteal mmHg >brachial pressure • DeMussets- Head bobbing • Quincke pulses – nail bed pulsations		• Narrow AP diameter • Low Body weight (thin) • Hypotension • Scoliosis, Pectus Excavatum
HEART SOUNDS	• ***Paradoxically split S_2*** (If severe) • S_4 if LVH	• ***Prominent S_1**** *"closing snap"* ± diminish with ↑severity • ***OPENING SNAP**** (OS)	• ***Water hammer pulse*** • Pistol shot over fem art.	• ***Widely split S_2*** • ± S_3, decreased S_1	
MANAGEMENT	***Aortic valve replacement (AVR) once sxatic**** Severe AS is preload dependent ⇨ avoid exertion, venodilators & negative inotropes (CCB, B-blockers)	• ***Valvotomy in young patients*** if rheumatic dz is cause, sxatic & valve orifice < 1.0 cm² • Repair preferred over replacement	**Meds: *Vasodilators*** (↓afterload increases forward flow) **Surgery:** acute or sxatic AR or ↓LV <55% (need hyperdynamic ventricle to maintain CO)	**Meds: *vasodilators:***↓Afterload increases forward flow ***(ACEI)*** **Surgery: *valve repair preferred vs. valve replacement**** (Acute/sxatic or ↓LV <55%)	- ***Reassurance good prognosis in asymptomatic patients or mild sx**** - ***Beta blockers for autonomic dysfunction****
MURMUR MANEUVERS	• ↓venous return (Valsalva/standing) DECREASES ALL MURMURS EXCEPT: ❶ ↑'es the murmur of hypertrophic cardiomyopathy* & ❷ causes earlier click of MVP • ↑venous return (lying supine, squatting, leg raise) INCREASES ALL MURMURS EXCEPT: ❶ ↓ murmur in hypertrophic cardiomyopathy* & ❷ later click of MVP • Inspiration ↑'es all R-sided murmurs, Expiration ↑'es all L-sided murmurs. AORTIC (AR,AS): ↑'es if sitting forward; MITRAL (MR,MS): ↑'es with left lateral decubitus				

ABDOMINAL AORTIC ANEURYSM (AAA)

- Focal aortic dilation > 1.5 normal (> 3.0 cm considered aneurysmal). **Infrarenal most common site.**
- Pathophysiology: *proteolytic degeneration of aortic wall* & connective tissue inflammation.

RISK FACTORS

- **Smoking (main modifiable risk factor), age >60 years, Caucasians, males,** hyperlipidemia, atherosclerosis, connective tissue disorder (eg, Marfan), Syphilis, Hypertension.
- Protective factors: female sex, Diabetes mellitus, non-Caucasian race, moderate alcohol consumption.

CLINICAL MANIFESTATIONS

- **Most patients are asymptomatic** - may be found to incidentally on imaging or in patients with an abdominal bruit or a palpable abdominal mass.
- Symptomatic (unruptured): presents with **abdominal, flank, or back pain**. On examination, an **abdominal bruit** may be auscultated and a **pulsatile abdominal mass** may be palpated.
- Symptomatic (ruptured): abdominal, flank or back pain, abdominal bruit, pulsatile mass, **hypotension or syncope. Flank ecchymosis.**
- Aortoenteric fistula: presents as acute GI bleed in patients who underwent prior aortic grafting.

DIAGNOSIS

- **CT scan with IV contrast: best initial test in symptomatic, hemodynamically stable patients** to determine presence, size, & extent.
- **Focused bedside ultrasound:** may be initial study of choice in **hemodynamically unstable** patients with suspected AAA.
- Patients with known AAA who present with classic symptoms or signs of rupture can be taken to the operating room for surgical repair without preoperative imaging.

Asymptomatic with suspected AAA:

- Abdominal ultrasound: **initial test in asymptomatic patients & to monitor progression.**

MANAGEMENT

- **Symptomatic or ruptured: immediate surgical repair** (endovascular stent graft or open repair).
- β-blockers reduces shearing forces, ↓'es expansion & rupture risk.

AAA SCREENING

- **One-time screening via abdominal ultrasound in men 65-75 years of age who ever smoked.**

≥5.5 cm OR > 0.5 cm expansion in 6 months	**IMMEDIATE SURGICAL REPAIR (even if asymptomatic), symptomatic patients or patients with acute rupture.**
>4.5 cm	Vascular surgeon referral.
4 - 4.5 cm	Monitor by ultrasound every 6 months.
3 - 4 cm	Monitor by ultrasound every year.

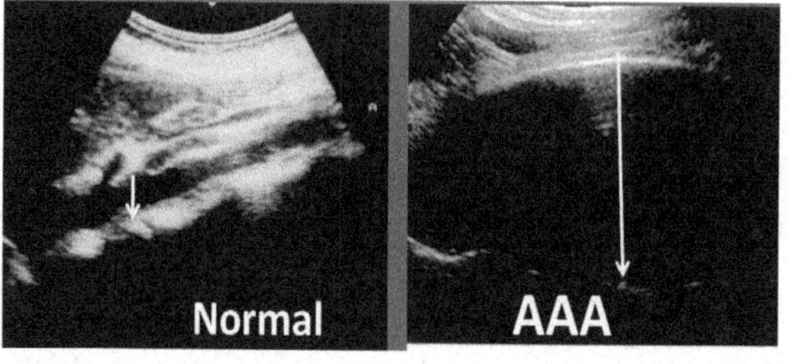

AORTIC DISSECTION

- Tear through the innermost layer of the aorta (intima) due to cystic medial necrosis.
- **Ascending most common** near the aortic arch or left subclavian (65%), 20% descending, 10% aortic arch. **Ascending = high mortality.**

RISK FACTORS
- **Hypertension (most important)**, age > 50 years (20-30 years of age in patients with Marfan syndrome), men, vasculitis (rare), trauma, family history of aortic dissection, Turner's syndrome, Collagen disorders: (eg, Marfan syndrome, Ehlers-Danlos), pregnancy.

CLINICAL MANIFESTATIONS
- **Chest Pain**: sudden onset of **severe, tearing (ripping, knife-like) chest/upper back pain may radiate between the scapulae.**
  - ascending aorta ⇨ anterior chest pain (especially Type A).
  - aortic arch ⇨ neck/jaw pain.
  - descending aorta ⇨ **interscapular pain** (especially with Type B).
- **Unequal blood pressure in both arms**: variation in pulse & blood pressure (>20mmHg difference) between right & left arms. Decreased peripheral pulses (radial, carotid, femoral).
- May be hypertensive or hypotensive. Back pain, spine ischemia, altered mental status.
- New onset of aortic regurgitation if ascending.

DIAGNOSIS
- **CT angiogram**, MR angiogram, and Transesophageal echocardiogram are the **most commonly used first-line imaging** modalities in suspected Aortic dissection.
- Chest radiograph: **widened mediastinum classic** (may be normal in 10% so a normal CXR does not rule out dissection).

MANAGEMENT:
- **Surgical: used in acute proximal** (Stanford A/ DeBakey I and II) OR acute distal with complications (vital organ involvement, impending rupture, etc). Preoperative blood pressure control.
- **Medical: descending/distal** (Stanford B/Debakey III). **Nonselective beta blockers (eg, Labetalol)** with **Sodium nitroprusside added if needed**; Nicardipine. Systolic blood pressure is rapidly lowered to a goal of 100-120 mmHg within 20 minutes.

AORTIC DISSECTION CLASSIFICATION

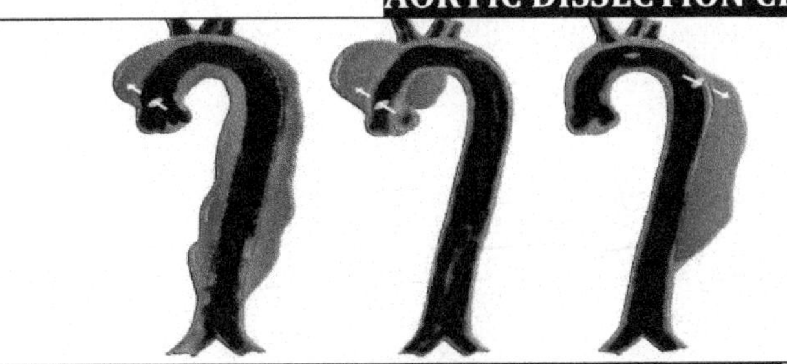

Type	DeBakey I	DeBakey II	DeBakey III
	Stanford A		Stanford B
	Proximal		Distal

DeBakey

Type I – Originates in ascending aorta, propagates at least to the aortic arch and often beyond it distally.

Type II – Originates in and is confined to the ascending aorta.

Type III – Originates in descending aorta, rarely extends proximally but will extend distally.

Stanford

A – Involves ascending aorta and/or aortic arch, & possibly descending aorta.

B – Involves the descending aorta (distal to left subclavian artery origin), without involvement of the ascending aorta or aortic arch.

PERIPHERAL ARTERIAL DISEASE

- Atherosclerotic disease of the arteries of the lower extremities.

CLINICAL MANIFESTATIONS

- **Intermittent claudication – most common symptom** (lower extremity pain with ambulation).

VESSEL INVOLVED	AREA OF CLAUDICATION	PERCENTAGE
AORTIC BIFURCATION/COMMON ILIAC	**Buttock, hip, groin.**	25-30%
	Leriche's syndrome: triad: ❶ claudication (buttock, thigh pain) ❷ impotence & ❸ decreased femoral pulses.	
FEMORAL ARTERY OR BRANCHES	**Thigh, upper calf**	**80 -90%**
POPLITEAL ARTERY	**Lower calf,** ankle and foot	
TIBIAL AND PERONEAL ARTERIES	Foot	40-50%

- Ischemic rest pain: in advanced disease. Most common at night and relieved with foot dependency.

PHYSICAL EXAMINATION

- Pulses: **decreased or absent pulses.** Bruits (>50% occlusion). Decreased capillary refill.
- Skin: **atrophic skin changes** – muscle atrophy, thin/shiny skin, hair loss, thickened nails, cool limbs, and areas of necrosis. Usually no edema. Ulcers, especially **lateral malleolar ulcers.**
- Color: **pale on elevation, dependent rubor** (dusky red with dependency).

DIAGNOSIS

- **Ankle-brachial index: most useful screening test** (simple, quick noninvasive).
  - **⊕ PAD if ABI <0.90** (0.50 is severe). Rest pain if < 0.4. Normal ABI 1-1.2.
  - >1.2 ⇨ possible noncompressible (calcified) vessels – may lead to a false reading.
- Arteriography: gold standard. Usually only performed if revascularization is planned.

MANAGEMENT

- Supportive: **first-line therapy - exercise** (fixed distance walking), decreasing risk factors (eg, **smoking cessation associated with greatest benefit**, hyperlipidemia, DM), foot care.
- Platelet inhibitors: **Cilostazol most effective medical therapy.** Aspirin, Clopidogrel, Pentoxifylline.
- Revascularization: Percutaneous transluminal angioplasty (first-line revascularization procedure), bypass grafts, endarterectomy (last-line).

ACUTE ARTERIAL OCCLUSION

- Acute limb ischemia - rapidly developing or sudden decrease in limb perfusion. **Vascular emergency**.
- Etiologies: **thrombotic occlusion most common** (with preexisting Peripheral arterial disease) – **most common in the superficial femoral** or popliteal artery.

CLINICAL MANIFESTATIONS:

- 6 Ps – **paresthesias (often early), pain,** pallor, pulselessness, poikilothermia, **paralysis (late finding associated with a worse prognosis)**. Symptoms usually distal to the occlusion.
- Decreased capillary refill, decreased or absent pulses, cool temperature.

WORKUP

- **Bedside arterial Doppler** to assess for pulses. **CT angiography** (quicker) or catheter angiography.
- An immediately threatened limb may undergo further evaluation and treatment in a surgical suite.

MANAGEMENT

- **Reperfusion mainstay of treatment – surgical bypass, surgical or catheter based thromboembolectomy**, endarterectomy. Thrombolytic therapy or Percutaneous angioplasty.
- Supportive: pain control, fluid resuscitation, unfractionated Heparin.

THROMBOANGIITIS OBLITERANS (BUERGER's DISEASE)

- Nonatherosclerotic inflammatory **small and medium vessel vasculitis,** leading to vasocclusive phenomena.
- **Suspect in young smokers/tobacco users with distal extremity ischemia/ischemic ulcers or gangrene of the digits.**

RISK FACTORS
- **Strong association with tobacco use.**
- Most commonly seen in **young men 20-45 years of age** especially in India, Asia, and the Middle East.

CLINICAL MANIFESTATIONS
- Triad: **distal extremity ischemia both upper and lower extremities** (eg, claudication in the lower calf or arch of the foot, ischemic ulcers), **Raynaud's phenomenon,** and **superficial migratory thrombophlebitis** - due to decrease blood flow in the medium and small arteries and veins:

DIAGNOSIS
- Abnormal Allen test: delayed perfusion of the radial and ulnar arteries.
- **Aortography: corkscrew collaterals**.
- Biopsy: segmental vascular inflammation.

MANAGEMENT:
- **Smoking/tobacco use cessation cornerstone of management**.
- Wound care – debridement, moist dressings, negative pressure wound therapy.
- Amputation if gangrene occurs or to avoid the spread of infection in severe ischemic cases.
- Iloprost: prostaglandin analog that may help with critical limb ischemia while smoking cessation is in progress.
- Calcium channel blockers for Raynaud's phenomenon.

ATRIAL MYXOMA

- Most common primary cardiac tumor. Rare.
- **80% occur in the left atrium** (most are found near the fossa ovalis).

PATHOPHYSIOLOGY
- Because many are pedunculated, some can cause a **"ball-valve" obstruction of the mitral orifice, mimicking Mitral stenosis.**

CLINICAL MANIFESTATIONS
- Dyspnea, weight loss and syncope (from mitral valve obstruction). Triad of embolic phenomenon, Mitral stenosis-like symptoms and constitutional "flu-like" symptoms (fever, weight loss).
- Physical examination: classically also associated **Mitral-stenosis like findings** (eg, **Prominent S1, low-pitched diastolic murmur**).

DIAGNOSIS
- **Transesophageal echocardiogram** - pedunculated mass with **"ball-valve"** obstruction of the mitral valve orifice.

MANAGEMENT
- Surgical removal.

GIANT CELL (TEMPORAL) ARTERITIS

- Large & medium vessel **granulomatous vasculitis** of the **extracranial branches of the carotid artery** (temporal artery, occipital artery, ophthalmic artery, & posterior ciliary artery).
- **Same clinical spectrum as Polymyalgia Rheumatica**.
- Risk factors: **women, >50y,** Northeastern Europeans.

CLINICAL MANIFESTATIONS

- Classic symptoms: **headache, jaw claudication with mastication, visual changes** (eg, anterior ischemic optic neuritis most common, monocular vision loss, amaurosis fugax, CRAO).
  - The headache is new in onset, localized, often unilateral, & lancinating in the temporal area.
- May have **scalp tenderness**. The temporal artery may be tender, pulseless, or normal.
- Constitutional symptoms: fever, fatigue, weight loss, night sweats, malaise.

DIAGNOSIS

- **GCA is primarily a clinical diagnosis –** headache, jaw claudication, fever, and visual changes.
- Labs: **increased ESR** & CRP. Normocytic normochromic anemia.
- Temporal biopsy: definitive diagnosis (not always positive).
- Temporal artery ultrasound may show thickening (halo sign), stenosis, or occlusion.

MANAGEMENT:

- **Initiate high-dose corticosteroids once GCA is suspected to prevent blindness** (do not delay treatment to biopsy or for biopsy results). **Blindness most common complication.**
- Steroid-sparing agents or steroid-refractory agents – Methotrexate, Azathioprine.
- Low-dose Aspirin.

SUPERFICIAL THROMBOPHLEBITIS

- Inflammation and/or thrombosis of a superficial vein.
- **Most commonly associated with IV catheterization, pregnancy, varicose veins,** venous stasis.
- **Trousseau sign: migratory thrombophlebitis associated with malignancy** (eg, Pancreatic cancer). May be seen with other vasculitic disorders.

CLINICAL MANIFESTATIONS

- Local phlebitis: **tenderness, pain, induration, edema, & erythema along the course of the vein** under the skin. May feel a **palpable cord.**

DIAGNOSIS

- Mainly a clinical diagnosis
- **Venous Duplex ultrasound: noncompressible vein** with clot and wall thickening.
- Hypercoagulability workup: **Factor V Leiden (most common cause)**, prothrombin gene mutations, Protein C and S, antiphospholipid antibodies, lupus anticoagulant, factor VII, homocysteine.
- Migratory phlebitis: malignancy workup: carcinoembryonic antigen (CEA), prostate specific antigen (PSA), colonoscopy, CT scan, mammography (as indicated based on suspicion).

MANAGEMENT

- **Supportive mainstay – NSAIDs, extremity elevation, warm compresses.**
- Vein ligation/excision (phlebectomy): if extensive varicose veins, septic phlebitis, or persistent symptoms despite supportive measures.
- Septic: IV antibiotics (eg, Penicillin + Aminoglycoside) – suspect if febrile.
- If the clot is near the saphenofemoral junction, consider anticoagulation.

DEEP VENOUS THROMBOSIS

- *Most important consequence is pulmonary embolism (50%);* both are manifestations of a single entity.
- **Most DVTs originate in the calf.**

RISK FACTORS (Virchow's triad)

- **Intimal damage:** trauma, infection, inflammation
- **Stasis:** eg, Immobilization or prolonged sitting >4hours.
- **Hypercoagulability:** eg, Protein C or S Deficiency, Factor V Leiden mutation, antithrombin III deficiency, oral contraceptive use, malignancy, pregnancy, smoking.

CLINICAL MANIFESTATIONS

- **Unilateral swelling & edema of the lower extremity > 3cm most specific sign.**
- **Calf pain & tenderness.** May be warm to palpation.
- Homan sign (deep calf pain with foot dorsiflexion while squeezing the calf) is not reliable.

DIAGNOSIS

- **Venous Duplex Ultrasound:** usually **first-line imaging.**
- D-dimer: highly sensitive but not specific. There are 2 main uses of D-dimer: **negative D-dimer with a low-risk for DVT can exclude DVT as the diagnosis.** In a patient with moderate risk, a positive D-dimer and a negative initial ultrasound, serial ultrasounds are recommended. In general, any positive DVT should be followed by ultrasonography.
- Contrast venography: definitive diagnosis (gold standard). It is invasive, difficult to perform, and rarely used. CT venography and MR venography rarely used.

MANAGEMENT

- **Anticoagulation: first-line treatment for most patients with DVT.** Options include Low molecular weight heparin + Warfarin, LMWH + either Dabigatran or Edoxaban or monotherapy with Rivaroxaban or Apixaban.
- **IVC filter:** 3 main reasons for IVC filter placement: **recurrent DVT/PE despite adequate anticoagulation** OR **stable patients in whom anticoagulation is contraindicated** OR right ventricular dysfunction with an enlarged RV on echocardiogram.
- Thrombolysis or Thrombectomy: generally not performed (reserved for massive DVT or severe cases).

RISK FACTORS VENOUS THROMBOEMBOLISM (VTE)	RECOMMENDED DURATION OF THERAPY
1st event with reversible or time-limiting RF for VTE	**at least 3 months** (Risk factors: trauma, surgery, OCPs etc).
1st episode of IDIOPATHIC DVT (no malignancy) - Proximal DVT or PE - Distal DVT	Long-term anticoagulation 3 months if severely symptomatic distal DVT No tx & surveillance (ultrasound) if asymptomatic distal DVT
Pregnancy	LMWH preferred as initial & long-term therapy.
Malignancy	LMWH as initial & long-term therapy. Warfarin or direct oral anticoagulants are alternatives to LMWH in these patients.

2016 ACCP guidelines: novel oral anticoagulants (Apixaban, Dabigatran, Edoxaban, Rivaroxaban) are preferred over Warfarin therapy in the management of DVT/PE (if no cancer is present).

WELL'S CRITERIA FOR DVT

Clinical feature	Points	
Active cancer (including treatment within 6 months, or palliation)	1	
Paralysis, paresis, or immobilization of lower extremity	1	
Bedridden for more than 3 days because of surgery (within 4 weeks)	1	
Localized tenderness along distribution of deep veins	1	
Swelling of entire leg	1	
Unilateral calf swelling of greater than 3 cm (below tibial tuberosity)	1	
Unilateral pitting edema	1	
Collateral superficial veins	1	
Alternative diagnosis as likely or more likely than DVT	-2	
Total points		

erpretation:

- Low probability of DVT: -2 to 0 points
- Moderate probability: 1- 2 points
- High probability: 3 – 8 points

LOW MOLECULAR WEIGHT HEPARIN (LMWH)	UNFRACTIONATED HEPARIN (UFH)
• **MOA: potentiates antithrombin III -** works more on factor Xa than thrombin (Factor IIa). • **SQ injection. Compliant, low-risk patients can be discharged home during bridging therapy.** • **Duration of Action ~12 hours.** • **No need to monitor PTT** (weight based – more predictable dosing). • **Protamine Sulfate is the antidote** (not as effective as it is for UFH). • **Lower risk of HIT** (higher anti Xa-IIa ratio means less potential binding with platelets). • **CI: Renal failure** (Cr >2.0) because LMWH excreted by kidneys, **Thrombocytopenia.**	• **MOA: potentiates antithrombin III, inhibits thrombin & other coagulation factors.** • Continuous IV drip – requires hospitalization for bridging therapy. • **Duration of Action: 1h after IV drip is discontinued.** • **Must monitor PTT 1.5-2.5x normal value.** • **Protamine Sulfate is the antidote.** • **Heparin Induced Thrombocytopenia** – Heparin acts as a hapten (stimulates the immune response when attached to platelet factor 4). This complex activates platelets, causing simultaneous thrombocytopenia & thrombosis. **Management:** other anticoagulants: ex: Argatroban or Bivalirudin. DO NOT use Warfarin (may develop necrosis)

Peripheral VENOUS disease	Peripheral ARTERIAL disease
• **Leg pain:** **Worse c leg dependency, standing/prolonged sitting.** **IMPROVES with walking, elevation of leg.** • **Cyanotic leg with dependency.**	• **Leg pain:** **Better with leg dependency, rest.** **WORSE with walking, elevation of leg, cold.** • **Redness leg with dependency - DEPENDENT RUBOR & cyanotic leg with elevation.**
• **Leg ulcers:** **Esp @ MEDIAL malleolus, uneven ulcer margins**	• **Leg ulcers:** **Esp @ LATERAL malleolus, clean margins**
• **Skin Findings:** **Stasis dermatitis:** eczematous rash, thickening of skin **BROWNISH PIGMENTATION.** **Pulses & temperature usually normal.** **Prominent edema common.**	• **Skin Findings:** **Atrophic skin changes:** thin shiny skin, loss of hair, muscle atrophy, pallor, thick nails. Livedo reticularis (mottled appearance). **↓pulses & temperature usually cool.** Minimal to no edema.

VARICOSE VEINS

- **Dilation of superficial veins due to failure of the venous valves in the saphenous veins**, leading to retrograde flow, venous stasis, and pooling of blood.

RISK FACTORS

- Family history, female gender, increased age, standing for long periods, obesity, increased estrogen (eg, OCP use, pregnancy), chronic venous insufficiency.

CLINICAL MANIFESTATIONS

- **Most are asymptomatic** but may present due to cosmetic issues.
- Dull ache or pressure sensation. Pain is worse with prolonged standing or sitting with the leg dependent and is relieved with elevation.
- Physical examination: dilated visible veins, telangiectasias, swelling, discoloration, Venous stasis ulcers: severe varicosities resulting in skin ulcerations. ± Mild ankle edema.

MANAGEMENT

- **Conservative: compression stockings, leg elevation, pain control**.
- Ablation: catheter-based endovenous thermal ablation (laser or radiofrequency).
- Ligation and stripping, sclerotherapy.

CHRONIC VENOUS INSUFFICIENCY

- Changes due to venous hypertension of the lower extremities as a result of **venous valvular incompetency**.
- Most commonly occurs after superficial thrombophlebitis, after DVT or trauma to the affected leg.

CLINICAL MANIFESTATIONS

- **Leg pain worsened with prolonged standing**, prolonged sitting with the feet dependent
- **Leg pain improved with ambulation and leg elevation.**
- Pain classically described as a burning, aching, throbbing, cramping or "heavy leg".

PHYSICAL EXAM FINDINGS

- Stasis Dermatitis: itchy **eczematous rash** (inflammatory papules, crusts or scales), excoriations, weeping erosions & **brownish or dark purple hyperpigmentation of the skin** (hemosiderin deposition).
- **Venous stasis ulcers** (especially at the **medial malleolus)** may be seen.
- **Dependent pitting leg edema**, increased leg circumference, varicosities & erythema with normal pulse and temperature.
- Atrophie blanche: atrophic, hypopigmented areas with telangiectasias & punctate red dots.

MANAGEMENT

- **Conservative: initial management of choice for most.** Includes **leg elevation, compression stockings, exercise,** & weight management.
- Treat the underlying cause. Surgical intervention usually reserved for patients not responsive to conservative therapy.
- Ulcer management: compression bandaging systems (eg, zinc impregnated gauze), wound debridement if needed, Aspirin (accelerates ulcer healing)

SALICYLATE (ACETYLSALICYLIC ACID), ASPIRIN

MECHANISM OF ACTION

- Non-selectively and irreversibly inhibits cyclooxygenase (COX-1 & COX-2), decreasing prostaglandin and thromboxane A2 synthesis, producing anti-inflammatory, analgesic, antipyretic effects, and reducing platelet aggregation.

INDICATIONS

- Pain, fever arthritis (anti-inflammatory at high doses), anti-platelet aggregation (eg, ACS, MI, TIA, thromboembolic stroke prevention, rheumatic fever, Kawasaki disease.

CONTRAINDICATIONS/CAUTIONS

- **Renal injury** (eg, acute renal failure, interstitial nephritis), gastric mucosal injury (eg, gastritis, gastric ulcer, GI bleed) due to loss of the protective effect of prostaglandins, pill-induced esophagitis, decreased uric acid excretion (cautious use in patients with Gout).
  - Increased risk of Reye syndrome if used in children with viral infection.
  - Asthma exacerbation (arachidonic acid is converted to leukotrienes, leading to bronchoconstriction).
  - Possible hemolytic anemia in patients with G6PD deficiency.
  - Contraindicated in hemophiliacs, increased bleeding with Von Willebrand disease.
  - Enhances the effect of Lithium, Warfarin, Heparin, Digoxin.

ACUTE TOXICITY OR OVERDOSE

- **Ototoxicity:** hearing loss, tinnitus, vertigo, cranial nerve VIII toxicity.
- GI symptoms: nausea, vomiting, and diarrhea are early symptoms of toxicity.
- Neurologic symptoms: altered mental status changes, lethargy, seizures.
- Noncardiogenic pulmonary edema (ARDS)
- Respiratory alkalosis (early on from respiratory center stimulation, leading to hyperventilation) followed by high anion-gap metabolic acidosis (inhibits oxidative phosphorylation and Krebs cycle, leading to accumulation of lactic acid).
- Renal insufficiency, hypokalemia, liver injury.

MANAGEMENT OF TOXICITY OR OVERDOSE

- Supportive care, IV hydration.
- Alkalinization of the urine and serum with IV sodium bicarbonate to increase salicylate excretion and decrease CNS toxicity.
- Activated charcoal to block salicylate absorption in those who ingested salicylate within the past 2 hours (used in those who are alert with a secured airway).
- Dialysis – severe cases (eg, salicylate concentration > 100 mg/dL).

CARDIOLOGY PHOTO CREDITS

Aortic Dissection
By J. Heuser (Own work) [GFDL (http://www.gnu.org/copyleft/fdl.html) or CC-BY-SA-3.0 (http://creativecommons.org/licenses/by-sa/3.0/)], via Wikimedia Commons
Sinus tachycardia & bradycardia
Andrewmeyerson [CC BY-SA 3.0 (https://creativecommons.org/licenses/by-sa/3.0)]
ST depressions
By Bron766 (Own work) [CC-BY-SA-3.0 (http://creativecommons.org/licenses/by-sa/3.0)], via Wikimedia Commons
ST MI evolution
By Келладин (Own work) [CC-BY-SA-3.0 (http://creativecommons.org/licenses/by-sa/3.0)], via Wikimedia Commons
De winter T waves
By Bron766 (Own work) [CC-BY-SA-3.0 (http://creativecommons.org/licenses/by-sa/3.0)], via Wikimedia Commons
Hyperkalemia
By Jer5150 (Own work) [CC-BY-SA-3.0 (http://creativecommons.org/licenses/by-sa/3.0)], via Wikimedia Commons
Sick Sinus Syndrome
By CardioNetworks: [ ] (CardioNetworks: SSS_ecg_001.jpg) [CC-BY-SA-3.0 (http://creativecommons.org/licenses/by-sa/3.0)], via Wikimedia Commons
Wenckeback
By CardioNetworks: Googletrans (CardioNetworks: De-Rhythm_Mobitz.png) [CC-BY-SA-3.0 (http://creativecommons.org/licenses/by-sa/3.0)], via Wikimedia Commons
Second degree AV Block
By Dr. Alberto Giniger, ICBA, Buenos Aires, Argentina (Dr. Alberto Giniger, ICBA, Buenos Aires, Argentina) [CC-BY-SA-3.0 (http://creativecommons.org/licenses/by-sa/3.0)], via Wikimedia Commons
Electric Alternans
By James Heilman, MD (Own work) [CC-BY-SA-3.0 (http://creativecommons.org/licenses/by-sa/3.0) or GFDL (http://www.gnu.org/copyleft/fdl.html)], via Wikimedia Commons
Atrial Flutter
By Atrial_flutter34.JPG: James Heilman, MD derivative work: Mysid (using Perl and Inkscape) (This file was derived from: Atrial_flutter34.JPG) [CC-BY-SA-3.0 (http://creativecommons.org/licenses/by-sa/3.0) or GFDL (http://www.gnu.org/copyleft/fdl.html)], via Wikimedia Commons
Multifocal Atrial tachycardia
By Jer5150 (Own work) [CC-BY-SA-3.0 (http://creativecommons.org/licenses/by-sa/3.0)], via Wikimedia Commons
Torsades
By Displaced (Own work) [Public domain], via Wikimedia Commons
WPW
By CardioNetworks: Googletrans (CardioNetworks: De-Rhythm_WPW.png) [CC BY-SA 3.0 (http://creativecommons.org/licenses/by-sa/3.0)], via Wikimedia Commons
WPW
By James Heilman, MD (Own work) [CC BY-SA 3.0 (http://creativecommons.org/licenses/by-sa/3.0)], via Wikimedia Commons
Bigeminy
By James Heilman, MD (Own work) [CC-BY-SA-3.0 (http://creativecommons.org/licenses/by-sa/3.0) or GFDL (http://www.gnu.org/copyleft/fdl.html)], via Wikimedia Commons
VTach
By Glenlarson (Own work) [Public domain], via Wikimedia Commons
Ventricular Fibrillation
By CardioNetworks: Googletrans [CC-BY-SA-3.0 (http://creativecommons.org/licenses/by-sa/3.0)], via Wikimedia Commons
Kerley B Lines
By Braegel (Own work) [GFDL (http://www.gnu.org/copyleft/fdl.html) or CC-BY-SA-3.0-2.5-2.0-1.0 (http://creativecommons.org/licenses/by-sa/3.0)], via Wikimedia Commons
Batwing Pulmonary Edema
By CDC/ D. Loren Ketai, M.D. (http://phil.cdc.gov, #6077) [Public domain], via Wikimedia Commons
Pericarditis
By CardioNetworks: Googletrans (CardioNetworks: De-Stadia_pericarditis.png) [CC-BY-SA-3.0 (http://creativecommons.org/licenses/by-sa/3.0)], via Wikimedia Commons
DeBakey Classification
By J. Heuser (Own work) [GFDL (http://www.gnu.org/copyleft/fdl.html) or CC-BY-SA-3.0 (http://creativecommons.org/licenses/by-sa/3.0/)], via Wikimedia Commons

Abdominal Aorta
By Nevit Dilmen (Own work) [GFDL (http://www.gnu.org/copyleft/fdl.html), CC-BY-SA-3.0 (http://creativecommons.org/licenses/by-sa/3.0/) or CC-BY-SA-2.5-2.0-1.0 (http://creativecommons.org/licenses/by-sa/2.5-2.0-1.0)], via Wikimedia Commons

Aortic Dissection CT scan
By J. Heuser JHeuser (own patient) [GFDL (http://www.gnu.org/copyleft/fdl.html) or CC-BY-SA-3.0 (http://creativecommons.org/licenses/by-sa/3.0/)], via Wikimedia Common

Junctional Rhythm
By Steven Fruitsmaak (Own work) [CC BY-SA 3.0 (http://creativecommons.org/licenses/by-sa/3.0)], via Wikimedia Commons

CHAPTER 2 - PULMONARY SYSTEM

LUNG VOLUMES:

- **Tidal volume (TV):** the volume of air moved into or out of the lungs during quiet breathing.
- **Residual Volume (RV):** the volume of air remaining in the lungs after maximal expiration. This residual volume functions to maintain alveolar patency, especially during end expiration.
- **Expiratory reserve volume (ERV):** the volume of air that can be further exhaled at the end of normal expiration.
- **Inspiratory reserve volume (IRV):** the volume of air that can be further inhaled at the end of normal inspiration.
- **Vital Capacity (VC):** maximum volume of air that can be exhaled following maximum inspiration (IRV + TV + ERV).
- **Total Lung Capacity (TLC):** the volume in the lungs at maximum inspiration (VC + RV).
- **Functional residual capacity (FRC):** volume of gas in the lungs at normal tidal volume end expiration (ERV + RV). This is the air in which gas exchange takes place.
  - ↑FRC seen in disorders with hyperinflation (due to loss of elastic recoil, PEEP).
  - ↓FRC seen in restrictive lung diseases.
- **FEV_1 Forced Expiratory Volume in 1 second**: the volume of air that has been exhaled at the end of the first second of forced expiration.
- **Forced Vital Capacity (FVC):** measurement of the volume of air that can be expelled from a maximally inflated lung, with the patient breathing as hard & fast as possible.

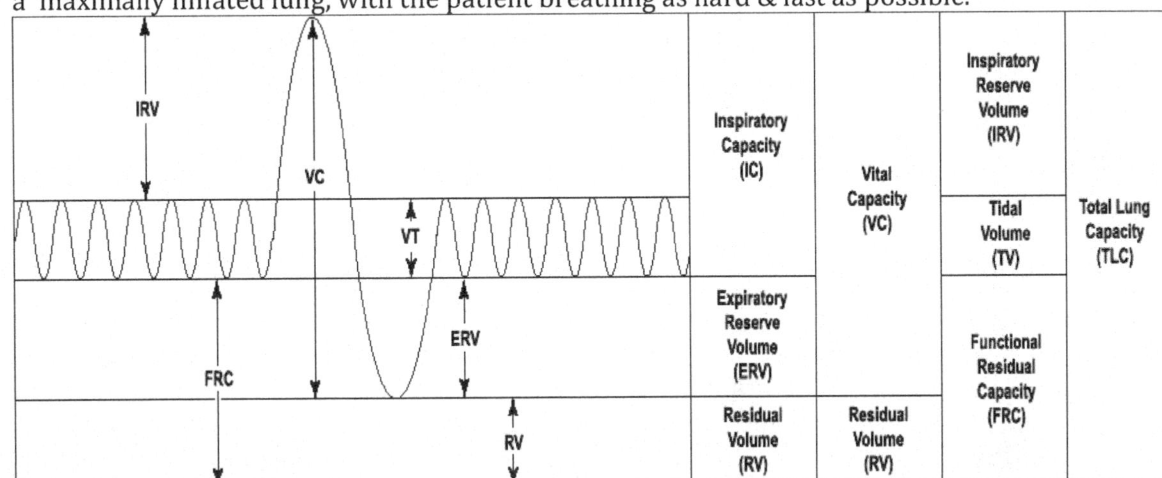

4 MAIN ATYPICAL SOUNDS

1. **WHEEZING:** high-pitched, **whistling, continuous**, musical sound (**usually louder during expiration** compared to inspiration) **produced by narrowed/obstructed airways.** Seen with obstructive lung diseases (Asthma, COPD) Bronchiectasis, Bronchiolitis, Lung cancer, Sleep apnea, CHF, GERD, anaphylaxis, foreign body etc.
2. **RHONCHI:** continuous, rumbling (rattling), coarse, **low-pitched sounds** (sounds like snoring) that **may clear with cough** or suctioning. Rhonchi are caused by increased secretions or obstruction in the bronchial airways.
3. **CRACKLES (RALES):** discontinuous high-pitched sounds **heard during inspiration** (usually not cleared by cough). Due to the "popping" open of collapsed alveoli & small airways (from fluid, exudates or lack of aeration). Seen with pneumonia, atelectasis, bronchitis, bronchiectasis, pulmonary edema & pulmonary fibrosis.
4. **STRIDOR:** monophonic sound usually loudest over the anterior neck due to **narrowing of the larynx or anywhere over the trachea**. Can be heard during inspiration, expiration or throughout the respiratory cycle.

CHRONIC OBSTRUCTIVE PULMONARY DISEASE (COPD)

- **COPD:** progressive, **largely irreversible airflow obstruction** due to ❶ **loss of elastic recoil** & ❷ **increased airway resistance**. COPD includes: ❶ **EMPHYSEMA** & ❷ **CHRONIC BRONCHITIS.**
- **Common >55y.** Chronic bronchitis usually episodic; Emphysema usually has a steady decline.
- Both usually coexist with one being more dominant.

RISK FACTORS

- **Cigarette smoking/exposure most important risk** (90%). Only 15% of smokers develop COPD.
- **Alpha-1 antitrypsin deficiency: only genetic disease linked to COPD** in **younger patients <40y.**
- Occupational/environmental exposures, recurrent airway infections.

EMPHYSEMA – Pink puffer

- **Permanent enlargement of the terminal airspaces** (distal to the terminal bronchioles) with no obvious fibrosis.

ETIOLOGIES

- **Smoking most common.** Air pollution, hazardous dust.

PATHOPHYSIOLOGY

- Chronic inflammation, decreased protective enzymes (eg, alpha-1 antitrypsin) & increased damaging enzymes (eg, elastase release from macrophages & neutrophils) cause **alveolar capillary destruction + alveolar wall destruction.** Matched V/Q defects & decreased gas exchange surface area. **Loss of elastic recoil** & airway collapse makes expiration an active process & **increased compliance** leads to **airway obstruction** (increased air trapping).

- **Centrilobar (proximal acinar) involvement is most commonly associated with smoking.**

- Panacinar (diffuse) is associated with Alpha-1 antitrypsin deficiency.

- Paraseptal (distal acinar) can be seen with the above 2 or with spontaneous Pneumothorax (if isolated).

CLINICAL MANIFESTATIONS

- **Dyspnea (hallmark of Emphysema),** chronic cough (with or without sputum production).

- Physical examination: Hyperinflation: **decreased breath sounds, increased anteroposterior diameter (barrel chest),** hyperresonance to percussion, wheezing. Cachectic and non-cyanotic = **"pink puffers".**

- Severe disease = **pursed-lip expiration** (increases airway pressure & prevents airway collapse) & semi-tripod positioning (sitting forward) to improve breathing.

DIAGNOSIS

- **Pulmonary function test: gold standard.** Obstructive pattern that is not fully reversible:
  Airway obstruction: **decreased FEV1, decreased FEV1/FVC <70%** predicted, decreased FVC.
  Hyperinflation: increased volumes (eg, RV, TLC, RV/TLC, FRC). **Decreased DLCO in Emphysema.**

- Chest radiograph: hyperinflation: **flattened diaphragms, increased AP diameter, decreased vascular markings; bullae.**

CHRONIC BRONCHITIS

- Defined as **productive cough for at least 3 months a year for 2 consecutive years.**
- ETIOLOGIES: **smoking most common.** Air pollution, hazardous dust.

PATHOPHYSIOLOGY

- Chronic inflammation leads to **mucous gland hyperplasia**, goblet cell mucus production, dysfunctional cilia, & infiltration of neutrophils and CD8+ cells.
- These changes increase susceptibility to infections (eg, *S. pneumoniae, H. influenzae*).

CLINICAL MANIFESTATIONS

- 3 cardinal symptoms: **chronic cough, sputum production, and dyspnea.** May have prolonged expiration.

PHYSICAL EXAMINATION

- **Crackles (rales), rhonchi, wheezing.** Signs of cor pulmonale include an enlarged tender liver, jugular venous distention, and peripheral edema.
- Cyanosis and obesity **"blue bloaters".**

DIAGNOSIS

- **Pulmonary function test: gold standard.** Obstructive pattern that is not fully reversible:
  Airway obstruction: **decreased FEV1, decreased FEV1/FVC <70%** predicted, decreased FVC.
  Hyperinflation: increased volumes (eg, RV, TLC, RV/TLC, FRC). Normal DLCO.
- Chest radiograph: pulmonary hypertension (eg, enlarged right heart border, increased AP diameter and vascular markings).
- ECG: **cor pulmonale** (eg, RVH, right atrial enlargement, right axis deviation).
  May see Multifocal atrial tachycardia.
- CBC: **increased hemoglobin and hematocrit** (chronic hypoxia).
- ABG: **respiratory acidosis** (severe hypoxemia and hypercapnia).

	EMPHYSEMA	CHRONIC BRONCHITIS
CLINICAL MANIFESTATIONS	• **Dyspnea most common symptom.** • Accessory muscle use, tachypnea, prolonged expiration. Mild cough.	• **Productive cough hallmark** symptom, prolonged expiration.
PHYSICAL EXAMINATION	**Hyperinflation:** • **Hyperresonance** to percussion • **↓/absent breath sounds, ↓fremitus** • **Barrel chest (↑AP diameter),** quiet chest. • Pursed-lip breathing.	• **Rales (crackles), rhonchi, wheezing** ±change in location with cough. • ± Signs of cor pulmonale (**peripheral edema, cyanosis**)
ABG/LABS	Can develop respiratory acidosis if severe	• **Respiratory acidosis.** • **↑Hematocrit/RBC** (hypoxia stimulates erythropoiesis)
V/Q MISMATCH	• Matched V/Q defects • Mild to moderate hypoxemia • CO2 often normal initially	• **Severe V/Q mismatch,** • Severe hypoxemia • **Hypercapnia**
APPEARANCE	**Pink puffers:** cachectic, pursed lip breathing- noncyanotic	**Blue bloaters:** obese & cyanotic

MANAGEMENT OF COPD

FACTORS THAT REDUCE MORTALITY

- **Smoking cessation is the most important step in the management of COPD** (immediate effects).
- **Oxygen therapy** for those with paO2 ≤55 mmHg or saturation ≤88%; mortality benefit is directly proportional to the number of hours that oxygen is used.
- Pneumococcal vaccinations and annual Influenza vaccinations.

GENERAL MANAGEMENT

- Regular physical activity
- Pulmonary rehabilitation
- Regular review/correction of inhaler technique.
- **Antibiotics for acute exacerbations of Chronic bronchitis –** Macrolides (eg, Azithromycin, Clarithromycin); Cephalosporins (eg, Cefuroxime, Cefixime), Amoxicillin-clavulanate, Fluoroquinolones.

The GOLD criteria looks at FEV1 and FEV1/FVC ratio.
The revised GOLD criteria also looks at additional factors, such as risk of exacerbations.

Minimally symptomatic, low risk of exacerbation (Category A):

- **Short-acting bronchodilator**: beta agonist (SABA) or anticholinergic agent (SAMA) as needed.
- A combination SABA-SAMA can be used if single agent is insufficient.

More symptomatic, low risk of exacerbation (Category B):

- Add a long-acting bronchodilator (LAMA or LABA) to the short-acting bronchodilator.
- **LAMA may be slightly more efficacious than a LABA** (reduced exacerbation rate).

Minimally symptomatic on a day-to-day basis (Category C):

- **LAMA**
- Alternatives include: LAMA + LABA OR 2) LABA + inhaled glucocorticoid.
- **In general, combination of LAMA + LABA is more efficacious than monotherapy. As monotherapy, LAMA slightly more efficacious than LABA.**

Higher symptom burden:

- LAMA + LABA (preferred) or LABA + inhaled glucocorticoid.
- If persistent, triple inhaler therapy is recommended (LAMA + LABA + glucocorticoid).

OXYGEN THERAPY IN COPD

Rationale:

- Patients develop Pulmonary hypertension and subsequent right-sided Heart failure (cor pulmonale) as a result of hypoxic vasoconstriction, which increases right-sided arterial pressure.
- Oxygen can lead to a reduction of right atrial pressure.
- **Long-term use of oxygen reduces mortality** & improves quality of life in **severe COPD.**

Indications of O2 therapy:

- Cor pulmonale
- O2 saturation ≤88%
- PaO2 ≤55 mmHg

  - Lung reduction surgery: improves dyspnea by removing damaged lung, which allows the remaining lung to expand & function more efficiently.
  - Lung transplantation. Replacement of α-1 antitrypsin in some patients.

BRONCHODILATORS	Improve symptoms but do not decrease progression or reduce mortality.
LAMA **Tiotropium** (inhaled powder)	Mechanism of action • Long-acting anticholinergic (antimuscarinic) LAMA that leads to bronchodilation (M1 and M3 selectivity) Benefits: • Improves lung function, decreases hyperinflation, improves quality of life. • As long-term monotherapy, **may be slightly more efficacious than LABAs.** Adverse effects • **Anticholinergic:** dry mouth, thirst, blurred vision, urinary retention, difficulty swallowing.
SAMA **Ipratropium**	Mechanism of action • Short-acting anticholinergic (antimuscarinic) SAMA that leads to bronchodilation (M1, M2, and M3 receptors) Indications: • As-needed relief of intermittent increases in dyspnea (may combined with a short-acting beta agonist). Adverse effects • **Anticholinergic:** dry mouth, thirst, blurred vision, urinary retention, difficulty swallowing.
LABA: **Salmeterol** Formoterol	Mechanism of action • Long-acting beta-2 agonist. Indications: • Decreases exacerbation rates, improved quality of life, and lung function.
SABA: **Albuterol**	Mechanism of action • Short-acting beta-2 agonist. Indications: • As-needed relief of intermittent increases in dyspnea (may combined with a short-acting antimuscarinic agent). Adverse reactions • Beta-1 cross reactivity: tachycardia, palpitations, tremors, CNS stimulation.
INHALED GLUCOCORTICOIDS **Fluticasone**	Indications: • Can be added to a LABA and/or LAMA for severe or persistent disease. Adverse reactions • Oral candidiasis.

COPD RADIOLOGIC FINDINGS

NORMAL PA CXR

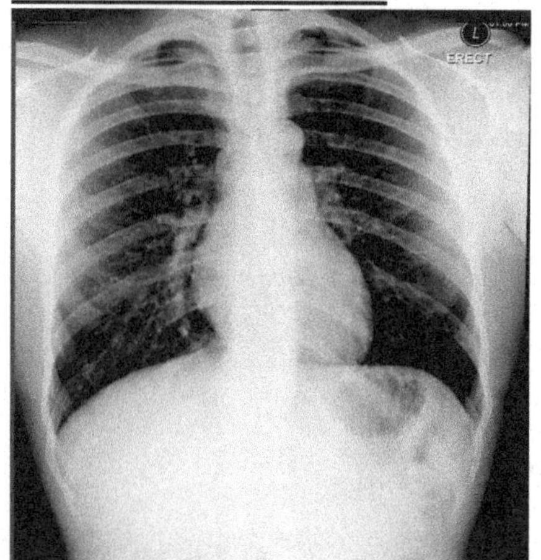

Note roundness of the diaphragms.

EMPHYSEMA

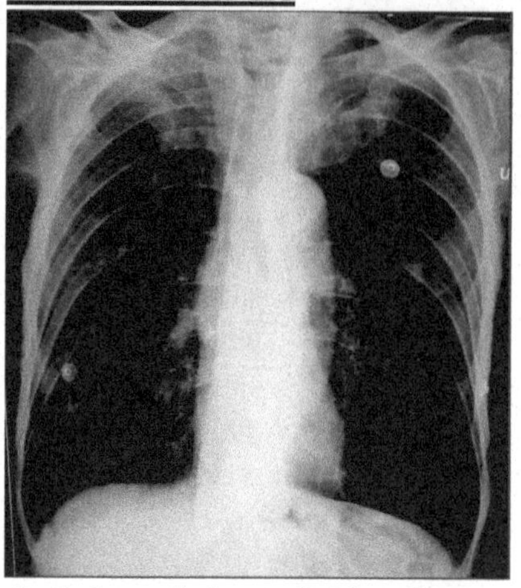

1. **Enlarged lung fields, flattened diaphragms.**
2. **Trapped air** (darker lung areas).
3. **Decreased vascular markings.**
4. **Bullae** seen (right side).

CHRONIC BRONCHITIS

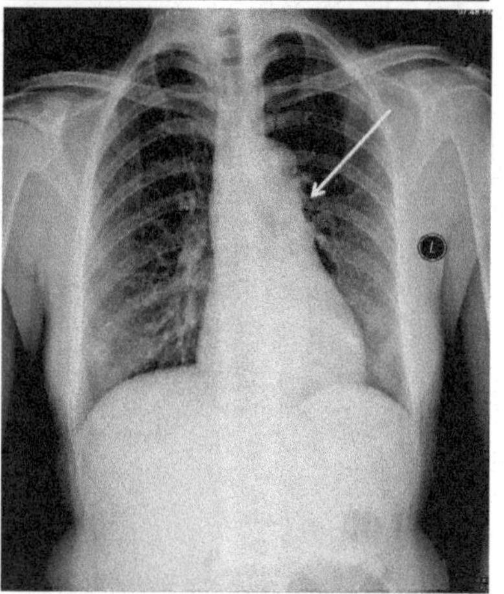

1. **Increased vascular markings, normal diaphragms.**
2. Prominent pulmonary artery & pulmonary hypertension (arrow), horizontal heart.
3. Right heart enlargement.

NORMAL LATERAL CXR

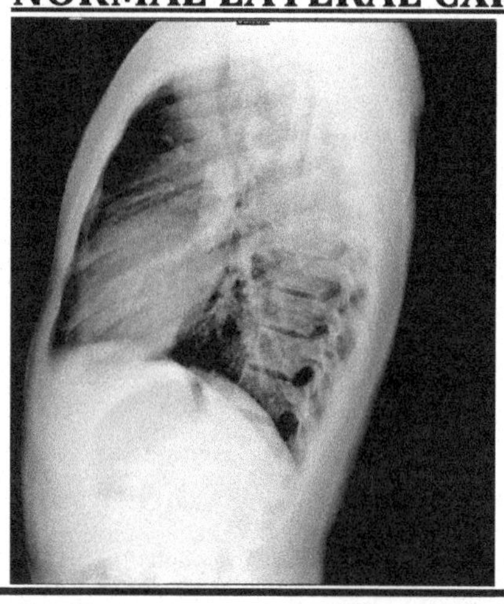

EMPHYSEMA

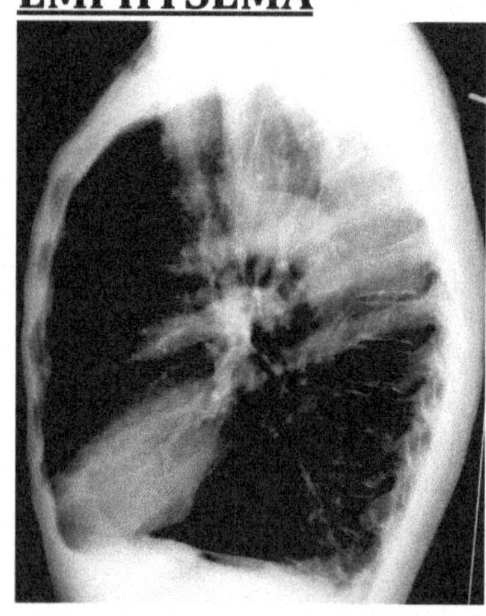

EMPHYSEMA LATERAL CXR:

1. **barrel chest**
2. **increased AP diameter**

NORMAL CT SCAN

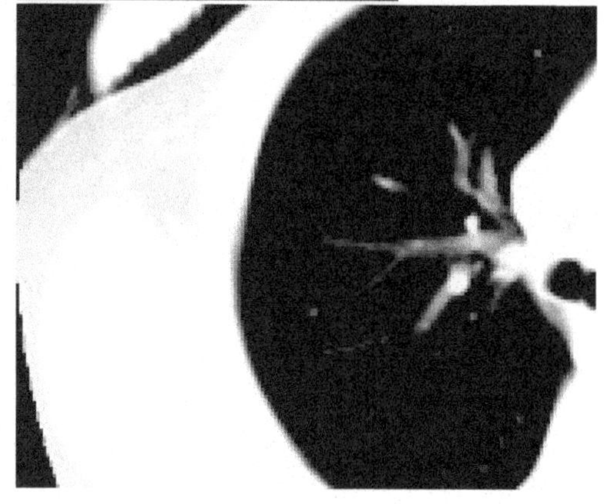

EMPHYSEMA

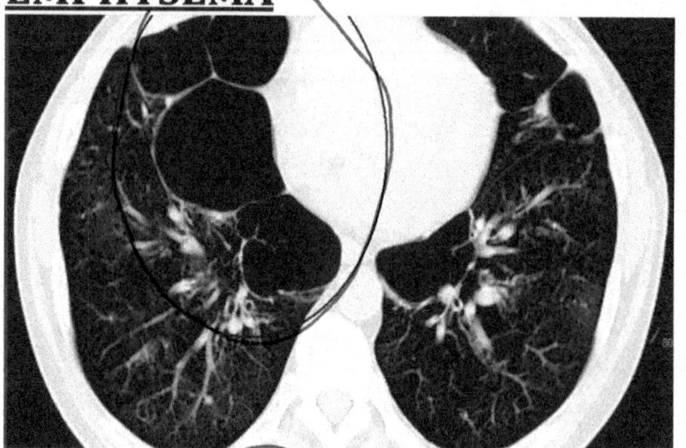

Emphysema: **bullae** (circular areas of darkness), which signifies airspace loss.

CYSTIC FIBROSIS

- Autosomal recessive exocrinopathy.
- Most common in **Caucasians & Northern Europeans**.

PATHOPHYSIOLOGY

- Mutation in the Cystic fibrosis transmembrane conductance receptor (CFTR) gene leads to **abnormal chloride and water transport** across exocrine glands throughout the body, leading to **thick, viscous secretions of the lungs,** pancreas, sinuses, intestines, liver, and genitourinary tract.

CLINICAL MANIFESTATIONS

- Infancy: **meconium ileus**, failure to thrive, diarrhea from malabsorption (may lead to rectal prolapse).
- Pulmonary: CF is the **most common cause of Bronchiectasis in US**
- GI: malabsorption especially of fat-soluble vitamins A, D, E, & K, steatorrhea, diarrhea, recurrent pancreatitis (may lead to pancreatic insufficiency), distal intestinal obstruction, biliary cirrhosis.
- Infertility due to azoospermia. Sinusitis.

DIAGNOSIS

- **Elevated sweat chloride: test of choice (most accurate).** Chloride levels 60 mmol/L or greater on 2 occasions after Pilocarpine administration (Pilocarpine is a cholinergic drug that induces sweating).
- Chest radiographs: Bronchiectasis common, hyperinflation of the lungs.
- Pulmonary function test: obstructive pattern (usually irreversible).
- DNA analysis – genotyping is not as accurate as sweat chloride testing because there are more types of mutations than those tested with genotyping.

MANAGEMENT

- **Antibiotics are often needed** – Macrolides (eg, Azithromycin, Clarithromycin); Cephalosporins (eg, Cefuroxime, Cefixime), Amoxicillin-clavulanate, Fluoroquinolones. Inhaled Aminoglycosides.
- Airway clearance treatment - eg, inhaled bronchodilators, decongestants, mucolytics, inhaled recombinant human deoxyribonuclease (breaks down large amounts of DNA in the respiratory mucus that clogs up the airways).
- Supportive: pancreatic enzyme replacement, supplementation of fat soluble vitamins (A, D, E, K), vaccinations (eg, Pneumococcal, Influenza).
- Lung and pancreatic transplantation in selected cases.

	OBSTRUCTIVE DISORDERS	RESTRICTIVE DISORDERS
PULMONARY FUNCTION TESTS (PFT)	**INCREASED lung volumes** **Hyperinflation: ↑TLC, RV, RV/TLC, FRC** **Obstruction: ↓FEV1, ↓FVC; ↓FEV1/ FVC** FEV1 decreases more than the FVC	**DECREASED lung volumes** **↓TLC, RV, RV/TLC, FRC, FVC** **Normal or ↑FEV_1/FVC**, ↓FEV1
COMPLIANCE	**↑ compliance with Emphysema**	↓ compliance
EXAMPLES	• Asthma • COPD (Chronic bronchitis, Emphysema) • Bronchiectasis • Cystic Fibrosis • **Coal Workers Pneumoconiosis often presents with an obstructive pattern**	• Sarcoidosis • Pneumoconiosis • Idiopathic Pulmonary Fibrosis • ↓Muscular effort: Myasthenia Gravis, Polio • Scoliosis, Mesothelioma

BRONCHIECTASIS

- Permanent and irreversible dilatation of the bronchial airways.

ETIOLOGIES

- **Cystic fibrosis most common cause in US** (50%).

- **Recurrent lung infections:**
  Pseudomonas aeruginosa **most common cause if due to Cystic fibrosis.**
  H. influenzae the most common cause if not due to Cystic Fibrosis.

- Airway foreign body, tumors, Alpha-1 antitrypsin deficiency, collagen vascular disease (eg, Rheumatoid arthritis, Aspergillosis, panhypogammaglobulinemia, and immune deficiency.

PATHOPHYSIOLOGY

- Dilatation of the airways and impairment of the mucociliary escalator leads to repeat infections, airway obstruction, and peribronchial fibrosis.

- Increased risk for *Pseudomonas aeruginosa*, *Mycobacterium avium* complex, and Aspergillus.

CLINICAL MANIFESTATIONS

- **Persistent productive cough with thick sputum,** dyspnea, pleuritic chest pain.

- **Hemoptysis** (bronchial artery erosion).

- Physical examination: nonspecific – crackles (most common), wheezing, rhonchi.

DIAGNOSIS

- **High-resolution CT scan: preferred imaging of choice.**
  Findings include thickened bronchial walls, airway dilatation, and lack of tapering of the airway (**tram-track appearance**), **signet ring sign** (increased airway diameter > adjacent vessel diameter).

- Chest radiographs: usually abnormal but nonspecific. Findings include linear atelectasis, tram-track appearance, opacities, and increased bronchial markings.

- **Pulmonary function test: gold standard.** Obstructive pattern that is not fully reversible:
  Airway obstruction: **decreased FEV1, decreased FEV1/FVC <70%** predicted, decreased FVC.
  Hyperinflation: increased volumes (eg, RV, TLC, RV/TLC, FRC).

MANAGEMENT

- Conservative: chest physiotherapy (mucus clearance), mucolytics, bronchodilators.

- **Antibiotics are often needed** – Macrolides (eg, Azithromycin, Clarithromycin); Cephalosporins (eg, Cefuroxime, Cefixime), Amoxicillin-clavulanate, Fluoroquinolones. Inhaled Aminoglycosides. Antibiotic cycling often used (eg, 1 weekly each month).

- Surgery: resection or transplantation in severe or refractory cases.

BRONCHIECTASIS

NORMAL CXR

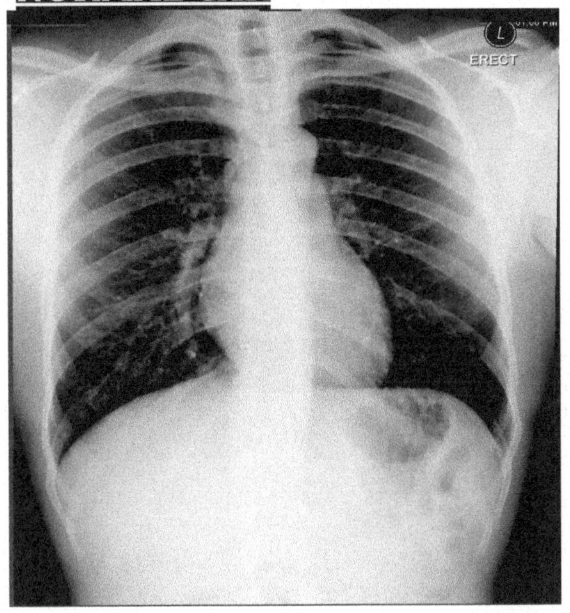

BRONCHIECTASIS

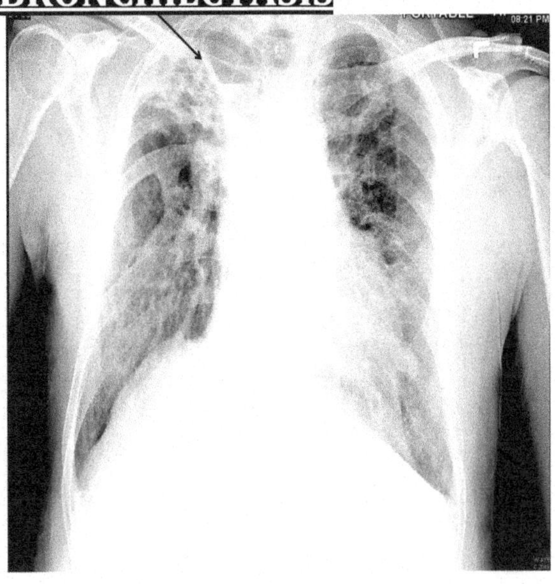

Bronchiectasis: irregular opacities, crowded bronchial markings, "tram track" markings.

NORMAL CT SCAN

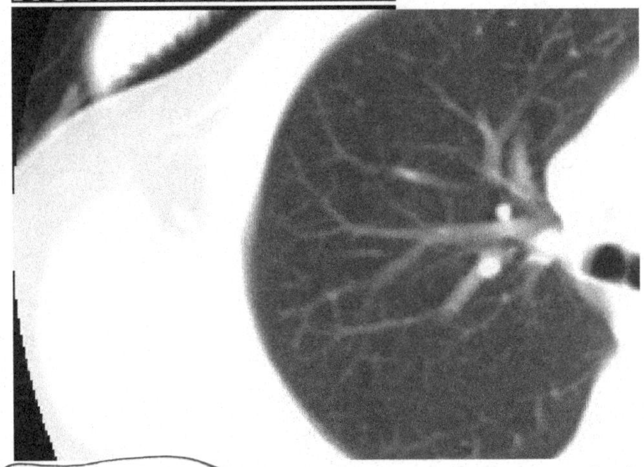

Signet ring sign: pulmonary artery coupled with a dilated bronchus (white arrow).

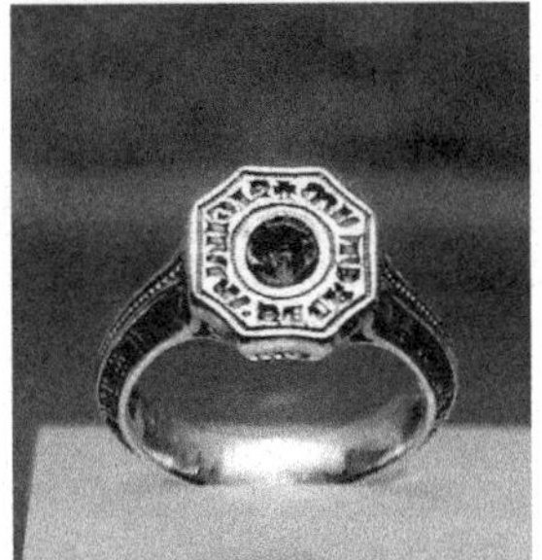

BRONCHIECTASIS

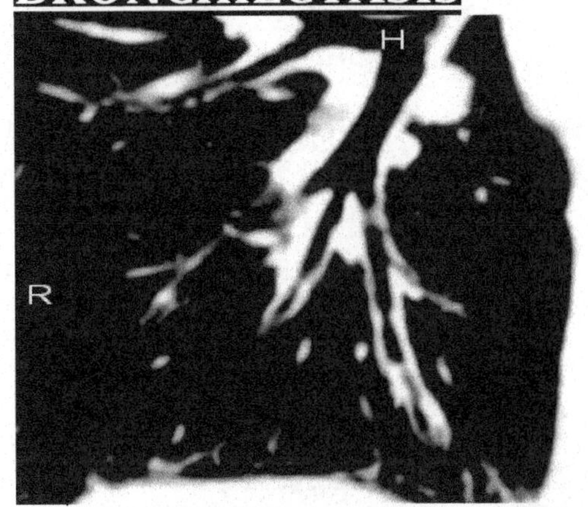

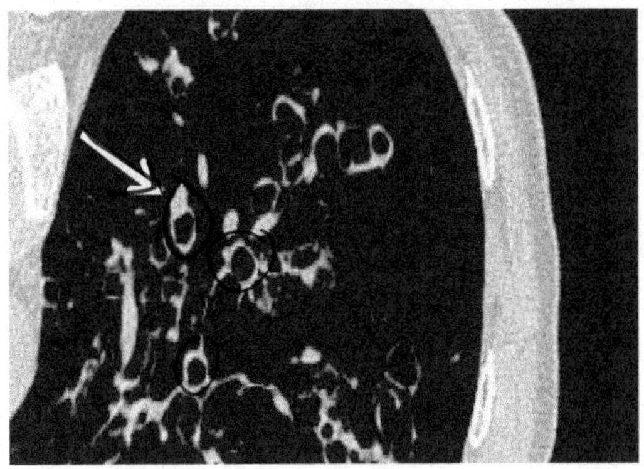

- Proximal airway dilation with thick walls, lack of airway tapering giving a "tram-track" appearance (above photo).
- Signet ring sign (arrow).

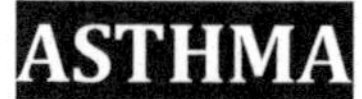

ASTHMA

- **Reversible,** often **intermittent**, obstructive disease of the small airways.

PATHOPHYSIOLOGY

- 3 components - **airway hyperreactivity, bronchoconstriction, and inflammation.** Increased IgE binds to mast cells, initiating an inflammatory response, including increased Leukotrienes.
- Can present at any age but initial occurrence most common in childhood.

RISK FACTORS

- **Atopy strongest risk factor,** family history, air pollution, obesity, environmental tobacco smoke, male gender.
- **Samter's triad (Aspirin-exacerbated respiratory disease)** consists of Asthma + chronic rhinosinusitis with nasal polyps + sensitivity to Aspirin and/or NSAIDs
- **Atopic triad** (patients with one condition are likely to develop one or two of the other) - Asthma, Atopic dermatitis (Eczema), & Allergic rhinitis

TRIGGERS

- Intrinsic (non-allergic): anxiety, stress, exercise, cold air, dry air, hyperventilation, & viral infections.
- Extrinsic (allergic): animal dander, pollen, mold, dust mites, cockroaches etc. Associated with **increased IgE.**
- Other: medications (eg, Aspirin, NSAIDs, Beta blocker, histamine), GERD.

CLINICAL MANIFESTATIONS

- **Classic triad: dyspnea, wheezing and cough (especially at night).** May have chest tightness & fatigue.
- Clues to severity include previous intubations, hospital admissions, or ICU admission.

PHYSICAL EXAMINATION

- **Prolonged expiration with wheezing,** hyperresonance to percussion, decreased breath sounds, tachycardia, tachypnea, use of accessory muscles.
- Severe Asthma and Status asthmaticus: inability to speak in full sentences, "tripod" positioning, **silent chest** (no air movement), **altered mental status** (ominous), pulsus paradoxus (inspiratory blood pressure drop > 10 mmHg), PEFR < 40% predicted.
- Findings of longstanding disease: Nasal polyps or Atopic dermatitis may be seen.

DIAGNOSIS OF ASTHMA IN THE OFFICE

- **Pulmonary function tests: gold standard in making the diagnosis of Asthma. Reversible obstruction (decreased FEV1,** decreased FEV1/FVC; increased RV, TLC, and RV/TLC).
  - Bronchoprovocation: **Methacholine challenge** (≥20% decrease on FEV1) followed by bronchodilator challenge (increase of FEV1 ≥12% is expected).

DIAGNOSIS OF AN ACUTE ASTHMA EXACERBATION

- **Peak expiratory flow rate: best & most objective way to assess exacerbation severity & patient response** to treatment.
  - Discharge criteria: PEFR >70% predicted or PEFR > 15% initial attempt, subjective improvement.
- Pulse oximetry: SaO2 <90% indicative of respiratory distress.
- ABG: not usually ordered in most exacerbations. **Respiratory alkalosis is expected** (from tachypnea). Pseudonormalization (normal CO2) or respiratory acidosis may indicate impending respiratory failure.
- Chest radiograph: usually normal. Generally not helpful in the diagnosis of Asthma but may be used to rule out other causes of symptoms (eg, Pneumonia).

Asthma Pharm.

QUICK RELIEF FOR ACUTE EXACERBATION (RESCUE DRUGS)

β2 AGONISTS SHORT-ACTING (SABA)

Albuterol, Levalbuterol, **Terbutaline**, **Epinephrine**

- Indications: **first-line treatment for acute exacerbation – most effective & fastest** (2-5 minutes).
- MOA: **bronchodilator** (especially **peripherally**), decreases bronchospasm, inhibits the release of bronchospastic mediators, increases ciliary movement, ↓'es airway edema & resistance.
- Administration: MDI, nebulizer. **Nebulizers most common used in ED** (MDI ±slightly more efficacious). Generally given every 20 minutes x 3 doses (or continuous) + reevaluation after 3 doses (at least q 1-2 hours).
- S/E: **β-1 cross reaction**: **tachycardia/arrhythmias, muscle tremors, CNS stimulation**, hypokalemia.

ANTICHOLINERGICS (ANTIMUSCARINICS)

Ipratropium

- MOA: **central bronchodilator** (inhibits vagal-mediated bronchoconstriction) & inhibits nasal mucosal secretions. ⊕ synergy between β2 agonists & anticholinergics. Most useful in the first hour.
- S/E: **thirst, blurred vision, dry mouth, urinary retention, dysphagia, acute glaucoma, BPH.**

CORTICOSTEROIDS

Prednisone, Methylprednisolone, Prednisolone

- MOA: **anti-inflammatory**. **All but the mildest exacerbations should be discharged on a short course of oral corticosteroids** (eg, 3-5 days) unless contraindicated. **Steroids decrease relapse** & reverse the late pathophysiology. Short courses don't need tapering (unless on chronic steroids, or recent treatment with repeated short courses in a short period). Onset of action 4-8 hours for both oral & IV.
- S/E: **immunosuppression, catabolic, hyperglycemia, fluid retention, osteoporosis, growth delays.**

LONG-TERM (CHRONIC, CONTROL) MAINTENANCE

INHALED CORTICOSTEROIDS (ICS)

Beclomethasone, Flunisolide, Triamcinolone

- Indications: **first-line long term, persistent (chronic maintenance).** Effective long-term control with very low incidence of systemic side effects. MOA: cytokine & inflammation inhibition.
- S/E: **oral candidiasis** (using spacer & rinsing mouth after inhaler use decreases risk), dysphonia.

LONG-ACTING β2 AGONISTS (LABA)

Salmeterol, ICS/LABA: Budesonide/**Formoterol**, Fluticasone/Salmeterol

- Mechanism: bronchodilator that prevents symptoms (especially nocturnal asthma).
- Indications: **long-acting β2 agonists added to steroids** (or other long term asthma medications) **ONLY if persistent asthma is not controlled with ICS alone** (the option of increasing the ICS dose = addition of LABA). Once asthma control is maintained (>3 months), step down off LABA is recommended.
- CI: **NOT used as a rescue drug in acute exacerbations or as monotherapy for long-term Asthma.**

MAST CELL MODIFIERS

Cromolyn, Nedocromil

- MOA: inhibits mast cell & leukotriene-mediated degranulation. Used as prophylaxis only.
- Indications: improved lung function, ↓airway reactivity (**inhibits acute response to cold air, exercise, sulfites). Minimal side effects** (throat irritation). Effective prophylaxis may take several weeks.

LEUKOTRIENE MODIFIERS/RECEPTOR ANTAGONISTS (LTRA)

Montelukast, Zafirlukast, Zileuton

- MOA: blocks leukotriene-mediated neutrophil migration, capillary permeability, smooth muscle contraction via leukotriene receptor inhibition. Zileuton does so via 5-lipoxygenase inhibition.
- Indications: useful in asthmatics with **allergic rhinitis/aspirin-induced Asthma.** Prophylaxis only.
- Adverse effects: minimal side effects (increased LFTs, headache, GI myalgias). Zafirlukast has been associated with Churg-Strauss syndrome.

THEOPHYLLINE

- MOA: methylxanthine (similar to caffeine) - **bronchodilator** that **improves respiratory muscle endurance,** phosphodiesterase inhibitor which inhibits leukotriene synthesis & inflammation. Not used often due to narrow therapeutic index (TI). Smoking decreases Theophylline levels so **higher doses of Theophylline are needed in smokers.** It is a nonselective adenosine receptor antagonist.
- Ind: long-term asthma prophylaxis in selected patients. NOT used in acute asthma exacerbations.
- Adverse effects: **nervousness,** nausea, vomiting, anorexia, **headache,** CNS/respiratory stimulant, diuresis, tachycardia. Many drug interactions. **Narrow TI: toxicity causes arrhythmias & seizures.**

IV MAGNESIUM: **bronchodilator** (↓Ca^{+2}-mediated smooth muscle contraction) used in severe Asthma.
HELIOX: decreases airway resistance because helium + oxygen is lighter than room air.
KETAMINE: IV anesthetic that has sedative, analgesic & bronchodilator effects. May be useful as an induction/sedation agent in young otherwise healthy population of intubated patients.

OMALIZUMAB: anti-IgE antibody (inhibits IgE inflammation). Used in severe, uncontrolled asthma.

CLASSIFICATION OF ASTHMA SEVERITY				
	INTERMITTENT	PERSISTENT		
		MILD	MODERATE	SEVERE
Symptoms	≤2 x /day ≤2/ week	>2days/week (but not daily)	Daily	Throughout the day
SABA use for sx	**≤2x/day** **≤2x/week**	>2days/week (but not >1x/day)	Daily	Several times a day
Nighttime awakenings	**≤2x/month**	3-4 x/month	>1x/week (but not nightly)	Often Usually nightly
Interference with normal activity	None	Minor limitation	Some limitation	Extremely limited
Lung Function	• Normal FEV1 between exacerbations • FEV1 >80% predicted • FEV1/FVC normal	• FEV1 ≥80% predicted • FEV1/FVC normal	• **FEV1 60 – 80% predicted** • FEV1/FVC reduced by 5%	• **FEV1 <60% predicted** FEV1/FVC reduced >5%
Recommended Management	• Inhaled SABA as needed	• Inhaled SABA as needed + **Low-dose ICS**	• **Low ICS + LABA** OR • **Increase ICS dose (medium)** or • Add LTRA	• High dose ICS + LABA • **± Omalizumab** (Anti-IgE drug)
Exacerbations requiring PO steroids	0-1/year	≥2/year		

ICS=Inhaled Corticosteroid; LABA=Long Acting β_2 Agonist; SA = short, LTRA + Leukotriene Receptor Antagonists

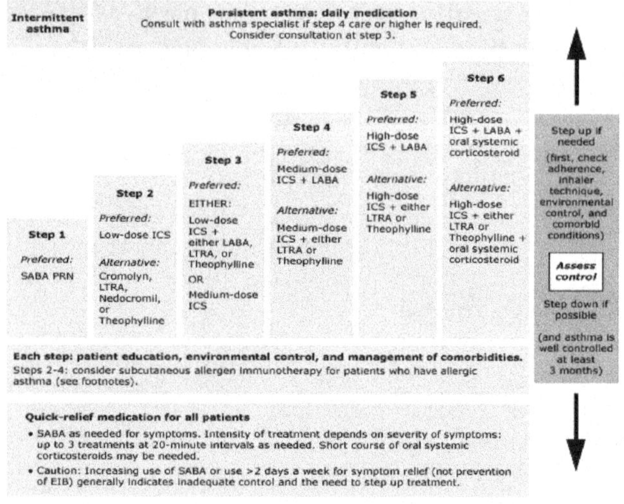

Step down if symptoms controlled >3 months

SARCOIDOSIS

- Idiopathic, chronic multisystemic inflammatory granulomatous disease.

RISK FACTORS
- **Females, African-Americans, Northern Europeans.**

PATHOPHYSIOLOGY
- Exaggerated T cell response to a variety of antigens or self-antigens, leading to central immune system activation, granuloma formation, and peripheral immune depression.

CLINICAL MANIFESTATIONS
- **50% are asymptomatic** (incidentally found on imaging)
- Pulmonary: **dry (nonproductive) cough, dyspnea**, chest pain, & **rales** on examination.
- Lymphadenopathy: intrathoracic lymphadenopathy (*hilar nodes*, paratracheal).
- Skin: **erythema nodosum (classic), lupus pernio (most specific),** maculopapular rash (most common). Parotid gland enlargement.
- Eyes: anterior uveitis.
- Cardiac: restrictive cardiomyopathy, arrhythmias, heart blocks.
- Rheumatologic: arthralgias, fever, malaise, weight loss, hepatosplenomegaly.
- Neurologic cranial nerve palsies (especially facial nerve - CN VII), Diabetes insipidus.
- Löfgren syndrome: triad of erythema nodosum + bilateral hilar LAD + polyarthralgias with fever.

DIAGNOSIS
- Based on compatible clinical/radiologic findings, noncaseating granulomas & excluding other causes.

- **Chest radiographs: best initial test - bilateral hilar lymphadenopathy classic.**
  Interstitial lung disease: reticular opacities, ground glass appearance. Eggshell calcifications, fibrosis.
  Stage I: BHL (no sx or mild pulmonary sx).
  Stage II: BHL + ILD (moderate pulmonary sx).
  Stage III: ILD only.
  Stage IV: fibrosis (restrictive disease).

- Pulmonary function tests: **restrictive pattern is classic**:
  - Normal or increased FEV_1/FVC, normal or decreased FVC, decreased FEV1.
  - Decreased lung volumes (eg, VC, RV, FRC, TLC).
  - PFTs primarily used to monitor response to treatment.

- Tissue Biopsy: most accurate - **noncaseating granulomas** classic nonspecific histological finding.

- Labs: **increased ACE levels**, hypercalciuria, hypercalcemia, increased vitamin D. Cutaneous anergy.

MANAGEMENT
- **Asymptomatic: observation** - spontaneous remission within 2 years in most without treatment.
- Symptomatic: **oral corticosteroids first-line management** of choice when treatment is needed.
- Methotrexate. Hydroxychloroquine can be used for severe skin lesions.

PROGNOSIS
- Prognosis good overall. 40% spontaneously resolve; 40% improve with treatment; 20% progress to irreversible lung injury.
- Good prognosis: Stage I, erythema nodosum.
- Interstitial lung disease & lupus pernio associated with poorer prognosis.

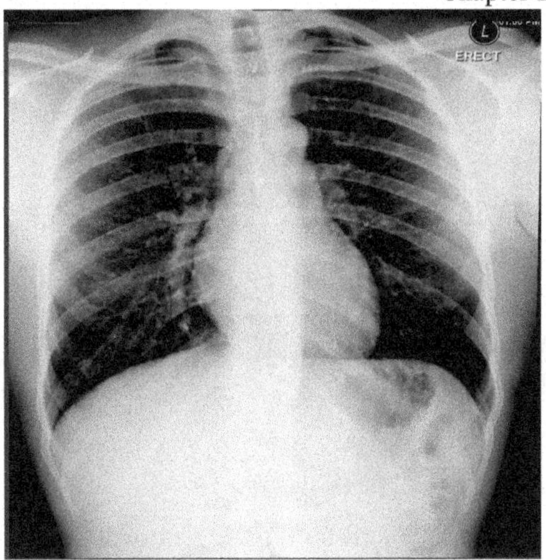

Normal

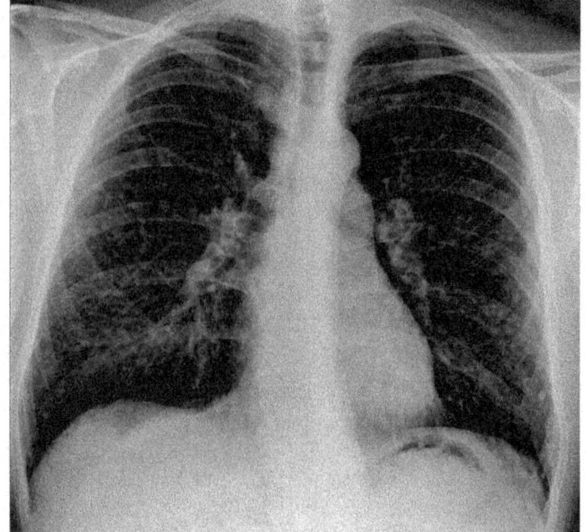

Sarcoidosis: bilateral hilar lymphadenopathy

IDIOPATHIC FIBROSING INTERSTITIAL PNEUMONIA (PULMONARY FIBROSIS)

- Progressive scarring of the lungs due to an unknown cause.
- Most common in **men >40 years of age**, smokers.

CLINICAL MANIFESTATIONS

- Progressive dyspnea, nonproductive cough.
- Physical examination: fine, dry, bibasilar inspiratory crackles. Clubbing of the fingers may be seen.

DIAGNOSIS

- Chest radiographs: basal predominant **reticular opacities (honeycombing).**
- Chest CT: preferred imaging modality - **reticular honeycombing, focal ground-glass opacification**, traction Bronchiectasis or Bronchiolectasis.

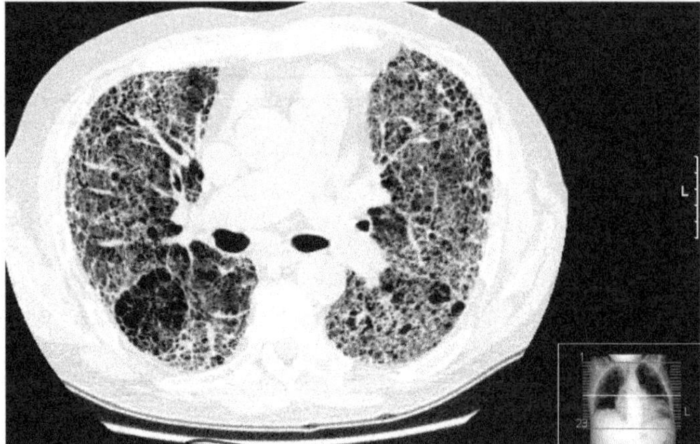

- Pulmonary function test: **restrictive pattern** - normal or **increased FEV1/FVC**, normal or decreased FVC, **decreased lung volumes** (eg, VC, RV, FRC, TLC), decreased DLCO.
- Biopsy: honeycombing (large cystic airspaces from cystic fibrotic alveolitis).

MANAGEMENT

- No effective medical management. **Lung transplant only possible cure** (poor prognosis without transplant). Strategies include smoking cessation, oxygen.
- Pirfenidone and Nintedanib are antifibrotic agents that may slow progression but does not significantly benefit mortality

PNEUMOCONIOSES/ENVIRONMENTAL LUNG DISEASES

PNEUMOCONIOSIS: chronic fibrotic lung disease secondary to **inhalation of mineral dust.**

SILICOSIS

- Occupational pulmonary disease caused by inhalation of silicon dioxide.
- Silicosis greatly increases the risk for Tuberculosis and non TB mycobacterium infections.
- Pathophysiology: silica deposits activate alveolar macrophages, which stimulate fibrogenesis.

RISK FACTORS

- Silica dust inhalation: coal mining, **quarry work** with **granite, slate, quartz,** pottery makers, **sandblasting**, glass & cement manufacturing, masonry, hydraulic fracturing.

CLINICAL MANIFESTATIONS

- Chronic: often asymptomatic, dyspnea on exertion, nonproductive cough. Crackles (rales).
- Acute: dyspnea, cough, weight loss, fatigue.

DIAGNOSIS:

- Chest radiographs:
  - Multiple small (<10mm) round nodular opacities (miliary pattern) **primarily in the upper lobes.**
  - **Eggshell calcifications of hilar & mediastinal nodes** (only seen in 5-20%).
  - Bilateral nodular densities progress from periphery to the hilum.

- Lung Biopsy.

MANAGEMENT:

- Removal from exposure mainstay of management.
- Nonspecific supportive management - corticosteroids, oxygen, rehab. Nonspecific treatment.

COAL WORKER'S PNEUMOCONIOSIS (black lung disease)

- Lung disease from inhalation and deposition of coal dust particles.

CLINICAL MANIFESTATIONS

- Dyspnea, cough. Fine crackles (rales) often heard.
- **Caplan syndrome: Coal worker pneumoconiosis + Rheumatoid Arthritis** (serologic positive).

DIAGNOSIS

- Chest radiograph: **small nodules** predominantly in the **upper lung** with **hyperinflation of lower lobes in an obstructive pattern** (resembles Emphysema).

- Pulmonary function test: **obstructive pattern.**

- Lung biopsy: shows dark "black" lungs (not needed for diagnosis).

MANAGEMENT

- Supportive.

BERYLLIOSIS

- Granulomatous pulmonary disease caused by beryllium exposure.
- Beryllium is often alloyed with nickel, aluminum, and copper so people working in those industries are at increased exposure.

RISK FACTORS

- **Aerospace, electronics**, ceramics, tool & dye manufacturing, jewelry making, fluorescent light bulbs.

CLINICAL MANIFESTATIONS

- Dyspnea, cough, joint pain, fever, weight loss.

DIAGNOSIS

- Chest radiograph: normal 50%, hilar lymphadenopathy & increased interstitial lung markings (similar to Sarcoidosis).
- Beryllium lymphocyte proliferation test to assess lymphocyte uptake of thymidine.
- Pulmonary function test: restrictive lung pattern.
- Biopsy: noncaseating granulomas.

MANAGEMENT

- **Corticosteroids,** oxygen.
- Methotrexate if Corticosteroids fail.

COMPLICATIONS

- Associated with increased risk of lung, stomach, and colon cancer.

BYSSINOSIS

- Lung disease due to **cotton exposure** in those employed in the **textile industry** (may be caused by flax or hemp dust exposure).

CLINICAL MANIFESTATIONS:

- Dyspnea, wheezing, cough, chest tightness.
- The symptoms tend to get worse at the beginning of the work week then improve later in the week or on the weekend "Monday fever'. May be progressive in some patients.

ASBESTOSIS

- Slow, progressive diffuse pulmonary fibrosis as a result of inhalation of asbestos fibers.
- Seen 15-20 years after lengthy exposure to asbestos.

RISK FACTORS
- **Destruction, repair or renovation of old buildings, insulation** and fire-resistant products, ship building.
- Asbestos was commonly used due to its fire-resistant, thermal, & electrical insulation attributes.

CLINICAL MANIFESTATIONS
- Dyspnea on exertion, cough.
- Physical examination: bibasilar crackles.

DIAGNOSIS
- Chest radiographs:
  - **Pleural plaques** pleural thickening or calcification of the parietal pleura) especially involving the **lower lobes.**
  - Interstitial fibrosis (honeycomb lung) **–** irregular linear opacities especially in the lower lobes.
  - **"Shaggy heart" sign** – indistinct heart border, "ground glass" appearance of the lung fields.
- Pulmonary function tests: **restrictive lung pattern** - normal or **increased FEV1/FVC**, normal or decreased FVC, **decreased lung volumes** (eg, VC, RV, FRC, TLC).
- Biopsy: may show **linear asbestos bodies** in the lung tissue (ferruginous bodies).

MANAGEMENT
- No specific therapy. Management includes: bronchodilators, O_2, corticosteroids, ± lung transplant.

COMPLICATIONS
- **Bronchogenic carcinoma (most common)**
- **Malignant mesothelioma of the pleura (most specific).**

ALPHA-1 ANTITRYPSIN DEFICIENCY

- **Genetic disorder that leads to panacinar Emphysema**, hepatomegaly, and Cirrhosis.

CLINICAL MANIFESTATIONS
- Lung: emphysema (eg, dyspnea), Bronchiectasis.
- Liver: hepatomegaly, signs and symptoms of Cirrhosis

DIAGNOSIS
- Chest radiographs: bullous changes more prominent at the lung bases.
- CT scan: panacinar emphysema (dilation of terminal airways)
- PFTs: obstructive pattern. Liver biopsy: PAS-positive globules in hepatocytes.

MANAGEMENT
- Medical: IV pooled alpha-1 antitrypsin
- Surgical: lung transplant

HYPERSENSITIVITY PNEUMONITIS / EXTRINSIC ALLERGIC ALVEOLITIS

PNEUMONITIS: ***generalized lung inflammation of the alveoli & respiratory bronchioles due to organic dusts, molds, foreign proteins & chemicals.***

- MC seen in 30s – 50s.
- **PATHOPHYSIOLOGY:** ***inflammatory reaction to an ORGANIC ANTIGEN**** ⇨ sensitization to the antigen. Subsequent, heavy exposure ⇨ neutrophil activation in small airways & alveoli with mononuclear cell invasion. Release of proteolytic enzymes contributes to the hypersensitivity reaction.

DISEASE	ANTIGEN	SOURCE
FARMER'S LUNG **CATTLE WORKER'S LUNG**	Thermophilic actinomycetes (gram positive bacteria), Saccharopolyspora rectivirgula, Micropolyspora faeni	Moldy hay
VENTILATION WORKER'S LUNG	Thermophilic actinomycetes, Mycobacterium Avium Complex	Water related contamination: humidifiers, air conditioners, heating/cooling systems
BIRD BREEDER'S LUNG	Avian proteins	Bird feces, feathers, or serum proteins of bird
SEQUOIOSIS **"SAW MILL WORKER" LUNG**	Graphium Auerobasidium Other fungi	Sawdust from moldy redwood (seen in lumbar mill workers).
METAL WORKER'S LUNG	Mycobacterium immunogenium	Contaminated metalworking fluids
MUSHROOM LUNG	Actinomycetes	Moldy spores
GRAIN WORKER'S LUNG	Sitophilus granaries	Exposure to wheat infested c weevils
CHEMICAL WORKER'S LUNG	Diisocyanate chemical	Manufacture of plastics, polyurethane

CLINICAL MANIFESTATIONS

1. **ACUTE HYPERSENSITIVITY PNEUMONITIS:** ***rapid onset: fevers, chills***, dyspnea, productive cough, chest tightness, malaise ***occurring 4-8 hours after prolonged exposure to antigen***. ***Inspiratory crackles on physical exam.***
   Biopsy: micronodular interstitial involvement with poorly formed noncaseating granulomas. May be normal.

2. **SUB ACUTE (INTERMITTENT):** ***gradual development*** of ***dyspnea, productive cough***, anorexia, weight loss, pleuritis. Similar to acute but longer duration & less severe (***usually no fevers, chills***). Associated c more organized granulomas CXR: micronodular opacities especially in the lower lung fields. **Biopsy:** noncaseating granulomas (more organized than in acute) may be fibrotic.

3. **CHRONIC HYPERSENSITIVITY PNEUMONITIS:** progressive worsening of symptoms. No history of acute episodes. Slow onset of progressive dyspnea, weight loss, clubbing, tachypnea. Associated with only partial recovery after agent exposure is eliminated.

DIAGNOSIS:

1. **CXR:** Acute: diffuse micronodular interstitial pattern. Subacute & chronic: micronodular opacities especially in the lower lung fields.
2. **PFT's:** ***restrictive component***, ↓DL_{CO}, hypoxemia. CBC: leukocytosis with left shift. Positive hypersensitivity panel

MANAGEMENT

1. ***Avoidance of allergen, Corticosteroids***

SILO FILLER DISEASE

- **HYPERSENSITIVITY PNEUMONITIS** from **NITROGEN DIOXIDE GAS EXPOSURE RELEASED FROM PLANT MATTER** stored in silos as they ferment (especially at the chute & base of the silo).
- The gas is converted to nitric acid in the lungs when inhaled.
- Also seen with combustion exposure (eg, fires, diesel fume).

CLINICAL MANIFESTATIONS
- Cough, dyspnea, fatigue, cardiopulmonary edema. May develop bronchiolitis obliterans.

MANAGEMENT
- Occupational reduction of exposure - not entering recently filled silos for 2 weeks, entering at the top of the silo, use of respiratory N95 masks.

DIFFERENTIAL DIAGNOSIS
- Farmer's lung (allergic alveolitis/pneumonitis specifically due to moldy hay exposure).

PARROT FEVER (PSITTACOSIS)

- Infection with ***Chlamydophila psittaci*** due to exposure to **infected birds** (eg, parrot ducks, etc.).

TRANSMISSION
- Inhalation of organism in dried feces (eg, cleaning cages, mouth to beak contact, bird exposure).
- 5-14 day incubation period.

CLINICAL MANIFESTATIONS
- **Flu-like symptoms** (eg, dry cough, fever, myalgias, headache).

PHYSICAL EXAMINATION
- Rales, may have pleural rub. May develop hepatitis, respiratory failure, encephalitis, or endocarditis.

DIAGNOSIS
- Chest radiograph: atypical pneumonia, lobar changes, ground-glass opacities.
- Serologic testing: microimmunofluorescent antibody testing. Culture not routinely performed as it can be hazardous to lab personnel.

MANAGEMENT
- **Tetracyclines first-line**.
- Macrolides.

INFLUENZA

- **Influenza A associated with more severe outbreaks** compared to B.

TRANSMISSION

- Primarily via airborne respiratory secretions (eg, sneezing, coughing, talking, breathing), contaminated objects.

INCREASED RISK

- Age > 65 years, pregnancy, immunocompromised.

- Children are important vectors for the disease (**the highest rates of infection are seen among children but individuals 65 or older are at the highest risk for complications**).

- Complications include pneumonia, respiratory failure, death, meningitis, myocarditis, encephalitis, rhabdomyolysis, and kidney failure.

CLINICAL MANIFESTATIONS

- **Abrupt onset** of a wide range of symptoms including headache, fever, chills, malaise, URI symptoms, pharyngitis, pneumonia.

- **Myalgias most commonly involving the legs & lumbosacral areas.**

DIAGNOSIS

- Rapid influenza nasal swab or viral culture.

MANAGEMENT

- Mild disease & healthy: **supportive mainstay of treatment in healthy patients** (eg, Acetaminophen or Salicylates), rest.

- **Antivirals recommended in patients that are hospitalized or at high risk of complications** – eg, **65 years of age or older**, cardiovascular disease (except isolated hypertension), pulmonary disease, immunosuppression (eg, malignancy, Diabetes mellitus, HIV infection, post-transplant), chronic liver disease, and hemoglobinopathies (eg, Sickle cell disease, Thalassemia).
  - Neuraminidase inhibitors: **Oseltamivir best if initiated within 48 hours of symptom onset.** Works against both A and B. Zanamivir and Peramivir are alternatives.
    Adverse reactions: skin reactions, nausea, vomiting and transient neuropsychiatric events. Egg allergy is a contraindication to Zanamivir.

  - Adamantane derivatives: Amantadine & Rimantadine are effective against influenza A only (high level of resistance) so not recommended for treatment or prophylaxis vs. Influenza A.

CHEMOPROPHYLAXIS

- Oseltamivir can be used in high-risk groups one year or older in cases of outbreaks & exposure.

- **During Influenza outbreaks in long-term facilities, all residents should receive chemoprophylaxis, regardless of immunization status.**

- For the general population, only individuals who did not receive the annual influenza vaccine should be given chemoprophylaxis.

INFLUENZA VACCINE

INDICATIONS:

- **Inactivated vaccine: annual influenza vaccination for all individuals 6 months of age or older (including pregnancy).** High-dose used in patients >65 years of age.
- Live attenuated (intranasal): can be used for annual vaccination in ages 2 to 49 years of age.

TIMING:

- The Influenza vaccine should be administered annually to everyone 6 months or older, **ideally before the onset of Influenza activity in the community (by the end of October in the northern hemisphere** and by April in the southern hemisphere).

ADVERSE REACTIONS

- Injection site reaction, fever, myalgia, irritability.
- Nasal spray may cause upper or lower respiratory tract symptoms.
- Allergic reaction and anaphylaxis rare.

CONTRAINDICATIONS & PRECAUTIONS:

- Contraindications to both: anaphylaxis to the influenza vaccine, **Guillain-Barré syndrome** within 6 weeks after a previous influenza vaccination, **high fever, infants < 6 months of age.**
- Although allergy to protein egg used to be a contraindication, **patients with egg allergy of any severity (including anaphylaxis) can safely receive the egg-based inactivated Influenza vaccine in a medical setting supervised by a health care provider.**

- **Contraindications to live attenuated vaccine only: immunocompromised patients** (including HIV), **pregnancy, adults age 50 or older**, individuals who have taken an influenza antiviral medication within the last 48 hours, close contacts and caregivers of severely immunocompromised persons who require a protected environment.

ACUTE BRONCHITIS

- Inflammation of the bronchi.

ETIOLOGIES

- **Most commonly caused by viruses** (eg, Adenovirus, Parainfluenza, Influenza, Coronavirus, Coxsackie, Rhinovirus, Respiratory syncytial virus.
- Bacterial: *S. pneumoniae, H. influenzae, M. catarrhalis, Mycoplasma.*

CLINICAL MANIFESTATIONS

- **Hallmark is cough** (may be productive, present for at least 5 days but usually lasts last 1-3 weeks).
- Malaise, dyspnea, wheezing, URI symptoms (runny nose, sore throat, low-grade fever, malaise).
- May have **hemoptysis** (Acute bronchitis & Bronchogenic carcinoma are the 2 most common causes of Hemoptysis).
- Physical examination: often normal but may have wheezing and rhonchi.

DIAGNOSIS

- **Usually a clinical diagnosis without the need for imaging**.
- Chest radiographs: **usually normal or nonspecific.** Radiographs only indicated if Pneumonia is suspected.

MANAGEMENT

- **Symptomatic management** (eg, fluids, antitussives, antipyretics, analgesics).
- Antibiotics are not usually indicated in most patients.

PERTUSSIS (WHOOPING COUGH)

- Highly contagious infection 2ry to ***Bordetella pertussis***, a gram-negative coccobacillus.
- Rarely seen due to widespread vaccination. Most common in children < 2 years of age.
- Transmission: respiratory droplets during coughing fits.
- 7-10 day incubation period.

CLINICAL MANIFESTATIONS
- Catarrhal phase: URI symptoms lasting 1-2 weeks. Most contagious during this phase.
- Paroxysmal phase: **severe paroxysmal coughing fits** with **inspiratory whooping sound after cough fits.** May have **post coughing emesis**. Often lasts 2-4 weeks.
- Convalescent phase: resolution of the cough (coughing stage may last for up to 6 weeks).

DIAGNOSIS
- Clinical diagnosis. When available, order both **throat culture** & PCR. **Lymphocytosis** common.
- Throat culture: cultures most sensitive during the first 2 weeks of illness.
- PCR of nasopharyngeal swab: sensitive up to 4 weeks of illness.

MANAGEMENT
- **Supportive mainstay of treatment:** oxygenation, nebulizers, mechanical ventilation as needed. Droplet precautions if admitted.
- **Antibiotics** are used to decrease contagiousness of the affected patient. **Macrolides drug of choice** (eg, **Azithromycin**, Erythromycin). Azithromycin better tolerated and is preferred in children < 1 month of age. Trimethoprim-sulfamethoxazole second-line.

Bactrim

COMPLICATIONS
- Include **pneumonia**, encephalopathy, otitis media, sinusitis, and seizures. ↑mortality in infants due to apnea/cerebral hypoxia associated with coughing fits.

PERTUSSIS PREVENTION
- In the US, 5 doses of DTaP is typically recommended at 2 months, 4 months, 6 months, 15-18 months, and 4-6 years of age.
- A booster dose is administered between 11-18 years of age.

BRONCHIOLITIS

BRONCHIOLITIS OBLITERANS (CONSTRICTIVE)

- Patchy chronic inflammation & fibrosis of the bronchioles ⇨ collapse/obliteration of the bronchioles. Granulation tissue in the bronchiole lumen ⇨ obstructive lung disease. Mosaic pattern on CT scan.
- MC seen with post lung transplant rejection, inhalation injuries (eg, silo filler's dz), drug reactions, RA.
  Mgmt: high-dose Corticosteroids & immunosuppression. Lung transplant definitive treatment.

CRYPTOGENIC ORGANIZING PNEUMONIA (COP)

- Formerly known as Bronchiolitis Obliterans with Organizing Pneumonia (BOOP).
- Persistent alveolar exudates ⇨ inflammation & scarring **(fibrosis) of the bronchioles AND alveoli.** Resembles pneumonia on CXR but does not respond to antibiotics. CXR findings that persist despite clinical improvement of the patient. Often idiopathic or occurs after pneumonia.
  Management: Corticosteroids.

ACUTE BRONCHIOLITIS

- Infection and inflammation of the bronchioles (smaller passages)

ETIOLOGIES

- **Respiratory syncytial virus (RSV) most common cause,** Rhinovirus, Adenovirus, Influenza virus, Parainfluenza virus, etc.

RISK FACTORS

- **Infants 2 months to 2 years most commonly affected.** <6months in age, exposure to cigarette smoke, lack of breastfeeding, prematurity (<37 weeks' gestation) & crowded conditions (eg, day care).

CLINICAL MANIFESTATIONS

- **Viral prodrome** (eg, fever, URI symptoms) for 1-2 days **followed by respiratory distress** (eg, wheezing, tachypnea, nasal flaring, cyanosis, retractions, rales).
- Signs of severity: hypoxemia, apnea, respiratory failure.

DIAGNOSIS

- **Mainly a clinical diagnosis.**
- Chest radiograph: nonspecific: hyperinflation, peribronchial cuffing or thickening, atelectasis etc. Not routinely performed but may be used to rule out other causes.
- Nasal washings using monoclonal antibody testing.
- Pulse oximetry single best predictor of disease in children.

MANAGEMENT

- **Supportive measures mainstay of treatment - humidified oxygen, IV fluids,** nebulized saline, cool mist humidifier, antipyretics (eg, Acetaminophen).
- Mechanical ventilation may be indicated if severe.
- Medications play a limited role: beta-agonists, nebulized racemic epinephrine; Corticosteroids not indicated unless history of underlying reactive airway disease.
- Ribavirin may be administered if severe lung or heart disease or in immunosuppressed patients.

PREVENTION IN HIGH-RISK:

- **Palivizumab** during the first year of life for children < 29 weeks, symptomatic chronic lung disease of prematurity, congenital heart disease, neuromuscular difficulties, immunodeficiency.
- **Handwashing is preventative.**

ACUTE EPIGLOTTITIS (SUPRAGLOTTITIS)

- Severe, potentially life-threatening inflammation of the epiglottis.
- Most common in children 3 months – 6 years. Males 2 times more common. Occurs in any season. Diabetes mellitus is a risk factor in adults.

ETIOLOGIES

- ***Haemophilus influenzae B* historically was the most common cause** (reduced incidence in US due to Hib vaccination). Hib epiglottitis still occurs especially in *unvaccinated children or foreign immigrants.*
- **If immunized, suspect Streptococcal species** (*eg,* ***Group A streptococcus,*** *S. pneumoniae*), other *H. influenzae, S. aureus.* May occur with cocaine use in adults.

CLINICAL MANIFESTATIONS

- "3 Ds" – **Dysphagia, Drooling, & Distress.**
- Fever, **odynophagia, inspiratory stridor**, dyspnea, hoarseness, muffled "hot potato" voice, **tripoding:** sitting leaned forward with the elbow on the lap (refuses to lie supine).

DIAGNOSIS:

- **Laryngoscopy: definitive diagnosis** (cherry-red epiglottis with swelling) performed when securing the airway.
- Soft tissue lateral cervical radiographs: **thumb or thumbprint sign:** swollen, enlarged epiglottis (not necessary for diagnosis).
- Do not attempt to visualize using a tongue depressor in children.

MANAGEMENT

- **Maintaining the airway most important component of management** - place child in a comfortable position and keep the child calm to avoid airway issues. **The OR is best setting for intubation.**
- Dexamethasone for airway edema in some.
- **Antibiotics:** second or third-generation cephalosporin (eg, **Ceftriaxone or Cefotaxime).** Penicillin, Ampicillin or anti-staphylococcal coverage may be added (eg, Vancomycin).

PREVENTION

- **Rifampin given to all close contacts.**
- Routine use of *Haemophilus influenzae* type B (Hib) vaccine.

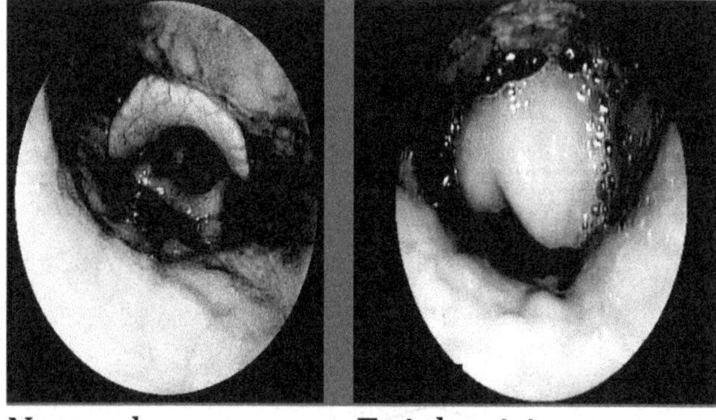

Normal Epiglottitis

Laryngoscopy definitive – cherry-red swollen epiglottis

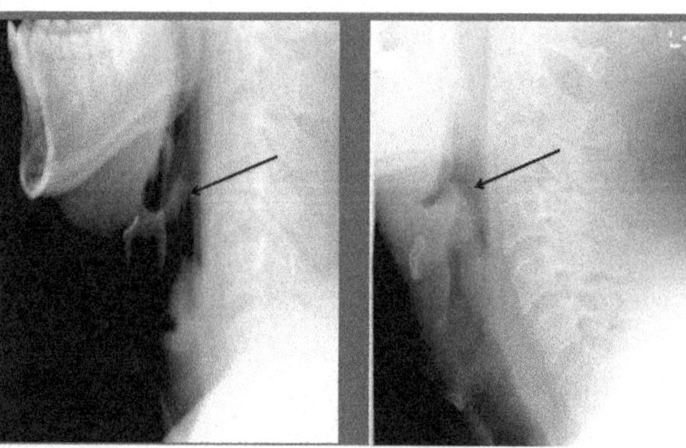

Normal Epiglottitis

Lateral views: Thumb or thumprinting sign

LARYNGOTRACHEITIS (CROUP)

- Inflammation of the larynx and subglottic airway.
- Most commonly occurs between 6 months – 6 years; especially in the fall & winter.

ETIOLOGIES

- **Parainfluenza virus type I most common cause.** RSV (2nd), Adenovirus, & Rhinovirus.

CLINICAL MANIFESTATIONS

- **Upper airway involvement**: harsh, **"seal-like barking" cough** – hallmark of the disease in infants & young children, **inspiratory stridor, hoarseness** (especially in older children and adults), dyspnea, low-grade fever. Symptoms often worse at night.

- URI symptoms (eg, **coryza**) prior during or after the acute presentation.
- Significant upper airway obstruction, respiratory distress, and rarely death.

DIAGNOSIS

- **Clinical diagnosis** (once Epiglottitis & foreign body aspiration are excluded).
- Frontal cervical radiograph: **steeple sign** (subglottic narrowing of the airway) - 50%. Rarely done.

MANAGEMENT

- **Mild** (no stridor at rest, no respiratory distress): **supportive** (eg, cool humidified air mist, hydration). Supplemental oxygen in patients with SaO2 <92%. **Dexamethasone provides significant relief** as early as 6 hours after single dose (oral or IM), results in faster resolution of symptoms, decreased length of stay, and decreased relapse. Patients can be discharged home.

- **Moderate** (stridor at rest with mild to moderate retractions): **Dexamethasone** PO or IM + supportive treatment. Nebulized Epinephrine. Should be observed for 3-4 hours after clinical intervention. May be discharged home if improvement is seen.

- **Severe** (stridor at rest with marked retractions): **Dexamethasone + nebulized Epinephrine & hospitalization.**

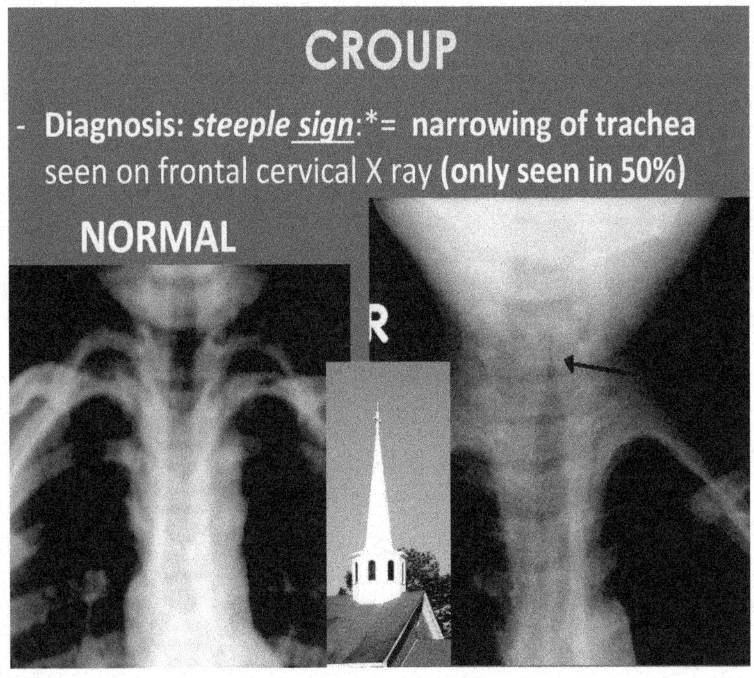

CROUP
- Diagnosis: steeple sign:*= narrowing of trachea seen on frontal cervical X ray (only seen in 50%)
NORMAL
R

PNEUMONIA

ETIOLOGIES

- Typical: ***Streptococcus pneumoniae* (most common),** *Haemophilus influenzae, Klebsiella pneumoniae, Staphylococcus aureus.*
- Atypical: *Mycoplasma pneumoniae, Chlamydophila pneumoniae, Legionella pneumophila,* viruses.

CLINICAL MANIFESTATIONS

- Typical: fever, productive cough, pleuritic chest pain, dyspnea. Rigors (severe chills with violent shaking) is classically associated with *Streptococcus pneumoniae.*
- Atypical: low-grade fever, dry nonproductive cough, extrapulmonary symptoms (eg, myalgias, malaise, pharyngitis, nausea, vomiting, diarrhea).

PHYSICAL EXAMINATION

- Typical: tachypnea, tachycardia, signs of consolidation: **bronchial breath sounds, dullness to percussion, increased tactile fremitus, egophony,** inspiratory rales (crackles).
- Atypical: **pulmonary exam often normal** (signs of consolidation usually absent). May have crackles (rales).
- Elderly, diabetic and immunocompromised patients may have minimal exam findings even with typical pneumonia.

	PERCUSSION	FREMITUS	BREATH SOUNDS
PNEUMONIA	Dullness	**INCREASED**	**Bronchial, EGOPHONY**
PLEURAL EFFUSION	Dullness	Decreased	Decreased
PNEUMOTHORAX or OBSTRUCTIVE LUNG DISEASE	**HYPERRESONANCE**	Decreased	Decreased

MICROBIOLOGY

Streptococcus pneumoniae

- **Most common cause of Community-acquired pneumonia** (65%).
- Classic presentation: sudden onset of one time **chills & rigors** (violent shivering), fever, productive cough with **blood-tinged (rusty) sputum.**
- Gram stain: **gram-positive diplococci.**

Haemophilus influenzae

- Second most common cause of Community-acquired pneumonia.
- Increased risk: **extremes of age** (<6y, elderly), **immunocompromised** (eg, Diabetes mellitus, HIV, chemotherapy), **underlying pulmonary disease** (eg, Asthma, **COPD, Bronchiectasis, Cystic fibrosis**), alcoholism.
- Often a colonizer of the respiratory tract. Gram-negative rod.

Staphylococcus aureus

- Commonly associated as a **superimposed infection after a viral infection** (eg, post influenza bacterial pneumonia), **hospital-acquired pneumonia** (eg, MRSA).
- Chest radiograph: classically associated with bilateral, multilobar infiltrates or abscesses (cavitary lesions).
- Sputum gram stain: **gram-positive cocci in clusters**.

Klebsiella pneumoniae
- Severe illness in **chronic alcoholism,** sick patients, patients with chronic illnesses (eg, Diabetes).
- May present with **purple-colored (currant jelly) sputum**.
- Chest radiograph: **cavitary lesions** are hallmark (nonspecific) or lobar consolidations.
- Sputum gram stain: gram-negative rods.

MYCOPLASMA PNEUMONIAE
- **Most common cause of atypical** (walking) **Pneumonia.**
- Risk factors: **young & healthy** (eg, school-aged children, college students, military recruits).
- Outbreaks often occur in the late summer & early fall.

CLINICAL MANIFESTATIONS
- Extrapulmonary symptoms: commonly presents with **pharyngitis & URI prodrome** (rhinorrhea, headache, malaise, fever) followed by persistent **dry (nonproductive) cough.** Physical examination often normal.
- Bullous myringitis (fluid-filled blisters on the tympanic membrane) is a rare, nonspecific finding.
- Complications include Stevens-Johnson syndrome, TEN, Erythema multiforme, **Cold autoimmune hemolytic anemia (IgM).**

DIAGNOSTIC TESTS
- Chest radiograph: atypical pattern: **reticulonodular pattern most common**, diffuse, patchy or interstitial infiltrates.
- PCR (test of choice), **cold agglutinins**, serology, special culture media (because it is a short rod without a cell wall, gram-stain not useful).

MANAGEMENT
- **Macrolides** (eg, **Azithromycin**, Clarithromycin) or **Doxycycline**
- **Lacks a cell wall** so naturally resistant to beta-lactams.

LEGIONELLA PNEUMOPHILA
- Aerobic, pleomorphic intracellular Gram-negative bacterium.
- Transmission: **outbreaks related to contaminated water sources** (eg, air conditions, potable water, cooling towers, ventilation systems etc.). No person to person transmission.
- Risk factors: immunosuppressed patients, smokers, elderly, chronic lung disease.

CLINICAL MANIFESTATIONS
- Fever, chills, dyspnea, dry cough, chest pain, malaise, myalgias.
- Extrapulmonary symptoms: **GI symptoms prominent: diarrhea** (watery and non-bloody), nausea, vomiting. Higher incidence of **Hyponatremia and increased liver function tests. Neurologic symptoms:** headache, confusion, altered mental status.
- Although "atypical", patients can be very ill.

DIAGNOSIS
- Nucleic acid detection (eg, **PCR preferred, urine antigen**, culture)

MANAGEMENT
- **Macrolides** (eg, Azithromycin, Clarithromycin) or **respiratory Fluoroquinolones** (eg, **Levofloxacin**, Moxifloxacin, and Gemifloxacin).

COMMUNITY ACQUIRED PNEUMONIA: ❶ **acquired OUTSIDE of the hospital setting** & patient is not a resident of a long-term care facility (eg, nursing home) OR ❷ patient that was ambulatory prior to admission who develops pneumonia **within 48 hours of initial hospital admission**.

HOSPITAL ACQUIRED (NOSOCOMIAL) PNEUMONIA: pneumonia occurring **>48 hours after hospital admission.** Often caused by **Pseudomonas, MRSA,** & other organisms found in the hospital.

	TYPICAL PNEUMONIA	ATYPICAL PNEUMONIA
ORGANISMS	***S. pneumoniae*** *H. influenzae* *Klebsiella pneumoniae* *S. Aureus*	***Mycoplasma pneumoniae*** *Chlamydophila pneumoniae* *Legionella pneumophila* Viruses
CHEST X RAY	Lobar pneumonia	Diffuse, patchy interstitial or reticulonodular infiltrates.
CLINICAL MANIFESTATIONS	• Sudden onset of fever • Productive cough + purulent sputum • Pleuritic chest pain • **Rigors (especially *S. pneumoniae*)** • Tachycardia, tachypnea	• Low grade fever • Dry, nonproductive cough • **Extrapulmonary symptoms:** myalgias, malaise, sore throat, headache, N/V/D.
PHYSICAL EXAMINATION	**Signs of consolidation:** • **bronchial breath sounds** • **dullness on percussion** • **↑TACTILE FREMITUS, EGOPHONY** • Inspiratory rales (crackles)	**Often normal**. ± crackles, rhonchi. Signs of consolidation usually absent.

ANTIBIOTIC MANAGEMENT OF PNEUMONIA

CLINICAL SCENARIO	EMPIRIC TREATMENT GUIDELINES
COMMUNITY-ACQUIRED, OUTPATIENT	**Macrolide or Doxycycline first line.** Fluoroquinolones only used first line if comorbid conditions/recent antibiotic use.
COMMUNITY-ACQUIRED, INPATIENT	[**β-lactam + either Macrolide** or Doxycycline] **OR broad spectrum FQ**
HOSPITAL ACQUIRED (*Pseudomonas* infection risk)	**Anti-PSEUDOMONAL β lactam + either anti-PSEUDOMONAL AG or FQ** • Add **Vancomycin** or Linezolid **if MRSA is suspected.** • Add **Levofloxacin** or **Azithromycin** if **Legionella** is suspected. • Add Trimethoprim/sulfamethoxazole ±corticosteroids if PCP suspected. *If documented β-lactam allergy: Fluoroquinolone ± Clindamycin. Aztreonam, Aminoglycoside
ASPIRATION (anaerobes)	• **Ampicillin-Sulbactam first-line** (parenteral) or **Amoxicillin-clavulanate** (oral). • Hospital-acquired : Imipenem, Meropenem, Piperacillin-tazobactam
DRUG RESISTANCE SUSPECTED	• **One of the following** (Piperacillin-tazobactam, Cefepime, Ceftazidime, Imipenem, Meropenem, Aztreonam) **plus one of the following:** Aminoglycoside, Antipseudomonal fluoroquinolone (eg, Ciprofloxacin, Levofloxacin) or a Polymyxin.

Inpatients therapy is IV antibiotics. Change to oral when clinically responding, able to take PO.

- **β-lactams: Ceftriaxone**; Cefotaxime, Ampicillin/sulbactam, or Ertapenem.
- **Anti-Pseudomonal β-lactams: Piperacillin/tazobactam, Ceftazidime, Cefepime**. Imipenem, Meropenem.
- **Macrolides:** Clarithromycin, Azithromycin.
- **Respiratory FQ (Fluoroquinolone): Levofloxacin, Moxifloxacin.** Gemifloxacin.
  Ciprofloxacin is NOT a respiratory Fluoroquinolone (may be used for Pseudomonas or Legionella).
- **Aminoglycosides (AG):** Amikacin, Gentamicin, Tobramycin.
- Supplemental oxygen, IV fluids, respiratory isolation (if suspect tuberculosis).

CURB65 admission if at least 2 (1 point each)
Confusion, **U**remia (>30 mg/dL), **R**espiratory rate ≥30, **B**P low (SBP <90 or DBP < 60), Age >**65**

ASPIRATION PNEUMONIA

- **Most commonly caused by anaerobes** (eg, *Peptostreptococcus, Bacteroides, Fusobacterium*, etc.). Increased incidence: periodontal disease.
- In chronically ill, gram-negative rods and Staphylococcus aureus may also be a cause.

PATHOPHYSIOLOGY

- Inhalation of oropharyngeal & gastric microbes.

RISK FACTORS

- Reduced consciousness, protracted vomiting, etc.
- **Most common in the right lower lobe** (due to vertical angle of the right mainstem bronchus).
- Associated with **foul-smelling sputum ("rotten egg" smell)**, pulmonary abscesses, & Empyema.

MANAGEMENT

- **Ampicillin-Sulbactam first-line** (parenteral) or **Amoxicillin-clavulanate** (oral).
- Alternative: Metronidazole plus either Amoxicillin or Penicillin G.
- Hospital-acquired aspiration: Imipenem, Meropenem, Piperacillin-tazobactam.

HISTOPLASMOSIS

- ***Histoplasma capsulatum*** - dimorphic oval yeast (not encapsulated despite its name).

TRANSMISSION

- Inhalation of **soil containing bird & bat droppings** in the **Mississippi & Ohio river valleys.** Also seen with demolition, people who explore caves (spelunkers), or excavators in those areas.

RISK FACTORS

- Immunocompromised states - AIDS-defining illness especially if CD4+ is ≤150.

CLINICAL MANIFESTATIONS

- **Asymptomatic: most patients**. Flu-like symptoms if they become symptomatic.
- **Pneumonia** (atypical). Fever, nonproductive cough, myalgias.
- **Dissemination:** if immunocompromised: hepatosplenomegaly, fever, oropharyngeal ulcers, bloody diarrhea, adrenal insufficiency. *Can mimic Tuberculosis.*

DIAGNOSIS

- Labs: increased alkaline phosphatase & LDH. Pancytopenia
- Chest radiographs: pulmonary infiltrates, hilar or mediastinal lymphadenopathy.
- **Antigen testing via sputum (PCR) or urine highly specific**.
- **Cultures: most specific test.** Sputum. Blood culture positivity if disseminated/HIV.

MANAGEMENT

- **Asymptomatic: no treatment required** (eg, patients with pulmonary symptoms < 4 weeks).
- **Mild-moderate disease: Itraconazole 1st line treatment.**
- **Severe disease: Amphotericin B.** Also used if Itraconazole therapy is ineffective.

PNEUMOCOCCAL VACCINES

Pneumococcal conjugate vaccine (PCV) 13

- Protects against 13 serotypes that account for 85% of the serotypes causing invasive pneumococcal infections, including meningitis and bacteremia.
- Administration: in patients 6 weeks through 5 years of age, it is administered as a part of a **4-dose immunization series (eg, given at 2, 4, 6, and 12 to 15 months of age).** May be indicated in older high-risk patients.

Pneumococcal Polysaccharide vaccine (PPSV23)

INDICATIONS:

- **All adults 65 years and older,** as well as **younger patients with conditions that increase the risk for developing complications from pneumococcal infection** (eg, pneumococcal Pneumonia or invasive pneumococcal disease).
- All patients who received PPSV23 before the age of 65 years should be revaccinated at age 65 unless the vaccine is given < 10 years prior to the patient turning 65 years old (in which the patient should be revaccinated 10 year following the first dose).
- If both vaccines are recommended then the patient should receive them as follows: 1) if the patient has had no prior vaccination with either vaccine, the patient should receive a single dose of PCV13 followed 8 weeks later by PPSV23 2) if the patient has received PPSV23 in the past, a single dose of PCV13 should be given 1 year after the administration of PPSV23.

CONTRAINDICATIONS

- Severe allergic or anaphylactic reaction to any component of the formulation of the vaccine or any diphtheria toxoid-containing vaccine.
- Pregnancy is not a contraindication to vaccination.

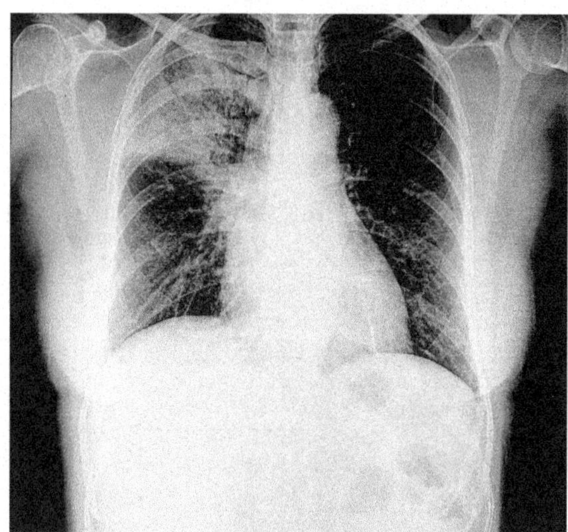

Typical (lobar) pneumonia

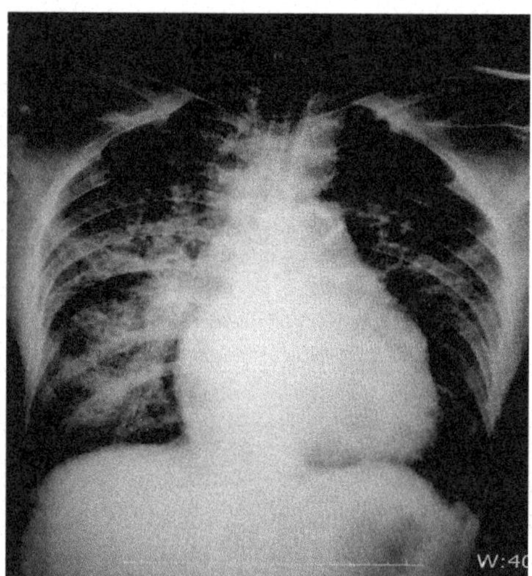

Atypical pneumonia

PNEUMOCYSTIS (PCP) PNEUMONIA

- ***Pneumocystis jirovecii*** (formerly *carinii*) is a yeast-like fungus (doesn't respond to antifungals).
- Transmission: inhalation.

RISK FACTORS

- Immunocompromised states (eg, HIV, malignancy, chemotherapy, transplant recipients) - **most common opportunistic infection in HIV** – especially if **CD4+ ≤ 200**.

CLINICAL MANIFESTATIONS

- Classic triad: progressive **dyspnea on exertion (most common), fever, & nonproductive cough.**
- **Oxygen desaturation with ambulation.**

DIAGNOSIS

- Chest radiographs: **diffuse bilateral interstitial infiltrates.** May be normal.
- Labs: **increased LDH** (>200 U/L), increased beta-D-glucan.
- Bronchoalveolar lavage specimen or induced sputum: Direct fluorescent antibody staining of the sample to see both trophic & cyst forms most common technique used.
  - Trophic forms: Wright-Giemsa stain. Cysts: methenamine silver & toluidine blue stains. If induced sputum is negative, bronchoscopy should be performed.
- Lung biopsy: definitive diagnosis (rarely performed).

MANAGEMENT

- **Trimethoprim-sulfamethoxazole drug of choice** x 21 days.
- **If HIV+, add Prednisone if hypoxic** (eg, PaO2 <70 mmHg, A-a gradient ≥ 35mmHg) to decrease mortality.
- IV Pentamidine in some severe cases.
- Sulfa allergy: Dapsone-Trimethoprim, Clindamycin-Primaquine, Atovaquone, IV Pentamidine.

G6PD deficiency:

- Mild disease: Atovaquone in sulfa-intolerant patients with G6PDD.
- Moderate disease: in sulfa-intolerant patients - Atovaquone, desensitize to TMP-SMX or switch to IV Pentamidine are options. **Avoid Dapsone or Primaquine.**

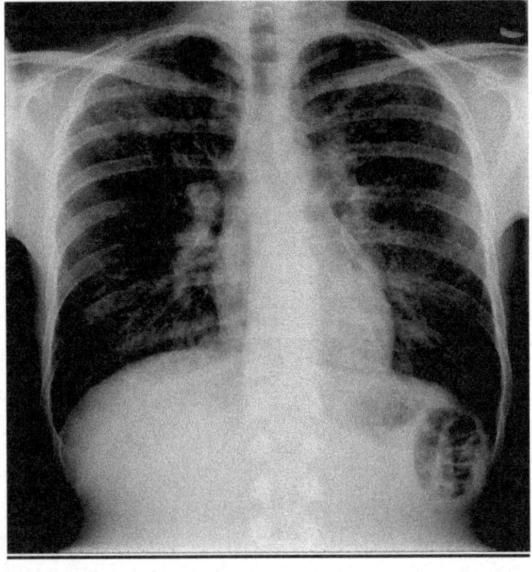

PCP Pneumonia:

- May have normal CXR 10-40% of cases.
- When ⊕, CXR findings classically show **bilateral diffuse symmetric finely granular opacities/reticular-interstitial airspace disease** 80%.
- Often with central location (can resemble non cardiogenic pulmonary edema).

PCP PROPHYLAXIS IN HIV

CD4 ≤200 cells/μL ⇨ **Trimethoprim-sulfamethoxazole.**

TUBERCULOSIS

- Infection of the respiratory system by ***Mycobacterium tuberculosis.***
- Transmission: **inhalation of airborne droplets.**
- Pathophysiology: after inhalation, Mtb goes to the alveoli, gets incorporated into macrophages and can disseminate from there.

RISK FACTORS
- Close contact with someone infected with TB, immigrants from highly endemic regions, crowded conditions (eg, prisons, shelters), healthcare workers, immunosuppression (eg, Diabetes mellitus).
- **TB & HIV infection: 7-10% yearly chance of reactivation** of latent TB infection.

OUTCOMES OF INFECTION WITH TUBERCULOSIS:

Primary TB
- The outcome of initial infection (usually self-limiting).
- Primary Rapidly Progressive TB: active initial infection with clinical progression ⇨ these patients are contagious. Common in children (especially <4 years of age) in endemic areas.

Chronic (Latent infection):
- **~90% control initial primary infection via caseating granuloma formation.** These granulomas may become caseating (central necrosis & acidic with low oxygen, making it hostile for Mtb to grow). Usually PPD ⊕ 2-4 weeks after infection. Need ALL 3 things to show infected with TB but not infectious: **1) ⊕ PPD + 2) no symptoms of infection + 3) no imaging findings of active infection.**

Secondary (Reactivation) TB:
- **Reactivation of latent TB with waning immune defenses** (elderly, HIV, steroid use, malignancy). 5-10% lifetime incidence. **Most commonly** localized in **apex/upper lobes with cavitary lesions** (due to ↑O_2 content of lung apices). **These patients are contagious.**

CLINICAL MANIFESTATIONS
- Pulmonary: cough (productive or nonproductive), hemoptysis, fever, chills, night sweats, chest pain.
- Extrapulmonary: can affect any organ - **cervical lymph nodes (Scrofula),** meningitis, **Pott's disease (vertebrae),** Miliary TB, pericarditis, adrenal gland involvement, & genitourinary.

DIAGNOSIS:
- **Chest radiograph: often initial test** ordered.
  - **Reactivation: apical (upper lobe)** fibrocavitary disease most common.
  - **Primary TB: middle/lower lobe** consolidation.
  - **Miliary TB:** CXR shows small **millet-seed** like nodular lesions (2-4mm).
  - TB pleurisy: pleural effusion caused by tuberculosis infection.
  - Granuloma: residual evidence of healed primary TB. Ghon's complex: calcified primary focus + lymph node. Ranke's complex: healed fibrocalcific Ghon complex seen on CXR.
- Sputum acid-fast staining: 3 samples taken on 3 consecutive days must be negative to rule out TB. Only one ⊕ sample is needed to rule in TB. Early AM gastric specimens if unable to give sputum.
- Sputum cultures: at least 3 samples on 3 consecutive days (preferably early morning specimens).
- Nucleic acid amplification testing: more sensitive than sputum smears.

MANAGEMENT OF ACTIVE TB
- **Initiate 4-drug therapy: RIPE (Rifampin, Isoniazid, Pyrazinamide, Ethambutol)** for 2 months followed by 4 month continuation phase with Rifampin and Isoniazid (pending sensitivity) – **6 month total treatment duration.**
- Streptomycin can be used instead of Ethambutol (RIPE or RIPS).

DRUG	ADVERSE EFFECTS	CONSIDERATIONS
RIFAMPIN (RIF)	**Thrombocytopenia,** flu-like symptoms. **Orange colored secretions** (eg, tears, urine). GI upset, hypersensitivity, fever, hepatitis.	MOA: inhibits RNA synthesis CI: in patients taking protease inhibitors, NNRTIs
ISONIAZID (INH)	**Hepatitis (especially ↑35y of age).** **Peripheral neuropathy.** Drug-induced lupus, rash. Abdominal pain, high anion gap acidosis. Cytochrome P450 inhibition.	MOA: inhibits mycolic acid synthesis **Peripheral neuropathy prevented by pyridoxine (B_6).** Baseline LFTs recommended.
PYRAZINAMIDE (PZA)	**Hepatitis & hyperuricemia.** GI symptoms, arthritis. **Photosensitive dermatologic rash.**	Can be given after 1st trimester. **Caution in gout & liver disease.**
ETHAMBUTOL (EMB)	**Optic neuritis** ⇨ scotoma, color perception problems (red-green), visual changes. **Peripheral neuropathy**, GI symptoms, rash.	
STREPTOMYCIN (STM)	**Ototoxicity (CN 8), nephrotoxicity.**	Streptomycin is an aminoglycoside.

TREATMENT OF LATENT TB INFECTION (LTBI)

SCENARIO	REGIMEN
Likely INH sensitive	**INH + Pyridoxine** (Vitamin B6) **x 9 months.** Alternatives: RIF x 4 months or INH+ Rifapentine (DOT).
Contact case INH-resistant	RIF + PZA x 4 months (consult with ID specialist).

- **Latent TB diagnosis** must meet all 3 criteria:
  ❶ **asymptomatic** person who is ❷ **PPD ⊕** & ❸ **NO evidence of active infection on CXR/CT scan (these patients are NOT contagious).**
- Treatment of latent TB reduces the lifetime reactivation risk from 10% to 1%.

TB SCREENING FOR INFECTION

- **Purified Protein Derivative (PPD):** examine 48-72h for **TRANSVERSE INDURATION** (redness not considered positive). **Any positive PPD should be followed by CXR to rule out active disease.**

REACTION SIZE	PERSONS CONSIDERED TO HAVE ⊕ TEST
≥5 mm	**- HIV ⊕ or immunosuppressed** (eg, Prednisone 15mg/day >1 month). **- Close contacts of patients with active TB.** **- CXR consistent with old/healed TB (calcified granuloma).**
≥10 mm	**- All other high-risk populations/high prevalence populations.** - Recent conversion = ↑induration by >10 mm in the past 2 years.
≥15 mm	Everyone else (no known risk factors for TB)
False negative	**Anergy** (HIV, Sarcoidosis), **Faulty application** (if given SQ instead of TD), acute TB (normally takes 2-10 weeks to convert), acute non-TB infections, malignancy.
False ⊕	**Improper reading, cross reaction with an atypical** (eg, Mycobacterium avium complex), **within 2-10 years of BCG vaccination** (although usually <10mm).
Booster effect	Infected person's immune system "forgets" about TB until years later when testing "reminds" the immune system. Next PPD will be ⊕ because of initial infection (years ago) NOT because recently converted. Confirmed by 2-step PPD testing.

History of a previous BCG vaccine has no impact or effect on recommendations for the screening and treatment of Latent tuberculosis infection in adults.

- **Interferon Gamma Release Assay:** blood test with improved specificity, no reader bias, no booster phenomenon, & not affected by prior BCG vaccination (eg, Quantiferon-TB Gold assay).
- Chest radiograph: used in PPD+ patients who require yearly screening (eg, healthcare workers).

NORMAL CXR

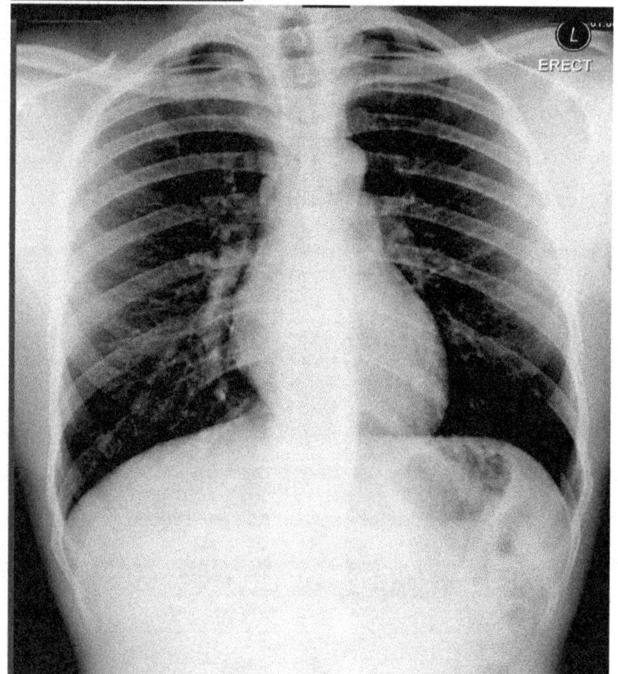

MILIARY TUBERCULOSIS

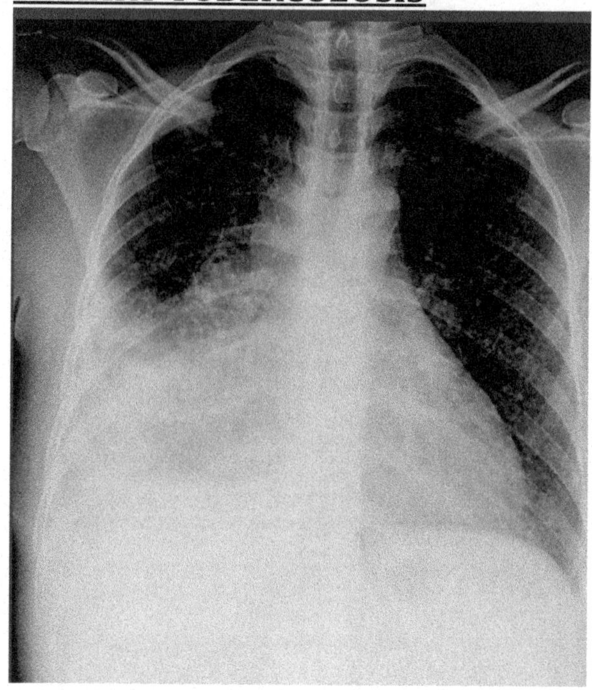

CLASSIC MILIARY TB: diffuse millet seed size infiltrates throughout the lung fields.

CLASSIC PRIMARY TB

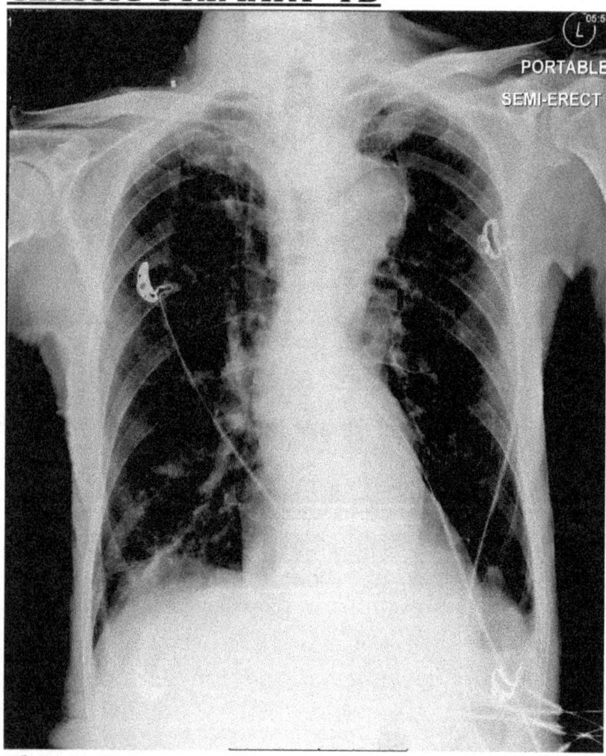

Classic Primary TB:
Lower lobe consolidation.
Right-sided hilar consolidation also seen here.

CLASSIC REACTIVATION TB

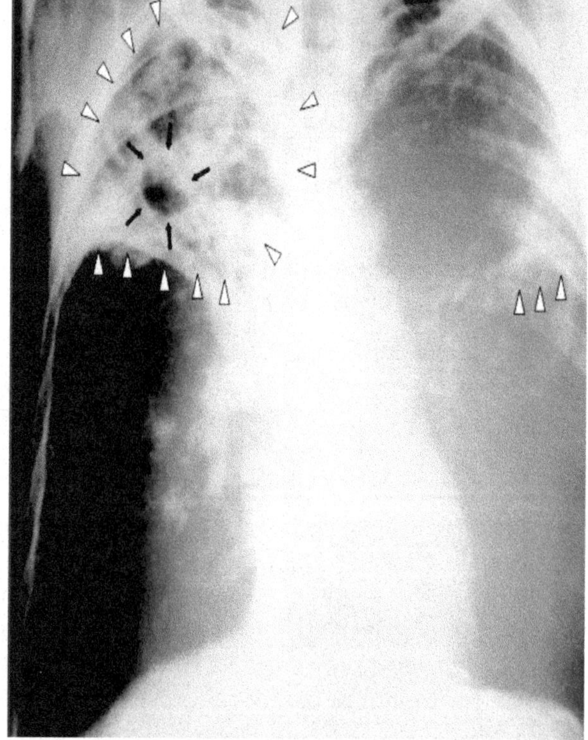

CLASSIC REACTIVATION TB:
Infiltrates and **cavitation** in the **upper lobe/apices.**

SOLITARY PULMONARY NODULE

- Single, small (30 mm or less), usually well-circumscribed lesion that is surrounded entirely by pulmonary parenchyma.

ETIOLOGIES

- **Infectious granulomas most common** (>75% of all benign nodules), especially Mycobacteria (eg, Tuberculosis) and fungi (eg, Histoplasmosis, Coccidioidomycosis).
- May be benign or malignant tumors (eg, lung cancer, metastasis, carcinoid tumors). Thymoma most common mediastinal tumor.

RISK OF MALIGNANCY

- **Increased risk**: **spiculated** nodule, large (>2 cm), irregular borders, asymmetric calcification, upper lobe location, >40 years of age, smoker, enlarging lesions, abnormal PET scan.
- **Decreased risk**: well circumscribed smooth borders, small (<1cm), **dense diffuse calcification, <30 years of age**, nonsmoker, no change in size, normal CT scan.

DIAGNOSTIC WORKUP

- **Chest radiograph: usually the initial test** that revealed the pulmonary nodule.
- CT chest: **imaging of choice to determine the likelihood of malignancy of a nodule found incidentally on chest radiographs**.
- PET scan may be used to determine to determine metabolic functioning of the nodule.

MANAGEMENT

- Low probability: active surveillance with monitoring for changes.
- Intermediate: bronchoscopy if central lesion. Transthoracic needle aspiration for peripheral lesion.
- High: resection with biopsy.

BRONCHIAL CARCINOID TUMORS

- Rare neuroendocrine (enterochromaffin cell) tumors characterized by slow growth, low metastasis and are usually well-differentiated.
- GI tract is the most common site of carcinoid tumors. Lung is the second most common.
- May secrete serotonin, ACTH, ADH, or melanocyte stimulating hormone. Most common <60y.

CLINICAL MANIFESTATIONS

- Most are asymptomatic.
- Focal wheezing, cough, hemoptysis. SIADH, Cushing's syndrome, obstruction.
- **Carcinoid syndrome:** (rare but classic) - periodic episodes of **diarrhea** (serotonin release), **flushing, tachycardia, and bronchoconstriction** (histamine release) and hemodynamic instability (eg, hypotension).

DIAGNOSIS

- Bronchoscopy: **pink to purple well-vascularized centrally-located tumor.**
- Tumor localization: CT scan & Octreotide scintigraphy.
- Biopsy is definitive.

MANAGEMENT

- Surgical excision definitive management. Tumors are often resistant to radiation and chemotherapy.
- Octreotide may be used to reduce symptoms (decreases secretion of the active hormones).

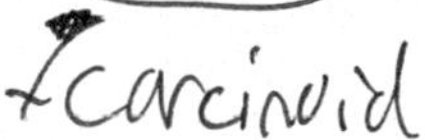

BRONCHOGENIC CARCINOMA

- Second most common cancer diagnosed in the US (after prostate in men & breast in women).
- **Most common cause of cancer-related deaths in the US.**
- Greatest tendency to METS to the brain, bone, liver, lymph nodes, & adrenals.

RISK FACTORS

- **Cigarette smoking most common cause** (including second-hand). Smoking associated with >90% (exception is lepidic pattern). Asbestosis second most common cause.
- **Asbestosis & smoking are synergistic.**
- Radon exposure (eg, uranium miners). Idiopathic Pulmonary Fibrosis, Tuberculosis, & COPD associated with increased lung cancer incidence. Genetic susceptibility is also a factor.

DIVIDED INTO 2 MAIN TYPES

- **Non-small cancer:** includes Adenocarcinoma, Large cell, Squamous cell, Lepidic pattern. **Usually treated with surgical resection.**
- **Small cell cancer:** because it usually metastatic at the time of presentation, **chemotherapy is the initial management of choice for most** (with or without radiation).

LUNG CANCER SCREENING

- The US Preventative Services Task Force recommends **annual low-dose CT screening** for those **55-80 who have no symptoms of lung cancer + a 30 PPY smoking history who currently smoke or have quit within 15 years.**
- Screening should be discontinued once a person has not smoked for 15 years or develops a health condition that substantially limits life expectancy or the ability or willingness to undergo curative surgery.

ADENOCARCINOMA OF THE LUNG

- **Most common primary lung cancer in smokers, women, men, & nonsmokers.**

RISK FACTORS

- **Smoking strongest risk factor**. Exposure to silica, asbestos, radon, heavy metals.

CHARACTERISTICS

- **Typically peripheral.** Arises from bronchial mucosal glands. It is a type of non-small cell lung cancer.
- With the new classification, bronchioloalveolar carcinoma and mixed subtypes Adenocarcinoma are eliminated. "Lepidic" has been used to describe non-invasive growth along intact alveolar septae (formerly bronchioloalveolar).
- Lepidic pattern: a rare low-grade subtype (has the best prognosis). Classically presents with voluminous sputum & an interstitial lung pattern on CXR.

CLINICAL MANIFESTATIONS

- Asymptomatic in early disease. Cough, dyspnea, hemoptysis, weight loss.

DIAGNOSIS

- Histology: **gland formation, mucin production**.

MANAGEMENT

- **Surgical resection in most cases.**

SQUAMOUS CELL LUNG CARCINOMA

- Tumor arises from proximal portions of the tracheobronchial epithelium. Most are bronchial in origin.
- Classified as a type of non-small cell lung carcinoma.
- Second most common cause of lung carcinoma (after Adenocarcinoma).

RISK FACTORS

- **Smoking strongly associated.**

CHARACTERISTICS

- "CCCP" **typically centrally located** and may be associated with a widened mediastinum. Associated with **cavitary lesions, hypercalcemia,** & **Pancoast syndrome.**

DIAGNOSIS

- May be detected in the sputum since it is commonly central.
- Biopsy: keratinization and/or intracellular desmosomes (bridges).

SMALL CELL (OAT CELL) CARCINOMA

- Aggressive type of lung cancer associated with **early metastasis.**
- Comprises about 15% of all lung cancers.

RISK FACTORS:

- **Cigarette smoking** has the strongest association with Small cell lung cancer (SCLC) and Squamous cell carcinoma. Males.

CLINICAL MANIFESTATIONS

- Cough, chest pain, dyspnea, hemoptysis, wheezing, weight loss.
- **Paraneoplastic syndromes:** SVC syndrome, SIADH (hyponatremia), Cushing syndrome, & Lambert-Eaton syndrome. SCLC is the most common solid tumor to present with paraneoplastic syndromes.

DIAGNOSIS

- Chest radiograph: mass often **centrally located.** CT scan gives more information.
- Biopsy: usually CT-guided or via bronchoscopy (if central).
- Histology: sheets of small dark blue cells with rosette formation (about 2x the size of lymphocytes). The size of the cells primarily distinguish small cell from NSCLC.

MANAGEMENT

- **Chemotherapy is the treatment for most** (with or without radiation) because they are **often metastatic at the time of presentation.**

PARANEOPLASTIC SYNDROMES

- Set of systemic symptoms and/or signs due to tumor release of hormones & cytokines or by an immune response against the tumor.
- Examples: SVC syndrome, SIADH (hyponatremia), Cushing syndrome & Lambert-Eaton syndrome.
- Small cell lung carcinoma is the most common solid tumor to present with paraneoplastic syndromes.

SUPERIOR VENA CAVA SYNDROME

- Signs and symptoms due to partial or complete extrinsic obstruction of blood flow through the superior vena cava.

ETIOLOGIES

- **Small cell bronchogenic carcinoma most common**, Hodgkin lymphoma, metastatic tumors, SVC stenosis.

CLINICAL MANIFESTATIONS

- Face and/or neck swelling, facial plethora, headache, **dilated & prominent neck & chest veins**.

DIAGNOSIS

- Chest radiograph: may show right hilar mass or widening of the mediastinum.
- CT scan provides better imaging and can assess the degree of obstruction.

MANAGEMENT

- Supportive: elevation of the head. Endovascular management.

LAMBERT-EATON MYASTHENIC SYNDROME

- **Antibodies against presynaptic voltage-gated calcium channels** prevent acetylcholine release, leading to muscle weakness.
- **Most commonly associated with Small cell lung cancer** & other malignancies.

CLINICAL MANIFESTATIONS

- **Proximal muscle weakness that improves with repeated muscle use** (unlike Myasthenia gravis). The weakness may cause difficulty arising from a chair, gait alteration or managing stairs.
- **Autonomic symptoms: dry mouth most common,** postural hypotension, & erectile dysfunction.
- Physical examination: **Hyporeflexia.** Sluggish pupillary response. No muscle atrophy.

DIAGNOSIS

- Voltage-gated calcium channel antibody assay.
- Electrophysiology: reproducible post exercise increase in compound muscle activation on repetitive nerve stimulation testing.
- CT scan to assess for underlying malignancy.

MANAGEMENT

- **Treat the underlying malignancy.**
- Initial medical management: **Pyridostigmine**. 3,4-diaminopyridine.
- Second-line: Plasmapheresis, IVIG, oral immunosuppressants.

SUPERIOR SULCUS (PANCOAST) TUMORS

- **Tumors located in the superior sulcus** (near the apex) characterized by a distinct pattern of signs and symptoms.
- The diagnosis of Pancoast tumor is determined by the location not the histology.

ETIOLOGIES

- Non-small cell lung carcinoma > 95% of all cases (eg, **Squamous cell lung carcinoma**).

PATHOPHYSIOLOGY

- Tumor compression of the lower brachial plexus, ulnar nerve and/or cervical sympathetic nerve chain.

CLINICAL MANIFESTATIONS

- **Shoulder and arm pain most common initial symptom** (in the distribution of the C8, T1, and T2 dermatomes).
- **Horner syndrome:** the triad of **ipsilateral ptosis, miosis, and anhidrosis**. May be preceded by ipsilateral flushing and facial diaphoresis.
- **Weakness atrophy of the muscles of the hand** and/or arm.
- May have **ulnar neuropathy.**
- Because the tumors are usually peripheral, pulmonary symptoms (eg, cough, dyspnea, hemoptysis) are uncommon until the disease is advances.

DIAGNOSIS

- **Chest radiograph often initial test ordered** but MRI is better to assess the extent of infiltration of adjacent tissues.
- Needle biopsy definitive diagnosis.

MANAGEMENT

- Options include combination of induction chemotherapy/radiotherapy followed by radical surgical resection.

Pancoast tumor (labeled as P, non-small cell lung carcinoma, right lung),

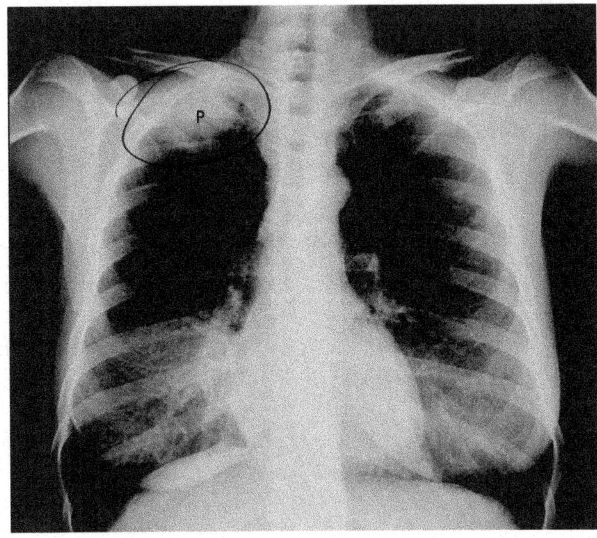

Horner's syndrome: miosis, ptosis, anhidrosis (due to cervical cranial nerve sympathetic compression.

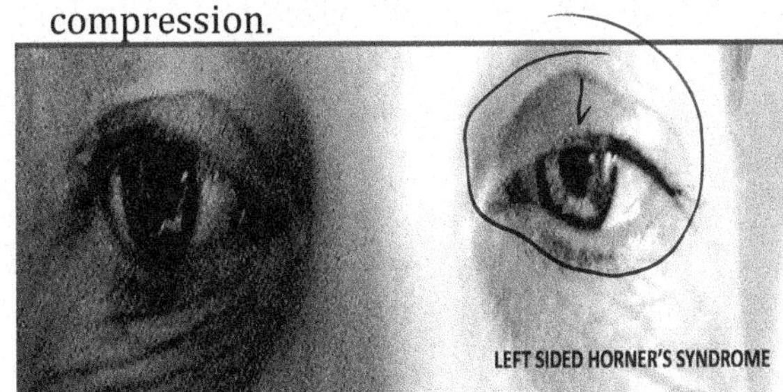

MESOTHELIOMA

- **Tumor originating from the pleura** (80%), peritoneum (2nd most common), tunica vaginalis, or pericardium. ¾ are malignant (poor prognosis if malignant).
- **80% due to chronic asbestos exposure.**

CLINICAL MANIFESTATIONS
- Pleural mesothelioma: pleuritic chest pain, dyspnea, fever, night sweats, weight loss, hemoptysis.

DIAGNOSIS
- Chest radiograph: **unilateral pleural thickening,** bloody pleural effusions are common.
- Pleural biopsy: closed, via video-assisted thoracoscopy (VATS), or open thoracotomy.

MANAGEMENT
- Combined approach may include chemotherapy (eg, a platinum agent plus pemetrexed), macroscopic complete resection with either pleurectomy/decortication or radical extrapleural pneumonectomy, and radiation therapy.
- Not surgical candidate: systemic chemotherapy and/or palliative radiation therapy.

FOREIGN BODY ASPIRATION

- Aerodigestive foreign body causing varying amounts of obstruction to the airway.
- Common items include food, coins, toys food and balloons **(peanuts are the most common foreign body aspirated in children).**
- **Mean age is 2** (incisors are used to bite the food but absence of molars make it difficult to grind food).
- The main cause of death is due to hypoxic-ischemic brain injury and less commonly, pulmonary hemorrhage.
- Complications include bronchiectasis, pneumonia, lung abscess, and atelectasis.
- **Most common on the right side** (due to wider, more vertical, & shorter right main bronchus).
  Position may influence location:
  Supine: most common in superior segment of the right lower lobe.
  Sitting/standing: most common in posterobasal segment of the right lower lobe.
  Lying on right side: most common in right middle lobe or posterior segment of the right upper lobe.

CLINICAL MANIFESTATIONS
- Asymptomatic or **sudden onset of choking, cough, and dyspnea**.
- Physical examination: **wheezing or asymmetric breath sounds.** May be normal.

DIAGNOSIS
- Chest radiographs: **air trapping most common finding in children,** atelectasis, pneumothorax. A normal chest radiograph does not rule out FB aspiration. May order additional neck films.
- CT chest: may be indicated in symptomatic patients with negative radiographs.
- **Rigid bronchoscopy definitive diagnostic test** (also therapeutic because object can be removed). Flexible rather than rigid bronchoscopy may be used for diagnostic purposes in cases when the diagnosis is not clear or if the FBA is known but the location is unclear.

MANAGEMENT
- **Removal of foreign object via rigid bronchoscopy.** Thoracotomy if refractory to bronchoscopy.
- In acute choking, the Heimlich maneuver should be performed. Emergency tracheostomy performed if Heimlich maneuver is not successful.

COSTOCHONDRITIS & TIETZE SYNDROME

COSTOCHONDRITIS

- Acute inflammation of the costal cartilages or costochondral junctions.

ETIOLOGIES
- Often idiopathic but can occur postviral or posttraumatic (eg, physical strain, excessive coughing).

CLINICAL MANIFESTATIONS
- **Pleuritic chest pain** that may be worse with inspiration, coughing, or certain body movements.

PHYSICAL EXAMINATION
- **Reproducible point chest wall tenderness** with palpation, most commonly involves the third, fourth & fifth sternocostal joints.
- The **absence of palpable edema** helps to distinguish Costochondritis from the less common Tietze syndrome.

DIAGNOSIS
- Usually a diagnosis of exclusion. Labs, ECG, and radiographs are usually within normal limits.

MANAGEMENT
- NSAIDs

TIETZE SYNDROME

- Acute inflammation of the costal cartilages or costochondral junctions.

ETIOLOGIES
- Often idiopathic but can occur postviral or posttraumatic (eg, physical strain, excessive coughing).

CLINICAL MANIFESTATIONS
- **Pleuritic chest pain** that may be worse with inspiration, coughing, or certain body movements.

PHYSICAL EXAMINATION
- **Reproducible point chest wall tenderness with palpable edema.** Most commonly involves the second and third costochondral junctions.
- The presence of palpable edema distinguishes Tietze from Costochondritis.

DIAGNOSIS
- Usually a diagnosis of exclusion. Labs, ECG, and radiographs are usually within normal limits.

MANAGEMENT
- NSAIDs

PLEURAL EFFUSION

- Abnormal accumulation of fluid in the pleural space (not a disease itself but a sign of a disease).

TYPES

- Parapneumonic: **noninfected pleural effusion** secondary to bacterial pneumonia.
- Empyema: **direct infection of the pleural space** - grossly purulent/turbulent effusion.
- Hemothorax: gross blood (eg, chest trauma or malignancy).
- Chylothorax: increased lymph. Associated with persistent turbidity after centrifuge (if not ⇨ empyemic).

ETIOLOGIES

- **Transudate: CHF most common cause (> 90%), Nephrotic syndrome, Cirrhosis,** Atelectasis, Hypoalbuminemia. Due to either increased hydrostatic pressure or decreased oncotic pressure.
- **Exudate: any condition associated with infection or inflammation.** Contains plasma, proteins, WBCs, platelets, & RBCs. **Pulmonary embolism** (rarely transudative), malignancy.

PRESENTATION

- Clinical manifestations: asymptomatic, dyspnea, pleuritic chest pain, cough.
- Physical examination: **dullness to percussion, decreased fremitus, decreased breath sounds.** May have a pleural friction rub.

DIAGNOSIS:

- Chest radiographs: **initial test of choice - blunting of the costophrenic angles (meniscus sign).** Lateral decubitus also helpful to differentiate loculations from empyema and detect smaller effusions. In extreme cases, it may cause lung collapse or mediastinal shift to the contralateral side.
  - PA/lateral: >175cc can obscure the lateral costophrenic sulcus. 500cc (for the diaphragm). **Blunting of costophrenic angles (⊕ menisci sign)** ± loculations (due to pleural adhesions).
  - **Lateral decubitus films: best** - detects smaller effusions, differentiates loculations & empyema from new effusions or scarring.

- **Thoracentesis: diagnostic gold standard.** Can be diagnostic and therapeutic. Helps to distinguish between transudate and exudate. Not usually performed if the cause is clear.

  Light's criteria: an exudate is present if any of these 3 are present
  1) pleural fluid protein : serum protein >0.5 or
  2) Pleural fluid LDH: serum LDH >0.6 or
  3) Pleural fluid LDH >2/3 the upper limit of normal LDH
- CT scan or US: may be helpful for additional information (eg, if an Empyema is present).

MANAGEMENT

- **Treat the underlying disease mainstay of treatment** (pleural effusion is a sign of an underlying disease).

- Thoracentesis: diagnostic and therapeutic. Not always needed. Don't remove > 1.5 liters during any one procedure.

- Chest tube fluid drainage: if **empyema (eg, pleural fluid pH < 7.2, glucose < 40 mg/dL, or positive gram stain** of pleural fluid). May inject with streptokinase to facilitate breakup of loculations.

- Pleurodesis: if malignant or chronic effusions. Talc most commonly used, Doxycycline, Minocycline. Bleomycin rarely used due toxicity.

PLEURAL EFFUSION

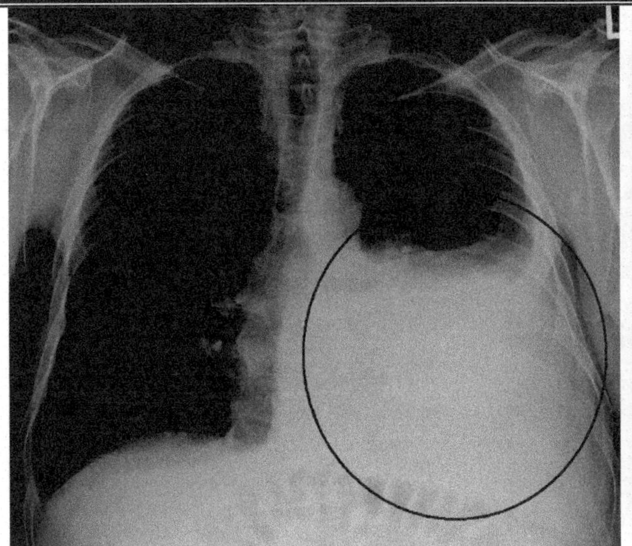

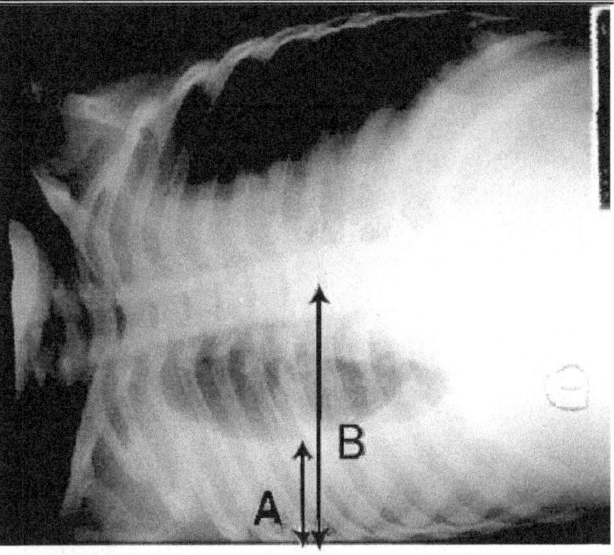

Pleural Effusion PA Film: notice the clear costophrenic angle on the right side with **blunting of the costophrenic angle** on the left side.

Pleural Effusion (Lateral Decubitus Film): layering of the fluid.

PNEUMOTHORAX

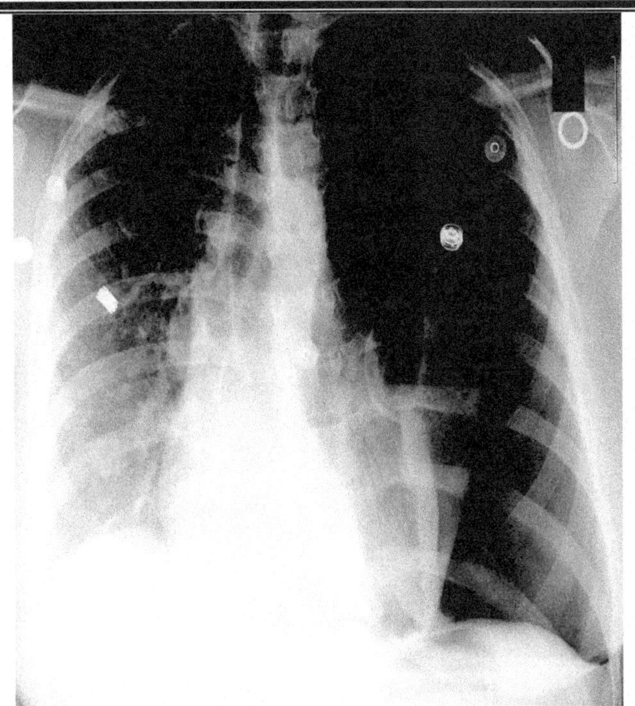

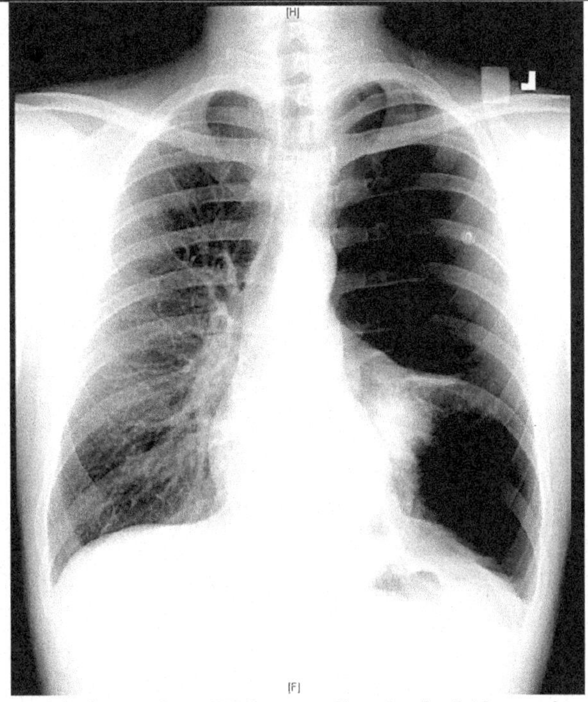

Linear shadow of visceral pleura with **decreased peripheral lung markings on the left side**

L-sided tension PTX: **mediastinal shift** to the right side.

PNEUMOTHORAX

- Air in the pleural space, leading to collapse of the lung from the positive intrapleural air pressure.

TYPES

- Primary spontaneous (PSP): atraumatic and idiopathic with **no underlying lung disease**. Due to bleb rupture. Mainly affects **tall, thin men 20- 40 years of age, smokers,** family history of Pneumothorax.
- **Secondary spontaneous (SSP): underlying lung disease** (eg, COPD, Asthma).
- Traumatic: iatrogenic (eg, during CPR, thoracentesis, PEEP ventilation, subclavian line placement). Car accidents etc.
- **Tension:** any type in which **positive air pressure pushes the trachea, great vessels, & heart to the contralateral side.**
- Catamenial: occurs during menstruation (ectopic endometrial tissue in the pleural space).

CLINICAL MANIFESTATIONS

- **Chest pain** - usually **pleuritic, unilateral,** non-exertional, sudden. Dyspnea.

PHYSICAL EXAMINATION

- **Hyperresonance to percussion, decreased fremitus**, & **decreased breath sounds** over the affected area. Unequal respiratory expansion.
- Tension: **increased JVP, systemic hypotension,** pulsus paradoxus.

DIAGNOSIS

- **Chest radiograph: initial test of choice (expiratory upright view preferred).**
  - Decreased peripheral markings (collapsed lung tissue)
  - **Companion lines** (visceral pleural line running parallel with the ribs).
  - Deep sulcus sign on supine film.

MANAGEMENT

Small PSP < 3 cm from chest wall at the apex:

- **Observation + supplemental oxygen** if small & first episode (<15-20% the diameter of the hemithorax or less than 3 cm between the chest wall & the lung on CXR). May be discharged if stable & repeat films after 6 hours excludes progression. Chest tube thoracostomy if worse on repeat films.

Large PSP (>3 cm from chest the wall at the apex):

- Needle or catheter aspiration vs. chest tube or catheter thoracostomy.

Stable, SSP:

- **Chest tube or catheter thoracostomy + hospitalization**

Tension:

- **Needle aspiration followed by chest tube** thoracostomy.

Other:

- Thoracoscopy: may be indicated if there is persistent leak after chest tube placement or no regression with chest tube.
- Persistent or recurrent: video-assisted thoracoscopic surgery or thoracotomy.

PATIENT EDUCATION

- Avoid pressure changes for a minimum of 2 weeks (eg, high altitudes, smoking, unpressurized aircrafts, scuba diving).

PULMONARY HYPERTENSION

- **Elevated mean pulmonary arterial pressure ≥20 mmHg** with a pulmonary vascular resistance > 3 Wood units.

PATHOPHYSIOLOGY
- Increased pulmonary vascular resistance leads to right ventricular hypertrophy, increased RV pressure and eventually right-sided Heart failure.
- Primary: **Idiopathic. Most common in middle-aged or young women** (mean age of diagnosis 50 years). BMPR2 gene defect. BMPR2 gene normally inhibits pulmonary vessel smooth muscle growth and vasoconstriction.
- Secondary: pulmonary HTN due to pulmonary disease, sleep apnea, PE, cardiac, metabolic, or systemic disease.

CLASSIFICATION

I:	**Idiopathic pulmonary arterial hypertension (Primary).** Diagnosis of exclusion.
II:	Pulmonary HTN due to left heart disease
III:	Pulmonary HTN due to hypoxemic or chronic lung disease (eg, COPD)
IV:	Pulmonary HTN due to chronic thromboembolic disease

CLINICAL MANIFESTATIONS
- **Dyspnea,** fatigue, chest pain, weakness, cyanosis, edema. Exertional syncope if severe.

PHYSICAL EXAMINATION
- **Accentuated S2:** due to prominent P2. May have a fixed or paradoxically split P2.
- **Signs of right-sided Heart failure:** increased JVP, peripheral edema, ascites.
- Pulmonary regurgitation, right ventricular heave, systolic ejection click.

DIAGNOSIS
- Chest radiograph: enlarged pulmonary arteries, interstitial or alveolar edema, signs of right-sided heart failure.
- ECG: **cor pulmonale** (eg, RVH, right axis deviation, right atrial enlargement, right BBB).
- Echocardiogram: large right ventricle, RVH.
- **Right heart catheterization: definitive diagnosis (gold standard)** – elevated pulmonary artery pressure, RV pressure, and increased pulmonary vascular resistance.
- CBC: **polycythemia** with **increased hematocrit.**

MANAGEMENT
- Correct the underlying cause if identified.

- Primary: vasoreactivity trial with inhaled Nitric oxide, IV Adenosine or Calcium channel blocker.
  - **If vasoreactive, Calcium channel blockers are first-line.**
  - **Prostacyclins** (eg, Epoprostenol, Iloprost)
  - **Phosphodiesterase-5 inhibitors** (eg, Sildenafil, Tadalafil)
  - Endothelin receptor antagonists (eg, Bosentan)
  - **Oxygen therapy**, especially if associated with COPD.
  - Long-term anticoagulation in some.

- Heart-lung transplant definitive.

PULMONARY EMBOLISM (PE)

- Obstruction of the pulmonary blood flow due to a blood clot (usually a thromboembolism from a DVT).
- **70% arise from deep vein in the legs** (the majority of the rest are from the pelvic veins).

RISK FACTORS: Virchow's triad:
- **Intimal damage** - eg, trauma, infection, inflammation.
- **Stasis** - eg, immobilization, surgery, prolonged sitting >4 hours.
- **Hypercoagulability** - eg, Protein C or S Deficiency, Factor V Leiden mutation, antithrombin III deficiency, oral contraceptive use, malignancy, pregnancy, smoking.

CLINICAL MANIFESTATIONS
- Symptoms: classic triad of sudden onset of **dyspnea (most common symptom), pleuritic chest pain**, hemoptysis (classic but rare); cough.
- PHYSICAL EXAMINATION: **tachypnea (most common sign)**, tachycardia, low-grade fever. Positive Homan sign (not specific). Lung exam is usually normal.
- If massive PE, may present with syncope, hypotension and/or pulseless electrical activity.

ANCILLARY TESTS IN PE:
Chest radiographs: most common initial test to evaluate chest pain. CXR often normal in PE.
- **A normal CXR (most common finding) in the setting of hypoxia is highly suspicious for PE.**
- Atelectasis is the most common abnormal finding.
- Classic but rare findings include:
  - **Westermark's sign** - avascular markings distal to the PE.
  - **Hampton's hump** - wedge-shaped infiltrate due to infarction.

ECG:
- **Nonspecific ST/T changes & sinus tachycardia most common.**
- Right heart dysfunction (5%) may show **S1Q3T3 - most specific for PE** (wide deep S in lead I; both an isolated Q as well as T wave inversion in lead III), right ventricular strain, right bundle branch block, or inferior Q waves.

- ABG: **initially respiratory alkalosis** (2ry to hyperventilation) **+ hypoxemia**. Respiratory acidosis may occur with time or massive PE. Increased A-a gradient.

- D dimer: **helpful ONLY if negative & low suspicion for PE** (high sensitivity, poor specificity).

Confirmatory tests for PE:
- **Helical (spiral) CT angiography: best initial test confirm the presence of PE** in most patients (>95% specificity, sensitivity 95-98%).

- **V/Q scan:** used in patients when CT scan can't be performed (eg, **pregnancy, increased creatinine**). Interpreted based on clinical suspicion. A normal one rules out PE. If indeterminate, then test for DVT. If DVT negative, may proceed to angiography. If high probability, treat as if positive for PE.

- Pulmonary angiography: *gold standard (definitive).* Not usually performed (associated with 0.5% mortality). May be ordered if high suspicion & negative CT or VQ scan.

- Venous Doppler ultrasound of the lower extremities: may be used if VQ scan or CT does not give a clear diagnosis. Serial ultrasounds may be performed to increase diagnostic specificity in patients with a negative PE.

MANAGEMENT OF PE

Hemodynamically stable:

- **Anticoagulation: first-line therapy in most patients -** eg, Heparin bridge plus Warfarin or a novel oral anticoagulant (eg, Dabigatran, Rivaroxaban, Apixaban, or Edoxaban).

- **IVC filter:** indicated in stable 3 patients:
  1) **anticoagulation is contraindicated** (eg, recent bleed, bleeding disorders).
  2) **anticoagulation is unsuccessful -** PE despite anticoagulation (eg, INR 2-3 on Warfarin).
  3) if RV dysfunction is seen on echocardiogram (the next embolus, even if small can be fatal).

Hemodynamically unstable:

Hypotension SBP < 90 mmHg), acute RV dysfunction

- Thrombolysis: hemodynamically unstable patients or severe PE (eg, right-sided Heart failure).
  - Contraindicated if bleed, CVA, recent intracranial bleed, or bleeding disorder.
  - Relative contraindications: uncontrolled hypertension, surgery, or trauma within 6 weeks.

- Thrombectomy or embolectomy: unstable or massive PE if thrombolysis is contraindicated or ineffective.

SBP < 90 = Hypotension

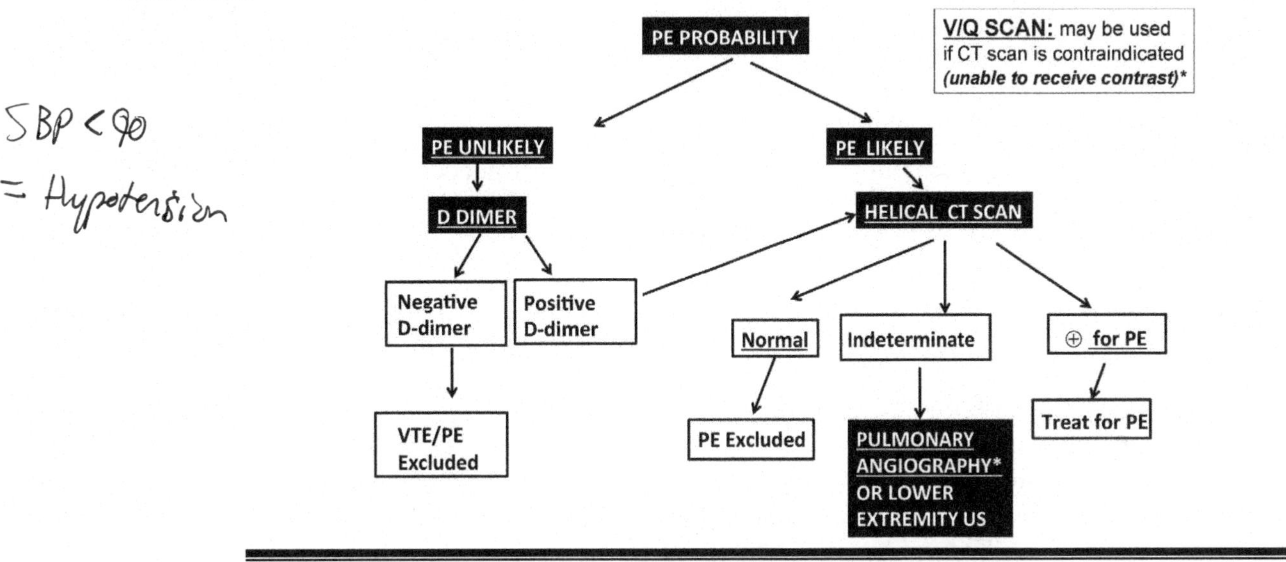

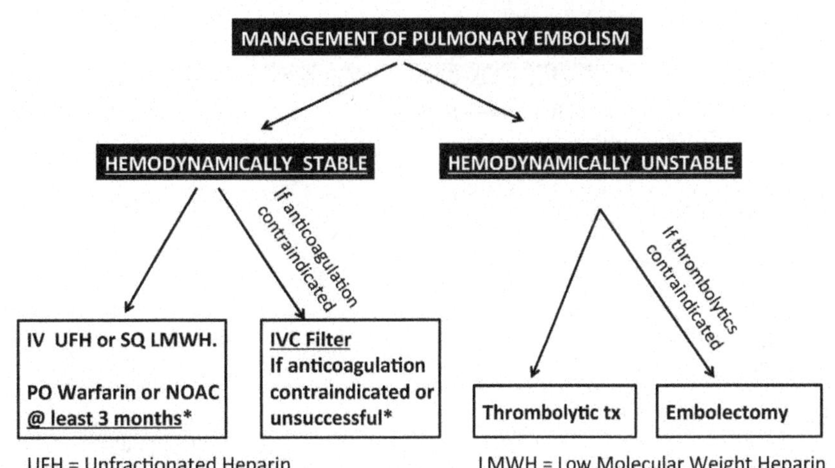

UFH = Unfractionated Heparin
LMWH = Low Molecular Weight Heparin
NOAC = Novel Oral Anticoagulants

- Factor Xa inhibitors (Rivaroxaban, Edoxaban, Apixaban); Direct thrombin inhibitor: Dabigatran

WELLS' CRITERIA FOR PE

Used to determine clinical probability of PE

3 points are added for the following:

- Clinical signs and symptoms of DVT
- PE is #1 diagnosis OR equally likely

1.5 points are added for the following:

- Heart rate > 100 bpm
- Immobilization at least 3 days OR surgery in the previous 4 weeks
- Previous, objectively diagnosed DVT or PE

1 point added:

- Hemoptysis
- Malignancy with treatment within 6 months of palliative

Interpretation:

- Low probability of PE: < 2 points. May consider D-dimer or use PERC criteria.
- Moderate probability: 2-6 points. Consider CT angiography (CTA) or high-sensitivity D-dimer.
- High probability: >6 points. Consider CTA

PERC

The Pulmonary Embolism Rule Out Criteria (PERC) is used in patients with a low clinical probability of PE. The following 8 are part of the PERC criteria:

1. Age <50 years
2. Heart rate <100 beats/minute
3. Oxyhemoglobin saturation 95 percent or greater
4. No hemoptysis
5. No estrogen use
6. No prior DVT or PE
7. No unilateral leg swelling
8. No surgery/trauma requiring hospitalization within the prior four weeks

- In patients with low risk who meet all 8 criteria, no further testing for PE is needed.
- In patients with low risk but do not fulfill all of the criteria, D-dimer testing is indicated.

LOW MOLECULAR WEIGHT HEPARIN (LMWH)	UNFRACTIONATED HEPARIN (UFH)
• **MOA: potentiates antithrombin III -** works more on factor Xa than thrombin (Factor IIa).	• **MOA: potentiates antithrombin III, inhibits thrombin & other coagulation factors.**
• **SQ injection. Compliant, low-risk patients can be discharged home during bridging therapy.**	• Continuous IV drip – requires hospitalization for bridging therapy.
• **Duration of Action ~12 hours.**	• **Duration of Action: 1h after IV drip is discontinued.**
• **No need to monitor PTT** (weight based – more predictable dosing).	• **Must monitor PTT 1.5-2.5x normal value.**
• **Protamine Sulfate is the antidote** (not as effective as it is for UFH).	• **Protamine Sulfate is the antidote.**
• **Lower risk of HIT** (higher anti Xa-IIa ratio means less potential binding with platelets).	• **Heparin Induced Thrombocytopenia** – Heparin acts as a hapten (stimulates the immune response when attached to platelet factor 4). This complex activates platelets, causing simultaneous thrombocytopenia & thrombosis. **Management:** other anticoagulants: ex: Argatroban or Bivalirudin. DO NOT use Warfarin (may develop necrosis)
• **CI: Renal failure** (Cr >2.0) because LMWH excreted by kidneys, **Thrombocytopenia.**	

PE PROPHYLAXIS

The single most important step in managing PE. Prophylaxis is warranted preoperatively in patients undergoing surgery with prolonged immobilization, pregnant women, h/o prior DVT/PE.

- **Early ambulation:** low risk, minor procedures in patients <40y.
- **Elastic stockings/pneumatic compression devices/venodyne boots:** moderate risk.
- **Low molecular weight heparin:** patients undergoing orthopedic or neurosurgery, trauma.

CXR FINDINGS IN PULMONARY EMBOLISM

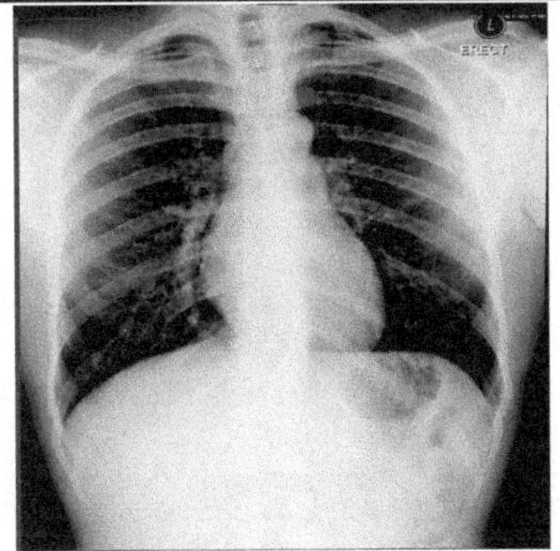

Normal CXR: MC finding in PE

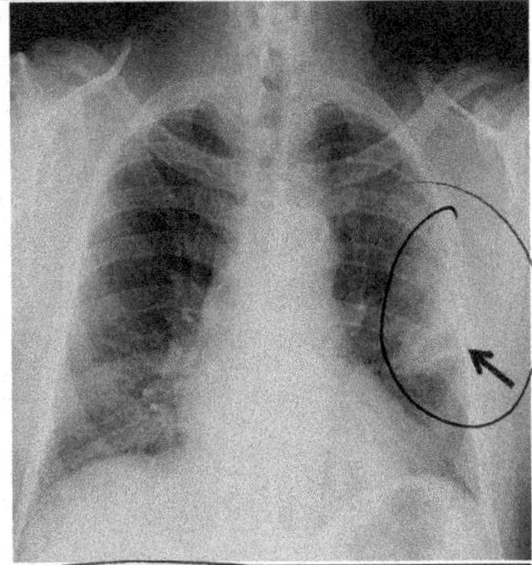

Hampton's Hump: Wedge-shaped infiltrate/infarction (arrow). Classic (not common)

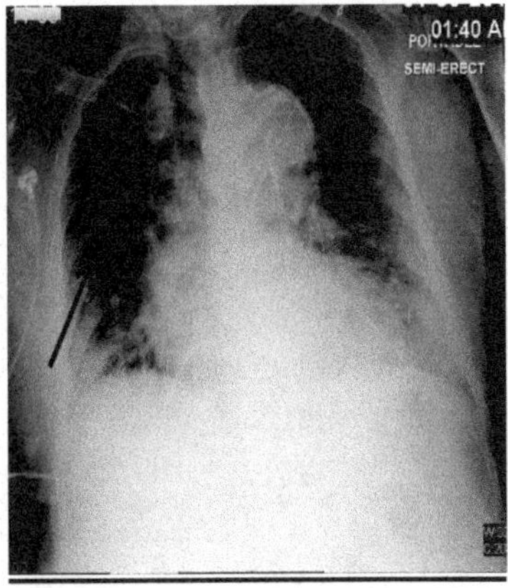

Westermark sign: Avascular markings distal to the area of the embolus. Classic (not common)

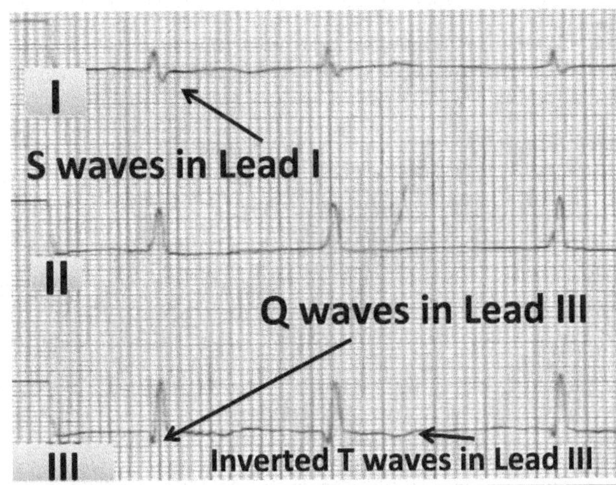

ECG FINDINGS:

❶ **Nonspecific ST/T wave changes and sinus tachycardia are the most common ECG findings.**

❷ **S1Q3T3:** more specific:
- Deep S in lead I
- Pathological Q wave & T wave inversion in lead III.

S1Q3T3 due to the presence of cor pulmonale with a large Pulmonary embolus. Classic (not common).

ACUTE RESPIRATORY DISTRESS SYNDROME

- Acute, diffuse inflammatory form of lung injury and respiratory failure due to a variety of causes.
- **Associated with a high mortality rate** due to acute hypoxemic respiratory & organ failure.

PATHOPHYSIOLOGY

- Diffuse alveolar damage & surfactant leads to increased permeability of the capillary-alveolar barrier, leading to noncardiogenic pulmonary edema, shunting & **hypoxemia without hypercarbia.**

RISK FACTORS

- Most commonly develops in **critically ill patients** (eg, **Gram-negative sepsis – most common**, severe trauma, severe Pancreatitis, aspiration of gastric contents, near drowning etc.).

CLINICAL MANIFESTATIONS

- Acute dyspnea & hypoxemia. Multi-organ failure if severe.

DIAGNOSIS

3 main components:

- **Severe hypoxemia refractory to supplemental oxygen.**

HYPOXEMIA	PaO_2/FIO_2 ratio (mmHg)	VENTILATION
Mild:	201 – 300	PEEP or CPAP ≥5cm H_20 (formerly Acute Lung Injury).
Moderate:	101 - 200	PEEP ≥5 cm H_20
Severe:	100 or less	PEEP ≥5 cm H_20

- Chest radiographs: **bilateral diffuse pulmonary infiltrates** (similar to CHF but ARDS **classically spares the costophrenic angles**).

ADULT RESPIRATORY DISTRESS SYNDROME

Pulmonary Capillary Wedge Pressure:

- *CXR of ARDS & cardiogenic pulmonary edema looks the same*
- *PCWP <18mmHg→ ARDS**
- *PCWP >18mmHg→ Cardio Pul. Edema*

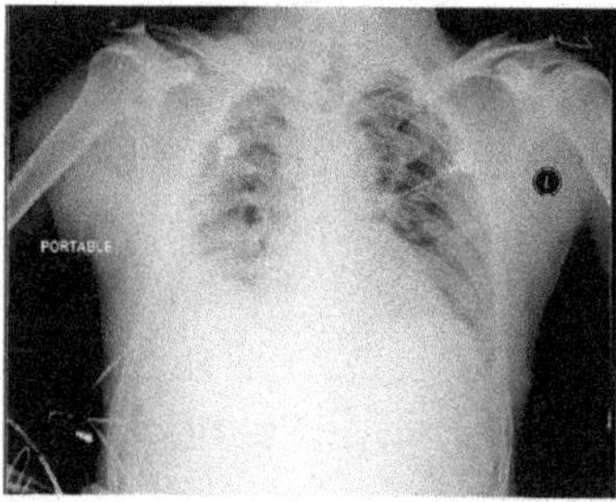

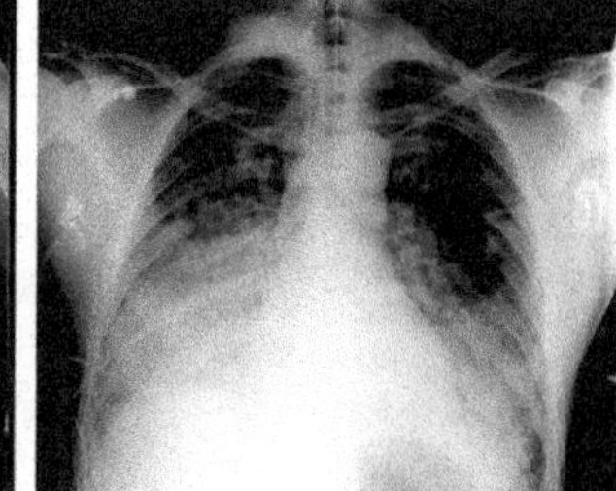

Cardiogenic Pulmonary Edema **ARDS**

- Absence of cardiogenic pulmonary edema (CHF): **pulmonary capillary wedge pressure <18 mm Hg** with right heart catheterization. Normal left atrial pressure.

MANAGEMENT

- **Noninvasive or mechanical ventilation + treat the underlying cause:** CPAP with full face mask, PEEP, & low tidal volume.
  - **Low tidal volume** has been shown to decrease non-pulmonary organ failure and weaning.
  - **Positive end-expiration pressure (PEEP) improves hypoxemia** by preventing alveolar collapse, which improves the ventilation-perfusion mismatch as well as increases functional residual capacity (the volume of air remaining in the lungs at end expiration).

SLEEP APNEA

- Involuntary cessation of breathing during sleep.
- Complications include Pulmonary hypertension & arrhythmias.

RISK FACTORS
- **Obesity strong risk factor,** age (most common in the sixth and seventh decades), males.

TYPES
- Central sleep apnea: reduced CNS respiratory drive leads to decreased respiratory effort.
- Obstructive sleep apnea: physical airway obstruction (may be due to external airway compression, decreased pharyngeal muscle tone, increased tonsil size or deviated septum).

CLINICAL MANIFESTATIONS
- Snoring, unrestful sleep (which may lead to chronic daytime sleepiness). Nocturnal choking.
- Physical examination: large neck circumference, crowded oropharynx, micrognathia.

DIAGNOSIS
- **In-laboratory polysomnography: first line diagnostic test.**
  15 or more events/hour: obstructive or mixed apneas, hypopneas, respiratory effort arousals etc.
- Labs: polycythemia (due to chronic hypoxemia).
- Epworth sleepiness scale: used to quantify patient's perception of fatigue and sleep.

MANAGEMENT
- Behavioral changes include weight loss, abstaining from alcohol, & changes in sleep positioning.
- **CPAP (continuous positive airway pressure) is the mainstay of treatment.**
- Oral appliances can be tried if CPAP is unsuccessful or as an alternative.
- Surgical correction. Tracheostomy is considered the definitive treatment for obstructive sleep apnea. Other interventions include: nasal septoplasty & uvulopalatopharyngoplasty.

NORMAL BREATH SOUNDS

BRONCHIAL	Loud high-pitch sounds heard over trachea and larynx (manubrium).	**Expiration (longer) > inspiration**
BRONCHOVESICULAR	Medium-pitched sounds heard over the primary bronchus and posteriorly between the scapula.	Expiration = Inspiration
VESICULAR	Soft, gentle sounds over all the areas.	Inspiration > expiration

ABNORMAL BREATHING

1. **CHEYNE-STOKES: cyclic breathing in response to hypercapnia.** Smooth increases in respirations & then gradual decrease in respirations with a period of apnea 15-60 seconds.
   Due to **decreased brain blood flow** slowing the impulses to the respiratory center.

2. **BIOT'S BREATHING: irregular respirations (quick shallow breaths of equal depth)* with irregular periods of apnea** (usually of equal depth in comparison to Cheyne-Stokes breathing).
   Can be seen with damage to the medulla oblongata or opioid use.

3. **KUSSMAUL'S RESPIRATION:** (hyperpnea): **deep, rapid, continuous respirations** as a result of **metabolic acidosis** - deep breaths with large tidal volumes (body's attempt to compensate by blowing off excess CO_2). No expiratory pause (no stopping between inhalation & exhalation).

NEONATAL RESPIRATORY DISTRESS SYNDROME

- Atelectasis and pulmonary perfusion without ventilation due to **insufficiency of surfactant production by an immature lung**. Primarily a disease of **preterm infants**.
- Most common single cause of death in the first month of life.
- Surfactant production begins 24 – 28 weeks. By 35 weeks, enough surfactant is produced.

RISK FACTORS

- **Caucasians, males, multiple births, maternal Diabetes,** C-section delivery, perinatal infections.

CLINICAL MANIFESTATIONS

- Usually presents **at birth or shortly after birth with respiratory distress** (eg, tachypnea > 60/min, tachycardia, chest wall retractions, expiratory grunting, nasal flaring, cyanosis).

DIAGNOSIS

- CXR: bilateral diffuse **reticular (ground-glass) opacities + air bronchograms,** poor lung expansion, domed diaphragms.
- ABG: hypoxia (often unresponsive to oxygen supplementation). Normal or slightly increased PCO2.
- Postmortem histopathology: waxy-appearing layers lining the collapsed alveoli. Airway distention.

MANAGEMENT

- **Exogenous surfactant via endotracheal tube** to open the alveoli. Continuous positive airway pressure (CPAP).
- Clinical course is 2-3 days with or without treatment.
- 90% survival rate with treatment and normal return of lung function within 1 month.

PREVENTION

- Antenatal glucocorticoids given to mature lungs if premature delivery expected (between 24-36 wks).

MECONIUM ASPIRATION

- Entrance of meconium-containing amniotic fluid into the respiratory tract ⇨ respiratory distress, hypoxia & acidosis.
- Increased incidence in **postterm infants** & infants small for gestational age. May occur with **fetal distress & hypoxia.**

CLINICAL MANIFESTATIONS

- **Signs of respiratory distress** usually after birth – cyanosis, severe tachypnea, use of accessory muscles, intercostal retractions, nasal flaring.

DIAGNOSIS

- Evidence of meconium-stained amniotic fluid. May be present in the trachea, vernix or umbilical cord.
- CXR: coarse, irregular infiltrates with lung **hyperinflation** (flattened diaphragms, increased AP diameter). May show pneumothorax.

MANAGEMENT

- **Prevention is the most effective therapy – prevention of postterm delivery** (>41 weeks) via labor induction & prevention of fetal hypoxia.
- Supportive management: maintain adequate oxygenation & ventilation, empirical antibiotic therapy, correction of electrolyte abnormalities.

PULMONARY PHOTO CREDITS

Asbestosis
By LT John R. Dryden, MD, MC, USN, Naval Medical Center San Diego. Used with permission.

Asthma step up chart

By National Heart, Blood, and Lung Institute [CC-BY-2.5 (http://creativecommons.org/licenses/by/2.5)], via Wikimedia Commons
Lung Volumes
By Vihsadas at en.wikipedia (Transferred from en.wikipedia) [Public domain], from Wikimedia Commons

Asthma step up chart
By National Heart, Blood, and Lung Institute [CC-BY-2.5 (http://creativecommons.org/licenses/by/2.5)], via Wikimedia Commons
Emphysema CXR
By James Heilman, MD (Own work) [CC-BY-SA-3.0 (http://creativecommons.org/licenses/by-sa/3.0) or GFDL (http://www.gnu.org/copyleft/fdl.html)], via Wikimedia Commons
Lateral CXR Emphysema
By James Heilman, MD (Own work) [CC-BY-SA-3.0 (http://creativecommons.org/licenses/by-sa/3.0) or GFDL (http://www.gnu.org/copyleft/fdl.html)], via Wikimedia Commons
Emphysema CT scan
By PLoS Medicine [CC-BY-3.0 (http://creativecommons.org/licenses/by/3.0)], via Wikimedia Commons
Sarcoidosis
By Jmh649 (Own work) [CC-BY-SA-3.0 (http://creativecommons.org/licenses/by-sa/3.0) or GFDL (http://www.gnu.org/copyleft/fdl.html)], via Wikimedia Commons
Sarcoidosis
Erythema Nodosum
By James Heilman, MD (Own work) [CC-BY-SA-3.0 (http://creativecommons.org/licenses/by-sa/3.0) or GFDL (http://www.gnu.org/copyleft/fdl.html)], via Wikimedia Commons
Lupus Pernio
By M. Sand, D. Sand, C. Thrandorf, V. Paech, P. Altmeyer, F. G. Bechara [CC-BY-2.0 (http://creativecommons.org/licenses/by/2.0)], via Wikimedia Commons
Schaumann Bodies
By Yale Rosen [CC-BY-SA-2.0 (http://creativecommons.org/licenses/by-sa/2.0)], via Wikimedia Commons
Asteroid Bodies
By Nephron (Own work) [CC-BY-SA-3.0 (http://creativecommons.org/licenses/by-sa/3.0) or GFDL (http://www.gnu.org/copyleft/fdl.html)], via Wikimedia Commons
Sarcoid
By Yale Rosen [CC-BY-SA-2.0 (http://creativecommons.org/licenses/by-sa/2.0)], via Wikimedia Commons
Silicosis
By Gumersindorego (Own work) [CC-BY-SA-3.0 (http://creativecommons.org/licenses/by-sa/3.0)], via Wikimedia Commons
Pancoast Tumor
By Jmarchn (Own work) [CC-BY-SA-3.0-2.5-2.0-1.0 (http://creativecommons.org/licenses/by-sa/3.0) or GFDL (http://www.gnu.org/copyleft/fdl.html)], via Wikimedia Commons
Bronchial Carcinoma
Lange123 at the German language Wikipedia [GFDL (http://www.gnu.org/copyleft/fdl.html) or CC-BY-SA-3.0 (http://creativecommons.org/licenses/by-sa/3.0/)], from Wikimedia Commons
Horner's syndrome
By Waster [CC-BY-2.5 (http://creativecommons.org/licenses/by/2.5)], via Wikimedia Commons
Pneumothorax
By Photographed by User Clinical Cases 00:42, 7 November 2006 [CC-BY-SA-2.5 (http://creativecommons.org/licenses/by-sa/2.5) or CC-BY-SA-2.5 (http://creativecommons.org/licenses/by-sa/2.5)], via Wikimedia Commons
Tension Pneumothorax
By James Heilman, MD (Own work) [CC-BY-SA-3.0 (http://creativecommons.org/licenses/by-sa/3.0)], via Wikimedia Commons

Pleural Effusion
By User InvictaHOG on en.wikipedia Edited by InvictaHOG, all edits released into public domain Commons upload by Magnus Manske 13:26, 28 April 2006 (UTC) [Public domain], via Wikimedia Commons

Pleural effusion
By James Heilman, MD (Own work) [CC-BY-SA-3.0 (http://creativecommons.org/licenses/by-sa/3.0) or GFDL (http://www.gnu.org/copyleft/fdl.html)], via Wikimedia Commons

Hampton's Hump
By Thomas C Alewine. Used with direct permission from Mr Alewine. Special Thanks to Mr. Alewine

LATERAL CXR

By Stillwaterising (Own work) [CC0], via Wikimedia Commons

Lobar Pneumonia
By Hellerhoff (Own work) [CC-BY-SA-3.0 (http://creativecommons.org/licenses/by-sa/3.0) or GFDL (http://www.gnu.org/copyleft/fdl.html)], via Wikimedia Commons

Left lower lobe pneumonia
By James Heilman, MD (Own work) [CC-BY-3.0 (http://creativecommons.org/licenses/by/3.0)], via Wikimedia Commons

Pneumonia
By Hellerhoff (Own work) [CC-BY-SA-3.0 (http://creativecommons.org/licenses/by-sa/3.0) or GFDL (http://www.gnu.org/copyleft/fdl.html)], via Wikimedia Commons

Lingula Pneumonia
By James Heilman, MD (Own work) [CC-BY-SA-3.0 (http://creativecommons.org/licenses/by-sa/3.0) or GFDL (http://www.gnu.org/copyleft/fdl.html)], via Wikimedia Commons

Tuberculosis – Reactivation
This image is a work of the Centers for Disease Control and Prevention, part of the United States Department of Health and Human Services, taken or made as part of an employee's official duties. As a work of the U.S. federal government, the image is in the public domain.

Miliary TB
ErikH from nl [GFDL (http://www.gnu.org/copyleft/fdl.html), GFDL (http://www.gnu.org/copyleft/fdl.html) or CC-BY-SA-3.0 (http://creativecommons.org/licenses/by-sa/3.0/)], from Wikimedia Commons

Epiglottitis
By Med Chaos (Own work) [CC-BY-SA-3.0 (http://creativecommons.org/licenses/by-sa/3.0)], via Wikimedia Commons

Epiglottitis
By 藤澤孝志 (Own work) [CC-BY-SA-3.0 (http://creativecommons.org/licenses/by-sa/3.0)], via Wikimedia Commons

Bronchiolitis
By Matteo Di Nardo, Daniela Perrotta, Francesca Stoppa, Corrado Cecchetti, Marco Marano and Nicola Pirozzi [CC-BY-2.0 (http://creativecommons.org/licenses/by/2.0)], via Wikimedia Commons

CROUP
By Frank Gaillard (Own work) [GFDL 1.3 (www.gnu.org/licenses/fdl-1.3.html), GFDL 1.3 (www.gnu.org/licenses/fdl-1.3.html), CC-BY-SA-3.0 (http://creativecommons.org/licenses/by-sa/3.0), CC-BY-SA-3.0 (http://creativecommons.org/licenses/by-sa/3.0) or GFDL

Multilobar pneumonia
By Christaras A (Converted from anonymized dicom image) [GFDL (http://www.gnu.org/copyleft/fdl.html), CC-BY-SA-3.0 (http://creativecommons.org/licenses/by-sa/3.0/) or CC BY 2.5 (http://creativecommons.org/licenses/by/2.5)], via Wikimedia Commons

PCP Pneumonia
By -- Samir धर्म 06:38, 14 January 2007 (UTC) (http://en.wikipedia.org/wiki/Image:PCP_CAP_CXR.JPG) [GFDL (http://www.gnu.org/copyleft/fdl.html) or CC-BY-SA-3.0 (http://creativecommons.org/licenses/by-sa/3.0/)], via Wikimedia Commons

Pulmonary fibrosis
Drriad [CC BY-SA 3.0 (https://creativecommons.org/licenses/by-sa/3.0)]

Other images: Shutterstock (used with permission)

CHAPTER 3 - GASTROINTESTINAL/NUTRITION

TOXINS	CLINICAL EXAM	WORKUP	ANTIDOTES/MGMT
ACETAMINOPHEN	Toxicity overwhelms the enzyme capability of the liver ⇨ ↓glutathione ⇨ **hepatic necrosis** • Anorexia, N/V, diaphoresis ⇨ RUQ pain, jaundice, coagulation abnormalities.	• APAP levels Follow nomogram • LFTs • PT/PTT/INR • UA, ECG	• **N-acetylcysteine antidote** (glutathione substitute). • **Activated charcoal** especially within 1 hour of ingestion.
SALICYLATES - **Aspirin** - **Pepto Bismol** - Ben Gay - Oil of Wintergreen	• **Respiratory alkalosis** due to respiratory stimulation ⇨ **high anion gap metabolic acidosis** occurs later. Fever. • **CNS:** seizures, coma, encephalopathy. • Renal failure, pulmonary edema.	• Salicylates levels • Metabolic acidosis • ***Hypokalemia*** (from ↑urinary K+ loss)	• Resuscitation (ABCs) • GI decontamination: Activated charcoal, gastric lavage • Alkalinization: sodium bicarbonate • Glucose helps with CNS sx • IV fluids • Hemodialysis (if severe).
BASES **- Oven cleaner** **- Drain cleaner** **- Bleach**	• Esophageal or gastric perforation, epiglottitis. • Respiratory distress. • Irritated mucous membranes.	• EGD to assess for damage.	• Supportive care • Emesis prevention • ±small amount of H_2O or milk as a diluent. • *Gastric lavage or acids contraindicated!* (will worsen symptoms).
HYDROCARBONS - Gasoline - Benzene - Petroleum - Kerosene, Motor oil	• **Aspiration pneumonitis** • Tachycardia, fever • CNS depression • Mucosal irritation • Vomiting, bloody diarrhea	• CXR: ± pneumonia, pneumothorax of pleural effusion). • UA • ECG	• Supportive treatment • ±antibiotics if pneumonia • *Avoid emetics or lavage*
ANTICHOLINERGICS - **Antihistamines** - Atropine - **Tricyclic antidepressants (TCA's)** **Anticholinergics have antimuscarinic effects**	**Sympathetic Stimulation:** • **Hyperthermia (no sweating)** • **Tachycardia**, **HTN** • **Hot, flushed, dry skin & mucous membranes.** • **Mydriasis,** visual changes • Urinary retention, ileus **CNS** • Confusion, seizure, coma, respiratory depression,	• ECG with TCA: **wide QRS, prolonged QT,** heart block, asystole, brady & tachyarrhythmias, ventricular arrhythmia (due to **Na channel blocker effects of TCA's)**	• Activated charcoal • Whole bowel irrigation • **Physostigmine** (acetylcholinesterase inhibitor) • **TCA toxicity:** supportive. **Sodium bicarbonate antidote.** Diazepam for seizures.
CHOLINERGICS - **Organophosphates** - **Insecticides & Pesticides** Chlorthion, Diazinon, Malathion - Sarin gas	**Muscarinic S/E: "SLUDD-C":** ↑**s**alivation, **l**acrimation, **u**rination, ↑GI: **d**iarrhea, **emesis, miosis.** CV: bradycardia, hypotension, Respiratory: bronchospasm and rhinorrhea. **Nicotinic S/E:** mydriasis, tachycardia, weakness, HTN, fasciculations. **Children usually present with nicotinic S/E** "Garlic" breath (also seen with arsenic).	• RBC cholinesterase levels • Blood glucose levels	• **Atropine + Pralidoxime** - Atropine (anticholinergic) - Pralidoxime reactivates the cholinesterase enzyme • Remove contaminated clothes

Miosis = Constricted pupils

Mydriasis = Dilated pupils

IRON	**GI:** nausea, vomiting, abdominal pain, shock, coagulopathy, red urine.	• RBC indices. LFTs • Metabolic acidosis • UA: assess for renal damage	• Emesis with gastric lavage • Whole bowel irrigation • **Deferoxamine** • Hemodialysis

POISONS	TREATMENT	NOTES
Tricyclic antidepressants	**Sodium bicarbonate** may be used for cardiotoxicity.	Cardiotoxicity = prolonged QT interval.
Amphetamines	Ammonium chloride	
Opioids	**Naloxone, Naltrexone**	May be needed if severe (ex. respiratory depression).
Benzodiazepines	**Flumazenil**	Only used in severe cases.
Beta blockers	**Glucagon**	Usually given as an IM injection.
Theophylline	**Beta blockers**	Overdose symptoms usually due to ↑sympathetic activity.
Digitalis	**Digibind**	May need IV Magnesium.
Methemoglobin	Methylene blue, Vitamin C	
tPA, streptokinase	Aminocaproic acid	
Warfarin	**Vitamin K & fresh frozen plasma** Cryoprecipitate if continued bleeding	Especially if INR >10
Heparin	**Protamine sulfate**	
Ethylene glycol (Antifreeze)	**IV ethanol infusion** Fomepizole	

ACUTE CHOLECYSTITIS

- Inflammation and infection of the gallbladder due to obstruction of the cystic duct by gallstones.
- ***E. coli* most common,** *Klebsiella,* and other gram-negative enteric organisms.

CLINICAL MANIFESTATIONS
- **Continuous RUQ or epigastric pain** - may be **precipitated by fatty foods or large meals.**
- May be associated with **nausea** & guarding, anorexia.

PHYSICAL EXAMINATION
- **Fever** (often low-grade). **Enlarged, palpable gallbladder**
- **⊕ Murphy's sign:** RUQ pain or inspiratory arrest with palpation of the gallbladder.
- **⊕ Boas sign:** referred pain to the right shoulder or subscapular area (phrenic nerve irritation).

DIAGNOSIS
- **Ultrasound: initial test of choice** - thickened or distended gallbladder, pericholecystic fluid, sonographic Murphy's sign.
- CT scan: alternative to ultrasound & can detect complications.
- Labs: **increased WBCs** (leukocytosis with left shift), increased bilirubin, increased alkaline phosphatase, & increased LFTs.
- **HIDA scan: most accurate test** - Cholecystitis present if there is no visualization of the gallbladder.

MANAGEMENT
- **NPO, IV fluids, antibiotics** (eg, Ceftriaxone + Metronidazole) **followed by cholecystectomy** (usually within 72 hours). Laparoscopic cholecystectomy preferred whenever possible.
- Cholecystostomy (percutaneous drainage of the gallbladder) if patient is nonoperative.

ACUTE ACALCULOUS CHOLECYSTITIS

- Acute necroinflammatory disease of the gallbladder not due to gallstones.
- Accounts for 10% of Acute cholecystitis.

PATHOPHYSIOLOGY
- **Gallbladder stasis and ischemia** leading to a local inflammatory reaction in the gallbladder wall; leads to concentration of bile salts, gallbladder distention, secondary infection, perforation, or necrosis of gallbladder tissue.

RISK FACTORS: current hospitalization, **critically-ill** patients.

CLINICAL MANIFESTATIONS: fever, leukocytosis, jaundice, sepsis, vague abdominal discomfort.

DIAGNOSIS
- Based on clinical symptoms in the setting of supportive imaging and the exclusion of alternative diagnosis.
- **Ultrasound initial test of choice –** distended gallbladder with thickened walls and pericholecystic fluid without calcifications.
- Contrast-enhanced abdominal CT scan If diagnosis remains uncertain after Ultrasound.
- HIDA scan performed if diagnosis remains uncertain after CT scan.

MANAGEMENT
- **Supportive care -** IV fluids, bowel rest, pain control, correction of electrolytes, broad-spectrum antibiotics.

CHRONIC CHOLECYSTITIS

- Fibrosis and thickening of the gallbladder due to chronic inflammatory cell infiltration of the gallbladder evident on histopathology.
- The presence of Chronic cholecystitis does not correlate with symptoms.
- Almost always associated with gallstones.

ACUTE ASCENDING CHOLANGITIS

- **Biliary tract infection secondary to obstruction of the common bile duct (CBD)** - eg, **gallstones**, malignancy.

ETIOLOGIES
- Most due to Gram-negative enteric organisms that ascend from the duodenum - ***E. coli* most common**, *Klebsiella* (second most common), *Enterobacter, B. fragilis*. Anaerobes or Enterococcus.

CLINICAL MANIFESTATIONS
- **Charcot's triad: fever/chills + RUQ pain + jaundice.**
- Reynold's pentad (add hypotension or shock + altered mental status).

DIAGNOSIS
- Labs: **leukocytosis** (may have left shift). **Cholestasis: increased alkaline phosphatase & GGT, increased bilirubin >** increased ALT & AST.

- **Ultrasound: initial imaging test of choice.**

- MRCP most accurate imaging test.

- Cholangiography: **gold standard** via **ERCP** or PTC (percutaneous transhepatic cholangiography) – usually performed once the patent has been afebrile/stable for 48 hours after IV antibiotics.

INITIAL MANAGEMENT
- **IV antibiotics followed by CBD decompression & stone extraction once stable (eg, ERCP).**

- **Antibiotics**: Ampicillin/sulbactam, Piperacillin/tazobactam; Ceftriaxone + Metronidazole. Fluoroquinolone + Metronidazole; Ampicillin + Gentamicin.

COMMON BILE DUCT DECOMPRESSION & STONE EXTRACTION
- **ERCP** (sphincterotomy). Usually performed once the patent has been afebrile/stable for 48 hours after IV antibiotics.

- Percutaneous transhepatic cholangiogram (PTC) catheter drainage or percutaneous cholecystostomy tube patients or if unable to do ERCP.

- Open surgical decompression + T-tube insertion.

Eventually, the patient should undergo elective cholecystectomy.

CHOLELITHIASIS

- Gallstones in the biliary tract (usually in the gallbladder) without inflammation.
- Complications include Choledocholithiasis, Acute cholangitis, & Acute cholecystitis.

TYPES OF GALLSTONES
- **Cholesterol most common** (mixed & pure) 90%; Pigmented 10%.
- Black stones: hemolysis or ETOH-related Cirrhosis.
- Brown stones: increased in Asian population, parasitic, or bacterial infections.

RISK FACTORS
- **5Fs (fat, fair, female, forty, fertile):** OCPs (increased estrogen), Native Americans, bile stasis, chronic hemolysis, Cirrhosis, infection, rapid weight loss, Inflammatory bowel disease, total parenteral nutrition (TPN), fibrates, increased triglycerides.

CLINICAL MANIFESTATIONS
- Most are asymptomatic. May be an incidental finding.
- **Biliary "colic": episodic, abrupt RUQ** or epigastric pain, resolves slowly, **lasting 30 minutes to hours.** May be associated with **nausea & precipitated by fatty foods or large meals.**

DIAGNOSIS
- **Ultrasound: initial test of choice.** CT or MRI may also be used.

MANAGEMENT
- Observation if asymptomatic.
- Symptomatic: Ursodeoxycholic acid may be used to dissolve the gallstones (takes 6-9 months). Elective cholecystectomy.

CHOLEDOCHOLITHIASIS

- **Gallstones in the common bile duct** (can lead to cholestasis due to blockage).

CLINICAL MANIFESTATIONS
- **Prolonged biliary colic**: right upper quadrant or epigastric pain, nausea, and vomiting. The pain is **usually more prolonged** due to the presence of the stone blocking the bile duct).
- Physical examination: RUQ or epigastric tenderness. **Jaundice.**

DIAGNOSIS
- Labs: elevated AST and ALT. **Increased alkaline phosphatase + GGT (cholestasis).**
- **Ultrasound:** often **initial imaging test ordered**.
- **ERCP: diagnostic test of choice.** ERCP can be diagnostic as well as therapeutic (allows for stone extraction). Often obtained after ultrasound.
- Magnetic resonance cholangiopancreatography (MRCP) and endoscopic ultrasound (EUS) may be used in patients with intermediate risk (determined by labs & transabdominal ultrasound).

MANAGEMENT
- **ERCP stone extraction preferred** over laparoscopic choledocholithotomy.

NEONATAL JAUNDICE

- **Yellowish discoloration of the skin, sclera, and the conjunctiva** due to elevated plasma bilirubin in a newborn.

- Usually a transient and mild condition but in severe cases, may lead to kernicterus (cerebral dysfunction & encephalopathy).

- **Physiologic jaundice presents on days 3-5 of life** & bilirubin levels fall in about 50% of the neonates during the first week of life.

ETIOLOGIES

- Physiologic: transient decrease in UGT enzyme activity (UGT is the enzyme that conjugates bilirubin). Breastfeeding failure – caused by insufficient breast milk consumption (inadequate amounts of bowel movements to excrete bilirubin from the body). Breast milk jaundice – infant liver is not mature enough to process lipids, occurs around 4th and 7th day of life (mother should continue to breastfeed).

- Pathologic: Crigler-Najjar syndrome, Gilbert syndrome, Cretinism, Hemolytic anemia, Dubin-Johnson syndrome. Pathologic causes may occur in the first 24 hours of life, persists > 10-14 days, bilirubin increase > 5mg/dL/day, associated with a bilirubin > 12 mg/dL in a term infant, conjugated bilirubin > 2 mg/dL or >20% of total bilirubin.

CLINICAL MANIFESTATIONS

- **Jaundice**: yellowing of the skin, sclera and the conjunctiva. In neonates, jaundice usually progresses from head to toe with increasing bilirubin levels. Associated with **bilirubin levels > 5.0 mg/dL.**

- **Kernicterus – cerebral dysfunction and encephalopathy** due to bilirubin deposition in brain tissue. This can manifest as seizures, lethargy, irritability, hearing loss, mental developmental delays. Associated with **bilirubin levels > 20 mg/dL.**

WORKUP

- Bilirubin, Coombs test distinguishes between immune-mediated (eg, ABO incompatibility) from non-immune-mediated hemolytic disorders, blood smear if hemolysis, LFTs, alkaline phosphatase.

MANAGEMENT

- No management needed in physiologic jaundice.

- **Phototherapy initial management of choice** of all types. For term infants (38 weeks GA or longer) without risk factors, phototherapy is initiated based on total bilirubin: 24 hours of age >12 mg/dL, 48 hours of age > 15 mg/dL or 72 hours of age > 18 mg/dL. Values lower can be used in preterm or at-risk infants.

- **Exchange transfusion in severe cases** (eg, hemolysis, ABO incompatibility. Rh isoimmunization). IV immunoglobulin may be needed with iso-immune hemolysis.

DUBIN-JOHNSON SYNDROME

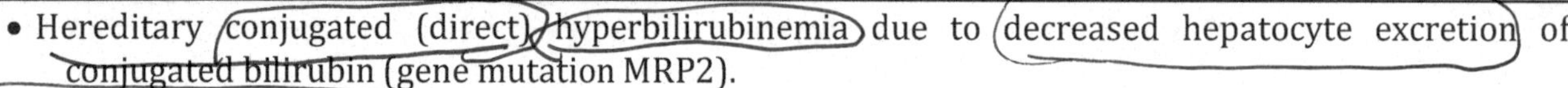

- Hereditary conjugated (direct) hyperbilirubinemia due to decreased hepatocyte excretion of conjugated bilirubin (gene mutation MRP2).
- Think Ds **D**ubin, **Direct** bilirubinemia, **Dark liver**

CLINICAL MANIFESTATIONS
- Usually asymptomatic.
- May present with generalized constitutional symptoms. Mild icterus

DIAGNOSIS
- Mild, **isolated conjugated (direct) hyperbilirubinemia** (often between 2 – 5 mg/dL) but can increase with concurrent illness, pregnancy or OCPs.
- Biopsy: **grossly black liver** & dark granular pigment in the hepatocytes.

MANAGEMENT
- None needed.

Rotor's syndrome: similar to Dubin-Johnson but milder in nature, associated with conjugated & unconjugated hyperbilirubinemia and not associated with grossly black liver on biopsy.

CRIGLER-NAJJAR SYNDROME

- **Hereditary unconjugated (indirect) hyperbilirubinemia.**
- Pathophysiology: decreased activity of the glucuronosyltransferase (UGT) enzyme needed to convert indirect bilirubin to direct bilirubin.

TYPES:
- Type I: **no UGT activity**. Autosomal recessive.
- Type II (Arias Syndrome): very little UGT activity (10% or less of normal).

CLINICAL MANIFESTATIONS
- **Type I: neonatal jaundice with severe progression in the second week, leading to kernicterus** (bilirubin-induced encephalopathy) - hypotonia, deafness, lethargy, oculomotor palsy. Potentially fatal.
- Type II: usually asymptomatic. Often an incidental finding on routine lab testing.

DIAGNOSIS:
- **Isolated indirect (unconjugated) hyperbilirubinemia** + otherwise **normal liver function tests.**
- Type I: serum indirect bilirubin often between 20-50 mg/dL.
- Type II: serum indirect bilirubin often between 7-10 mg/dL. May increase during illness/fasting.
- Liver looks normal on biopsy.

MANAGEMENT OF TYPE I:
- **Phototherapy mainstay of treatment.**
- Plasmapheresis may be used in acute elevations of bilirubin levels (eg, crisis).
- Liver transplant definitive.

MANAGEMENT OF TYPE II:
- Treatment usually isn't necessary but if required, **Phenobarbital** has been shown to increase UGT activity. Type I is not responsive to Phenobarbital.

GILBERT'S SYNDROME

- Hereditary unconjugated (indirect) hyperbilirubinemia.
- Relatively common (5 – 10% of US population).

PATHOPHYSIOLOGY

- **Reduced UGT activity** (10-30% of normal) & decreased bilirubin uptake, leading to increased indirect bilirubin. Glucuronosyltransferase (UGT) is the enzyme responsible for the conjugation of bilirubin.

CLINICAL MANIFESTATIONS

- Asymptomatic in most cases.
- May develop **transient episodes of jaundice during periods of stress, fasting, alcohol, or illness.**

DIAGNOSIS

- Usually an incidental finding: slight **increase in isolated Indirect bilirubin level with otherwise normal LFTs.**

MANAGEMENT

- No treatment needed (mild, benign disease).

- Hereditary unconjugated (indirect) hyperbilirubinemia. Relatively common (5 – 10% of US population).

PATTERNS OF LIVER INJURY

❶ **HEPATOCELLULAR DAMAGE:** ↑ALT & AST primarily. ALT more sensitive for liver disease than AST.

❷ **CHOLESTASIS:** **↑levels of alkaline phosphatase with ↑GGT.** ↑**bilirubin** greater than ↑ALT & AST.

❸ **LIVER "SYNTHETIC" FUNCTION:**

PROTHROMBIN TIME (PT): depends on synthesis of coagulation factors (vitamin K dependent): Factors 2,7,9,10. **PT is an earlier indicator of severe liver injury/prognosis than albumin.** Prolonged PT is seen when 80% of the liver's protein synthesizing ability is lost.

ALBUMIN: useful marker of overall liver protein synthesis. Levels decreases with liver failure.

DISORDERS	LABORATORY PATTERN OF LIVER INJURIES
ETOH HEPATITIS	**AST:ALT>2 ⇨ alcohol hepatitis** "S = Scotch" (AST levels usually <500). AST is found primarily in the mitochondria. ETOH causes direct mitochondrial injury ⇨ ↑AST
VIRAL/TOXIC/INFLAMMATORY PROCESSES	• **ALT >AST ⇨ usually.** Think ALT for Liver. • **AST & ALT >1,000** ⇨ usually **acute viral hepatitis** (A, B & rarely C) • Chronic viral hepatitis B, C, D ⇨ mildly ↑ALT & AST (usually <400)
BILIARY OBSTRUCTION OR INTRAHEPATIC CHOLESTASIS	• **↑alkaline phosphatase (ALP) ⇨ ↑ALP with ↑GGT suggests hepatic source or biliary obstruction.** • GGT most sensitive indicator of biliary injury (nonspecific). • If ↑ALP without ↑GGT, look for sources other than the liver (eg, bone, gut).
AUTOIMMUNE HEPATITIS	• **↑ALT >1,000, ⊕ANA, ⊕ smooth muscle antibodies, ↑IgG. Responds to Corticosteroids,** Azathioprine.

CONSTIPATION

- Infrequent bowel movements (<2/week), straining, hard stools, feeling of incomplete evacuation).

ETIOLOGIES

- Disordered movement of stool through colon/anus/rectum (usually the proximal GI tract is intact).
- Slow colonic transit: idiopathic, motor disorders (colorectal CA, DM, hypothyroid), adverse effects of many drugs **eg, Verapamil, opioids.** Outlet delay: Hirschsprung's disease.

DRUG/INTERVENTION	COMMENTS
FIBER	**MOA: retains water & improves GI transit.**
BULK FORMING LAXATIVES Psyllium Methylcellulose Polycarbophil Wheat Dextran	• Mechanism: **absorbs water & increases fecal mass**. Increases the frequency & softens the consistency of stool with minimal effects. • Dietary fiber & bulk forming laxatives the most physiologic & effective approach to constipation. • Adverse effects: flatulence, bloating.
OSMOTIC LAXATIVES Polyethylene Glycol (PEG)	• MOA: causes H_2O retention in stool (osmotic effect pulls H_2O into gut). • Adverse effects: flatulence, bloating.
Lactulose	Synthetic disaccharide (sugar) not absorbed (pulls water into gut). Adverse effects: bloating, flatulence. Also used in hepatic encephalopathy.
Sorbitol	Synthetic sugar (cheap). Adverse effects: bloating, flatulence.
Saline Laxatives - Milk of Magnesia - Magnesium Citrate	Adverse effects: hypermagnesemia (especially with chronic renal disease).
STIMULANT LAXATIVES Bisacodyl Senna	• Mechanism: increases **acetylcholine-regulated GI motility (peristalsis)** & alters electrolyte transport in the mucosa. • Adverse effects: diarrhea, abdominal pain

FECAL IMPACTION

- Copious amount of an immovable solid bulk of stool in the rectum.
- Due to decreased mobility & inability to sense and respond to the presence of stool in the rectum.

DIAGNOSIS

- Digital rectal examination (copious amounts of stool).
- Abdominal radiographs if digital rectal examination is nondiagnostic.

MANAGEMENT

Disimpaction and colon evacuation, followed by a routine bowel regimen to reduce recurrence:

- **Digital disimpaction followed by warm-water enema with mineral oil** – disimpaction allows for manual fragmentation of the fecal bolus to ease passage through the anal canal. Warm-water enema with mineral oil is used to soften the impaction and facilitate passage.
- **Polyethylene glycol** can be employed after disimpaction of the distal colon (either orally or via nasogastric tube).
- Other options if disimpaction is unsuccessful include water-soluble contrast enema (under fluoroscopy), Local anesthesia to relax the anal canal & pelvic floor muscles + abdominal massage or Colonoscope with a snare to fragment the fecal bolus (after preparation with mineral oil enemas).
- Identify and reduce or eliminate causes of constipation.

ANORECTAL ABSCESS & FISTULAS

ABSCESS

- Often results from bacterial infection of anal ducts or glands.
- ***Staphylococcus aureus* most common**, *E. coli, Bacteroides, Proteus, Streptococcus.*
- **Posterior rectal wall most common site.**

FISTULA

- Open tract between two epithelium-lined areas. Seen especially with deeper abscesses.

CLINICAL MANIFESTATIONS

- Abscess: anorectal swelling, rectal pain that is worse with sitting, coughing, & defecation. May be febrile. Focal edema, induration, and fluctuance on examination. Deeper abscess may only be palpated on digital rectal exam or seen on imaging studies.
- Fistula: may cause anal discharge & pain

MANAGEMENT

- **Incision & drainage: mainstay of treatment** followed by **WASH** – **W**arm-water cleansing, **A**nalgesics, **S**itz baths, **H**igh-fiber diet.
- Antibiotics are not usually required in simple cases.

ANAL FISSURES

- **Painful linear tear/crack** in the distal anal canal.

ETIOLOGIES

- Low-fiber diets, passage of large, hard stools, constipation, or other anal trauma.

CLINICAL MANIFESTATIONS

- **Severe painful rectal pain & bowel movements** causing the **patient to refrain from defecating**, **bright red blood per rectum**.

PHYSICAL EXAMINATION

- **Longitudinal tear** in the anoderm that usually extends no more proximally than the dentate line. **Most common at the posterior midline** (99% men, 90% women).
- **Skin tags** seen in chronic.

MANAGEMENT

- **>80% resolve spontaneously.**
- **Supportive measures: first line management:** warm water Sitz baths, analgesics, high fiber diet, increased water intake, stool softeners, laxatives, & mineral oil.
- Second line treatment: topical vasodilators: Nitroglycerin (Adverse effects: headache & dizziness); Nifedipine ointment.
- Botox injections to reduce spasm of the internal sphincter (may be more effective than topical dilators).
- Surgery: eg, lateral internal sphincterotomy reserved for refractory cases.

HEMORRHOIDS

- Engorgement of venous plexuses.

Internal hemorrhoids
- Originate from superior hemorrhoid vein & are proximal (above) the dentate line.
- **Internal hemorrhoids tend to bleed & are usually painless.**

Based on the degree of prolapse from the anal canal:

I	does not prolapse (confined to anal canal). May bleed with defecation.
II	prolapses with defecation or straining but spontaneously reduce.
III	prolapses with defecation or straining, requires manual reduction.
IV	Irreducible & may strangulate.

External hemorrhoids
- Originate from the inferior hemorrhoid vein & are distal (below) the dentate line.
- **External hemorrhoids tend to be painful and don't usually bleed.**

RISK FACTORS
- Increased venous pressure: straining during defecation (eg, constipation), pregnancy, obesity, prolonged sitting, cirrhosis with portal hypertension.

CLINICAL MANIFESTATIONS

Internal hemorrhoids:
- **Intermittent rectal bleeding most common - painless bright red blood per rectum** (hematochezia) - seen on toilet paper, coating the stool, or dispersed in toilet water.
- May have rectal itching & fullness, or mucus discharge.
- Uncomplicated internal are usually not tender and not palpable (unless they are thrombosed). Rectal pain with internal suggests a complication.

External hemorrhoids:
- **Perianal pain aggravated with defecation**.
- May have tender palpable mass. May have skin tags.

DIAGNOSIS
- Visual inspection, digital rectal examination, fecal occult blood testing.
- Anoscopy for internal allows for direct visualization and diagnosis of internal.
- Proctosigmoidoscopy or colonoscopy may be indicated in patients with hematochezia to rule out proximal sigmoid disease.

MANAGEMENT
- **Conservative treatment: high-fiber diet, increased fluids. Warm Sitz baths** & topical rectal corticosteroids (analgesics like lidocaine) may be used for pruritus & discomfort or thrombosis.
- Procedures: if failed conservative management, debilitating pain, or strangulation. Options include **rubber band ligation (most commonly used)**, sclerotherapy, or infrared coagulation. Excision of thrombosed external hemorrhoids may be performed.
- Hemorrhoidectomy: for stage IV or those not responsive to the aforementioned therapies. Surgical management used for external hemorrhoids.

DIVERTICULOSIS

- Diverticula: outpouchings due to herniation of the mucosa into the wall of the colon along natural openings at the vasa recta of the colon.
- Left colon most common in incidence, Right colon most common location for bleeding.
- Risk factors: **low fiber diet, constipation, & obesity.**

CLINICAL MANIFESTATIONS
- Usually asymptomatic – incidental finding.
- Lower GI bleeding: **Diverticulosis is the most common cause of acute lower GI bleeding (painless hematochezia)** in adults.

DIAGNOSIS
- **Colonoscopy test of choice** (once upper GI bleed has been ruled out). Diagnostic and therapeutic.
- Radionuclide imaging (eg, technetium-99 tagged red blood cell scan) usually followed by arteriography is the next step if the bleeding is not visualized on colonoscopy.

MANAGEMENT
- In most cases, the bleeding stops spontaneously.
- Resuscitation (2 large bore IVs, fluids and/or blood products if needed, correction of coagulopathies).
- Endoscopic therapy to control bleeding if active (eg, Epinephrine injection, tamponade).
- Asymptomatic diverticulosis can be followed on a high fiber diet, use of Bran, or psyllium.

DIVERTICULITIS

- Microscopic perforation of a diverticulum leads to inflammation & focal necrosis.
- Considered complicated if it leads to bowel perforation, abscess, fistula, or bowel obstruction.
- **Sigmoid colon most common area** (due to high intraluminal pressure). Onset usually > 40y of age.

CLINICAL MANIFESTATIONS
- **LLQ abdominal pain (most common),** LLQ tenderness, **low-grade fever.** May have nausea, vomiting, constipation, diarrhea, flatulence, bloating, or changes in bowel habits.
- Physical examination: often normal. A tender mass may be present due to inflammation or abscess.

DIAGNOSIS
- **CT scan initial imaging test of choice.** Colonoscopy & Barium enema not used (perforation risk).
- Labs: **leukocytosis.**

MANAGEMENT
- **Uncomplicated: treated as an outpatient with oral antibiotics** (eg, **Metronidazole + either Ciprofloxacin or Levofloxacin**) for 7-10 days and clear liquid diet (or diet as tolerated). Trimethoprim-sulfamethoxazole plus Metronidazole is an alternative.
- Surgery: indicated if refractory to medical therapy, frequent recurrences, perforation, or strictures.

CRITERIA FOR ADMISSION
- Patients with complicated diverticulitis (perforation, abscess, obstruction, or fistula). CT-guided percutaneous drainage may be needed in Acute diverticulitis with abscesses >3 cm for resolution.
- Uncomplicated diverticulitis with high-risk (high fever >102.5F, sepsis, immunosuppression, increased age, unable to tolerate oral intake etc.).

TOXIC MEGACOLON

- Nonobstructive, extreme **colon dilation > 6 cm + signs of systemic toxicity.**
- ETIOLOGIES: complications of IBD (eg, **Ulcerative colitis**), infectious colitis (eg, ***C. difficile***, CMV), ischemic colitis, volvulus, diverticulitis, radiation, & obstructive Colorectal cancer.

CLINICAL MANIFESTATIONS

- **Profound bloody diarrhea,** abdominal pain & distention, nausea, vomiting, tenesmus.

Physical examination:

- Lower abdominal tenderness & **distention.**
- **Signs of toxicity:** altered mental status, fever, tachycardia, hypotension, dehydration. May have signs of peritonitis (rigidity, guarding, rebound tenderness).

DIAGNOSIS

- Radiologic evidence of colon >6 cm: **abdominal radiographs usually the initial imaging of choice.** CT scan may be used to assess for complications.
- 3 or more of the following: fever >38C, pulse >120, neutrophilic leukocytosis >10,500/microL, anemia PLUS
- At least 1: hypotension, dehydration, electrolyte abnormalities or altered mental status.

MANAGEMENT

- **Supportive mainstay** - bowel rest, bowel decompression with NG tube, broad-spectrum antibiotics (eg, Ceftriaxone + Metronidazole), fluid and electrolyte replacement.
- Management of the underlying cause (eg, Corticosteroids in Ulcerative colitis).

OGILVIE SYNDROME

- **Colonic pseudo-obstruction** (acute dilation of the colon in the absence of any mechanical obstruction).
- Usually involves the cecum and the right colon.

ETIOLOGIES

- Similar to Adynamic ileus - **postoperative state**, medications (eg, **opiates,** anticholinergics), metabolic (eg, **hypokalemia, hypercalcemia**), severe medical illness, metabolic (eg, **Hypothyroidism**, diabetes).

CLINICAL MANIFESTATIONS

- **Abdominal distention main feature.**
- Nausea, vomiting, abdominal pain, constipation. May have paradoxical diarrhea.
- Physical examination: distention and tympanitic abdomen.

DIAGNOSIS

- Abdominal radiographs: dilated right colon often from the cecum with cutoff at the splenic flexure.
- Abdominal CT scan or contrast enema: proximal right colonic dilation. CT Most accurate test.

MANAGEMENT

- **Conservative:** **IV fluid & electrolyte repletion** if colon dilation <12 cm & absence of severe symptoms or peritonitis.
- Medical decompression: **Neostigmine** used in patients at risk for perforation (eg, cecal diameter >12 cm) or if **failed 24-48 hours of conservative therapy**.
- Colonoscopic decompression: for failure of conservative treatment & Neostigmine.
- Surgical decompression: (with cecostomy or colectomy) used if all the other therapies fail.

INFLAMMATORY BOWEL DISEASE (IBD)

- Includes both Ulcerative colitis and Crohn disease.

RISK FACTORS

- **Race & Ethnicity:** more common Jewish population (especially **Ashkenazi Jews**), increased in Caucasians compared to Blacks & Hispanics.
- **Age & Gender:** classically onset is seen between **15 – 35 years**. UC seen slightly more in males, CD slightly more seen in females.
- Genetics: 10-30% patients have a first-degree relative with IBD.
- **Smoking:** smoking is associated with an increased incidence of Crohn. **Smoking may be protective in UC** (smokers who stop smoking who have a history of UC have increased incidence of flares).
- **Diet:** Western style diet is associated with increased incidence of IBD.
- Infections: alteration in bowel microbes (eg, during viral or bacterial infections) may trigger inflammatory process that goes unchecked.
- Medications: NSAIDs, oral contraceptives, or hormone replacement therapy may be associated with an increased risk.

EXTRA-INTESTINAL MANIFESTATIONS

These manifestations can be seen with Crohn disease or Ulcerative colitis

- Rheumatologic: musculoskeletal pain, arthritis, ankylosing spondylitis, osteoporosis.
- Dermatologic: erythema nodosum, pyoderma gangrenosum.
- Ocular: conjunctivitis, **anterior uveitis/iritis** (ocular pain, headache, blurred vision, headache). Episcleritis: mild ocular burning.
- Hepatobiliary: fatty liver, primary sclerosing cholangitis.
- Hematologic: B12 and Iron deficiency especially with CD. Increased risk of thromboembolism.

	ULCERATIVE COLITIS (UC)	**CROHN DISEASE (CD)**
AREA AFFECTED	• **Limited to colon** (**begins in rectum** with **CONTIGUOUS SPREAD PROXIMALLY** to colon. • **RECTUM ALWAYS INVOLVED**	• **ANY SEGMENT OF THE GI TRACT** from mouth to anus. • **MC in TERMINAL ILEUM ⇨ RLQ pain**
DEPTH	• Mucosa & submucosa only	• **TRANSMURAL**
CLINICAL MANIFESTATIONS	• Abdominal pain: **LLQ MC**, colicky • **Tenesmus, urgency** • **BLOODY DIARRHEA hallmark** (stools with mucus/pus), hematochezia	• Abdominal Pain: **RLQ pain MC** (crampy) & weight loss more common with Crohn • Diarrhea with no visible blood usually
COMPLICATIONS	• Primary Sclerosing Cholangitis, Colon ca, Toxic megacolon (More common in UC). • **Smoking decreases risk for UC.**	• **Perianal disease**: fistulas, strictures, abscesses, **GRANULOMAS.** • Malabsorption: Fe & **B_{12} deficiency**
COLONOSCOPY	• **Uniform inflammation** • ±ulceration in rectum and/or colon. • **PSEUDOPOLYPS.**	• **"SKIP LESIONS"** = normal areas interspersed between inflamed areas, **COBBLESTONE appearance.**
BARIUM STUDIES	**"STOVEPIPE SIGN"** - loss of haustral markings).	• **"STRING SIGN":** barium flow through narrowed inflamed/scarred area due to transmural strictures.
LABS	• **⊕ P-ANCA (more common in UC)**	• ⊕ **ASCA** (**antibodies vs *Saccharomyces cerevisiae***)
SURGERY	• **Curative**	• Noncurative

CROHN DISEASE

- Idiopathic autoimmune Inflammatory bowel disease.

- **Transmural inflammation** that **affects any part of the GI tract** (anywhere from mouth to anus). Transmural inflammation may lead to **fistulas, bowel strictures, perianal disease, abscesses,** fissures, fibrosis, & bowel obstruction.

- **Terminal ileum most commonly involved segment.** ~ 55% **ileocolitis**, ~ 40% affect the small bowel only; ~ 20% colitis only. Rectum is often spared in CD.

CLINICAL MANIFESTATIONS

- **Ileocolitis:** crampy abdominal pain (especially **right lower quadrant**), **diarrhea (not usually grossly bloody), weight loss,** fever.

- Jejunoileitis: malabsorption, steatorrhea, nutritional deficiencies & electrolyte disorders.

- Colitis & perianal disease: diarrhea, perirectal abscesses, anorectal fistula & fissure formation, bowel obstruction.

DIAGNOSIS

- Upper GI series: **initial test of choice - string sign** (barium flowing through narrowed inflamed/scarred areas), fistula formation.

- Endoscopy: **segmental "skip areas"** (normal areas in between damaged areas), **cobblestoning** of the mucosa, aphthous ulcerations, strictures.

- Biopsy: **transmural inflammation,** microscopic skip areas, **noncaseating granulomas.** Creeping fat on gross dissection is pathognomonic.

- Labs: **anti-Saccharomyces cerevisiae antibodies,** iron & **B12 deficiency** if severe, increased ESR & CRP.

MANAGEMENT

- Limited ileocolonic disease: **5-ASA** (eg, **Mesalamine**) **or oral Glucocorticoids.**

- Ileal & proximal colon disease: **Glucocorticoids** (eg, enteric coated Budesonide, Prednisone).

- Severe & refractory: Azathioprine, 6-Mercatopurine, Methotrexate and anti-TNF agents (eg, Adalimumab, Infliximab) are all options.

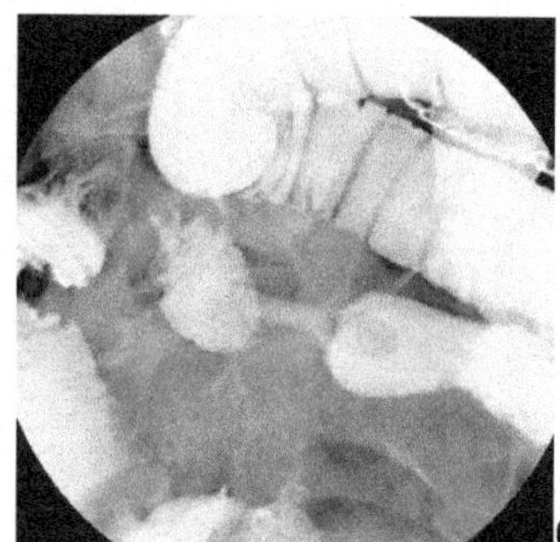

Crohn disease: **string sign** (narrowing of the lumen).

ULCERATIVE COLITIS

CLINICAL MANIFESTATIONS
- **Diarrhea (often bloody), crampy abdominal pain** (especially **left lower quadrant**), **& tenesmus.**
- Mild: 4 or less bowel movements/day (may be bloody). No signs of systemic toxicity. Episodes of constipation may also be seen. May have mild abdominal pain.
- Moderate: frequent loose bowel movements >4/day, abdominal pain, may be anemic from the bloody stools.
- Severe: 6 loose bowel movement/day, severe abdominal pain, signs of systemic toxicity (fever, anemia, elevated ESR & CRP), may have weight loss.

DIAGNOSIS
- Flexible sigmoidoscopy: nonspecific - pseudopolyps, **uniform erythema, & ulceration** (eg, friable mucosa, continuous, circumferential pattern). Diffuse and contiguous rectal involvement.
- Biopsy: nonspecific - crypt abscesses & atrophy, inflammation, basal plasmacytosis
- Barium enema: **stovepipe or lead pipe sign** (cylindrical bowel with loss of Haustral markings).
- Labs: **positive P-ANCA.** Increased ESR, CRP, leukocytosis, anemia of chronic disease. Fetal lactoferrin & calprotectin are sensitive for acute inflammation.

MANAGEMENT
- **Mild to moderate distal**: **topical 5-aminosalicylic acid (ASA) first-line.** Topical corticosteroids may be added. Oral 5-ASA can be added if needed.
- Mild to moderate pancolitis: combination therapy with oral 5-ASA, topical –ASA, & steroids.
- Severe: oral glucocorticoids + high dose 5-ASA + topical 5-ASA or steroids.
- Fulminant colitis: IV glucocorticoids, IV fluids, broad-spectrum antibiotics.
- Surgical resection in some cases.

MAINTENANCE THERAPY FOR CD & UC

6-Mercaptopurine & Azathioprine
- Mechanism purine analogues that inhibit immune response. Azathioprine is converted to 6-MP.
- Indications: used as **steroid-sparing agents**. May also be used as maintenance therapy.
- Adverse effects: rash, fever, pancreatitis, nausea, bone marrow suppression, risk of lymphoma.

Methotrexate
- Mechanism: anti-inflammatory that decreases interleukin production.
- Indications: used to induce remission & to reduce the use of corticosteroids.
- Adverse reactions: leukopenia, pneumonitis, hepatic fibrosis (evaluate with periodic CBCs & LFTs)

Cyclosporine:
- Mechanism: immunomodulator that reduces IL production by T cells & inhibits calcineurin (a chemical messenger that activates macrophages).
- Indications: used in UC refractory to IV glucocorticoids.

Tacrolimus:
- Mechanism: macrolide antibiotic with immunomodulatory properties. More effective than azathioprine. Used in refractory disease.

Anti-TNF agents:
- Inhibit proinflammatory cytokines (Adalimumab, Infliximab, Certolizumab).

Anti-integrins: Natalizumab

CHRONIC MESENTERIC ISCHEMIA

- Ischemic bowel disease due to mesenteric atherosclerosis - decreased supply during increased demand (eating).
- **Most patients have atherosclerotic disease** (eg, history of MI).

PATHOPHYSIOLOGY
- Episodic intestinal **hypoperfusion related to eating** (increased demand during eating + decreased blood supply).

CLINICAL MANIFESTATIONS
- Abdominal pain: chronic dull **abdominal pain worse after meals (intestinal angina).**
- Anorexia (**aversion to eating**) leading to **weight loss**.

DIAGNOSIS
- Angiography: definitive diagnostic test.

MANAGEMENT
- Revascularization is the definitive management (eg, angioplasty with stenting or bypass).

ACUTE MESENTERIC ISCHEMIA

- Abrupt onset of small intestinal hypoperfusion.

ETIOLOGIES
- **Acute arterial occlusion: embolism from Atrial fibrillation most common, thrombotic** (eg, Atherosclerosis). **Superior mesenteric artery occlusion most common.**
- Nonocclusive arterial ischemia: hypoperfusion due to shock, vasopressors (decreased blood flow), cocaine (due to vasospasm).
- Venous thrombosis: obstruction of the intestinal venous outflow.

CLINICAL MANIFESTATIONS
- Abdominal pain: **"severe abdominal pain out of proportion to physical findings"** - no peritoneal signs. Pain is usually poorly localized.
- May develop nausea, vomiting, diarrhea.
- Advanced disease: peritonitis (eg, rigidity, guarding & rebound tenderness), heme-positive stool or shock.

DIAGNOSIS
- **CT angiography:** often **initial test to assess ischemia** if stable. Done without oral contrast.
- **Conventional arteriography: definitive diagnosis.**
- Labs: **leukocytosis, lactic acidosis**, increased hematocrit (hemoconcentration), increased amylase & LDH.

MANAGEMENT

Depends on the cause
- **Surgical revascularization:** eg, embolectomy if due to embolism; angioplasty with stenting or bypass to treat arterial thrombosis.
- Surgical resection if the bowel is not salvageable.
- Anticoagulation or thrombolysis in venous thrombosis. Anticoagulation in patients with A fib.

ISCHEMIC COLITIS

- Decreased colonic perfusion, leading to inflammation.

ETIOLOGIES

- **Most commonly due to transient systemic hypotension or atherosclerosis** involving the superior & inferior mesenteric arteries.
- Most common at "watershed" areas (between 2 arteries with decreased collaterals) such as the **splenic flexure & rectosigmoid junction.**

RISK FACTORS

- Elderly, Diabetes mellitus, aortoiliac surgery or instrumentation, cardiac catheterization, myocardial infarction, constipation-inducing medications.

CLINICAL MANIFESTATIONS

- **Left-sided (LLQ) crampy, abdominal pain with tenderness, bloody diarrhea, or hematochezia** (due to colonic sloughing from ischemia).
- Pain usually is not as severe and is more lateral compared to Acute mesenteric ischemia.
- May develop bowel gangrene (associated with lactic acidosis & leukocytosis).

DIAGNOSIS

- **CT of the abdomen: often the first imaging test for acute colonic ischemia** - wall edema, **"thumbprinting"** = segmental bowel wall thickening (nonspecific).
- Colonoscopy: segmental ischemic changes in areas of low perfusion (splenic flexure). Edematous, friable mucosa. Not performed if signs of peritonitis or bowel perforation is suspected.

MANAGEMENT

- **Supportive care: restore perfusion, bowel rest, IV fluids,** & observe for signs of perforation is the management for most patients (usually resolves without specific therapy).
- May need empiric broad-spectrum antibiotics.

COLON POLYPS

- **Pseudopolyps/Inflammatory:** due to inflammatory bowel disease (eg, Ulcerative colitis or Crohn disease). **Not considered cancerous.**
- **Hyperplastic: low risk for malignancy**. Most common non-neoplastic polyp. They are a type of serrated polyps (saw tooth pattern).

Hamartomatous polyps

- Juvenile polyp: relatively more common during childhood. An isolated (solitary) juvenile polyp is not associated with increased cancer risk.
- Juvenile polyposis syndrome: autosomal dominant condition associated with multiple hamartomatous polyps. Associated with increased risk of colorectal and gastric cancer.
- Peutz-Jeghers polyps: usually associated with Peutz-Jeghers syndrome (STK11 mutation). Usually benign but may undergo malignant transformation so they are usually resected.

Adenomatous polyps: Most common neoplastic polyp. They comprise 2/3 of all colonic polyps. Average is 10-20 years before becoming cancerous (especially >1cm)

- **Tubular adenoma**: nonpedunculated (most common type of adenomatous polyp. Associated with the least risk of all the 3 types of adenomatous polyps).
- Tubulovillous (mixture). Intermediate risk.
- **Villous adenoma: highest risk of becoming cancerous**. Tends to be sessile.

COLORECTAL CANCER (CRC)

- **Most arise from adenomatous polyps.**

RISK FACTORS
- **Age >50 years** (peaks 65y), African-Americans, family history of colorectal cancer
- Inflammatory bowel disease: **Ulcerative colitis** > Crohn; The increased risk of Colon cancer begins about 8 to 10 years after the initial diagnosis of pancolitis, and at 15 to 20 years for colitis limited to the left colon.
- Diet & lifestyle: **diet (low fiber, high in red or processed meat,** animal fat), obesity, smoking, ETOH.

GENETICS
- **Familial adenomatous polyposis:** genetic mutation of the APC gene. Adenomas begin in childhood. Almost all will develop colon cancer by age 45y. Prophylactic colectomy best for survival.
- Turcot syndrome: FAP-like syndrome + CNS tumors (medulloblastoma, glial tumors).
- **Lynch syndrome (Hereditary nonpolyposis colorectal cancer):** autosomal dominant. Due to loss-of-function in DNA mismatch repair genes (MLH1, MSH2/6, PMS3). Has 40% risk of colon cancer (type I especially seen on the right side). Type II has increased risk of extra-colonic cancers: **endometrial** (especially), ovarian, small intestine, brain, & skin. Mean age is in the late 40s but can develop cancer in their 20s.
- **Peutz-Jehgers Syndrome:** autosomal dominant. Associated with **hamartomatous polyps, mucocutaneous hyperpigmentation** (lips, oral mucosa, hands), risk of breast & pancreatic cancer.

PROTECTIVE FACTORS
- Physical activity, regular use of aspirin, and NSAIDs are associated with a decreased risk.

CLINICAL MANIFESTATIONS
- Iron deficiency anemia (fatigue, weakness), rectal bleeding, abdominal pain, & change in bowel habits. **Colorectal cancer is the most common cause of large bowel obstruction in adults.**
- Advanced disease: ascites, abdominal masses, & hepatomegaly.

- **Right-sided (proximal)** lesions tend to cause **chronic occult bleeding (Iron deficiency anemia,** positive Guaiac) & diarrhea.

- **Left-sided (distal)** lesions tend to cause **bowel obstruction,** present later & cause **changes in stool diameter**. May develop ***Streptococcus bovis*** endocarditis.

DIAGNOSIS
- **Colonoscopy with biopsy: diagnostic test of choice.**

- Barium enema: **apple core lesion classic** (filling defect). Lesions seen on barium enema need a follow up colonoscopy or CT colonography.

- Laboratory: **iron deficiency anemia classic** (colorectal cancer is the most common cause of occult GI bleeding in adults).

- Tumor markers: **CEA is the most commonly monitored tumor marker** (not specific).

MANAGEMENT
- Localized: surgical resection (radical vs. endoscopic) followed by postoperative (adjuvant) chemotherapy to destroy residual cells and micrometastases.
- Metastatic: palliative chemotherapy.

COLON CANCER SCREENING GUIDELINES

	Fecal Occult Blood test	COLONOSCOPY
Average Risk	**Annually at 50y**	**Colonoscopy q 10y (or flex sig q5y)** up to 75y
1st-degree relative ≥60y	**Annually at 40y**	**Colonoscopy q 10y**
1st degree relative <60y	**Annually at 40y** (or 10y before the age relative was diagnosed)	**Colonoscopy q 5y**

- Patients are screened until at least 75 years.
- USPSTF guidelines recommends any of the 3 approaches: ❶ High Sensitivity fecal occult blood testing: annually ❷ Colonoscopy every 10y from age 50-75 (individualized after 75) ❸ Flexible sigmoidoscopy every 5 years along with fecal occult blood testing every 3 years.

Lynch syndrome (HNPCC):
- Screening beginning at 20-25 years of age via colonoscopy every 1-2 years

Familial adenomatous polyposis:
- Initiate screen at age 10-12 years with flexible sigmoidoscopy yearly.

ESOPHAGITIS

ETIOLOGIES
- **Gastroesophageal reflux disease (GERD) most common cause.**
- Infectious: Candida, CMV, HSV. Most commonly associated with immunocompromised states.
- Eosinophilic: due to allergic reaction
- Pill-induced: bisphosphonates, beta blockers, calcium channel blockers, NSAIDs
- Caustic (corrosive): due to acidic or basic substances

CLINICAL MANIFESTATIONS
- The three classic symptoms of esophagitis are **odynophagia (hallmark), dysphagia, and retrosternal chest pain.**

DIAGNOSIS
- **Upper endoscopy** allows for direct visualization. Double-contrast Esophagram.

MANAGEMENT
- Treat the underlying cause.

IRRITABLE BOWEL SYNDROME

- Chronic, functional idiopathic pain disorder with NO organic cause.

- Onset most common in late teens, early 20s. Most common in women.

PATHOPHYSIOLOGY OF IBS
- **Abnormal motility:** chemical imbalance in the intestine (including serotonin & acetylcholine) causing abnormal motility & spasm ⇨ abdominal pain. Altered gut microbiota.

- **Visceral hypersensitivity** patients have lowered pain thresholds to intestinal distention.

- **Psychosocial interactions** & altered central nervous system processing.

CLINICAL MANIFESTATIONS:
- Hallmark: **abdominal pain associated with altered defecation/bowel habits** (diarrhea, constipation or alternation between the two). **Pain often relieved with defecation.**

ALARM SYMPTOMS IN IBS
- Evidence of GI bleeding: occult blood in stool, rectal bleeding, anemia.
- Anorexia or weight loss, fever, nocturnal symptoms, family history of GI cancer, IBD or celiac sprue.
- Persistent diarrhea causing dehydration; severe constipation or fecal impaction; Onset >45y.

DIAGNOSIS
- Diagnosis of exclusion (after workup eg, colonoscopy & abdominal CT rule out other etiologies.
- **Rome IV Criteria:** recurrent abdominal pain on average at least 1 day/week in the last 3 months associated with at least 2 of the following 3:
  - ❶ **related to defecation**
  - ❷ onset associated with **change in stool frequency**
  - ❸ onset associated with **change in stool form (appearance)**

MANAGEMENT
- **Lifestyle & dietary changes first-line management.** This includes **low fat, high fiber, & unprocessed food diet.**
- Avoid beverages containing sorbitol or fructose (eg, apples, raisins), avoid gas-producing foods (eg, beans, some cruciferous vegetables. Sleep, smoking cessation & exercise.

CONSTIPATION SYMPTOMS:
- Prokinetics: **fiber, psyllium**. **Polyethylene glycol** may be added after fiber. Bulk-forming or saline laxatives.
- Lubiprostone & Linaclotide are usually reserved for people with no response to above.

DIARRHEA SYMPTOMS:
- **Loperamide**, Eluxadoline, Rifaximin. Bile acid sequestrants, Alosetron.
- Anticholinergics/antispasmodics (eg, **Dicyclomine,** Hyoscyamine).

INFECTIOUS ESOPHAGITIS

RISK FACTORS

- **Immunocompromised states** (eg, HIV, post-transplant, malignancy, chemotherapy) but can occur in healthy patients.
- **Candida is the most common cause**. In patients with classic symptoms, empiric treatment with Fluconazole can be initiated with upper endoscopy reserved if no response to initial therapy.

CLINICAL MANIFESTATIONS

- The three classic symptoms of esophagitis are **odynophagia (hallmark), dysphagia, and retrosternal chest pain.**

DISEASE	ENDOSCOPIC FINDINGS	1ST LINE MANAGEMENT	2ND LINE
CANDIDA	**linear yellow-white plaques**	**PO Fluconazole**	Voriconazole, Caspofungin
CMV	**large superficial shallow ulcers**	**Ganciclovir**	Valganciclovir, Foscarnet
HSV	**small, deep ulcers**	**Acyclovir**	Foscarnet

EOSINOPHILIC ESOPHAGITIS

- Allergic, inflammatory eosinophilic infiltration of the esophageal epithelium.
- Most commonly seen in children & associated with atopic disease (eg, Asthma, Eczema).

CLINICAL MANIFESTATIONS

- **Dysphagia (especially solids),** odynophagia. Reflux or feeding difficulties in children.

DIAGNOSIS

- Endoscopy: normal or **multiple corrugated rings**, white exudates.
- Biopsy: presence of abundance of eosinophils.

MANAGEMENT

- Remove foods that incite allergic response. PPIs may be needed in some.
- Inhaled topical corticosteroids (without using a spacer to allow for penetration).

PILL-INDUCED ESOPHAGITIS

- Esophagitis due to prolonged pill contact with the esophagus.

MEDICATIONS

- **NSAIDS, bisphosphonates,** beta blockers, calcium channel blockers, potassium chloride, iron pills, iron pills, vitamin C, beta blockers, & calcium channel blockers.

CLINICAL MANIFESTATIONS

- Odynophagia, dysphagia.

DIAGNOSIS

- Endoscopy: small, well-defined ulcers of varying depths.

MANAGEMENT

Take pills with at least 4 ounces of water, avoid recumbency at least 30-60 minutes after pill ingestion.

CAUSTIC (CORROSIVE) ESOPHAGITIS

- Ingestion of corrosive substances: alkali (drain cleaner, lye, bleach) or acids.

CLINICAL MANIFESTATIONS
- Odynophagia, dysphagia, hematemesis, dyspnea.

DIAGNOSIS
- Endoscopy is used to determine the extent of damage & look for complications (eg, esophageal perforation, stricture, & esophageal fistula).

MANAGEMENT
- Supportive, pain medications, IV fluids.

HIATAL HERNIA

- Herniation of structures from the abdominal cavity through the esophageal hiatus of the diaphragm.

Sliding:
- (Type I) - GE junction "slides" into the mediastinum (increases reflux). **Most common type** (95%).

Paraesophageal:
- (Type II) - "rolling hernia" – fundus of stomach protrudes through diaphragm with the GE junction remaining in its anatomic location.

CLINICAL MANIFESTATIONS
- Usually an asymptomatic incidental finding, may develop intermittent epigastric or substernal pain, postprandial fullness, retching or nausea.

MANAGEMENT
- Sliding: management of GERD – **PPIs + weight loss** (if indicated).
- Paraesophageal: surgical repair reserved for complications (eg, volvulus, obstruction, strangulation, bleeding, perforation, etc).

ESOPHAGEAL ATRESIA

- Complete absence or closure of a portion of the esophagus.
- **Most commonly associated with a tracheoesophageal fistula,** polyhydramnios.

CLINICAL MANIFESTATIONS
- **Presents immediately after birth with excessive oral secretions** that leads to **choking, drooling, inability to feed, respiratory distress, and coughing** (especially when attempting to feed).
- Gastric distention may occur. Aspiration pneumonia common.

DIAGNOSIS
- Inability to pass a nasogastric tube further than 10-15 cm (coiling in the esophagus).
- Fluoroscopy: small amount of water-soluble contrast may reveal it (but must be removed promptly to prevent aspiration). Barium should not be used.

MANAGEMENT
- Surgical ligation of the fistula with primary anastomosis of the esophageal segments may be done in stages of the distance between the 2 segments is large.

GASTROESOPHAGEAL REFLUX DISEASE (GERD)

- Reflux of gastric contents into the esophagus due to an **incompetent lower esophageal sphincter.**
- **Transient relaxation of LES** (incompetency) ⇨ gastric acid reflux ⇨ esophageal mucosal injury.

CLINICAL MANIFESTATIONS

- Typical: **heartburn (pyrosis) hallmark –** often retrosternal & postprandial, increased with supine position and may be relieved with antacids. Regurgitation: water brash, sour taste in the mouth, cough, sore throat.
- Atypical symptoms: hoarseness, aspiration pneumonia, wheezing, chest pain.
- **"Alarm" symptoms: dysphagia, odynophagia, weight loss, bleeding**.

COMPLICATIONS: 4 main complications may present with alarm symptoms

- Esophagitis - inflammation from acid.
- Stricture - narrowing from acidic damage.
- **Barrett's esophagus**: esophageal squamous epithelium replaced by precancerous metaplastic columnar cells from the cardia of the stomach.
- **Esophageal adenocarcinoma** as a result of Barrett's esophagus.

DIAGNOSIS OF TYPICAL GERD

- **Clinical diagnosis** based on history if presenting with classic, simple symptoms.
- **24-hour ambulatory pH monitoring: gold standard** if confirmation is needed.
- Esophageal Manometry: decreased LES pressure.

DIAGNOSIS IF PERSISTENT SYMPTOMS OR ALARM SYMPTOMS:

- **Endoscopy: first-line diagnostic test if persistent symptoms or complication of GERD is suspected** (eg, alarm symptoms, malignancy, symptoms >5-10 years, etc.).

MANAGEMENT

- Lifestyle modifications: - elevate the head of the bed 6-8 inches, avoid recumbency for 3 hours after eating, avoid food that delay gastric emptying (eg, fatty or spicy food, chocolate, peppermint, caffeinated products), smoking cessation, decreased alcohol intake, weight loss.
- Stage 2: intermittent or mild (< 2 episodes/week) - "as needed" pharmacologic therapy: antacids and H2 receptor antagonists.
- Stage 3: **Proton pump inhibitors in moderate to severe disease** (≥2 episodes/week).
- Nissen fundoplication in medication-refractory patients.

BARRETT'S ESOPHAGUS

- Esophageal squamous epithelium replaced by precancerous metaplastic columnar cells from the cardia of the stomach (precursor to Esophageal adenocarcinoma).
- A complication of longstanding GERD.

DIAGNOSIS

- Upper endoscopy with biopsy

Barrett's esophagus only (metaplasia)	PPIs and rescope every 3-5 years
Low-grade dysplasia	PPIs and rescope every 6-12 months
High-grade dysplasia	Ablation with endoscopy, photodynamic therapy, endoscopic mucosal resection, radiofrequency ablation

ESOPHAGEAL NEOPLASMS

MAJOR TYPES

Adenocarcinoma:
- **Most common cause in US** (50-80%). Seen in younger patients. Common in **Caucasian males.**
- **Most common in the distal esophagus, esophagogastric junction.**

Squamous cell:
- **Most common cause worldwide** (90-95%). Peaks 50-70 years of age.
- In the US, it is associated with **increased incidence in African-Americans.**
- Most common in the **mid to upper third** of the esophagus.

RISK FACTORS for **Adenocarcinoma:**
- **Major risk factors in the US are Barrett's esophagus** (a complication of **GERD), smoking & high body mass index.** Unlike Squamous cell, alcohol is not a risk factor for Adenocarcinoma.

RISK FACTORS for **Squamous cell carcinoma:**
- **Major risk factors in the US are smoking & alcohol.**
- Worldwide include poor nutritional status, low intake of fruits & vegetables, drinking beverages at high temperatures (thermal injury). HPV infection. N-nitroso compounds. Atrophic gastritis, Achalasia, Tylosis.

PROTECTIVE FACTORS
- Aspirin or NSAIDs may have protective effect of esophageal cancer, particularly in the setting of Barrett's esophagus.

CLINICAL MANIFESTATIONS
- Patients often have extensive disease by the time they become symptomatic.
- **Progressive dysphagia: hallmark - solid food dysphagia progressing to include fluids, odynophagia** (20%).
- **Weight loss,** anorexia. Iron deficiency anemia (chronic blood loss).
- Chest pain, anorexia, cough, hematemesis, reflux, hoarseness (recurrent laryngeal nerve).
- Horner's syndrome, tracheal-esophageal fistula. Hypercalcemia with Squamous cell carcinoma.

DIAGNOSIS
- **Upper endoscopy with biopsy: diagnostic study of choice.** Appearance - early lesions may appear as superficial plaques, nodules, or ulcerations. Advanced lesions may appear as strictures, ulcerated masses, circumferential masses, or large ulcerations.
- Double-contrast Barium esophagram.
- Pretreatment staging: **endoscopic ultrasound is the preferred method for locoregional staging.** Preoperative bronchoscopy with biopsy and brush cytology indicated for locally advanced lesions. CT neck chest abdomen, PET/CT scan.

MANAGEMENT
- Esophageal resection may be combined with chemotherapy.
- Radiation therapy, chemotherapy (eg, 5-FU).
- Palliative stenting to improve dysphagia may be needed in advanced cases.

ACHALASIA

- **Loss of peristalsis** and failure of relaxation of the lower esophageal sphincter **(LES)**.

PATHOPHYSIOLOGY

- Idiopathic proximal **degeneration of Auerbach's plexus** leads to increased LES pressure & impaired lower esophageal sphincter (LES) relaxation.
- Most commonly presents <50 years of age.

CLINICAL MANIFESTATIONS

- **Dysphagia to both solids and liquids** at the same time, regurgitation of undigested food, chest pain, cough. May develop malnutrition, weight loss, and dehydration.

DIAGNOSIS

- Barium esophagram: **"bird's beak" appearance of the LES** (LES narrowing) with proximal esophageal dilation & loss of peristalsis distally.
- **Manometry: most accurate test - increased LES pressure and lack of peristalsis**.
- Endoscopy: usually **performed in Achalasia prior to initiating treatment** to rule out Esophageal squamous cell carcinoma (Achalasia is a risk factor).

MANAGEMENT

- Decrease LES pressure: botulinum toxin injection (requires retreatment in 6-12 months); nitrates. Surgery more effective.
- Pneumatic dilation of LES
- Esophagomyomectomy (definitive)

ZENKER'S DIVERTICULUM

- **Pharyngoesophageal pouch (false diverticulum** – only involves the mucosa and possibly submucosa).
- Most common in males. Usually presents >60 years of age (often in the 70s).

PATHOPHYSIOLOGY

- Outpouching occurs due to weakness at the junction of Killian's triangle (between the fibers of the **cricopharyngeal muscle** & lower inferior pharyngeal constrictor muscle).

CLINICAL MANIFESTATIONS

- **Dysphagia**, regurgitation of undigested food, cough, feeling as if there is a lump in neck (neck mass), choking sensation, **halitosis** (due to food retention in the pouch).

DIAGNOSIS

- **Barium Esophagram** with video fluoroscopy **initial test of choice** - collection of dye behind the esophagus at the pharyngoesophageal junction.
- Upper endoscopy usually performed for surgical evaluation.

MANAGEMENT

- Observation if small & asymptomatic.
- Diverticulectomy, cricopharyngeal myotomy.

DISTAL (DIFFUSE) ESOPHAGEAL SPASM

- Esophageal motility disorder characterized by **severe non-peristaltic esophageal contractions** (uncoordinated contractions).

PATHOPHYSIOLOGY
- Impaired inhibitory innervation lead to premature and rapidly propagated contractions.

CLINICAL MANIFESTATIONS
- **Stabbing, chest pain worse with hot or cold liquids or food** (pain similar to Angina but not exertional).
- **Dysphagia to both solids and liquids** simultaneously, sensation of "object stuck in the throat"

DIAGNOSIS
- Esophagram: severe non-peristaltic contractions - **"corkscrew" esophagus**.
- **Manometry: (definitive) - increased simultaneous or premature contractions** in the distal esophagus with preservation of some peristaltic activity.
- Manometry often combined with Esophagram and Endoscopy to rule out malignancy.

MANAGEMENT
- **Anti-spasmodics first-line** (eg. **Calcium channel blockers**, Nitrates, Tricyclic antidepressants).
- Second-line: Botulinum toxin injection, Pneumatic dilation.
- Peroral endoscopic myotomy alternative if refractory to medical management.

HYPERCONTRACTILE (JACKHAMMER) ESOPHAGUS

- Esophageal motility disorder characterized by **increased pressure during peristalsis** (normally sequential contractions in the smooth muscle of the esophagus).
- Classically known as **Nutcracker esophagus.**

CLINICAL MANIFESTATIONS
- Dysphagia to both liquids & solids, chest pain similar to Distal (diffuse) esophageal spasm.

DIAGNOSIS
- **Manometry**: **(definitive) - increased pressure during peristalsis.**
- Upper endoscopy and Esophagram are usually normal.

MANAGEMENT
- Lower esophageal pressure: **Calcium channel blockers**, Nitrates, Botulinum toxin injection, Tricyclic antidepressants.

> - **Exam tip**
> - Distal (Diffuse) esophageal spasm and Hypercontractile esophagus have a similar presentation but manometry will show different peristaltic patterns to be able to distinguish between the two.

BOERHAAVE SYNDROME

- **Full thickness rupture** most commonly affecting the **left posterolateral wall of the lower esophagus.** 40% mortality.

ETIOLOGIES

- Associated with iatrogenic perforation of the esophagus during endoscopy (most common), **repeated, forceful retching or vomiting** (eg, Bulimia, alcoholism).

CLINICAL MANIFESTATIONS

- **Retrosternal chest pain worse with deep breathing & swallowing,** vomiting, hematemesis.

PHYSICAL EXAMINATION

- **Crepitus on chest auscultation** (subcutaneous emphysema).
- **Hamman's sign** (mediastinal "crackling" accompanying every heart beat) in the left lateral decubitus position.

DIAGNOSIS

- **Contrast esophagram: diagnostic test of choice** - leakage. **Gastrografin swallow preferred** (water soluble). Barium is caustic if it leaks through a perforation.
- Chest CT scan, CXR: left-sided hydropneumothorax (most common), **pneumomediastinum**, esophageal thickening.

MANAGEMENT

- Small & stable: IV fluids, NPO, broad-spectrum antibiotics, H2 receptor blockers.
- Large or severe: surgical repair.

MALLORY-WEISS SYNDROME (TEARS)

- **Longitudinal superficial mucosal lacerations** at the gastroesophageal junction or the gastric cardia.

PATHOPHYSIOLOGY

- Sudden rise in intraabdominal pressure or gastric prolapse into the esophagus (eg, **persistent retching or vomiting after ETOH binge**).
- May also be associated with Hiatal hernias.

CLINICAL MANIFESTATIONS

- **Upper GI bleeding** preceded by retching or vomiting: hematemesis, melena, hematochezia, syncope. 5-10% of all UGIB.
- May develop abdominal pain, back pain or hydrophobia.

DIAGNOSIS

- **Upper endoscopy test of choice - superficial longitudinal mucosal erosions.**

MANAGEMENT

- Not actively bleeding: **supportive mainstay of treatment** (eg, **acid suppression with PPIs** promotes healing). Most cases stop bleeding without intervention.
- Severe bleeding: options include thermal coagulation, hemoclips, endoscopic band ligation (with or without epinephrine), & balloon tamponade (eg, Sengstaken-Blakemore tube or Minnesota tube).

ESOPHAGEAL WEB

- Noncircumferential thin membrane in the **mid-upper esophagus**.
- May be congenital or acquired (eg, associated with Zenker's diverticulum).

CLINICAL MANIFESTATIONS
- Dysphagia especially to solids (eg, meat, bread). Many are asymptomatic.

DIAGNOSIS
- **Barium esophagram (swallow): diagnostic test of choice** (more sensitive than endoscopy).

MANAGEMENT
- Endoscopic dilation of the area if severe symptoms. PPI therapy after dilation may decrease the risk of recurrence.

Plummer-Vinson Syndrome:
- Triad of **dysphagia** + cervical **esophageal webs + iron deficiency anemia**. May also be associated with **atrophic glossitis**, angular cheilitis, koilonychia, & splenomegaly.
- Most common in Caucasian women 30-60y.
- Patients with Plummer-Vinson syndrome are at increased risk for Esophageal squamous cell carcinoma.

ESOPHAGEAL (SHATZKI) RING

- Circumferential diaphragm of tissue that protrudes into the esophageal lumen.
- **Most common at the lower esophagus (at the squamocolumnar junction).**

RISK FACTORS
- **Hiatal hernia present in most patients,** corrosive esophageal injury (eg, acid reflux), Eosinophilic esophagitis.

CLINICAL MANIFESTATIONS
- Most are asymptomatic.
- Episodic dysphagia, especially to solids (eg, meat, bread), bolus of food may get stuck in the lower esophagus ("Steakhouse syndrome").

DIAGNOSIS
- **Barium esophagram (swallow): more sensitive than endoscopy** - circumferential ridge a few cm above the hiatus of the diaphragm.
- Upper endoscopy: often performed in patients with Esophageal rings to biopsy the esophagus for associated Eosinophilic esophagitis.

MANAGEMENT
- **Symptomatic: dilation** (pneumatic or bougie); obliteration with biopsy forceps.
- Antireflux surgery if reflux is present.

ESOPHAGEAL VARICES

- Dilation of the gastroesophageal collateral submucosal veins as a complication of **portal vein hypertension** (including the left gastric vein).

RISK FACTORS
- **Cirrhosis most common cause in adults.**
- Portal vein thrombosis most common cause in children.

CLINICAL MANIFESTATIONS
- **Upper GI bleed: hematemesis, melena, hematochezia**. If severe, may develop signs and symptoms of hypovolemia.

DIAGNOSIS
- **Upper endoscopy: test of choice** (both diagnostic and therapeutic).

MANAGEMENT OF ACUTE VARICEAL BLEED
- Stabilize the patient: **2 large bore IV lines, IV fluids**. May need packed red blood cells if low hematocrit. If coagulopathy (increased INR and/or PT) may need fresh frozen plasma.

- **Endoscopic intervention: endoscopic variceal ligation initial treatment of choice.** Endoscopic sclerotherapy an option but has higher complication and rebleed potential.

- Pharmacologic vasoconstrictors:
  Octreotide first-line medical management. Can be used alone or as an adjunct to endoscopic treatment. Octreotide is a somatostatin analog that causes vasoconstriction of the portal venous flow, decreasing portal pressure and reducing bleeding.
  Second-line: Vasopressin second-line. Decreases portal venous pressure. Adverse effects: vessel constriction in other areas: coronary artery vasospasm, myocardial infarction, bowel ischemia.

- Balloon tamponade: used to stabilize bleeding not controlled by endoscopic or pharmacologic intervention or in rapid bleeds.

- Surgical decompression: transjugular intrahepatic portosystemic shunt (TIPS): indicated if bleeding despite endoscopic or pharmacologic treatment and in some advanced cases.

ANTIBIOTIC PROPHYLAXIS
- Fluoroquinolones (eg, Norfloxacin) or Ceftriaxone to prevent infectious complications (eg, Spontaneous bacterial peritonitis).

PREVENTION OF REBLEED:
- **Nonselective beta blockers (eg, Nadolol or Propranolol)** to prevent rebleeding one the patient has been stabilized.

- 90% of patients with cirrhosis develop esophageal varices, 30% of them bleed (mortality rate 30-50% with 1st bleed). 70% rebleed within 1st year of the initial bleed (1/3 of re-bleeds are fatal).

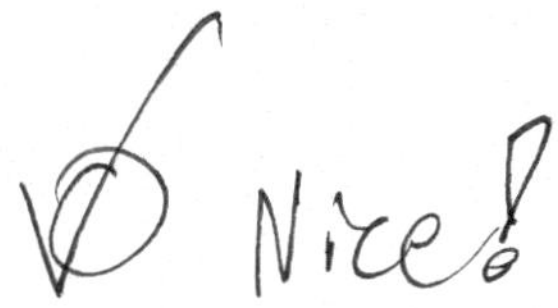

CELIAC DISEASE (SPRUE)

- **Autoimmune-mediated inflammation of the small bowel** due to reaction with alpha-gliadin in **gluten-containing foods** (eg, wheat, rye, barley).

PATHOPHYSIOLOGY
- Autoimmune damage leads to loss of villi with subsequent malabsorption.
- Increased incidence in females, European descent (Irish & Finnish).

CLINICAL MANIFESTATIONS
- **Malabsorption: diarrhea**, abdominal pain/distention, bloating, steatorrhea. Growth delays in children.

- **Dermatitis herpetiformis**: pruritic, papulovesicular rash most common on extensor surfaces, neck, trunk, & scalp.

DIAGNOSIS
- Clinical diagnosis: symptom improvement with a trial of gluten-free diet.

- Screening: **transglutaminase IgA antibodies initial test of choice.** Endomysial IgA antibodies.

- Definitive & confirmatory: **small bowel biopsy – atrophy of the villi** (most accurate).

MANAGEMENT
- Gluten-free diet - **avoid wheat, rye, barley**. Limit oat consumption. Rice, wine, & corn are safe.
- Vitamin supplementation.

LACTOSE INTOLERANCE

- Inability to digest lactose due to low levels of lactase enzyme.
- Lactase enzyme production normally declines in adulthood, especially in African Americans, Asians, & South Americans.

CLINICAL MANIFESTATIONS
- Loose stools, abdominal pain, flatulence, & borborygmi after ingestion of milk or milk-containing products.

DIAGNOSIS
- **Clinical diagnosis** – symptom improvement after a trial of lactose-free diet.

- **Hydrogen breath test: test of choice.** Hydrogen produced when colonic bacteria ferment the undigested lactose. Usually performed after a trial of a lactose-free diet if the diagnosis is uncertain.

MANAGEMENT
- Lactose-free diet or use of enzymes: lactase enzyme preparations
- Lactaid (prehydrolyzed milk).

PEANUT AND TREE NUT ALLERGY

- **Most are IgE mediated** but may be non Ig-E mediated or mixed.

RISK FACTORS
- **Genetics** - siblings of children with peanut allergy are at increased risk of developing a peanut allergy. Family history of personal history of atopic disease. Family history of peanut allergy
- Timing of exposure – **delayed introduction of nuts until > 3 years of age = increased risk**

CLINICAL MANIFESTATIONS
- Skin: pruritus, flushing, diaphoresis, urticaria & angioedema, contact urticaria
- Oropharyngeal: sneezing, nasal congestion, oral pruritus, rhinorrhea.
- Respiratory: wheezing, dyspnea, cough
- Cardiovascular: arrhythmias
- Eyes: conjunctival injection, lacrimation, pruritus, & periorbital edema
- GI: nausea, vomiting, abdominal pain, diarrhea
- Neurologic: dizziness, syncope, sense of doom

MANAGEMENT
- Patient education on avoiding products containing or cooked with the associated foods
- Complete avoidance of foods and similar foods
- Epinephrine autoinjectors should be prescribed in case of accidental exposure and reaction.

MANAGEMENT OF AN ACUTE ATTACK
- Antihistamines if mild.
- Epinephrine if severe

DUMPING SYNDROME

- Symptoms due to rapid gastric emptying & rapid fluid shifts when large amounts of carbohydrates (simple sugars) are ingested.
- **Often a complication of bariatric surgery.**

CLINICAL MANIFESTATIONS
- Early symptoms: GI symptoms - bloating, flatus, diarrhea, abdominal pain, nausea, & vasomotor symptoms (eg, diaphoresis, dizziness, tachypnea, hypotension, flushing). Often within 15 minutes.
- Late symptoms: hypoglycemia, syncope.

DIAGNOSIS
- Clinical diagnosis, modified oral glucose tolerance test.
- Barium fluoroscopy & radionuclide scintigraphy can be used to confirm rapid gastric emptying.

MANAGEMENT
- **Decreased carbohydrate intake** (especially simple sugars), eat more frequently with **smaller meals**, protein-rich foods, & separating solids from liquid intake by 30 minutes.

PEPTIC ULCER DISEASE (PUD)

- Gastric erosions > 0.5 cm on imaging.
- Duodenal ulcers: 4 times more common, usually benign.
- Gastric ulcers: 4% associated with Gastric adenocarcinoma.

PATHOPHYSIOLOGY

Imbalance between:

- **Increased aggressive factors in duodenal ulcers** (eg, Hydrochloric acid, *H. pylori*)
- **Decreased protective mechanisms with gastric ulcers** (eg, mucus, bicarbonate, prostaglandins).

ETIOLOGIES

- ***Helicobacter pylori*** **most common cause of gastritis.**
- **NSAIDs & Aspirin: second most common cause** - eg, **Gastric ulcers** (prostaglandin inhibition).
- Zollinger-Ellison Syndrome: gastrin-producing tumor. 1% of all cases of PUD.
- ETOH, smoking, stress (burns, trauma, surgery, severe medical illness); males, elderly, steroids, gastric cancer.

CLINICAL MANIFESTATIONS

- **Dyspepsia (burning, gnawing, epigastric pain)** hallmark; nausea, vomiting.
- **Duodenal ulcer:** dyspepsia **classically relieved with food**, antacids, or acid suppressants. Worse before meals or 2-5 hours after meals, nocturnal symptoms.
- **Gastric ulcer:** symptoms classically **worse with food** (especially 1-2 hours after meals), weight loss.
- Bleeding ulcer: hematemesis, melena, hematochezia. **PUD is the most common cause of upper GI bleed.**
- Perforated ulcer: sudden onset of severe abdominal pain (may radiate to the shoulder); peritonitis (**rebound tenderness, guarding, & rigidity**).

DIAGNOSIS

- **Upper endoscopy with biopsy: diagnostic test of choice.**
  All gastric ulcers need repeat upper endoscopy to document healing even if asymptomatic.
- H. pylori testing:
  - **Endoscopy with biopsy: gold standard in diagnosing *H. pylori* infection.** A rapid urease test and direct staining can be performed on the biopsy specimen.
  - **Urea breath test:** Noninvasive. *H. pylori* converts labeled urea into labeled carbon dioxide. Breathing out labeled urea = presence of *H. pylori*.
  - *H. Pylori* stool antigen (HpSA): >90% specific. Useful for diagnosing *H. pylori* & confirming eradication after therapy.
  - Serologic antibodies: only useful in confirming *H. pylori* infection NOT eradication (antibodies can stay elevated long after eradication of *H. pylori*).

MANAGEMENT if *H. pylori*-positive:

- **Bismuth quadruple therapy:** Bismuth subsalicylate + Tetracycline + Metronidazole + PPI x 14 days.
- Concomitant therapy: Clarithromycin + Amoxicillin + Metronidazole + PPI for 10-14 days.
- Triple therapy: Clarithromycin + Amoxicillin + PPI for 10-14 days (Metronidazole if Penicillin allergic). Alternative is Bismuth subsalicylate + Tetracycline + Metronidazole.

MANAGEMENT if *H. pylori*-negative:

- PPI; H_2 blocker, Misoprostol, antacids, Bismuth compounds, Sucralfate.

REFRACTORY

- Parietal cell vagotomy. Bilroth II (associated with Dumping syndrome).

	DUODENAL ULCERS (DU)	GASTRIC ULCERS (GU)
CAUSATIVE FACTORS	↑ **DAMAGING factors:** acid, pepsin, *H. pylori*	↓ **MUCOSAL PROTECTIVE factors:** ↓mucus, bicarb, prostaglandins; **NSAIDs**
INCIDENCE	• Most common in the duodenal bulb • **Almost always benign** • 4 times more common	• MC in the antrum of stomach. • **4% malignant:** all gastric ulcers need repeat endoscopy to document healing.
PAIN	• **Better with meals.** • Worse 2-5 hours after meals	• **Worse with meals** (especially **1-2 hours after meals)**
AGE	• MC in **younger patients:** 30-55y.	• MC in **older patients:** 55-70y.

MEDICAL MANAGEMENT OF PEPTIC ULCER DISEASE (PUD)

MEDICATION	COMMENTS
PROTON PUMP INHIBITORS **"AZOLES"** - **Omeprazole** - **Lansoprazole** - **Pantoprazole** - **Rabeprazole** - **Esomeprazole** - **Dexlansoprazole**	MOA: **block H+/K+ ATP-ase (proton pump) of parietal cell, reducing acid secretion.** More effective than H_2RA but of little clinical difference after 4 weeks in uncomplicated cases. Associated with faster symptom relief & healing. Usually taken **30 min before meals in AM.** Low risk in pregnancy. Indications: **most effective drug to treat PUD.** Gastritis, ZES. - 90% healing of duodenal ulcers after 4 weeks & gastric ulcers after 6 weeks. S/E: diarrhea, headache, hypomagnesemia, **B_{12} deficiency,** hypocalcemia. Omeprazole associated with *C. difficile* infections & hip fractures. DI: Omeprazole causes **CP450 inhibition** ⇨ ↑levels of Theophylline, Warfarin, Phenytoin, & other drugs.
H_2 RECEPTOR ANTAGONISTS **"TIDINES"** - **Cimetidine** - **Ranitidine** - **Famotidine** - **Nizatidine**	MOA: **histamine$_2$ receptor blocker** (indirectly inhibits proton pump) **reducing acid/pepsin secretion** (especially nocturnal). Ranitidine 6x more potent than Cimetidine. Usually taken at night. - 90% healing of duodenal ulcers after 6 weeks & gastric ulcers after 8 weeks. S/E: Ranitidine has few drug interactions. **B_{12} deficiency,** ↑LFTs. • Famotidine and Nizatidine may cause blood dyscrasias. Famotidine can prolong QT interval. CNS: confusion, dizziness, headache. • Many **drug interactions with Cimetidine: CP450 inhibition** ⇨ ↑levels of theophylline, warfarin, phenytoin, & other drugs. CNS: confusion, headache. Caution if renal/hepatic dysfunction. **Anti-androgen effects of Cimetidine: gynecomastia, impotence,** ↓libido.
MISOPROSTOL	MOA: **prostaglandin E_1 analog** that **increases bicarbonate & mucus secretion,** & reduces acid production. **Good for preventing NSAID-induced ulcers but not for healing already existing ulcers.** Also used to keep ductus arteriosus patent. S/E: diarrhea, abdominal cramping. CI: premenopausal women because it is **abortifacient** & causes cervical ripening.
ANTACIDS	**MOA:** neutralize acid, prevents conversion of pepsinogen to pepsin (active form). Systemic: Calcium carbonate (Tums). S/E: acid rebound, milk alkali syndrome. Nonsystemic: **Milk of Magnesia** (± cause **diarrhea**) **Amphogel (AlOH)** (± cause **constipation**, hypophosphatemia) Mg + ALOH + Simethicone (less S/E).
BISMUTH COMPOUNDS Pepto-Bismol Kaopectate	MOA: **antibacterial & cytoprotective** that inhibits peptic activity. Indications: limited role (used in quadruple therapy in H. pylori management). S/E: **darkening of tongue/stool, constipation,** neurotoxicity in high doses. Salicylate toxicity in overdose. Cautious use with renal insufficiency.
SUCRALFATE	MOA: **cytoprotective** (forms viscous adhesive ulcer coating that promotes healing, protects the stomach mucosa). Ind: usually used as an ulcer prophylactic measure than as for treatment of ulcers. S/E: metallic taste, constipation, nausea. Antacids may interfere with its action. Drug Interactions: **may reduce the bioavailability of H_2RAs, PPIs,** fluoroquinolones, when given simultaneously. Take on empty stomach.

GASTRITIS

ACUTE GASTRITIS

- Gastritis: superficial inflammation or irritation of the stomach mucosa with mucosal injury.
- Gastropathy: mucosal injury without evidence of inflammation.

PATHOPHYSIOLOGY

- **Imbalance between aggressive & protective mechanisms** of the gastric mucosa.

ETIOLOGIES

- ***Helicobacter pylori* most common cause of gastritis.**
- **NSAIDs & Aspirin: second most common cause**.
- Acute stress in critically ill patients.
- Other: heavy alcohol consumption, bile salt reflux, medications, radiation, trauma, corrosives, ischemia, pernicious anemia, portal hypertension.

CLINICAL MANIFESTATIONS

- Most commonly asymptomatic.
- If symptomatic symptoms are similar to Peptic ulcer disease (eg, dyspepsia, nausea, vomiting).

DIAGNOSIS

- Upper endoscopy with biopsy: diagnostic test of choice - thick, edematous erosions <0.5cm.
- *H. pylori* testing.

MANAGEMENT

- Similar to Peptic ulcer disease (eg, *H. pylori* eradication, acid suppression therapy with H2 receptor antagonist or PPIs, stop offending agents).
- Pharmacologic prophylaxis for patients at high risk for developing stress-related gastritis with IV proton pump inhibitors or H_2 blockers.

AUTOIMMUNE METAPLASTIC ATROPHIC GASTRITIS

- A form of **chronic gastritis** associated with chronic inflammation, gland atrophy, & epithelial metaplasia.
- Usually occurs in the **gastric fundus & body** (usually spares the antrum).
- Patients are at increased risk for developing Gastric adenocarcinoma.

PATHOPHYSIOLOGY

- T-cell mediated destruction of the oxyntic mucosa and **auto-antibodies against intrinsic factor & parietal cells.** The lack of intrinsic factor can lead to **B12 deficiency (Pernicious anemia).**
- The lack of parietal cells can lead to hypochlorhydria & hypergastrinemia.
- Iron deficiency can occur because gastric acid normally enhances iron absorption.

GASTRINOMA Zollinger-Ellison syndrome

- Gastrin-secreting neuroendocrine tumor, leading to severe Peptic ulcer disease & diarrhea.
- Most commonly seen in the **duodenal wall** (45%), pancreas (25%), lymph nodes (5-15%), other sites.

CLINICAL MANIFESTATIONS

- **Suspect Gastrinoma in patients if severe, recurrent, multiple, or refractory ulcers + diarrhea**.
- Severe peptic ulcer disease: multiple peptic ulcers, refractory ulcers, abdominal pain.
- Diarrhea: increased acidity inactivates the pancreatic enzymes, leading to malabsorption.

DIAGNOSIS

- Established by demonstrating **elevated basal or stimulated gastrin levels** once endoscopy confirms the presence of an ulcer.
- **Screening: elevated fasting gastrin levels best initial test** - >1,000pg/mL + gastric pH <2.
- **Confirmatory: Secretin test - persistent gastrin elevations in Gastrinomas**. Normally, gastrin release is inhibited by secretin. Other causes of hypergastrinemia are usually inhibited by secretin.
- Basal acid output: increased. Chromogranin A: increased in neuroendocrine tumors.
- Somatostatin receptor scintigraphy: most sensitive test for tumor localization and to detect primary or secondary lesions (may be combined with endoscopic ultrasound). Gastrinoma is associated with increased somatostatin receptors.

MANAGEMENT

- Local: tumor resection.
- Metastatic, unresectable: lifelong **high-dose PPIs** (blocks acid production).
- Surgical resection if liver involvement.
- The liver & abdominal lymph nodes are the MC sites for METS.

CARCINOID TUMORS

- Rare, Well-differentiated neuroendocrine tumor that arise from enterochromaffin cells.
- **55% occur in the GI tract**, 30% in the lungs.
- Carcinoid tumors are thought to arise from transformation of enterochromaffin-like cells (ECL cells, which are responsible for histamine secretion) due to chronic stimulation by gastrin. Autoimmune atrophic gastritis is associated with hypergastrinemia.

CLINICAL MANIFESTATIONS

- Many are asymptomatic (incidental finding on endoscopy). Local symptoms depends on the tumor location.
- **Carcinoid syndrome** - periodic episodes of **diarrhea** (serotonin release), **flushing, tachycardia, and bronchoconstriction** (histamine release) and hemodynamic instability (eg, hypotension).

DIAGNOSIS

- Many are asymptomatic (incidental finding on endoscopy).
- 24-hour urinary 5-hydroxyindoleacetic acid/5-HIAA excretion - the end product of serotonin metabolism.
- Radiolabeled somatostatin analogs can be used for tumor localization.
- Contrast-enhanced, triple-phase CT scans of the abdomen and pelvis. Contrast-enhanced MRI.

MANAGEMENT

- Depends on site. Options include surgical resection,

GASTRIC CARCINOMA

Types:
- **Adenocarcinoma most common** (90%).
- 4% lymphoma. Carcinoid tumors, stromal, sarcomas.

RISK FACTORS
- ***H. pylori* biggest risk factor** - associated with 90%.

- Most commonly occurs in males & >40 years of age.

- Dietary: **preserved foods** (eg, salted, cured, smoked, pickled food, food containing nitrites or nitrates). Diets low in raw fruits & vegetables. Obesity.

- Pernicious anemia, chronic atrophic gastritis, achlorhydria, smoking, blood type A, post antrectomy.

- Non-Hodgkin lymphoma: the stomach is the most common site of extranodal NHL.

DECREASED RISK
- Chronic Aspirin & NSAID use as well as increased intake of fruits and vegetables associated with a decreased risk. Wine consumption may be associated with decreased risk.

CLINICAL MANIFESTATIONS
- Most patients are advanced at the time of presentation.
- **Weight loss and persistent abdominal pain** (epigastric, vague, mild). **Early satiety,** abdominal fullness, nausea, post-prandial vomiting, dysphagia, melena, hematemesis. Iron deficiency anemia (chronic bleeding).

PHYSICAL EXAMINATION
- Palpable abdominal mass or signs of Metastasis:
  - Supraclavicular lymph nodes (Virchow's node)
  - Umbilical LN (Sister Mary Joseph's node)
  - Ovarian METS (Krukenburg tumor)
  - Palpable nodule on rectal exam (Blumer's shelf)
  - Left axillary lymph node (LN) involvement (Irish sign).
  - These nodes may be seen with other GI tumors.

DIAGNOSIS
- **Upper endoscopy with biopsy: initial test of choice for most gastric cancers.**

- Upper GI series: preferred if linitis plastica is suspected.

MANAGEMENT
- Endoscopic resection for early local disease.
- Gastrectomy, chemotherapy. Radiation for lymphoma.
- **Poor prognosis** (patients usually present late in the disease).

PYLORIC STENOSIS

- Hypertrophy & hyperplasia of the pyloric muscles, causing a **functional gastric outlet obstruction** (preventing gastric emptying into the duodenum).
- Most common cause of intestinal obstruction in infancy.

RISK FACTORS
- **Most common in the first 3-12 weeks of life**
- **Erythromycin use** (within the first 2 weeks of life)
- Caucasians, males 4:1, first-borns.

CLINICAL MANIFESTATIONS
- **Nonbilious, projectile vomiting** (especially after feeding) - hallmark.
- May have signs of dehydration, weight loss, & malnutrition.
- Physical examination: palpable pylorus (**"olive-shaped" nontender, mobile hard mass** to the right of the epigastrium) especially after emesis, hyperperistalsis, succussion splash on auscultation.

DIAGNOSIS
- **Abdominal ultrasound: initial test of choice** - elongated, thickened pylorus. More sensitive and no radiation risk.
- Upper GI series:
  String sign (thin column of barium through a narrowed pyloric channel), delayed gastric emptying.
  Railroad track sign: excess mucosa in the pyloric lumen resulting in 2 columns of barium
- Labs: **hypokalemia & hypochloremic metabolic alkalosis** from vomiting.

MANAGEMENT
- Initial: **rehydration (IV fluids)** & electrolyte repletion (eg, **potassium replacement**).
- Definitive: pyloromyotomy.

AUTOIMMUNE HEPATITIS

- Idiopathic chronic inflammation of the liver due to circulating autoantibodies.
- **Most common in young women.**
- Complications include Cirrhosis, Pericarditis, Myocarditis, proliferative Glomerulonephritis, Uveitis.

CLINICAL MANIFESTATIONS
- Asymptomatic, nonspecific symptoms (eg, fatigue, nausea, malaise, abdominal pain, arthralgia).

PHYSICAL EXAMINATION:
- May be normal. Hepatomegaly, splenomegaly and jaundice.

DIAGNOSIS
- Autoantibodies:
  Type I - **positive ANA, smooth muscle antibodies**
  Type II - anti-liver/kidney microsomal antibodies. Increased IgG.
- LFTs: hepatocellular pattern (increased ALT > 1,000)
- Liver biopsy: definitive diagnosis - bridging necrosis or multiacinar necrosis

MANAGEMENT
- **Corticosteroids;** Corticosteroids + **Azathioprine**; 6-Mercaptopurine

ACUTE HEPATITIS

ACUTE VIRAL HEPATITIS

CLINICAL MANIFESTATIONS

- Prodromal phase: malaise, arthralgia, fatigue, URI symptoms, anorexia, **decreased desire to smoke,** nausea, vomiting, abdominal pain, loss of appetite, acholic stools. Hepatitis A is associated with spiking fever.
- Icteric phase: **jaundice** (most don't develop this phase). If present, jaundice usually develops once the fever subsides.
- Fulminant: **encephalopathy, coagulopathy**, hepatomegaly, jaundice, edema, ascites, asterixis, hyperreflexia.

LABORATORY VALUES

- Increased ALT and AST (both usually >500 if acute & <500 if chronic). May have hyperbilirubinemia.

OUTCOMES

- Clinical recovery usually within 3-16 weeks; 10% HBV & 80% HCV become chronic.
- **Chronic Hepatitis:** disease >6 months duration. **Only HBV, HCV, HDV associated with chronicity.** Chronic may lead to end stage liver disease (ESLD) or hepatocellular carcinoma (HCC).
- **Fulminant:** encephalopathy, coagulopathy, jaundice, edema, ascites, asterixis, hyperreflexia.

FULMINANT HEPATITIS

- **Acute hepatic failure** in patients with Hepatitis.

ETIOLOGIES

- **Acetaminophen toxicity most common cause in the US.**
- **Viral hepatitis,** autoimmune hepatitis, drug reactions (eg, Tolcapone), sepsis.
- **Reye syndrome** - fulminant hepatitis in **children given Aspirin after a viral infection**.

CLINICAL MANIFESTATIONS

- **Encephalopathy:** vomiting, coma, AMS, seizures, **asterixis** (flapping tremor of the hand with wrist extension), hyperreflexia, cerebral edema, increased intracranial pressure.
- **Coagulopathy:** increased PT, INR (> or equal to 1.5) and eventually increased PTT due to decreased hepatic production of coagulation factors.
- Hepatomegaly. Jaundice (not usually seen in Reye syndrome).
- **Reye syndrome**: may develop rash (hands & feet), intractable vomiting, liver damage, encephalopathy, dilated pupils with minimal response to light, & multi-organ failure.

DIAGNOSIS

- Combination of symptoms, hepatic encephalopathy, abnormal LFTs, and increased INR 1.5 or greater.
- **Hypoglycemia common** (due to hepatic gluconeogenesis), **increased ammonia** (encephalopathy).
- Labs to look for cause (eg, Acetaminophen levels, viral serologies).

MANAGEMENT

- Supportive: IV fluids electrolyte repletion, Mannitol if ICP elevation, PPI stress ulcer prophylaxis. Blood products of platelets or cryoprecipitate reserved for active bleeding coagulopathy.
- **Liver transplant definitive.**

HEPATITIS A VIRUS (HAV)

- Acute viral infection of the liver due to HAV infection.

TRANSMISSION:

- **Fecal-oral (similar to HEV) – fecally contaminated food and water,** especially with **international travel,** close contact with an infected individual, day care workers, men who have sex with men, homelessness, shellfish, illicit drug use.

CLINICAL MANIFESTATIONS

- Most patients are asymptomatic or mildly symptomatic. **May be associated with spiking fever.**
- Malaise, anorexia, nausea, vomiting, abdominal pain. Physical examination: jaundice, hepatomegaly.

DIAGNOSIS

- LFT: elevated ALT, AST, bilirubin.
- **Acute: IgM anti-HAV**. Past exposure: IgG HAV Ab with negative IgM.

MANAGEMENT

- **No treatment needed** (self-limiting infection similar to HEV).
- Not usually associated with a chronic state (similar to HEV). Fulminant hepatitis is rare.

PREVENTION

- **Handwashing & improved sanitation greatest impact to reduce transmission,** food safety, immunization

PREEXPOSURE PROPHYLAXIS:

- Increased risk of HAV infection (see transmission risk). 2 doses given 6 months apart.
- HAV vaccination for international travelers 6 months of age or older.

POSTEXPOSURE PROPHYLAXIS:

- **Healthy individuals 1-40 years old: HAV vaccine preferred over immunoglobulin** (within 2 weeks of exposure).
- Healthy individuals > 40 years old: HAV vaccine (with or without immune globulin) rather than IG alone (within 2 weeks of exposure).
- Immunocompromised or chronic liver disease >1 year old: **HAV vaccine + HAV immunoglobulin** (within 2 weeks of exposure).

COAGULOPATHY OF LIVER DISEASE

- Decreased production of coagulation factor proteins associated with advanced liver disease.
- **Bleeding is the classic presentation** (eg, GI bleeding). May have signs of underlying liver disease.

DIAGNOSIS

- Function studies: **increased PT/INR and low albumin.** As the disease advances, **increased PTT will occur.** The coagulopathy corrects with mixing studies. Decreased fibrinogen.
- CBC: may have thrombocytopenia. Peripheral smear may show target cells.

MANAGEMENT

- **Cryoprecipitate if active bleeding or undergoing an invasive procedure.** Cryoprecipitate if decreased fibrinogen (replaces fibrinogen, factor VIII and VWF). Fresh frozen plasma may be used in select patients to replace deficient coagulation factors if no response to cryoprecipitate.
- Correct the underlying cause. Avoid alcohol consumption.
- Vitamin K does not correct the coagulopathy.

HEPATITIS E VIRUS (HEV)

- Acute viral infection of the liver due to HEV infection.

TRANSMISSION
- **Fecal-oral (similar to HAV) – fecally-contaminated food and water**, blood transfusions, and mother-to-child transmission.

CLINICAL MANIFESTATIONS
- Most patients are asymptomatic or mildly symptomatic.
- Malaise, anorexia, nausea, vomiting fever, abdominal pain.
- Physical examination: jaundice, hepatomegaly.
- Increased risk of fulminant hepatitis in pregnant women, malnourished, or patients with preexisting liver disease.

DIAGNOSIS
- LFTs: elevated ALT, AST, bilirubin.
- IgM anti-HEV

MANAGEMENT
- **No treatment needed** (self-limiting infection similar to HAV). Not associated with a chronic state (similar to HAV).
- **Highest mortality due to fulminant hepatitis during pregnancy,** especially during third trimester. In pregnancy the rate goes up between 10-25% (normal mortality rate is 1-3%).

HEPATITIS D VIRUS (HDV)

- Defective virus that **requires Hepatitis B virus** (HBsAg) **to cause co- or superimposed infection**.

PATHOPHYSIOLOGY
- HDV uses the HBsAg as its envelope protein. HDV has a direct cytopathic effect - more severe hepatitis & faster progression to Cirrhosis.

TRANSMISSION
- **Primarily parenteral** (eg, exposure to blood or blood products).

CLINICAL MANIFESTATIONS
- Most are asymptomatic.
- Fatigue, myalgia, nausea, RUQ pain, jaundice, dark urine, clay-colored stools.

DIAGNOSIS
- Screening: **Total anti-HDV.** Confirmed by immunochemical staining of liver biopsies for HDAg or RT-PCR assays for **HDV RNA in serum**.
- Hepatitis B serologies also performed.

MANAGEMENT
- No FDA approved management.
- Interferon alpha has been used in the management of Chronic HDV. Liver transplant definitive.

PREVENTION: **Hepatitis B vaccination**

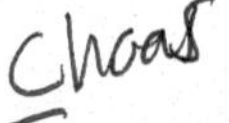

HEPATITIS C VIRUS (HCV)

- **85% of patients with HCV develop chronic infection.**

- Most common infectious cause of chronic liver disease, Cirrhosis, & liver transplantation in the US

TRANSMISSION
- **Parenteral: IV drug use most common in US**, needlestick injuries (0.3% conversion risk), increased risk if received blood transfusion before 1992.

- Sexual or perinatal not common. Not associated with breastfeeding.

CLINICAL MANIFESTATIONS
- Most are asymptomatic.

- Acute: fatigue, myalgia, nausea, RUQ pain, jaundice, dark urine, clay-colored stools

DIAGNOSIS
- Screening test: **HCV antibodies** usually becomes positive within 6 weeks. Does not imply recovery (may become negative after recovery). Increased LFTs.
- Confirmatory: **HCV RNA. HCV RNA more sensitive than HCV antibody** (may be positive in patients with negative antibody testing). HCV RNA is the best way to determine viral replication activity.

	HCV RNA	Anti-HCV
acute hepatitis	⊕	±
resolved hepatitis	Negative	±
chronic hepatitis	⊕	⊕

HCV RNA more sensitive than HCV antibody

- Genotyping is most effective to determine effective treatment options.

MANAGEMENT
- The newer regimens all have nearly equal efficacy (>95% cure rate with 12 weeks of oral therapy).
- Response to therapy is determined by PCR-RNA viral load at 12 and 24 weeks after therapy.
- Newer options can achieve a cure rate. Options include:
  Ledipasvir-Sofosbuvir
  Elbasvir-Grazoprevir
  Ombitasvir-Paritaprevir-Ritonavir plus Dasabuvir with or without Ribavirin
  Simeprevir plus Sofosbuvir
  Daclatasvir plus Sofosbuvir.

Older regimen:
- Pegylated interferon alpa-2b + Ribavirin.
- Adverse effects of Interferon: psychosis, depression thrombocytopenia, leukopenia, arthralgias.
- Adverse effects of Ribavirin: anemia

PROGNOSIS
- Some of the newer treatments may possibly reactivate Hepatitis B so perform HBV testing prior to initiating treatment.
- Increased risk for Cirrhosis (20% over a 20-30 year time period), Hepatocellular carcinoma (1-3%) and liver failure.

HEPATITIS B VIRUS (HBV)

TRANSMISSION

- Percutaneous, sexual, parenteral, perinatal.

CLINICAL MANIFESTATIONS OF ACUTE

Most are asymptomatic. 3 possible states:

- Subclinical (anicteric): constitutional symptoms (eg, malaise, arthralgia, fatigue, URI symptoms, nausea, vomiting, abdominal pain, anorexia, **decreased desire to smoke** in smokers).
- Icteric: jaundice (only seen in 30%).
- Fulminant: acute hepatic failure (eg, encephalopathy, coagulopathy, jaundice, edema, ascites).

CLINICAL MANIFESTATIONS OF CHRONIC

- Chronic hepatitis: persistent symptoms, elevated LFTs, and increased viral load.
- Chronic (carrier) state: asymptomatic, normal LFTs, low viral load, and undetectable HBeAg.

DIAGNOSIS

- Hepatitis B serologies: HB surface antigen, surface antibody, and core antibody.

Diagnosis	HBsAg	anti-HBs	anti-HBc	HbeAg	Anti-Hbe
WINDOW PERIOD	Negative	Negative	Ig**M**	Negative	Negative
ACUTE HEPATITIS	**POSITIVE**	Negative	Ig**M**	±	±
RECOVERY (RESOLVED)	Negative	**POSITIVE**	Ig**G**	Negative	Negative
IMMUNIZATION	Negative	**POSITIVE**	Negative	Negative	Negative
CHRONIC HEPATITIS REPLICATIVE	**POSITIVE**	Negative	Ig**G**	**POSITIVE**	Negative
CHRONIC HEPATITIS NONREPLICATIVE	**POSITIVE**	Negative	Ig**G**	Negative	**POSITIVE**

Chronic hepatitis = surface antigen positivity and failure to produce surface antibodies > 6 months

- LFTs: acute – AST and ALT in the thousands range; chronic: ALT and AST in the hundreds range or normal. Increased bilirubin especially in the icteric phase.
- HBV DNA: best way to assess viral replication activity.
- Liver biopsy can be used to determine the extent of damage.

MANAGEMENT OF ACUTE HBV

- **Supportive mainstay of treatment** (majority of patients will not progress to chronic infection).

MANAGEMENT OF CHRONIC HBV

- Antiviral therapy may be indicated if persistent, severe symptoms, marked jaundice (bilirubin >10 mg/dL), inflammation on liver biopsy, ↑ALT, or ⊕ HB envelope antigen persistence.
- Options include **Entecavir, Tenofovir**, Lamivudine, Adefovir, Telbivudine.
- Treatment can be stopped after confirmation (two consecutive tests four weeks apart) that the patient has cleared HBsAg.

HEPATITIS B VACCINATION

- The recombinant hepatitis B vaccine (non-adjuvanted) derived from yeast is most commonly used for vaccination.

Vaccination schedule:

- Infant: usually administered at birth, 1-2 months, and 6-18 months of age.
- Adult (no prior vaccination): 3 doses at 0, 1, and 6 months.
- Contraindicated if allergic to Baker's yeast.

HEPATITIS B SEROLOGIES

There are 5 variations of Hepatitis B you must know:

1. Window period: positive core IgM
2. Successful vaccination: positive surface antibody
3. Acute hepatitis: positive surface antigen, positive core IgM antibody
4. Chronic hepatitis: positive surface antigen, positive core IgG antibody
5. Distant resolved infection (recovery): positive surface antibody, positive core IgG antibody

ANTIBODY INTERPRETATION:

- **Positive HB surface Ag**: either acute or chronic. *HbsAg is usually the first positive serologic marker in acute.* The core antibody determines if acute or chronic (core IgM = acute, core IgG = chronic).
- **Positive HB surface Ab**: either recovery or vaccination
- **HB core Ab IgM**: window period or acute hepatitis
- **HB core Ab IgG**: resolved infection or chronic hepatitis

HEPATITIS B SEROLOGIES – 3 STEP APPROACH

STEP 1 – look at **Surface antigen** - if surface Ag is positive:
•⊕ = **acute** OR **chronic**

STEP 2 - if surface Ag (step 1) is positive, look at **Core antibody**:
•if **IgM** is ⊕ ⇨ **acute.** if **IgG** is ⊕ ⇨ **chronic.**

Step 3 is only needed if Surface antigen was negative in step 1

STEP 3 – If surface Ag was negative, look at **surface Ab.** If positive:
•Either **Vaccination** OR **recovery** (distant infection)

•If **surface Ab** is the **only thing positive** ⇨ **vaccination**

•If **core IgG Antibody** is **positive** ⇨ **recovery** (distant/resolved infection)

Another hack: If Envelope Ag is positive in either acute or chronic hepatitis, it doesn't help you determine their status. All Envelope Ag tells you if is highly replicating (if positive) or not highly replicative (if negative) so don't use it to determine status until the end if the question specifies replication or not.

In evaluating a patient, the following labs are obtained:
HB surface antigen: positive
HB surface antibody: negative
HB core antibody: positive IgG
Which of the following is the most likely diagnosis?

a. Window period
b. Successful vaccination
c. Acute Hepatitis B
d. Chronic Hepatitis B
e. Distant resolved infection (recovery)

STEP 1
Look at surface antigen (positive), so the answer has to be either acute or chronic.

STEP 2
Look at core antibody. If positive, it will either be IgG or IgM
Since it is IgG+, the answer is chronic hepatitis. You're done! ☺

HEPATOCELLULAR CARCINOMA

- Primary neoplasm of the liver.

RISK FACTORS
- **Chronic liver disease** (eg, chronic **HBV, HCV**, HDV, cirrhosis)
- Aflatoxin B1 exposure (*Aspergillus* spp).

CLINICAL MANIFESTATIONS
- Many are asymptomatic. Malaise, weight loss, jaundice, abdominal pain, hepatosplenomegaly.

DIAGNOSIS
- Contrast-enhanced CT scan or MRI tailored for liver lesion evaluation. Liver biopsy.

MANAGEMENT
- Surgical resection if confined to a lobe & not associated with cirrhosis.

SURVEILLANCE
- **Ultrasound primary modality every 6 months** (with or without **alpha-fetoprotein**).
- Performed in high-risk patients (eg, active hepatitis B with high AST and/or high viral load).

HEPATIC VEIN OBSTRUCTION (BUDD-CHIARI SYNDROME)

- **Hepatic venous outflow obstruction** leading to decreased liver drainage with subsequent portal HTN & cirrhosis.
- **Most common cause of Portal hypertension in children.**

TYPES
- **Primary: hepatic vein thrombosis (most common).**
- **Secondary hepatic vein or inferior vena cava occlusion** (eg, exogenous tumor compression).

RISK FACTORS
- Underlying thrombotic disorders (eg, malignancy, polycythemia, pregnancy, clotting disorders).

CLINICAL MANIFESTATIONS
- **Classic triad: ascites, hepatomegaly, & RUQ abdominal pain.**
- Rapid development of acute liver disease (eg, jaundice & hepatosplenomegaly).
- May have a subacute presentation.

DIAGNOSIS
- **Ultrasound: initial screening test of choice.**
- CT or MRI usually performed if US nondiagnostic.
- Venography gold standard. Not commonly performed
- Liver biopsy: usually not needed. Congestive hepatopathy classically described as **"nutmeg liver"**.

MANAGEMENT
- Options include Shunt decompression of the liver (eg, TIPS), angiography with stenting, anticoagulation (if thrombotic), thrombolysis (done if acute thrombus <3-4 weeks & not involving the inferior vena cava).
- Ascites: diuretics (removes excess fluid), low sodium diet, large volume paracentesis.

CIRRHOSIS

- **Mostly irreversible liver fibrosis with nodular regeneration** secondary to chronic liver disease.

PATHOPHYSIOLOGY
- Nodules cause increased portal pressure.
- Macronodules associated with higher risk of Hepatocellular carcinoma.

ETIOLOGIES
- **Chronic hepatitis C most common cause. Alcohol.** Chronic HBV, HDV.
- Nonalcoholic fatty liver disease (eg, obesity, DM, & hypertriglyceridemia).
- Hemochromatosis, autoimmune hepatitis, primary biliary cirrhosis, primary sclerosing cholangitis, drug toxicity.

CLINICAL MANIFESTATIONS
- General symptoms: fatigue, weakness, weight loss, muscle cramps, anorexia.
- Physical Exam: **ascites**, hepatosplenomegaly, **gynecomastia,** spider angioma, telangiectasias, caput medusa, muscle wasting, bleeding, palmar erythema, jaundice, Dupuytren's contractures.
- Hepatic encephalopathy: **confusion & lethargy** (**increased ammonia levels** toxic to the brain). PE: **asterixis (flapping tremor** with wrist extension) & fetor hepaticus. Esophageal varices

MANAGEMENT
- Avoidance of alcohol and hepatotoxic medications, weight reduction, vaccination for HAV and HBV.
- Treatment of the underlying cause when possible.
- Liver transplant: definitive management. Screening for HCC (ultrasound, alpha-fetoprotein).

Encephalopathy:
- **Lactulose or Rifaximin.** Neomycin second-line. Protein restriction.

Ascites:
- Sodium restriction. Diuretics (**Spironolactone, Furosemide**). Paracentesis.

Pruritus:
- **Cholestyramine** is a bile acid sequestrant that reduces bile salts in the skin, leading to less irritation from the bile salts.

Hepatocellular carcinoma surveillance:
- **Ultrasonography every 6 months** (with or without **alpha-fetoprotein**).
- Complications: end stage liver disease, hepatocellular carcinoma, esophageal varices, spontaneous bacterial peritonitis.

CIRRHOSIS STAGING CHILD-PUGH CLASSIFICATION

PARAMETERS	1 POINT	2 POINTS	3 POINTS
Total Bilirubin (mg/dL)	<2	2-3	>3
Serum albumin (g/dL)	>3.5	2.8 – 3.5	<2.8
PT INR	<1.7	1.71 – 2.30	>2.30
Ascites	None	Mild	Moderate to severe
Hepatic Encephalopathy	None	Grade I-II (or suppressed with medication)	Grade III-IV or refractory

POINTS	CLASS	1 YEAR SURVIVAL	2 YEAR SURVIVAL
5-6	A	100%	85%
7-9	B	81%	57%
	C	45%	35%

MODEL FOR END STAGE LIVER DISEASE: *slightly more accurate way to measure 3 month mortality*

MELD = 3.78×ln[serum bilirubin (mg/dL)] + 11.2×ln[INR] + 9.57×ln[serum creatinine (mg/dL)] + 6.43

LACTULOSE

Indications:

- Constipation: **osmotic laxative** - synthetic disaccharide sugar that is not absorbed (so it pulls water into the gut).
- **Hepatic encephalopathy:** bacterial flora converts lactulose into lactic acid, neutralizing ammonia in patients with Hepatic encephalopathy.

Adverse effects:

- bloating, flatulence, diarrhea.

SPONTANEOUS BACTERIAL PERITONITIS

- Infection of ascitic fluid without perforation of the bowel. A complication of Cirrhosis.

ETIOLOGIES

- ***E. coli* most common organism**. Streptococcus pneumoniae, anaerobes (rare).

CLINICAL MANIFESTATIONS

- Fever, chills, abdominal pain, increasing girth, diarrhea.
- Physical exam: findings of ascites (shifting dullness, fluid wave), abdominal tenderness.

DIAGNOSIS

- **Paracentesis: test of choice -** SAAG >1.1 (indicating portal hypertension), **cell count 250 cells/mm^3 or greater (determines need for treatment)**.
- Gram stain is often negative.
- Culture (most accurate test).

MANAGEMENT

- **Cefotaxime or Ceftriaxone.**

PROPHYLAXIS AFTER INITIAL OCCURRENCE

- Lifelong prophylaxis with Trimethoprim-sulfamethoxazole or Norfloxacin (SBP frequently recurs).

NONALCOHOLIC FATTY LIVER DISEASE

- NAFLD is an extremely common cause of mildly abnormal liver function tests.
- Etiologies: obesity, hyperlipidemia, glucocorticoid use, Diabetes mellitus.

Two types:

- Nonalcoholic fatty liver (NAFL): relatively benign. Not associated with fibrosis or malignant potential.
- Nonalcoholic steatohepatitis (NASH) is associated with inflammation and fibrosis and the potential to progress to cirrhosis (NASH is potentially premalignant).

DIAGNOSIS

- Biopsy: most accurate test - microvesicular fatty deposits similar to alcoholic liver disease without the history of heavy alcohol consumption.
- The most pertinent component is to exclude more serious causes of liver disease.

MANAGEMENT

- Correcting underlying causes.

PRIMARY BILIARY CIRRHOSIS/CHOLANGITIS (PBC)

- Idiopathic autoimmune disorder of **intrahepatic small bile ducts** that leads to decreased bile salt excretion, Cirrhosis, & End stage liver disease.
- **Most common in middle-age women (30-60 years).**

CLINICAL MANIFESTATIONS
- Most are asymptomatic - incidental finding of high alkaline phosphatase.
- **Fatigue (usually first symptom), pruritus**, RUQ discomfort.
- Physical examination: **hepatomegaly, jaundice,** xanthelasma, osteoporosis. Signs of Cirrhosis may occur late in the disease.

DIAGNOSIS
- Cholestatic pattern: **increased alkaline phosphatase & GGT**.
- **Antimitochondrial antibody hallmark.** Hypercholesterolemia.
- Ultrasound often initial imaging test.
- Liver biopsy: definitive diagnosis.

MANAGEMENT
- **Ursodeoxycholic acid first-line**. Obeticholic acid decreases fibrosis.
- Cholestyramine & UV light for pruritus.
- Liver transplant is definitive management

PRIMARY SCLEROSING CHOLANGITIS (PSC)

- Autoimmune, progressive cholestasis leading to **diffuse fibrosis of intra- and extrahepatic biliary ducts.**

RISK FACTORS
- **Most commonly associated with Inflammatory bowel disease - Ulcerative colitis** (90%).
- Men 20-40 years of age.
- Complications include Cirrhosis, liver failure, & Cholangiocarcinoma.

CLINICAL MANIFESTATIONS
- **Jaundice, pruritus,** fatigue, RUQ pain, **hepatomegaly, splenomegaly** (can present similar to Primary biliary cirrhosis).

DIAGNOSIS
- Cholestatic pattern: **increased alkaline phosphatase & GGT.** Increased ALT, AST, bilirubin, & IgM.
- **Positive P-ANCA hallmark.**
- **MRCP, ERCP: most accurate test - beaded appearance of the biliary ducts** (narrowing, strictures).
- Liver biopsy: rarely used - PSC is the only cause of Cirrhosis where liver biopsy isn't the most accurate test.

MANAGEMENT
- Stricture dilation for symptomatic relief. Cholestyramine for pruritus. Liver transplant definitive

- **Exam tip:**
- PBC vs PSC
- PBC – intrahepatic + anti-mitochondrial antibodies
- PSC: intra- & extrahepatic, +P-ANCA, history of UC

WILSON'S DISEASE (HEPATOLENTICULAR DEGENERATION)

- Rare autosomal recessive disorder leading to **copper accumulation in the body (eg, liver, brain, kidney, joints, & cornea).**

PATHOPHYSIOLOGY
- Defect in copper transporting protein (chromosome 13) leads to decreased biliary copper excretion due to **decreased ceruloplasmin**.

CLINICAL MANIFESTATIONS
- Liver: hepatitis, hepatosplenomegaly, cirrhosis, liver failure. Liver is the initial site of copper accumulation.

- CNS: **Dysarthria (most common)**, dystonia, Parkinson-like symptoms (bradykinesia, tremor, rigidity), hallucinations, hemiballismus, cognitive impairment, dementia, ataxia, seizures.

- Psychiatric: personality & behavioral changes, **psychosis, & delusions.**

- Joints: arthralgias from copper deposition.

PHYSICAL EXAMINATION
- Slit lamp examination: **Kayser-Fleischer rings** - brown or green pigmented rings due to copper deposition in the cornea (hallmark but not specific).

DIAGNOSIS
- **Decreased serum ceruloplasmin.**

- Increased 24-hour urinary copper excretion (also useful for monitoring treatment).

- Labs: elevated transaminases. Hemolytic anemia (Coombs negative).

- Molecular genetic testing for ATP7B

- **Liver biopsy: definitive** - more sensitive and specific (increased hepatic copper).

MANAGEMENT
- Copper-chelating agents: **Trientine** (less side effects) **or D-Penicillamine.** Pyridoxine (B6) is often given with Penicillamine to prevent B6 deficiency.

- Zinc supplementation (interferes with intestinal copper absorption).

INGUINAL HERNIAS

INDIRECT HERNIA

- Type of inguinal hernia with bowel protrusion at the internal inguinal ring.
- The origin of the sac is **LATERAL** to the inferior epigastric artery.
- **Most common type of hernia in both sexes** (more common in men), **young children, and young adults.**

PATHOPHYSIOLOGY

- Often congenital due to a **persistent patent process vaginalis.** An increase in abdominal pressure may force the intestines through the internal ring into the inguinal canal & may follow the testicle tract into the scrotum.

CLINICAL MANIFESTATIONS:

- Asymptomatic: swelling or fullness at the hernia site. Enlarges with increased intrabdominal pressure and/or standing. **May develop scrotal swelling.**
- **Incarcerated: painful, enlargement of an irreducible hernia** (unable to return the hernia contents back into the abdominal cavity). Nausea & vomiting if bowel obstruction present
- **Strangulated: ischemic incarcerated hernias** with **systemic toxicity** (irreducible hernia with compromised blood supply). Severe painful bowel movement (may refrain defecation).

DIAGNOSIS:

- Clinical. Groin ultrasound often the initial imaging of choice of an occult uncomplicated inguinal hernia. CT or MRI are alternatives.

MANAGEMENT

- Inguinal hernias often require surgical repair. Strangulated hernias are surgical emergencies.

DIRECT INGUINAL HERNIAS

- Type of inguinal hernia with bowel protrusion where the origin of the sac is **MEDIAL** to the inferior epigastric artery within Hesselbach's triangle. When you send a **D**irect **M**essage (DM – Direct is Medial).
- **Hesselbach's triangle: "RIP"** - **R**ectus Abdominis: medial border. **I**nferior epigastric vessels: lateral border. **P**oupart's (inguinal) ligament: inferior border.
- Pathophysiology: occurs as a result of weakness in the floor of the inguinal canal.
- Most commonly found on the right side.

CLINICAL MANIFESTATIONS

- Asymptomatic: swelling or fullness at the hernia site. Enlarges with increased intrabdominal pressure and/or standing.
- **Incarcerated: painful, enlargement of an irreducible hernia** (unable to return the hernia contents back into the abdominal cavity). Nausea & vomiting if bowel obstruction present
- **Strangulated: ischemic incarcerated hernias** with **systemic toxicity** (irreducible hernia with compromised blood supply). Severe painful bowel movement (may refrain defecation).

DIAGNOSIS

- Clinical. Groin ultrasound often the initial imaging of choice of an occult uncomplicated inguinal hernia. CT or MRI are alternatives.

MANAGEMENT

- Inguinal hernias often require surgical repair. Strangulated hernias are surgical emergencies.

FEMORAL HERNIAS

- Protrusion of the contents of the abdominal cavity through the femoral canal (below the inguinal ligament).
- **Most commonly seen in women.** They occur later in life compared to inguinal hernias.
- Because the femoral ring is smaller in women, they **often become incarcerated or strangulated** (femoral ring is smaller in women) compared to inguinal hernias.

UMBILICAL HERNIAS

- Hernia through the umbilical fibromuscular ring. Congenital (failure of umbilical ring closure).
- Usually due to loosening of the tissue around the ring in adults.

MANAGEMENT

- Observation: usually resolves by 2 years of age.
- Surgical repair may be indicated if still persistent in children 5 years of age or older to avoid incarceration or strangulation.

INCISIONAL (VENTRAL) HERNIAS

- Herniation through weakness in the abdominal wall.
- Incisional hernias most commonly occur with vertical incisions and in obese patients.

OBTURATOR HERNIAS

- Rare hernia through the pelvic floor in which abdominal/pelvic contents protrude through the obturator foramen.
- Most common in women (especially multiparous) or women with significant weight loss.

MANAGEMENT OF DIARRHEA

❶ FLUID REPLETION

Mainstay of management of gastroenteritis. Oral hydration preferred. Sports drinks, broths, IV saline. Pedialyte, Ceralyte.

❷ DIET

- **Bland low-residue diet** usually best tolerated (crackers, boiled vegetables, yogurts, soup). Eg, "BRAT" diet Bananas, Applesauce Rice Toast.

❸ ANTI-MOTILITY AGENTS

- Indications: Patients <65y with moderate to severe signs of volume depletion.
- CI: **DO NOT give anti-motility drugs to patients with invasive diarrhea (may cause toxicity).**

ANTI-DIARRHEALS	COMMENTS
BISMUTH SUBSALICYLATE Pepto-Bismol Kaopectate	MOA: **antimicrobial properties** against bacterial & viral pathogens, **Salicylate: anti-secretory & anti-inflammatory properties.** Ind: safe in patients with dysentery = significant fever, bloody diarrhea. S/E: **dark colored stools, darkening of tongue.** CI: children with viral illness (salicylate associated with ↑risk of Reye syndrome).
OPIOID AGONISTS **Diphenoxylate/**Atropine	**MOA:** binds to gut wall opioid receptors, inhibiting peristalsis (subtherapeutic Atropine added to discourage opioid overdose or misuse). **S/E: CNS (central opiate effects),** anticholinergic side effects. N/V/abdominal pain. **Constipation.**
Loperamide	Ind: **noninvasive diarrhea** (fever is absent or low grade & non bloody). MOA: binds gut wall **opioid receptors,** inhibiting peristalsis, ↑anal sphincter tone S/E: **avoid in patients with acute dysentery** or colitis.
ANTICHOLINERGICS **Phenobarbital/Hyoscyamine/ Atropine/ Scopolamine**	**MOA: anticholinergic** (Hyoscyamine, Atropine, Scopolamine) inhibits acetylcholine-related GI motility, relaxes GI muscles (***antispasmodic***), decreases gastric secretions; Phenobarbital slows down GI motility.

❹ ANTIEMETICS vomiting usually due to imbalance of serotonin, acetylcholine, dopamine, & histamine

Ondansetron **Granisetron** **Dolasetron**	**MOA: blocks serotonin receptors** (5-HT3) both peripherally & centrally in the chemoreceptor trigger zone. **S/E:** neurologic: headache, fatigue, sedation. GI bloating, diarrhea, constipation. Cardiac: prolonged QT interval, cardiac arrhythmias.
DOPAMINE BLOCKERS **Prochlorperazine** **Promethazine** **Metoclopramide**	**MOA: blocks CNS dopamine receptors (D_1 D_2).** Mild antihistaminic/muscarinic. Metoclopramide is also a prokinetic agent (increases GI motility). **S/E: QT prolongation, anticholinergic & antihistamine S/E (drowsiness),** hypotension, hyperprolactinemia. Extrapyramidal Sx (EPS): **rigidity, bradykinesia, tremor, akathisia** (restlessness) include: 1. **Dystonic Reactions (Dyskinesia):** reversible EPS hours-days after initiation → intermittent, spasmodic, sustained involuntary contractions (trismus, protrusions of tongue, forced jaw opening, facial grimacing, difficulty speaking, torticollis). **Mgmt: Diphenhydramine IV** or add anticholinergic agent (eg, Benztropine). 2. Parkinsonism: (due to ↓dopamine in nigrostriatal pathways) – rigidity, tremor

	NON-INVASIVE DIARRHEAS	INVASIVE DIARRHEAS
Pathophysiology:	Enterotoxins increase GI secretion of electrolytes ⇨ **secretory diarrhea** **No cell destruction/mucosal invasion.**	**Cytotoxins cause mucosal invasion & cell damage.**
Affected area:	**Small bowel ⇨ large voluminous** stool	**Large bowel ⇨ many small-volume stools, high fever.**
Vomiting	**Vomiting predominant symptom.**	Vomiting not as common.
Fecal Blood/WBC/mucus:	**Absent**	**⊕ Fecal blood/WBCs & mucus.**
Examples	Viral, S. Aureus, B. cereus, V. cholera, Enterotoxigenic E coli	Enterohemorrhagic E coli, Shigella, Salmonella, Yersinia, Campylobacter

NONINVASIVE (ENTEROTOXIN) INFECTIOUS DIARRHEA

- NONINVASIVE: vomiting, watery, voluminous (involves small intestine), no fecal WBCs or blood.

NOROVIRUS GASTROENTERITIS

- **Most common overall cause of gastroenteritis in adults in N. America and most common cause of viral gastroenteritis worldwide**.
- Peak incidence in the winter but can occur at any time of the year.

TRANSMISSION

- Fecal-oral route, contaminated food & water, fomite contamination. Often associated with **outbreaks** (eg, **cruise ships, hospitals, restaurants etc.**).

CLINICAL MANIFESTATIONS

- 24-48 hour incubation period. Symptoms last 2-3 days.
- **Vomiting predominant symptom**. Nausea, non-bloody diarrhea that lacks mucus, & fecal leukocytes (noninvasive). Generalized symptoms.

MANAGEMENT

- Fluid replacement (oral preferred).

ROTAVIRUS

- **Most commonly seen in young unimmunized children** between 6 months – 2 years of age.
- Transmission: fecal-oral route. IP <48 hours.

CLINICAL MANIFESTATIONS

- Children: vomiting, nonbloody diarrhea, & fever.
- Adults: symptoms usually less severe.

DIAGNOSIS

- PCR testing

MANAGEMENT

- **Oral rehydration mainstay of management.**

 Intestines like roots of a tree

STAPHYLOCOCCUS AUREUS GASTROENTERITIS

- Infection due to heat-stable enterotoxin B.
- Short incubation period **within 6 hours.**

SOURCES

- Food contamination most common source (eg, **dairy products, mayonnaise, meats, eggs, salads),** especially at room temperature.

CLINICAL MANIFESTATIONS

- **Prominent vomiting & nausea**, abdominal cramps are the usual symptoms.
- Fever, headache, & diarrhea are seen in a small amount of cases.

MANAGEMENT

- Fluid replacement (oral preferred). IV if unable to tolerate oral.

BACILLUS CEREUS GASTROENTERITIS

- Short incubation period **within 6 hours** (similar to *S. aureus*).
- Enterotoxin that can survive reheating.
- Sources: contaminated food **(eg, fried rice).**

CLINICAL MANIFESTATIONS

- **Prominent vomiting & nausea**, abdominal cramps are the usual symptoms.
- Fever, headache, & non-bloody diarrhea are seen in a small amount of cases.

MANAGEMENT

- Fluid replacement (oral preferred). IV if unable to tolerate oral.

ENTEROTOXIGENIC E. COLI

- **Most common cause traveler's diarrhea.**

RISK FACTORS

- **Contaminated food and water**. Contaminated water includes unpeeled fruits washed in the water, untreated drinking water/ice.
- Produces heat-stable toxins & heat-labile toxins. Incubation period 24-72 hours.

CLINICAL MANIFESTATIONS

- Abrupt onset of watery non-bloody diarrhea, abdominal cramping, vomiting.

DIAGNOSIS

- Gram stain & cultures.

MANAGEMENT

- **Oral rehydration therapy first-line.** Usually self-limiting.
- Loperamide. Bismuth subsalicylate.

VIBRIO CHOLERAE

- Gram-negative, comma-shaped rod transmitted via **contaminated food & water.**
- **Outbreaks may occur during poor sanitation & overcrowding conditions (especially abroad).**

PATHOPHYSIOLOGY

- **Exotoxin** causes a **secretory diarrhea** (inhibition of water, sodium and chloride absorption) which **may cause profound dehydration & hypovolemia.**

CLINICAL MANIFESTATIONS

- Vomiting, abdominal pain, borborygmi, cramping and **copious watery diarrhea = "rice water stools" (gray, with flecks of mucus & may have a "fishy odor" but no fecal odor, blood, or pus).**

DIAGNOSIS

- Clinical diagnosis. Stool cultures, PCR rapid testing

MANAGEMENT

- **Oral rehydration therapy and electrolyte replacement mainstay of treatment** (self-limited).
- Antibiotics: **Tetracyclines first-line antibiotic if needed.** Fluoroquinolones or Macrolides. Antibiotics may shorten the disease course in patients who are severely ill, other comorbid conditions, or with high fever.
- Prevention: in areas where it is endemic, use bottled water, wash hands often with soap and safe water, use chemical toilets, and cook food thoroughly.

VIBRIO PARAHAEMOLYTICUS & VULNIFICUS

- Gram-negative rods transmitted via **raw or undercooked shellfish consumption and seawater** (direct contact of water with wounds or shucking oysters), especially during warm summer months.
- *V. parahaemolyticus:* gastroenteritis
- *V. vulnificus:* gastroenteritis, **necrotizing fasciitis, cellulitis. Most common cause of death from seafood consumption in the US.**

RISK FACTORS FOR BACTEREMIA

- **Underlying liver disease** (eg, cirrhosis, alcoholism, hemochromatosis).
- **Immunocompromised** (eg, Diabetes mellitus).

CLINICAL MANIFESTATIONS

- Gastroenteritis: diarrhea, abdominal cramps, nausea, vomiting, fever.
- Cellulitis: due to exposure of wound to seawater or estuarine water.
- Necrotizing fasciitis: hemorrhagic bullae and may rapidly progress to shock.

DIAGNOSIS

- Clinical, stool studies, wound and blood cultures.

MANAGEMENT

- Gastroenteritis: rehydration therapy.
- Cellulitis: **Tetracyclines.**
- Necrotizing fasciitis: emergent surgical debridement + broad-spectrum antibiotics.

CLOSTRIDIOIDES DIFFICILE

- *Clostridioides difficile* (formerly Clostridium) is a spore-forming, toxin-producing, Gram-positive anaerobic bacterium.

RISK FACTORS

- **Recent antibiotic use** (eg, **Clindamycin**), **advanced age,** gastric suppression therapy (PPI, H_2 blockers).

PATHOPHYSIOLOGY

- Organism overgrowth secondary to alteration of the normal GI flora, most commonly seen after a course of antibiotics (eg, **Clindamycin classic in adults,** Amoxicillin in children) or chemotherapy. Can be a health-care associated infection.

CLINICAL MANIFESTATIONS

- Watery non-bloody diarrhea (noninvasive), abdominal cramps, fever, & abdominal tenderness.
- Complications include pseudomembranous colitis, bowel perforation, & **toxic megacolon.**

DIAGNOSIS

- ***C. difficile* toxin** (stool) – **initial test of choice.**
- **Leukocytosis** & increased WBC count classic.
- Sigmoidoscopy in select patients: **pseudomembranes.**

MANAGEMENT

- Discontinuing the offending antibiotic is the initial step in the management.
- **Contact precautions** & hand hygiene (**hand hygiene with soap & water may be more effective than alcohol-based hand sanitizers** in removing *C. difficile* spores - spores are resistant to killing by alcohol).
- **Oral Vancomycin** or **oral Fidaxomicin first-line agents. Metronidazole** is an alternative agent.
- Second recurrent CDI episode: pulse-tapered oral Vancomycin or Fidaxomicin.
- Recurrent disease treated with Metronidazole: oral Vancomycin.
- Frequently recurrent disease: (at least 3 recurrences) – fecal microbiota transplant.

INVASIVE INFECTIOUS DIARRHEA

- **INVASIVE: high fever, ⊕ blood & fecal leukocytes,** not as voluminous (large intestine), **mucus.**
- **DO NOT give anti-motility drugs with invasive diarrhea** (may cause toxicity).
- Includes: Campylobacter, Shigella, Salmonella, Yersinia, Enterohemorrhagic E coli, Campylobacter.

YERSINIA ENTEROCOLITICA

- Gram-negative coccobacillus with bipolar staining ("safety pin" appearance).
- Sources: **contaminated pork most common in the US,** milk, water, & tofu.

CLINICAL MANIFESTATIONS

- Fever, abdominal pain **mimic acute appendicitis** (can cause **mesenteric lymphadenitis,** producing abdominal tenderness or guarding).

DIAGNOSIS: cultures from stool, pharynx or mesenteric nodes.

MANAGEMENT

- **Fluid & electrolyte replacement mainstay of treatment.**
- Severe: Fluoroquinolones, Trimethoprim-Sulfamethoxazole.

Bactrim

CAMPYLOBACTER ENTERITIS

- *Campylobacter jejuni* most common cause of bacterial enteritis in the US.
- ***C. jejuni* most common antecedent event in post-infectious Guillain-Barré syndrome.**
- Most commonly affects children & young adults. 3-day incubation period.

SOURCES

- Contaminated food - **raw or undercooked poultry most common**, raw milk, contaminated water, dairy cattle. Puppies important source in children.

CLINICAL MANIFESTATIONS

- Fever, crampy periumbilical abdominal pain (**may mimic acute appendicitis**), nausea.
- Diarrhea initially watery progressing to bloody.

DIAGNOSIS

- Stool culture: gram-negative "**S, comma or seagull shaped**" organisms. Enzyme immunoassay or PCR.

MANAGEMENT

- **Fluid and electrolyte replacement mainstay of treatment** (usually mild & self-limiting with peak of illness lasting 24-48 hours).
- Severe or high-risk patients: **Macrolides first-line antibiotic of choice when needed** (eg, **Azithromycin**). Fluoroquinolones. Doxycycline.
- Loperamide & other anti-motility agents generally avoided in invasive diarrheas.

PREVENTION

- Proper food handling and handwashing can prevent spread.

ENTEROHEMORRHAGIC E. COLI 0157:H7

SOURCES

- Ingestion of **undercooked ground beef, unpasteurized milk or apple cider, day care centers, & contaminated water.**
- Incubation period average 4-9 days.

PATHOPHYSIOLOGY

- Shiga-like toxin (verotoxin) causes endothelial damage, leading to hemorrhage.
- Most commonly seen in **children** & elderly.

CLINICAL MANIFESTATIONS

- Watery diarrhea early on before becoming bloody. Crampy abdominal pain, vomiting.
- Fever usually absent or low-grade if present.

MANAGEMENT

- **Fluid replacement mainstay of treatment** & supportive measures. Avoid anti-motility drugs.
- **Avoid antibiotics in children due to increased incidence of Hemolytic uremic syndrome** (increased release of Shiga-like toxins).

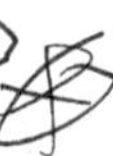

- Avoid anti-motility drugs (their use is associated with increased complications).

TYPHOID (ENTERIC) FEVER

- Diarrheal illness most caused by the gram-negative rod ***Salmonella typhi*** and *paratyphi.*
- More common in children & young adults. 5-21 day incubation period.

TRANSMISSION

- Fecal-oral, contaminated food or water.
- **History of travel to areas where sanitation is poor** (eg. South-Central Asia) or contact with carrier.

PATHOPHYSIOLOGY

- Crosses intestinal epithelium barrier through M cells overlying the lymphoid follicles of Peyer's patches.
- May colonize the gallbladder in chronic carriers.

CLINICAL MANIFESTATIONS

- **Headache, intractable fever, chills, abdominal pain,** constipation initially followed by non-bloody diarrhea (may be **"pea soup" green** in color), malaise, and anorexia.

PHYSICAL EXAMINATION

- **Fever with relative bradycardia** (classic but rare).
- **Rose spots** (faint pink or salmon-colored macular rash that spreads from trunk to extremities) occurs in the second week, abdominal tenderness.
- **Hepatosplenomegaly**, GI bleeding, signs of dehydration, and delirium may be seen in later stages.

DIAGNOSIS

- Culture of the stool and/or blood.

MANAGEMENT

- **Oral rehydration & electrolyte replacement first-line management.** Antibiotics often given.
- **Antibiotics: Fluoroquinolones first-line** (Ciprofloxacin, Ofloxacin), Macrolides, Ceftriaxone.

NONTYPHOIDAL SALMONELLA

- Other Salmonella species (eg, *S enteriditis, typhimurium*).
- **One of the most common causes of foodborne disease in US** (eg, **poultry, eggs,** milk products, fresh produce) and **contact with reptiles** (eg, turtles).
- 8-72 hour incubation period.

CLINICAL MANIFESTATIONS

- Nausea, vomiting, fever, abdominal cramping, diarrhea **(may be "pea soup" brown-green in color)** may be bloody, malaise, headaches.

DIAGNOSIS

- Stool cultures

MANAGEMENT

- **Oral rehydration & electrolyte replacement therapy mainstay of treatment.** Usually self-limited.
- Antibiotics: **Fluoroquinolones first-line when needed** (eg, severe disease).

ciprofloxacin, ofloxacin

SHIGELLOSIS

- Diarrheal illness most commonly caused by the gram-negative rods - ***Shigella sonnei* (most common in US),** *flexneri,* and *dysenteriae* (produces the most toxin).
- Children < 5 years in daycare at highest risk for Shigellosis.

PATHOPHYSIOLOGY

- *S. dysenteriae* produces a "Shiga" enterotoxin that is neurotoxic, cytotoxic, and enterotoxic.

TRANSMISSION

- Fecal-oral contamination, ingestion of contaminated food or water.
- **Highly virulent.** Incubation period 1-7 days.

CLINICAL MANIFESTATIONS

- **Lower abdominal pain**, abdominal cramps, high fever, tenesmus, **explosive watery diarrhea** that **progresses to mucoid & bloody diarrhea.**
- Neurologic manifestations especially in young children (eg, **febrile seizures**).
- Complications include reactive arthritis (Reiter syndrome), Hemolytic uremic syndrome (especially children), & Toxic megacolon.

DIAGNOSIS

- Stool cultures; Positive fecal WBCs & RBCs.
- CBC: **Leukemoid reaction (WBC >50,000**/microL).
- Sigmoidoscopy: punctate areas of ulceration.

MANAGEMENT

- **Oral rehydration and electrolyte replacement mainstay of treatment.**
- In general, anti-motility drugs should be avoided (can worsen the illness due to retained toxins).
- Antibiotics may be indicated if severe: Fluoroquinolones, third-generation Cephalosporins, Azithromycin, & Trimethoprim-sulfamethoxazole are options.

PROTOZOAN INFECTIONS

GIARDIA LAMBLIA

- *Giardia duodenalis* (also known as *G. lamblia* or *G. intestinalis*) is a protozoan parasite associated with sporadic or epidemic diarrheal illness.

SOURCES

- Ingestion of **contaminated water from remote streams/wells aka Beaver's fever** or **"Backpacker's diarrhea"**.
- Pathophysiology: Beavers are reservoirs for the protozoa. Outbreaks occur due to contaminated water, food, or fecal-oral transmission.

CLINICAL MANIFESTATIONS

- **Frothy, greasy, foul-smelling diarrhea** (steatorrhea) with **no blood** or pus, abdominal cramps, bloating. Malabsorption with chronic diarrhea.

DIAGNOSIS

- Antigen assays, trophozoites, & cysts on stool examination.

MANAGEMENT

- **Rehydration mainstay of treatment.**
- **Metronidazole,** Tinidazole, Albendazole, Quinacrine.
- Furazolidone may be used in children.

AMEBIASIS

- ***Entamoeba histolytica*** – protozoan most commonly transmitted by ingestion of cysts from fecally contaminated food and/or water.
- Not common in the US. Usually occurs in migrants from or travelers to endemic areas.
- May also be associated with **amebic liver abscess.**

CLINICAL MANIFESTATIONS

- Most infections are asymptomatic.
- GI symptoms: 1-3 week subacute onset of a range of **mild diarrhea to severe dysentery** (abdominal pain, diarrhea, bloody stools, mucus in stools weight loss, fever).
- Liver abscess: fever, RUQ pain, anorexia.

DIAGNOSIS

- Stool microscopy O&P (ova & parasites) – cysts with ingested RBCs. Because cysts are not constantly shed, at least 3 stool samples on different days should be examined.
- Antigen testing (eg, ELISA) – sensitive, easy to perform and rapid.
- Stool PCR – detects parasitic DNA or RNA in the stool.
- Liver abscess: ultrasound, CT or MRI

MANAGEMENT

- **Colitis: Metronidazole** or Tinidazole followed by an intraluminal parasitic (eg, **Paromomycin**, Diloxanide furoate or Diiodohydroxyquinoline).
- **Liver abscess:** Metronidazole or Tinidazole + intraluminal antiparasitic followed by Chloroquine. May need drainage if no response to medications after 3 days.
- Asymptomatic infections should be treated with an intraluminal agent alone.

SECRETORY DIARRHEA

ETIOLOGIES

- **Hormonal:** serotonin (carcinoid syndrome), calcitonin (medullary cancer of thyroid), gastrin (Zollinger-Ellison Syndrome).
- **Laxative abuse.**
- Vibrio cholerae.

WORKUP FINDINGS

- **Normal osmotic gap, large volume, no change in diarrhea with fasting.**

OSMOTIC DIARRHEA

ETIOLOGIES

- **Medications** (eg, Lactulose, Sorbitol, Antacids); Bacterial overgrowth (eg, Whipple's disease, Tropical sprue);
- **Malabsorption: Celiac disease,** pancreatic insufficiency, lactose intolerance.

WORKUP FINDINGS

- Decreased diarrhea with fasting, increased osmotic gap, increased fecal fat, deficiency in fat soluble vitamins.

WHIPPLE'S DISEASE

- ***Tropheryma whipplei:*** Gram-positive, non-acid-fast, periodic acid-Schiff-positive rod.

TRANSMISSION

- Contaminated soil (most commonly seen in farmers).

CLINICAL MANIFESTATIONS

- **Malabsorption:** chronic diarrhea, weight loss, steatorrhea, nutritional deficiency. Fever, lymphadenopathy, **nondeforming arthritis.**
- **Neurologic symptoms** including memory impairment & confusion. **Rhythmic motion of eye muscles while chewing.**

DIAGNOSIS

- **Duodenal biopsy: Periodic acid-Schiff (PAS)-positive macrophages,** non-acid-fast bacilli, **dilation of lacteals.**

MANAGEMENT

- Antibiotic therapy is usually prolonged (eg 1-2 years). **Penicillin** or Ceftriaxone followed by maintenance therapy with oral Trimethoprim-sulfamethoxazole.
- Doxycycline + Hydroxychloroquine is an alternative.

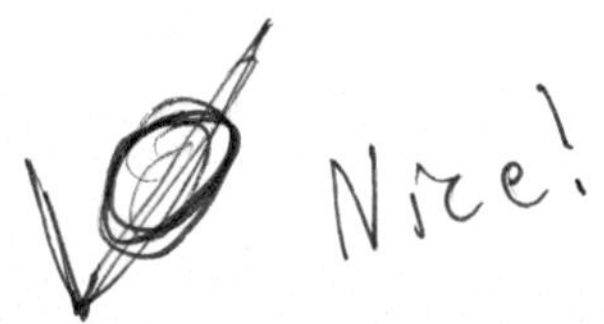

METABOLIC DISORDERS

G6PD DEFICIENCY

- **X-linked recessive** enzymatic disorder of RBCs that may cause **episodic hemolytic anemia.**

RISK FACTORS
- **Primarily males** (X-linked recessive).
- **10-15% of African-American males,** Mediterranean, African, Middle Eastern, SE Asian.

PATHOPHYSIOLOGY
- G6PD normally catalyzes NADP to NADPH, which protects the RBCs from oxidative injury.
- In G6PD deficiency, decreased G6PD activity during oxidative stress results in an oxidative form of Hb (methemoglobin). **The denatured hemoglobin precipitates as Heinz bodies.**
- RBC membrane damage and fragility causes extravascular RBC destruction (hemolysis) by reticuloendothelial macrophages in the spleen, marrow and liver as well as intravascular hemolysis.

EXACERBATING FACTORS
- **Infection most common cause** (eg, DKA), **Fava beans** (broad beans).
- Medications: eg, **Dapsone, Primaquine, Methylene blue, Nitrofurantoin, Phenazopyridine,** Rasburicase. Naphthalene mothball or henna exposure. "Sulfa" drugs at high doses.

CLINICAL MANIFESTATIONS
- **Most patients are asymptomatic until times of oxidative stress.**
- Episodic hemolytic anemia: symptoms begin 2-4 days after exposure. **Back or abdominal pain,** symptoms of **anemia, jaundice** (indirect bilirubin, dark urine), transient splenomegaly. Acute renal failure may occur in severe cases.
- Neonatal jaundice.

DIAGNOSIS
- Peripheral smear: **normocytic hemolytic anemia only during crises - schistocytes ("bite" or fragmented cells). +Heinz bodies hallmark.** Smear is usually normal when not in acute stage.
- Hemolytic anemia: increased reticulocytes, increased indirect bilirubin, decreased haptoglobin.
- Enzyme assay for G6PD: eg, Fluorescent spot test. DNA testing. Usually performed after episodes.

MANAGEMENT
- **Usually self-limited - avoid offending food & drugs,** treat underlying infection etc.
- Severe anemia: iron and folic acid supplementation. Blood transfusions if severe.
- Neonatal jaundice: phototherapy first-line. Exchange transfusion if refractory.

PAGET DISEASE OF THE BONE (OSTEITIS DEFORMANS)

- **Abnormal bone remodeling** seen in aging bone (increased osteoclastic bone resorption and increased osteoblastic bone formation). This leads to larger, weaker bones.
- Risk factors: persons of **Western European descent.** 40% autosomal dominant, >40y.

CLINICAL MANIFESTATIONS
- **Most are asymptomatic** (>70%). Found incidentally on radiographs or because of an incidentally **high alkaline phosphatase** on routine lab testing.
- **Bone pain is the most common symptom.** Bowing deformities.
- **Skull enlargement**: **deafness** (due to bony compression of CN VIII), headache.

DIAGNOSIS
- Labs: isolated **markedly elevated alkaline phosphatase.** Normal calcium, phosphate and parathyroid hormone levels. Increased urinary pyridinoline & N-telopeptide.
- Radiographs:
  Lytic phase: "blade of grass or flame shaped" lucency. Mixed phase (lucency + sclerosis).
  Sclerotic phase: increased trabecular markings.
  Skull radiographs: **cotton wool appearance –** sclerotic patches that are poorly defined & fluffy as a result of thickened, disorganized trabeculae, which leads to sclerosis in previously lucent bone.

MANAGEMENT
- Asymptomatic patients do not usually require treatment.
- **Bisphosphonates first-line medical management.** Vitamin D and calcium supplementation usually given to prevent hypocalcemia during bisphosphonate treatment. Normalization of alkaline phosphatase levels indicates response to treatment. NSAIDs for pain. Calcitonin.

BISPHOSPHONATES

- Newer nitrogen-containing bisphosphonates: IV: Zoledronate, Pamidronate. Zoledronate has greater efficacy than the other agents in severe Paget disease.
- **Oral: Alendronate, Risedronate.** Etidronate is a non-nitrogen bisphosphonate that is rarely used.

INDICATIONS
- **First-line medical management of Paget disease of the bone & Osteoporosis.**

MECHANISM OF ACTION
- **Inhibits osteoclast activity (decreasing bone resorption & turnover).** Alendronate & Risedronate inhibit both osteoclast & osteoblast activity.

CONSIDERATIONS:
- Taken with 8 ounces of plain water as well as 1-2 hours before meals (minimum 30 minutes), aspirin, Ca, Mg, Al & antacids. Poor oral absorption.
- **Calcium & vitamin D supplementation recommended.**

ADVERSE EFFECTS
- **Esophagitis** (especially Alendronate) so **must stay upright for at least 30 minutes**.
- Musculoskeletal pain, nephrotoxicity, thrombocytopenia, GI symptoms & Flu-like symptoms during initial treatment in naïve patients (IV forms).
- Rare but notable Adverse effects are **atypical femur fractures & osteonecrosis of the jaw.**

CONTRAINDICATIONS FOR ORAL BISPHOSPHONATES:
- Esophageal disorders, certain bypass procedures. Chronic kidney disease is a CI for both oral & IV.
- Alendronate contraindicated if esophageal stricture, dysphagia, or hiatal hernia.

PHENYLKETONURIA (PKU)

- Autosomal recessive disorder of amino acid metabolism associated with **phenylketone neurotoxicity** due to the accumulation of phenylalanine in the urine and the blood.

PATHOPHYSIOLOGY

- Decrease in the hepatic enzyme phenylalanine hydroxylase that metabolizes the amino acid phenylalanine into tyrosine.
- Neurotoxicity irreversible if not detected by 3 years old.

CLINICAL MANIFESTATIONS

- Presents after birth with **vomiting, mental delays**, irritability, convulsions, eczema, **increased deep tendon reflexes**. Intellectual disability. Children often **blonde, blue-eyed with fair skin.**

DIAGNOSIS

- Increased serum phenylalanine. Molecular analysis.
- **Urine with musty (mousy) odor** (from phenylacetic acid).
- Newborn screening routinely performed in US. Can be monitored during pregnancy (eg, 24 weeks GA).

MANAGEMENT

- **Lifetime dietary restriction of phenylalanine + increase tyrosine supplementation.** Phenylalanine levels are followed at regular intervals in neonates & less often in older children/adults. Some adults show improvement in behavior, symptoms, & sequelae when treated with a phenylalanine-restricted diet.
- **Avoid foods high in phenylalanine** (eg, milk, cheese, nuts, fish, chicken, meats, eggs, legumes, aspartame found in diet sodas).

VITAMIN C (ASCORBIC ACID) DEFICIENCY

RISK FACTORS

- Diets lacking raw citrus fruits & green vegetables (excess heat denatures vitamin C), smoking, illicit drug use, alcoholism, malnourished individuals, elderly. Symptoms can occur after 3 months of deficient intake.

CLINICAL MANIFESTATIONS

Scurvy 3 Hs

- **Hyperkeratosis:** hyperkeratotic follicular papules (often surrounded by hemorrhage). Coiled hairs.
- **Hemorrhage: vascular fragility** (due to abnormal collagen production) with **recurrent hemorrhages in gums, skin (perifollicular), & joints. Impaired wound healing.**
- **Hematologic**: anemia, glossitis, malaise, weakness. Increased bleeding time.

DIAGNOSIS

- Clinical. Serum ascorbic acid levels. Leukocyte ascorbic levels more accurate.

MANAGEMENT

- Ascorbic acid replacement. Hematologic symptoms improve within weeks, generalized symptoms can improve within days.

VITAMIN D DEFICIENCY

- Low bone turnover + decreased osteoid mineralization (Osteomalacia) and/or cartilage at the epiphyseal plates (Rickets)
- This is in contrast to osteoporosis, where mineral & matrix loss is proportional

OSTEOMALACIA

ETIOLOGIES

- **Severe vitamin D deficiency most common** - leads to decreased serum calcium & phosphate with subsequent **demineralization of the bone osteoid only ("soft bones").**
- Malabsorption (eg, chronic liver or kidney disease, gastric bypass celiac sprue etc.).
- **Disease in children = Rickets** & Osteomalacia. **Adults = Osteomalacia**

CLINICAL MANIFESTATIONS

- Asymptomatic initially. Diffuse **bone pain & tenderness, muscular weakness** (proximal). Hip pain may cause antalgic (waddling) gait.
- **Bowing of long bones.** Symptoms of hypocalcemia.

DIAGNOSIS

- Classic: **decreased calcium, phosphate, & 25-hydroxyvitamin D levels.**
- Increased alkaline phosphatase & PTH.
- Radiographs: **Looser lines (zones) –** transverse **pseudo-fracture lines** (narrow radiolucent lines from visible osteoid).

MANAGEMENT

- **Vitamin D supplementation first-line** (eg, **Ergocalciferol**).

RICKETS

- Low bone turnover + **decreased osteoid mineralization (Osteomalacia) and/or cartilage at the growth plates (Rickets).**
- Vitamin D deficiency most commonly seen between 3 months – 3 years when growth (calcium) needs are high + decreased sunlight exposure (eg, prolonged breastfeeding without vitamin D supplementation).

ETIOLOGIES

- Calcipenic (calcium deficiency &/or **vitamin D deficiency** including dietary deficiency, celiac disease, cystic fibrosis, or extensive bowel resection.
- Phosphopenic due to renal phosphate wasting (eg, Fanconi syndrome).

CLINICAL MANIFESTATIONS

- **Delayed fontanel closure,** growth delays, delayed dentition **& genu varum (lateral bowing** of the femur & tibia).

DIAGNOSIS

- Depends on the cause but classic labs are **decreased calcium, phosphate, & 25-hydroxyvitamin D levels** (calcipenic). Increased alkaline phosphatase & PTH.
- Radiographs: widening of the epiphyseal plate, **costochondral junction enlargement** (rachitic rosary), long bones appear to have a less distinct **"fuzzy" cortex.**

MANAGEMENT

- **Vitamin D supplementation first-line** (eg, **Ergocalciferol**).

VITAMIN A

- Vitamin A Function: vision, immune function, embryo development, hematopoiesis, skin, and cellular health (epithelial cell differentiation).
- Sources: found in the kidney, liver, egg yolk, butter, green leafy vegetables.

VITAMIN A EXCESS

- Acute toxicity: blurred vision, nausea, vomiting, vertigo, **Idiopathic intracranial hypertension.**
- Chronic toxicity: teratogenicity, alopecia, ataxia, visual changes skin disorders, hepatotoxicity

VITAMIN A DEFICIENCY

DEFICIENCY RISK FACTORS

- Patients with liver disease, ETOHics, fat-free diets (Vitamin A is a fat-soluble vitamin), fat malabsorption (eg, Cystic Fibrosis, Crohn ileitis, short bowel syndrome, bariatric surgery).

CLINICAL MANIFESTATIONS

- **Visual changes: especially night blindness,** xerophthalmia (dry eyes), retinopathy.
- Impaired immunity (poor wound healing, frequent infections), dry skin (follicular hyperkeratosis), poor bone growth, taste loss.
- **Squamous metaplasia** (conjunctiva, respiratory epithelium, urinary tract).
- **Bitot's spots:** white spots on the conjunctiva due to squamous metaplasia of the corneal epithelium.

DIAGNOSIS

- Clinical. Decreased serum retinol levels.

VITAMIN B DEFICIENCY

RIBOFLAVIN (B2) DEFICIENCY

CLINICAL MANIFESTATIONS

Oral, ocular, genital syndrome.

- Oral: lesions of mouth, **magenta colored tongue**, glossitis, angular cheilitis, stomatitis, pharyngitis.
- Ocular: photophobia, corneal lesions.
- Genital: scrotal dermatitis.

THIAMINE (B1) DEFICIENCY

ETIOLOGIES

- **Chronic alcoholism (most common),** weight loss surgery.

CLINICAL MANIFESTATIONS

- "Dry" Beriberi: **nervous system changes (eg, symmetric peripheral neuropathy,** paresthesias), sensory & motor neurons. Impaired coordination, impaired reflexes, anorexia, muscle cramps, & wasting.

- "Wet" Beriberi: **high output heart failure & Dilated cardiomyopathy.**

- Wernicke encephalopathy: triad of ataxia (difficulty walking & balance), global confusion, and ophthalmoplegia (paralysis or abnormalities of the ocular muscles). Considered a neurologic emergency. **Most common in chronic alcoholics.**

- Korsakoff dementia: memory loss **(especially short-term) & confabulation. Irreversible.** More of a chronic condition as a consequence of Wernicke's encephalopathy.

MANAGEMENT

- Beriberi: IV thiamine followed by oral thiamine.

NIACIN/NICOTINIC ACID (B3) DEFICIENCY

- Sources of B3 (Niacin/Nicotinic acid): meats, grains, legumes.

ETIOLOGIES

- Often due to **diets high in untreated corn** (lacks niacin & tryptophan), diets which **lack tryptophan,** alcoholism, anorexia or malabsorption. INH therapy.
- Carcinoid syndrome: increased tryptophan metabolism due to the production of serotonin.
- Hartnup disease: decreased tryptophan absorption in the kidneys & small intestine.

CLINICAL MANIFESTATIONS

- **Pellagra (3 Ds): dermatitis, diarrhea, & dementia.**
- Dermatitis: photosensitive hyperpigmented dermatitis (especially on sun-exposed areas); diarrhea and dementia (disorientation, delusions, & encephalopathy).

PYRIDOXINE (B6) DEFICIENCY

ETIOLOGIES

- Chronic alcoholism, **Isoniazid,** Penicillamine, Hydralazine, Levodopa + Carbidopa, oral contraceptives.

CLINICAL MANIFESTATIONS

- **Neurologic: peripheral neuropathy** (classic but rare), seizures, headache, mood changes.

- Stomatitis, cheilosis, glossitis, flaky skin, seborrheic dermatitis, **anemia**.

B12 (COBALAMIN) DEFICIENCY

- Sources of B12: natural sources **mainly animal in origin** (eg, meats, eggs, dairy products).

- Absorption: B12 is released by the acidity of the stomach and **combines with intrinsic factor, where it absorbed mainly by the distal ileum.**

ETIOLOGIES

- **Decreased absorption: Pernicious anemia most common cause** (lack of intrinsic factor due to parietal cell antibodies, leading to gastric atrophy). **Crohn disease** (affects the terminal ileum); Ileal resection, gastric bypass, post gastrectomy, gastritis, achlorhydria, tropical sprue, Zollinger-Ellison syndrome. **Chronic alcohol use.** Meds: H2 blockers, PPIs, decrease nucleic acid synthesis (**Metformin**, Zidovudine, Hydroxyurea), anticonvulsants. Fish tapeworm.

- Decreased intake: **vegans** (due to lack of consumption of meat and meat products).

CLINICAL MANIFESTATIONS

- Anemia symptoms **similar to Folate deficiency but associated with neurologic abnormalities.**

- Hematologic: fatigue, exercise intolerance, pallor.

- Epithelial: glossitis, diarrhea, malabsorption.

- **Neurologic symptoms: symmetric paresthesias most common initial symptom** (especially involving the legs), **lateral and posterior spinal cord demyelination & degeneration:** ataxia, weakness, **vibratory, sensory & proprioception deficits, decreased deep tendon reflexes** (hypotonia), +Babinski, seizures, psychosis.

DIAGNOSIS

- CBC with peripheral smear: **increased MCV (macrocytic anemia) +** megaloblastic anemia (**hypersegmented neutrophils, macro-ovalocytes,** mild leukopenia and/or thrombocytopenia**),** low reticulocytes.

- Decreased serum B12 levels, increased LDH, **increased homocysteine, increased methylmalonic acid** (distinguishes B12 from folate).

MANAGEMENT

B12 replacement

- Routes of administration: oral, sublingual, nasal and intramuscular/deep subcutaneous injection.

- **Symptomatic anemia or neuro findings: start with IM B12.** In adults, IM cyanocobalamin injection weekly until the deficiency is corrected and then once monthly. Patients can be switched to oral therapy after resolution of symptoms. **Patients with Pernicious anemia need lifelong monthly IM therapy** (or high-dose oral therapy).

- Dietary deficiency: oral B12 replacement.

ACUTE PANCREATITIS

- Acinar cell injury ⇨ **intracellular activation of pancreatic enzymes** ⇨ **autodigestion of pancreas.**

ETIOLOGIES

- **Gallstones & alcohol abuse are the 2 most common causes - gallstones most common** (40%), ETOH abuse second most common (35%).
- Medications: eg, **Thiazides, Protease inhibitors**, Estrogens, Didanosine, **Exenatide, Valproic acid**.
- Others: iatrogenic (ERCP), malignancy, scorpion sting, idiopathic, trauma, cystic fibrosis, hypertriglyceridemia, hypercalcemia, infection. Abdominal trauma or mumps in children.

CLINICAL MANIFESTATIONS

- **Epigastric pain** – constant, boring pain that often **radiates to the back** or other quadrant. Pain **exacerbated if supine,** eating **& relieved with leaning forward,** sitting or fetal position.
- **Nausea, vomiting, & fever common**. Shock in severe cases.
- Physical exam: **epigastric tenderness,** tachycardia. Decreased bowel sounds may be seen secondary to adynamic ileus. Dehydration or shock if severe.
- Necrotizing, hemorrhagic: **Cullen's sign** (periumbilical ecchymosis) and **Grey Turner sign** (flank ecchymosis).

DIAGNOSTIC CRITERIA

The diagnosis of Acute pancreatitis requires the **presence of 2 of the following 3** criteria:

- Acute onset of persistent, severe epigastric pain often radiating to the back,
- Elevation in serum lipase or amylase 3 times or greater the upper limit of normal
- Characteristic findings of Acute pancreatitis on imaging (CT, MRI, US).

No imaging is required if the patient meets the first 2 criteria.

DIAGNOSTIC LABS

- **Increased amylase & lipase: best initial tests.** Lipase more specific than amylase. Levels don't equal severity (not specific).
- ALT 3-fold increase highly suggestive of gallstone pancreatitis.
- **Hypocalcemia:** necrotic fat binds to calcium, lowering serum calcium levels (saponification).
- Leukocytosis; Elevated glucose, bilirubin, & triglycerides.

DIAGNOSTIC IMAGING

- **Abdominal CT: diagnostic imaging of choice.** Also recommended in patients who fail to improve or worsen after 48 hours of management to assess extent of necrosis. MRI alternative.
- Transabdominal US: recommended to assess for gallstones and bile duct dilation.
- Abdominal radiograph: **"sentinel loop" = localized ileus** of a segment of small bowel in the LUQ. **Colon cutoff sign:** abrupt collapse of the colon near the pancreas. Pancreatic calcification suggestive of chronic pancreatitis.
- MRCP useful to detect stones, stricture or tumor.
- Chest radiograph: left-sided, exudative pleural effusion in moderate to severe cases.

MANAGEMENT

- 90% recover without complications in 3-7 days & require supportive measures only - **"rest the pancreas".**
- **Supportive: NPO, high-volume IV fluid resuscitation** - Lactated ringers preferred (associated with decreased systemic inflammatory response compared to normal saline); **Analgesia** eg, Meperidine (Demerol).
- **Antibiotics: are not routinely used.** If severe infected pancreatic necrosis is seen (eg, >30% necrosis on CT or MRI), broad spectrum antibiotics (eg, Imipenem) may be used.

<u>RANSONS CRITERIA:</u> used to determine prognosis. APACHE score also used.

ADMISSION		WITHIN 48 HOURS	
<u>G</u>lucose	>200mg/dL	<u>C</u>alcium	<8.0 mg/dL
<u>A</u>ge	>55 years	<u>H</u>ematocrit fall	>10%
<u>LDH</u>	>350 IU/L	**<u>O</u>**xygen	P_{O2} <60 mmHg
<u>A</u>ST	>250 IU/dL	**<u>B</u>**UN	>5 mg/dL p IV fluids
<u>W</u>BC	>16,000/μL	**<u>B</u>**ase deficit	>4 mEq/L
		<u>S</u>equestration of fluid	> 6L

<u>Interpretation of Ranson's Criteria</u>

If the score ≥ 3, severe pancreatitis likely.
If the score < 3, severe pancreatitis is unlikely

Score 0 to 2 = 2% mortality
Score 3 to 4 = 15% mortality
Score 5 to 6 = 40% mortality
Score 7 to 8 : 100% mortality

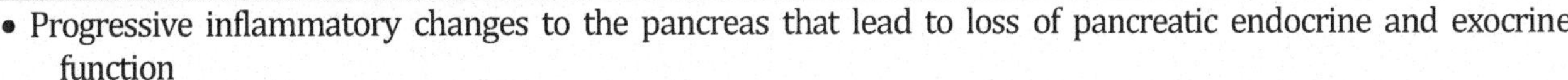

CHRONIC PANCREATITIS

- Progressive inflammatory changes to the pancreas that lead to loss of pancreatic endocrine and exocrine function

<u>ETIOLOGIES</u>

- **ETOH abuse most common** (70%), **idiopathic**, hypocalcemia, hyperlipidemia, islet cell tumors, familial, trauma, iatrogenic. Gallstones not significant as in acute.

<u>CLINICAL MANIFESTATIONS</u>

- **Triad of ❶ calcifications ❷ steatorrhea & ❸ Diabetes mellitus is hallmark** but seen in only 1/3 of patients.
- Weight loss. Epigastric and/or back pain may be atypical or completely absent.

<u>DIAGNOSIS</u>

- **Amylase & lipase usually normal** (or mildly elevated).
- **<u>CT scan</u>:** calcification of the pancreas. Often done in patients with acute pain to rule out other causes of abdominal pain.
- <u>Abdominal radiographs</u>: **calcified pancreas.**
- Endoscopic ultrasound or MRCP
- <u>Pancreatic function testing</u>: **fecal elastase most sensitive & specific.** Pancreatic stimulation with secretin & CCK (not usually done).

<u>MANAGEMENT</u>

- ETOH abstinence, pain control, low fat diet, vitamin supplementation.
- Oral pancreatic enzyme replacement
- Pancreatectomy only if retractable pain despite medical therapy

PANCREATIC CARCINOMA

- **70% found in the head of pancreas,** 20% body, 10% tail.

TYPES

- **Adenocarcinoma (ductal) most common** 90%, islet cell 5-10%.
- Ampullary & duodenal carcinomas; cystadenoma & cystocarcinoma.

RISK FACTORS

- **Smoking** (20%), **> 55 years of age,** chronic pancreatitis, Diabetes mellitus, males, obesity, African-Americans.

CLINICAL MANIFESTATIONS

- Usually presents late in the disease course - METS often present (eg, regional lymph nodes and liver).
- **Painless jaundice classic** (common bile duct obstruction); **weight loss**.
- Abdominal pain radiating to the back. May be relieved with sitting up & leaning forward. Tumors in body or tail produce symptoms later than in the head so usually more advanced at diagnosis. New onset diabetes mellitus. Depression.
- **Pruritus** (due to increased bile salts in skin), anorexia, acholic stools & dark urine (due to common bile duct obstruction).

PHYSICAL EXAMINATION

- Trousseau's malignancy sign = migratory phlebitis associated with malignancy. Nonspecific.
- **Courvoisier's sign palpable, NONtender, distended gallbladder** due to common bile duct obstruction (especially if head of the pancreas is involved).

DIAGNOSIS

- **CT scan: initial test of choice.**
  If CT is negative: the next step is an endoscopic ultrasound with biopsy of the pancreatic lesion.

  If CT is positive: the next step is simultaneous surgical removal/biopsy.
- Tumor markers: **CA 19-9** (often used to monitor after treatment), CEA.

MANAGEMENT

- Surgical: **Whipple procedure** (pancreaticoduodenectomy) if confined to the head or duodenal area. Tail (distal resection). Post-op chemotherapy (eg, 5-FU, Gemcitabine) or radiotherapy.
- Advanced or inoperative: ERCP with stent placement palliative for intractable itching.

PROGNOSIS

- Only 20% are resectable at the time of diagnosis.
- Overall 5-year survival rate is 5-15% (fourth leading cause of cancer-related deaths in the US).

MECKEL'S (ILEAL) DIVERTICULUM

- **Persistent portion of embryonic vitelline duct (yolk stalk, omphalomesenteric duct)** in the small intestine
- Most common congenital anomaly of the GI tract.
- **Rule of 2s:** 2% of population; within 2 feet from ileocecal valve, 2% symptomatic, 2 inches in length, 2 types of ectopic tissue (**gastric most common** or pancreatic), 2 years most common age at clinical presentation, 2 times more common in males.

PATHOPHYSIOLOGY
- Ectopic gastric or pancreatic tissue may secrete digestive hormones, leading to bleeding.

CLINICAL MANIFESTATIONS
- **Usually asymptomatic** – often an incidental finding during abdominal surgery for other causes.
- **Painless rectal bleeding or ulceration.** If present, pain is usually periumbilical.
- May cause intussusception, volvulus or obstruction. May cause diverticulitis in adults.

Diagnosis
- **Meckel scan:** looks for **ectopic gastric tissue** in the ileal area.
- Mesenteric arteriography or abdominal exploration

MANAGEMENT
- Surgical excision if symptomatic.

DUODENAL ATRESIA

- Complete absence or closure of a portion of the duodenum, leading to a **gastric outlet obstruction.**
- Risk factors: **polyhydramnios** (increased amniotic fluid), Down syndrome.
- Associated with other congenital defects.

CLINICAL MANIFESTATIONS
- **Neonatal intestinal obstruction:** shortly after birth (within the first 24-38 hours of life) with **bilious vomiting** (may be nonbilious), abdominal distention.

DIAGNOSIS
- Abdominal radiographs: **double bubble sign** (distended air-filled stomach + smaller distended duodenum separated by the pyloric valve).

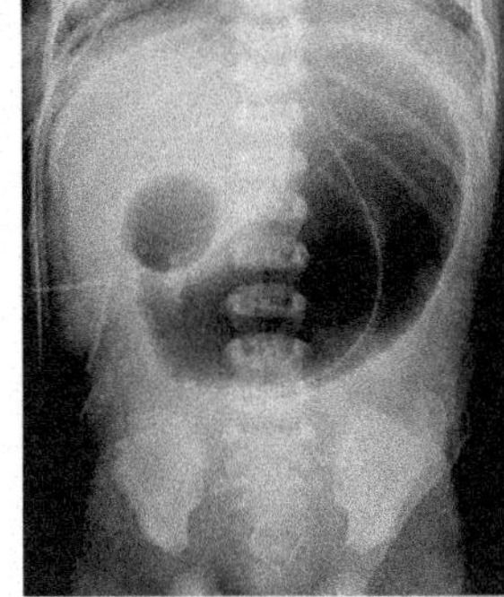

- Upper GI series: often performed preoperatively to assess the GI tract.

MANAGEMENT
- Decompression of the GI tract, electrolyte and fluid replacement
- Duodenoduodenostomy definitive management

VOLVULUS

- **Twisting of any part of the bowel** at its mesenteric attachment site.
- **Most commonly involves the sigmoid colon** & cecum in older adults.
- Midgut and ileum common in children.
- Complications obstruction and impaired vascular supply to the affected area.

CLINICAL MANIFESTATIONS

- **Obstruction:** crampy abdominal pain, distention, nausea, vomiting, constipation. **Tympanitic abdomen** with tenderness to palpation.
- Impaired vascular supply: fever, tachycardia, peritonitis (abdominal rigidity, guarding, rebound tenderness) and rarely sepsis.
- Neonates: bilious vomiting within the first week of life, colicky pain.

DIAGNOSIS

- Abdominal CT: dilated sigmoid colon, **"bird-beak" appearance at site of the volvulus.**
- Abdominal radiograph: **"bent inner tube" or "coffee bean" sign** – U-shaped appearance of the air-filled closed loop of distended colon with loss of haustral markings.

- Contrast enema: "bird's beak" appearance where the proximal and distal bowel rotate to form the volvulus. Not indicated if peritonitis is present.

MANAGEMENT

- **Endoscopic decompression (proctosigmoidoscopy) initial treatment of choice. Often a rectal tube is left in place** to decrease acute recurrence and decrease distention.
- **Decompression often followed by elective surgery** due to high rate of recurrence.
- Immediate surgical correction in patients with peritonitis, gangrene or if endoscopic decompression is unsuccessful. Includes: sigmoid resection with primary anastomosis or Hartmann's procedure.

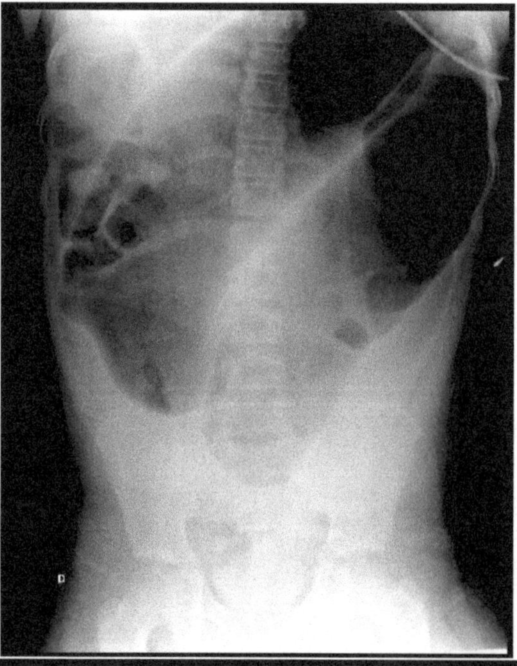

- Abdominal radiograph: **"bent inner tube" or "coffee bean" sign** – U-shaped appearance of the air-filled closed loop of distended colon with loss of haustral markings.

Photo credit: Mont4nha [CC0]

SMALL BOWEL OBSTRUCTION

- Partial or complete mechanical blockage of the small intestine.

ETIOLOGIES

- **Post-surgical adhesions most common** (60%), incarcerated hernias (2nd most common), Crohn disease, malignancy, intussusception. Malignancy is the most common cause of large bowel obstruction.

TYPES

- Closed loop vs. open loop: in closed loop, the lumen is occluded at two points, which can reduce the blood supply, causing strangulation, necrosis & peritonitis.
- Complete vs. partial: with complete, the patient usually has severe obstipation (unable to have bowel movements or pass gas).
- Distal vs. partial: distal presents more with abdominal distention & less vomiting.

CLINICAL MANIFESTATIONS

- 4 hallmark symptoms "CAVO" - **Crampy abdominal pain, Abdominal distention, Vomiting** & Obstipation (no flatus) usually a late finding.

PHYSICAL EXAMINATION

- Abdominal distention.
- Bowel sounds: **high-pitched tinkles on auscultation & visible peristalsis (early obstruction).** Hypoactive bowel sounds often heard in late obstruction.

DIAGNOSIS

- Abdominal radiographs: **multiple air-fluid levels** in a **"step-ladder" appearance**, **dilated bowel loops**. Minimal gas in colon if complete.
- CT scan: **transition zone** from dilated loops of bowel with contrast to an area of bowel with no contrast.

MANAGEMENT

- Nonstrangulated: **NPO (bowel rest), IV fluids. Bowel decompression** (NG suction) if severe vomiting.
- Strangulated: surgical intervention.

SPLENIC RUPTURE OR LACERATION

- The spleen is the most common organ injured during trauma (liver most common cause of bleeding).
- Associated with left-sided rib fractures, blunt abdominal trauma, infectious mononucleosis due to Epstein-Barr infection.

CLINICAL MANIFESTATIONS

- May have abdominal pain. May have signs of hypotension and shock.
- **Kehr sign**: referred left shoulder pain due to irritation of the diaphragm and the phrenic nerve.

DIAGNOSIS

- FAST abdominal examination, CT scan shows the extent of injury, exploratory laparotomy.

MANAGEMENT

- Incomplete rupture: endovascular embolization.
- Complete rupture or intractable bleeding: splenectomy.

PARALYTIC (ADYNAMIC) ILEUS

- **Decreased peristalsis WITHOUT structural obstruction** – nonmechanical factors affect & alter the normal coordination of the motor activity of the GI tract.

ETIOLOGIES

- **Postoperative state**
- Medications (eg, **opiates**)
- Metabolic (eg, **hypokalemia**, **hypercalcemia**)
- Severe medical illness, metabolic (**hypothyroidism**, diabetes)

CLINICAL MANIFESTATIONS

- Symptoms similar to small bowel obstruction - abdominal pain, nausea, vomiting, obstipation, abdominal distention, increased flatus, and inability to tolerate oral diet.

PHYSICAL EXAMINATION

- **Decreased or absent bowel sounds** (unlike early SBO that is classically associated with high-pitched sounds). No peritoneal signs.

DIAGNOSIS

- Plain radiographs: **dilated loops of bowel with no transition** zone, paucity of air in the colon and rectum.
- Labs: CBC, electrolytes, LFTs, amylase, lipase.
- CT of the abdomen if further testing needs to be performed.

MANAGEMENT

- **Supportive care: NPO or dietary restriction** - clear fluids with progression to liquid diet. **Electrolyte & fluid repletion**.
- Treat underlying cause.
- NG suction if moderate persistent nausea and/or vomiting.

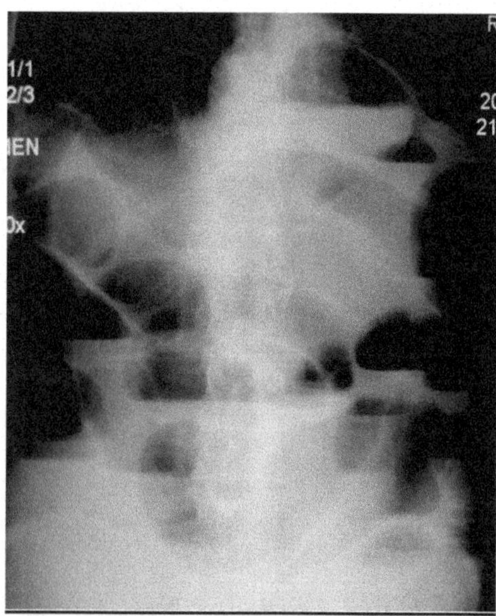

SMALL BOWEL OBSTRUCTION

- **Multiple air-fluid levels** in a **"step-ladder" appearance, dilated bowel loops**.

Photo: James Heilman, MD (Wikimedia commons)

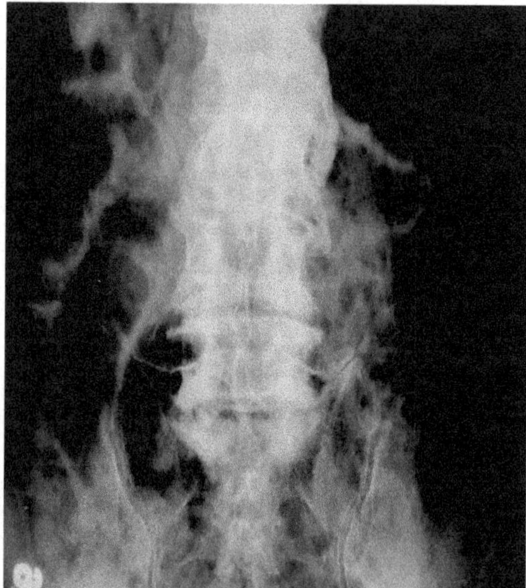

PARALYTIC ILEUS

- **Dilated loops of bowel with no transition zone.**

Photo: Nevit Dilmen (Wikimedia Commons)

INTUSSUSCEPTION

- **Telescoping (invagination) of an intestinal segment** into the adjoining distal intestinal lumen, leading to **bowel obstruction.** Most commonly occurs at the ileocolic junction.
- **Most common cause of bowel obstruction in children 6 months – 4 years of age.**

RISK FACTORS
- Children (2/3 seen between 6-18 months of age), males, commonly seen after viral infections.
- Lead points: **idiopathic most common,** Meckel diverticulum, enlarged mesenteric lymph nodes, hyperplasia of Peyer's patches, tumors, submucosal hematomas (HSP), foreign body.

CLINICAL MANIFESTATIONS
- Classic **triad: vomiting + abdominal pain + passage of blood per rectum – "currant jelly" stools** (stool mixed with blood & mucus). Abdominal pain is usually colicky in nature.
- Physical examination: **sausage-shaped mass in the right upper quadrant** or hypochondrium + **emptiness in the right lower quadrant (Dance's sign)** due to telescoping of the bowel.

DIAGNOSIS
- **Ultrasound: best initial test.** Donut or target sign. Abdominal radiographs: lack of gas in the bowels.
- **Air or contrast enema: both diagnostic and therapeutic. Air enema more commonly used** than barium enema, especially if peritonitis is present. Water-soluble contrast preferred over barium.

MANAGEMENT
- **Fluid and electrolyte replacement most important initial steps,** followed by NG decompression.
- Intussusception reduction: **pneumatic (air) or hydrostatic (saline or contrast) decompression (air is usually preferred). Admit for observation** (10% recurrence within 24 hours of treatment).
- Surgical resection if refractory to insufflation.

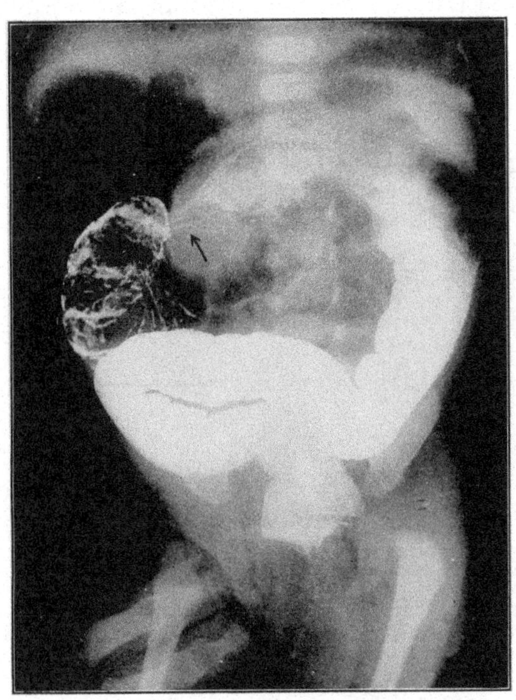

HIRSCHSPRUNG DISEASE

- **Congenital megacolon** due to an **absence of ganglion cells**, leading to a **functional obstruction.**
- Most common in the **distal colon and rectum** (80%).

RISK FACTORS

- **Males**: females 4:1, Down syndrome, Chagas disease, MEN II.

PATHOPHYSIOLOGY

- **Failure of complete neural crest** migration leads to an **absence of enteric ganglion cells** (**Auerbach** & Meissner plexuses).
- This leads to failure of relaxation of the aganglionic segment and subsequent functional obstruction.

CLINICAL MANIFESTATIONS

- **Neonatal intestinal obstruction:** **meconium ileus** (failure of meconium passage > 48 hours) in a full-term infant. **Bilious vomiting, abdominal distention.** No stool in rectal vault. Failure to thrive.
- Enterocolitis: vomiting, diarrhea, signs of Toxic megacolon (presents similar to sepsis).
- Chronic constipation in older children with milder disease.

DIAGNOSIS

- **Contrast enema**: **transition zone** (caliber change) between normal and affected bowel. Also helpful for presurgical planning.
- Anorectal manometry: may be used as a screening test. Increased anal sphincter pressure and lack of relaxation of the internal sphincter with balloon rectal distention.
- **Rectal biopsy: definitive. Rectal suction biopsy usually performed** with full thickness biopsy reserved if rectal suction biopsy is nondiagnostic.
- Abdominal radiographs: decreased or absence of air in the rectum + dilated bowel loops.

MANAGEMENT

- Resection of the affected bowel segment.

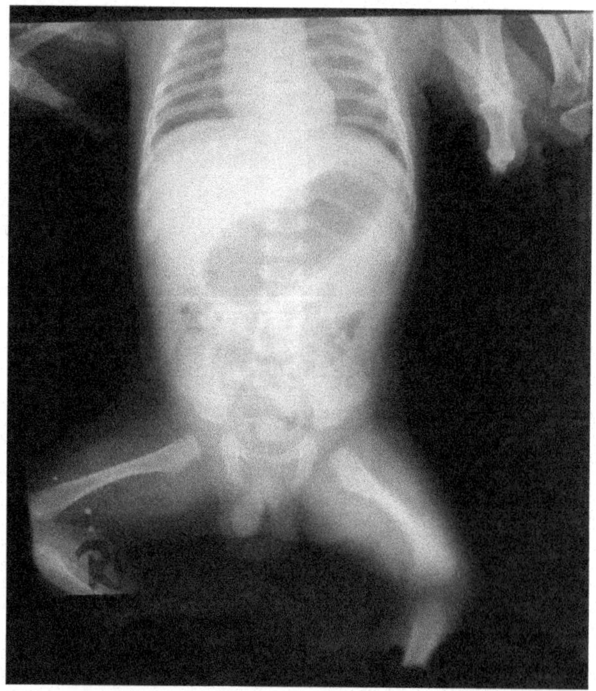

Photo: Shutterstock

APPENDICITIS

- Obstruction of the lumen of the appendix, resulting in inflammation & bacterial overgrowth.
- Most common 10 -30 years.
- Appendicitis is the most common cause of acute abdomen in children 12-18 years.

ETIOLOGIES

- **Fecalith & lymphoid hyperplasia most common,** inflammation, malignancy or foreign body. Lymphoid hyperplasia due to infection most common cause in children.

CLINICAL MANIFESTATIONS

- Classic presentation: **anorexia & periumbilical or epigastric pain followed by RLQ abdominal pain** (12-18 hours), nausea & vomiting **(vomiting usually occurs after the pain).**
- In patients with a retrocecal appendix, they may have an atypical pattern (eg, diarrhea) and positive rectal or gynecologic examination. Appendix may also be pelvic.
- Appendiceal inflammation stimulates nerve fibers around T8-T10, causing vague periumbilical pain. Once the parietal peritoneum becomes irritated, it radiates to the right lower quadrant.

PHYSICAL EXAMINATION

- Rebound tenderness, rigidity & guarding. Retrocecal appendix may have atypical findings.
- Tests for Appendicitis include:
  - **Rovsing sign:** RLQ pain with LLQ palpation.
  - **Obturator sign:** RLQ pain with internal & external hip rotation with flexed knee.
  - **Psoas sign:** RLQ pain with right hip flexion/extension (raise leg against resistance).
  - **McBurney's point tenderness:** point $^{1}/_{3}$ the distance from the anterior sup. iliac spine & navel

IMAGING

- In adults, CT scan is the preferred imaging of choice with ultrasound and MRI reserved for radiosensitive populations (eg, pregnant women, children).
- In children, a surgical consult is often obtained prior to imaging to determine if imaging is needed, depending on the risk.

MANAGEMENT

- Appendectomy (laparoscopic preferred when possible).

Photo credit: Paget disease of the bone
Jürgen Freyschmidt [Copyrighted free use]

Paget's skull
dr Laughlin Dawes [CC BY 3.0 (https://creativecommons.org/licenses/by/3.0)]

Small bowel obstruction
James Heilman, MD [CC BY-SA 3.0 (https://creativecommons.org/licenses/by-sa/3.0)]

Intussusception
Internet Archive Book Images [No restrictions]

Crohn disease
Hellerhoff [CC BY-SA 3.0 (https://creativecommons.org/licenses/by-sa/3.0)]

CHAPTER 4 – MUSCULOSKELETAL SYSTEM

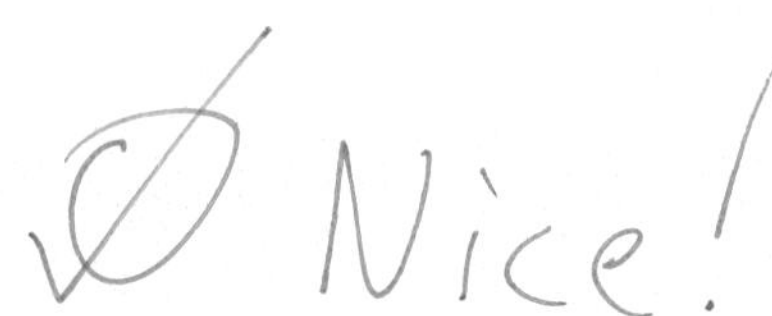

COMPARTMENT SYNDROME

- **Muscle & nerve ischemia (decreased tissue perfusion)** when the closed muscle compartment pressure > perfusion pressure.
- ETIOLOGIES: **trauma: most common after fracture of the long bones** (75%) especially involving the lower extremities, crush injuries, constriction (eg, tight casts, splints, & circumferential burns).

CLINICAL MANIFESTATIONS

- **Pain out of proportion to injury most specific.** Pain & paresthesia are the earliest symptoms.

PHYSICAL EXAMINATION

- **Pain with passive stretching** of the affected muscles is the **most sensitive earliest exam finding.**
- Tense compartment (**firm or "wood-like" feeling**).
- Pulselessness, pallor, decreased sensation & paresis (late findings); Capillary refill usually preserved.

DIAGNOSIS

- **Increased intracompartmental pressure** >30 mm Hg or Delta pressure <20-30 mm Hg indicates the need for fasciotomy. Δ pressure = Diastolic BP – measured compartment pressure.
- Increased creatinine kinase & myoglobin.

MANAGEMENT

- **Prompt decompression: emergency fasciotomy** to decompress the compartmental pressure.
- While awaiting decompression: place the limb at the level of the heart without elevation prior to decompression. Supportive management - removal of constrictive dressings, IV fluids, oxygen.

CHRONIC OSTEOMYELITIS

- Chronic infection of the bone (months to years).
- Etiologies: *S. aureus*, *Staph epidermis* (eg, prosthetic joint infections); Gram negative: *Pseudomonas* (IV drug abuse), Serratia, *E. coli*. May be polymicrobial.

SOURCES

- **Direct Inoculation:** infection close to bone s/p trauma, surgery, insertion of a prosthetic joint.
- **Contiguous spread with vascular insufficiency**: eg, Diabetes mellitus, Peripheral vascular disease.
- Acute hematogenous spread: Not a common cause in adults. Vertebral osteomyelitis is the most common cause of hematogenous Osteomyelitis in adults. Hematogenous spread in children.

CLINICAL MANIFESTATIONS

- Sinus tract drainage and nonspecific symptoms are hallmark.
- The involved limb may be edematous, warm, swollen, tender, with decreased ROM (due to pain).

DIAGNOSIS

- Radiographs: soft tissue swelling, periosteal reaction, osteopenia, bone destruction. **Sequestrum** (segments of necrotic bone that has become separated from normal bone), **Involucrum** = new periosteal bone formation that surrounds necrotic bone (sequestrum).
- MRI or CT scan: more sensitive than radiographs.
- Bone biopsy: essential to identify pathogens and obtain sensitivities.

MANAGEMENT

- **Surgical debridement + cultures initial treatment of choice for chronic Osteomyelitis.** Unlike acute Osteomyelitis, empiric antibiotics are generally not recommended.
- Antibiotic treatment is based on culture and sensitivity in chronic Osteomyelitis.

ACUTE OSTEOMYELITIS

- Infection of the bone. Most commonly seen in children.
- **Femur & tibia most common bones affected in children**.
- Vertebrae most common bone affected in adults.

RISK FACTORS
- Sickle cell disease, Diabetes mellitus, immunocompromised, preexisting joint disease.

SOURCES
- **Acute hematogenous spread: most common route in children.**
- Direct Inoculation: infection close to bone, post traumatic (eg, open fractures, puncture wounds), surgical (eg, insertion of a prosthetic joint).
- Contiguous spread with vascular insufficiency: eg, DM, peripheral vascular disease.

NOTABLE ORGANISMS
- ***Staphylococcus aureus*: most common organism overall.** Group A *Streptococcus* (S. pyogenes).
- ***Staphylococcus epidermis*** (coagulase-negative) - increased incidence after recent **prosthetic joint placement,** neonates, & children with indwelling catheters (eg, chronic hemodialysis).
- ***Salmonella* pathognomonic for Sickle cell disease.**
- ***Group B streptococcus*** – increased incidence in **neonates.**
- ***Pseudomonas aeruginosa*** - calcaneal osteomyelitis associated with **puncture wounds through tennis shoes.**

CLINICAL MANIFESTATIONS
- Nonspecific constitutional symptoms (eg, **fever,** chills, malaise), signs of **bone inflammation** (eg, **bone pain,** warmth, swelling, tenderness) & **limitation of function** (eg, restricted use of the extremity, decreased ROM, limp, refusal to bear weight).

DIAGNOSIS
- Labs: increased ESR & CRP (CRP more useful). WBC may be increased. Blood cultures + in 50%.
- **Radiographs:** usually the **initial imaging test** ordered. Evidence of bone infection may not be evident for up to 2 weeks after symptom onset.
  Early: soft tissue swelling & **periosteal reaction.** Later: lucent areas of cortical destruction.
- **MRI: most sensitive test in early disease.** CT scan often used for surgical planning.
- Radionuclide bone or Gallium scan: sensitive in early disease.
- **Bone Aspiration: gold standard (definitive).**

ACUTE OSTEOMYELITIS:
Antibiotics 4-6 weeks (at least 2 weeks via IV). May need debridement.

AGE	COMMON ORGANISMS	EMPIRIC THERAPY
Birth to 3 months	**Group B Strep,** Gram neg.	• Third-generation cephalosporin [eg, **Cefotaxime** (preferred) or Ceftazidime] **PLUS** anti-staphylococcal agent - **Vancomycin** (preferred), Nafcillin, or Oxacillin.
>3 months – adults	**Methicillin Sensitive (MSSA)** ***S. aureus***	• **Nafcillin, Oxacillin, Cefazolin**. (Clindamycin or Vancomycin if PCN allergic)
	Methicillin Resistant (MRSA)	• **Vancomycin,** Clindamycin, or Linezolid
Sickle cell	**Salmonella,** S. Aureus	**3rd gen Cephalosporin or FQ (Cipro** or Levofloxacin)
Puncture wound	**Pseudomonas**	• Ceftazidime of Cefepime. • Ciprofloxacin can be used in adults.

Puncture
Pseudomonas

OSTEOARTHRITIS (OA)

- Chronic disease due to loss of articular cartilage & joint degeneration; minimal/absent inflammation.
- Most common in **weight-bearing joints** (eg, knees, hips, spine, wrists).
- If the hand is affected, DIP involvement > PIP or MCP.

RISK FACTORS

- Modifiable: **obesity, trauma,** heavy labor.
- Nonmodifiable: **increasing age**, female gender, & family history.

CLINICAL MANIFESTATIONS

- Joint pain (usage related), stiffness and restriction of movement. The pain is usually worse in the late afternoon & evening.
- **Evening joint stiffness** – **worsens throughout the day** & with weather changes. If morning stiffness is present, it is of **short duration,** lasting <60 minutes (compared to RA).

PHYSICAL EXAMINATION

- Joint: **hard, bony joint**, decreased ROM, **crepitus.** No inflammatory signs.
- **Heberden node** (DIP enlargement) & **Bouchard nodes** (PIP enlargement).

DIAGNOSIS

- Radiographs: **asymmetric joint narrowing**, marginal **osteophytes, subchondral bone sclerosis,** bone cysts.
- Labs: lack of inflammatory markers - normal ESR, CRP, ANA, Rheumatoid factor.

MANAGEMENT

- Lifestyle modification: weight management, moderate exercise and use of assistive devices when needed.
- **Acetaminophen preferred initial analgesic if mild – moderate pain & in the elderly.**
- **NSAIDs:** topical or oral. Although **NSAIDs are more effective, NSAIDs are associated with increased adverse effects in the elderly** (eg, GI bleeding, renal injury). NSAIDs may be used if no relief with Acetaminophen and no risks or contraindications exist (eg, renal disease, Heart failure, Peptic ulcer disease, GI bleeds). Topical NSAIDs have a better safety profile and can be used if one or few joints are affected.
- Duloxetine in some patients with multiple joint involvement in whom NSAIDs are contraindicated.
- Topical Capsaicin (may cause local burning or irritation).
- Intraarticular corticosteroids provide temporary relief (usually about 4 weeks).
- Joint replacement if function is compromised.

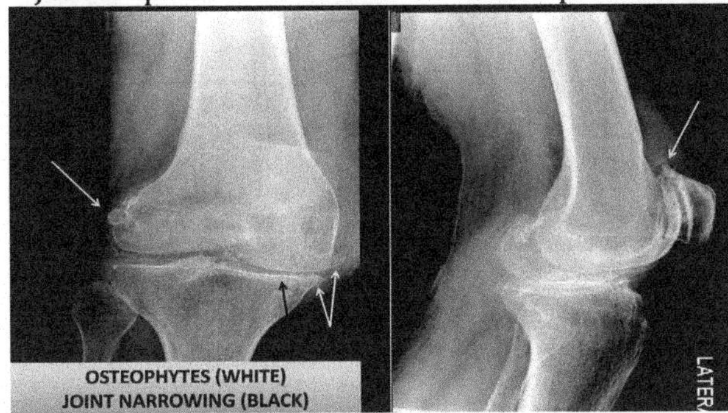

OSTEOARTHRITIS
- **Asymmetric joint narrowing**
- Marginal **osteophytes**
- **Subchondral bone sclerosis,** bone cysts.

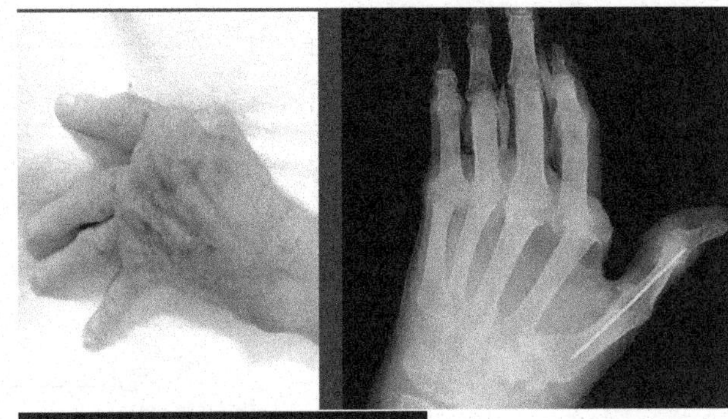

RHEUMATOID ARTHRITIS
- **Symmetric joint narrowing**
- **Osteopenia, bone & joint erosions.**
- Ulnar deviation in severe cases

RHEUMATOID ARTHRITIS (RA)

- Chronic systemic autoimmune inflammatory disease with symmetric polyarthritis, bone erosion, cartilage destruction & joint structure loss.

PATHOPHYSIOLOGY

- Hyperplastic synovial tissue (**pannus**) leads to joint destruction (T-cell mediated).
- Risk factors: women, 30-50y, smoking, HLA-DRB 1 & 4.

CLINICAL MANIFESTATIONS

- Systemic (constitutional) symptoms: fever, fatigue, weight loss, anorexia.
- Joint pain and stiffness: **morning stiffness >1 hour** after initiating movement, **improves later in the day.** Decreased ROM.
- Most commonly affects **small joints: wrist, MCP, PIP, MTP**, ankle. Characteristically **spares the DIP**.
- Felty syndrome: RA + splenomegaly + neutropenia
- Caplan syndrome: RA + Pneumoconiosis + pulmonary nodules

PHYSICAL EXAMINATION

- Joint: **symmetric** inflamed joints - **warm, erythematous, soft "boggy". Ulnar deviation** of the hand, swan neck & boutonniere deformities, rheumatoid nodules over bony prominences.

DIAGNOSIS

- Labs: **Rheumatoid factor (best initial test), Anti-cyclic citrullinated peptide antibodies** (Anti-CCP) **most specific**; Increased ESR & CRP.
- Radiographs: **symmetric joint narrowing, osteopenia, bone & joint erosions**. Severe is associated with joint subluxation. Plain radiographs are often normal in early disease.
- Cervical spine involvement can be seen, leading to subluxation (especially **C1-C2 subluxation**).

MANAGEMENT

- **Prompt initiation of DMARD to slow disease progression** (eg, **Methotrexate, Leflunomide**) + **NSAIDs** for **immediate symptom control**.
- Methotrexate or Leflunomide preferred in patients with high disease activity & advanced disease.
- Glucocorticoids second-line for symptom control (does not slow disease progression).

DISTINGUISHING BETWEEN RHEUMATOID ARTHRITIS AND OSTEOARTHRITIS

FEATURE	RHEUMATOID ARTHRITIS	OSTEOARTHRITIS
Primary joints affected	**Wrists, MCP, PIP** (DIP usually spared)	**DIP**, thumb (CMC)
Heberden's nodes	Absent	Frequently present
Joint Characteristics	Soft, warm, **BOGGY**, tender	**HARD & BONY**
Stiffness	• Worse after resting • Morning stiffness • **MORNING STIFFNESS ≥ 60 minutes**	• Worse after effort • **Evening stiffness.** • If morning stiffness present it is usually <60 minutes.
X ray findings	• **Osteopenia** • **SYMMETRIC joint narrowing**	• **Osteophytes** • **ASYMMETRIC joint narrowing** • Subchondral sclerosis
Laboratory findings	**Positive:** **RF, anti-CCP Ab**, ESR, CRP	Negative: RF, anti-CCP Ab, ESR, CRP

NON BIOLOGIC DMARDS

METHOTREXATE

- Mechanism: folic antagonist.
- Indications: **initial DMARD in most patients with RA**. Can be used in combination with biologic DMARDs. Methotrexate and Leflunomide good for severe disease or high disease activity.
- Adverse effects: **liver, lung, marrow: hepatitis, interstitial pneumonitis, & bone marrow suppression.**

LEFLUNOMIDE

- Alternative to Methotrexate with similar efficacy. T-cell inhibitor.

HYDROXYCHLOROQUINE

- Indications: can be used in mild disease or if the diagnosis is uncertain. Can also be used in combination with Methotrexate. Safe in pregnancy.
- Adverse effects: **retinal toxicity** (eye exams required while on therapy), ototoxicity.

SULFASALAZINE

- Indications: usually reserved for patients unable to take Methotrexate or Leflunomide.
- Adverse effects: **hemolysis** (especially if **G6PD deficient),** rash, hepatitis, & marrow suppression.

BIOLOGIC DMARDS

All patients on biologic DMARDs should have a PPD to rule out tuberculosis before initiating therapy.

TNF (TUMOR NECROSIS FACTOR)-INHIBITORS

- Etanercept, Infliximab, Adalimumab.
- Adverse effects: reactivation of Tuberculosis & other chronic infections, such as Hepatitis B and C. They should be avoided in patients with Multiple sclerosis.

ANAKINRA

- Mechanism: interleukin-1 receptor antagonist.
- Indications: often used when treatment with other DMARDs are not effective. Increased activity when used with Methotrexate.

RITUXIMAB

- Mechanism: **anti-CD20 B cell-depleting monoclonal antibody**.
- Indications: used with Methotrexate in patients not responding to TNF-inhibitors.
- Adverse effects: reactivation of chronic infections, such as Tuberculosis, HBV, HCV. Infusion reaction.

ABATACEPT

- Mechanism: T-cell inhibitor.
- Adverse effects: reactivation of chronic infections, such as Tuberculosis, HBV, HCV.

ANTIINFLAMMATORY MEDICATIONS FOR SYMPTOM CONTROL

NSAIDS

- Mechanism: analgesic & anti-inflammatory. **First-line for symptom control** but does not affect disease course so DMARD must also be initiated to slow down progression.
- Adverse effects: GI (gastritis, peptic ulcer disease), renal insufficiency, cardiovascular (↑ bleeding).

CORTICOSTEROIDS

- Mechanism: suppresses inflammation. Low-dose oral, IV, or intraarticular routes.
- Adverse effects: hyperglycemia, cataracts, weight gain, fluid retention, immunosuppression, hypertension, osteopenia (prevented with Calcium + Vitamin D).

SEPTIC ARTHRITIS

- Infection in the joint cavity. Medical emergency (can rapidly destroy the joint).
- **Knee most common joint involved in older children and adults** (>50%).
- **Hip joint most common in younger children**.
- Sternoclavicular joint seen in IV drug users.

RISK FACTORS
- Extremes of age, chronic medical condition, immunosuppression (eg, medications, HIV, IV drug use, Diabetes mellitus).
- Prosthetic joint/surgery, chronic arthropathies (eg, Rheumatoid arthritis, Gout, Osteoarthritis).

NOTABLE ORGANISMS
- **Staphylococcal species:** ***S. aureus* most common organism in all age groups** (>50%) including IV drug users (especially MRSA). *Staphylococcus epidermis* with increased incidence with recent prosthetic placement.
- **Streptococcal species:** second most common cause. Group A *Streptococcus*. Group B *Streptococcus*: neonates & infants < 3 months. *Streptococcus pneumoniae*.
- ***Neisseria gonorrhoeae*: sexually active young adults** – associated with tenosynovitis.
- Pseudomonas: increased incidence in immunocompromised (eg, IV drug use, older adults, neonates) or with trauma.
- Mycobacteria & fungi less common.

CLINICAL MANIFESTATIONS
- Joint involvement: **swollen warm, painful and tender joint with decreased ROM** (tenderness with micromotion).
- Constitutional symptoms: **fever,** chills, diaphoresis, myalgias, malaise.

DIAGNOSIS
- **Arthrocentesis: best initial and most accurate test - WBC ≥50,000 – primarily neutrophils.** WBC >1,100 considered positive in prosthetic joints. Aspirate also examined for crystals, gram stain, & culture.
- Increased ESR & CRP (nonspecific markers of inflammation). Although WBC, ESR, & CRP are usually monitored to assess response to treatment, **CRP is more useful**.
- Blood cultures positive in 50%.
- Radiographs may show soft tissue swelling. MRI/CT.

MANAGEMENT
- Prompt IV antibiotics, joint drainage, & debridement as needed.
- Joint drainage: arthrotomy (open surgical drainage), needle aspiration, or arthroscopic drainage.

GRAM STAIN	ANTIBIOTIC REGIMEN
NO ORGANISM SEEN (EMPIRIC)	**Ceftriaxone + Vancomycin** (±anti-Pseudomonas if suspected).
GRAM POSITIVE COCCI	**Vancomycin.** Nafcillin (if MSSA suspected)
GRAM NEGATIVE COCCI OR GONOCOCCUS SUSPECTED	**Ceftriaxone** (Gonococcal usually doesn't need arthrotomy). Cefotaxime, Ceftazidime. Fluoroquinolones.
GRAM NEGATIVE RODS	Ceftazidime + Gentamicin. Ciprofloxacin can be substituted if penicillin allergic.

HIP & PELVIS INJURIES

DEVELOPMENTAL DYSPLASIA OF THE HIP

- Abnormality in the shape and/or stability of the shape of the femoral head and acetabulum.
- Examination of the hip is performed during newborn assessment soon after birth and at every well-check visit until about 9 months of age and/or the child is walking independently.

RISK FACTORS
- **Breech presentation at delivery,** first-born children, females, positive family history.

PHYSICAL EXAMINATION

Assessed for hip instability, asymmetry, or limited abduction:
- Barlow maneuver: gentle adduction without downward pressure to feel for dislocatability, resulting in a "click", "clunk" or "jerk".
- Ortolani maneuver: abduction and elevation to feel for reducibility, resulting in a "click", "clunk" or "jerk".
- Other findings may include asymmetry (eg, skin folds, femur length, or gait) and restricted hip abduction.
- In infants > 3 months, the dislocation may become relatively fixed and the Galeazzi test can be used instead.

ORTOLANI MANEUVER:
Reduces the hip

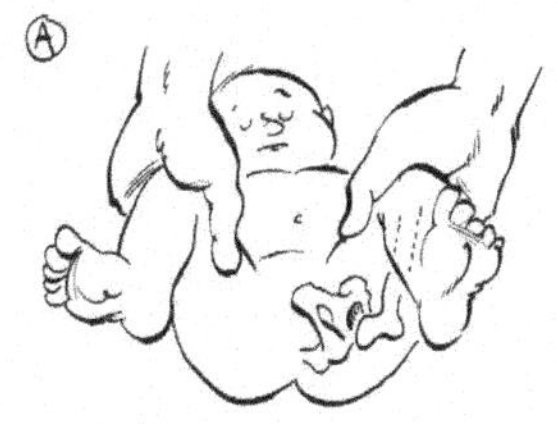

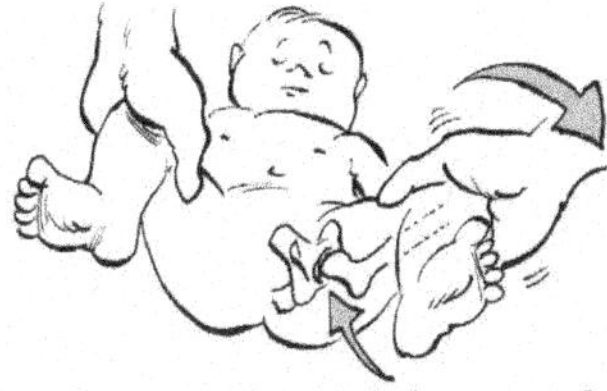

Examiner grasps the medial aspect of the knee & abducts the hips while applying anterior force to the femur, resulting in ***reduction of the hip joint*** (may feel a clunk).

BARLOW MANEUVER:
Dislocates the hip

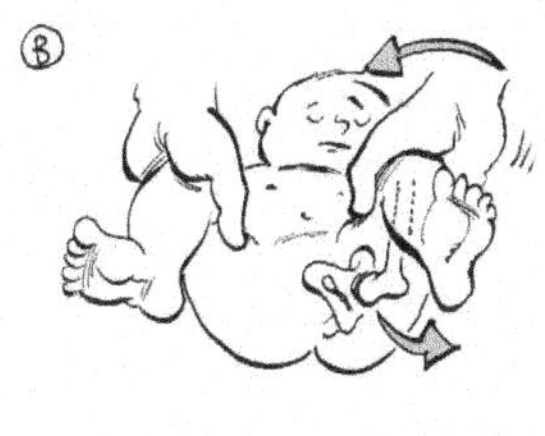

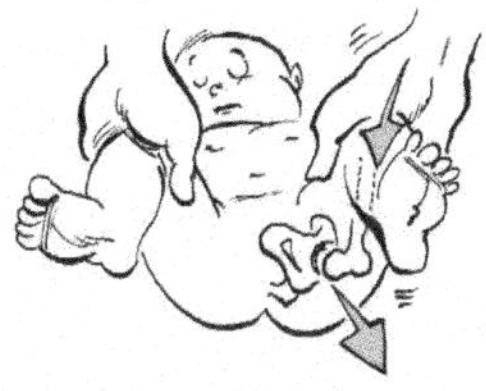

Examiner adducts the fully flexed hip while applying posterior force to the femur, ***resulting in dislocation of the hip.***

DIAGNOSIS
- Clinical with confirmation with imaging.
- Ultrasound: often used in children < 4 months of age
- AP radiographs in older children.

MANAGEMENT
- ≤ 6 months of age: Pavlik harness.
- 6 months – 2 years: closed reduction in the OR (may need athrogram).
- Monitoring with routine hip radiographs until the child is skeletally mature may be needed.
- **Hip dislocation assessment using the Barlow & Ortolani maneuvers.**
- In infants > 3 months, the dislocation may become relatively fixed and the Galeazzi test can be used instead.

PELVIC FRACTURES

- MECHANISM: high-impact injuries (eg, MVA). Low-impact injuries.

CLINICAL MANIFESTATIONS

- Symptoms can vary from pain with ambulation to inability to ambulate.
- Acetabular fractures most commonly occur with associated lower extremity, abdominal, or neurologic injuries. May have **perineal ecchymosis**.

DIAGNOSIS

- Imaging: radiographs. CT scan may be indicated if radiographs are negative or to get more details.
- Labs: CBC to monitor any blood loss, blood type and screen.

MANAGEMENT

- Depends on severity: weight bearing as tolerated for most pubic rami fractures, pelvic binder.
- ORIF for more severe fractures.
- For bleeding, a pelvic binder and IV fluid resuscitation is often used initially with vessel embolization if refractory.
- Complications include DVT, sciatic nerve damage, and vascular injury (bleeding).

HIP DISLOCATIONS

- Associated conditions: fractures of the hip or pelvis, knee injuries.

MECHANISM

- **Trauma most common cause** (eg, **MVA**, fall from height). Orthopedic emergency.
- **Posterior: most common type (90%).** Axial loading on an adducted femur.
- Anterior: axial loading on an abducted & externally rotated femur.
- Associated conditions: fractures of the hip & pelvis or knee injuries.

PHYSICAL EXAMINATION

- **Posterior:** (90%) - **hip pain with the leg shortened, internally rotated & adducted** with hip/knee slightly flexed.
- Anterior may be externally rotated & abducted.

RADIOGRAPHS

- Posterior: the femoral head appears smaller than the contralateral side and femur appears adducted.
- Anterior: the femoral head appears larger and the femur appears abducted.

MANAGEMENT

- Conservative: **closed reduction under conscious sedation**. Not performed if there is an associated ipsilateral femoral neck fracture.
- Open reduction.

COMPLICATIONS

- **Avascular necrosis** up to 13% (reduced with early closed reduction < 6 hours).
- **Sciatic nerve injury,** DVT, bleeding.
- In anterior hip dislocations, the femoral nerve is the most commonly injured nerve.

HIP FRACTURES

- Mechanism: minor or indirect trauma in the elderly. High-impact injuries in younger patients.
- Most common in osteoporotic women. Common in the elderly & patients with decreased bone mass.

3 MAIN TYPES:

- Femoral neck fractures: proximal (cephalad) to the trochanters. **Fractures of the femoral head and neck are associated with a higher incidence of avascular necrosis**.
- Intertrochanteric: between the greater and lesser trochanters.
- Subtrochanteric: distal (below) the trochanters.
- Intertrochanteric & subtrochanteric are extracapsular. Femoral head & neck fractures are intracapsular.

PHYSICAL EXAMINATION

- Hip, thigh or groin pain with the affected **leg shortened, abducted, & externally rotated.**

MANAGEMENT

- Operative: ORIF (open reduction & internal fixation) or arthroplasty are surgical options. Hip prosthesis may be used for femoral neck fractures. Pinning for some intertrochanteric fractures.
- May observe if high surgical risk, minimal pain or non-ambulatory prior to fracture.

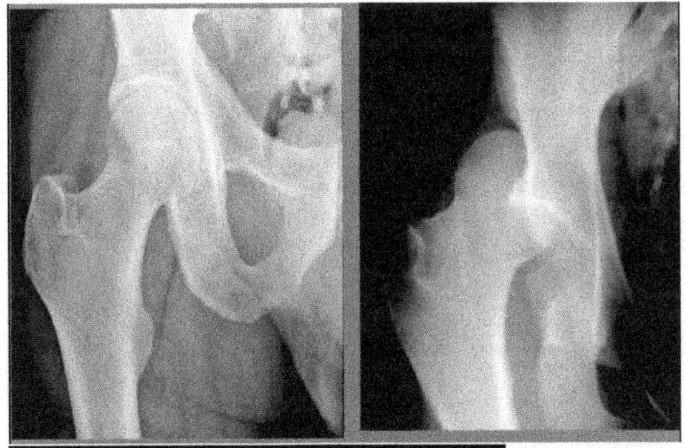

POSTERIOR HIP DISLOCATION

- **Hip pain with the leg shortened, internally rotated, & adducted** with hip/knee slightly flexed.

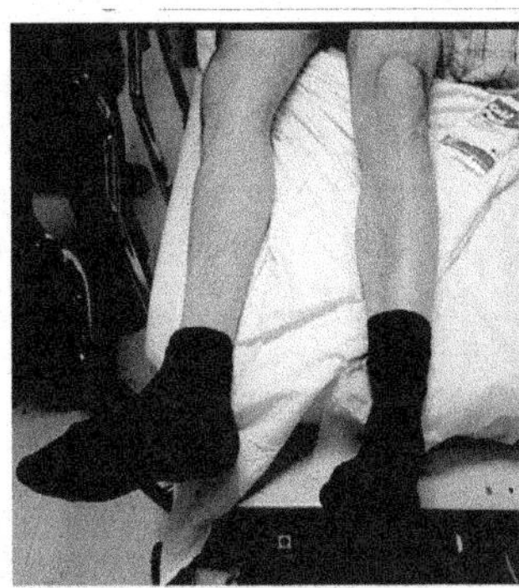

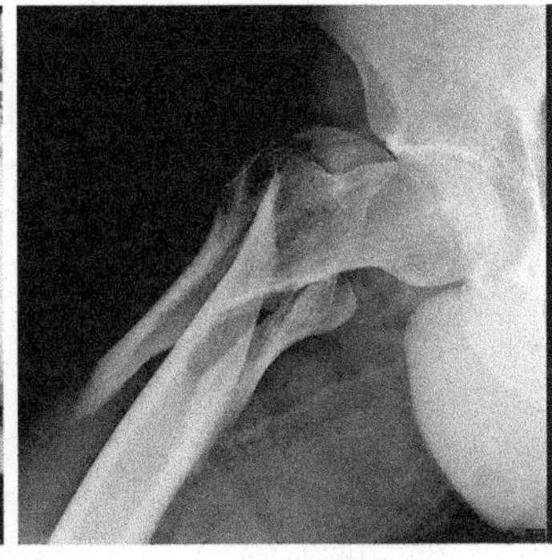

HIP FRACTURE

- Hip, thigh or groin pain with the affected **leg shortened, abducted, & externally rotated**

LEGG-CALVÉ -PERTHES DISEASE

- **Idiopathic avascular osteonecrosis of the femoral head in children** due to ischemia of capital femoral epiphysis. Usually unilateral.

RISK FACTORS

- Children **4-10 years,** 4 times more common in **males,** obesity, coagulation abnormalities (eg, Factor V Leiden).
- Decreased risk factors: low incidence in African-Americans.

CLINICAL MANIFESTATIONS

- **Painless limping** for weeks **(worsen with continued activity especially at the end of the day).**
- May have mild intermittent hip, thigh, knee, or groin pain. May have an antalgic or Trendelenburg gait.
- Restricted range of motion **(loss of abduction & internal rotation).** May have atrophy of the thigh muscles. Patients may lag in bone age & height.

RADIOGRAPHS

- Early: increased density of the femoral epiphysis, widening of the cartilage space.
- Advanced: deformity, **positive crescent sign** (microfractures with collapse of the bone).

MANAGEMENT

- **Observation**: **activity restriction** (non-weight bearing initially) with orthopedic follow up is initial treatment in most cases (usually self-limiting with revascularization within 2 years). May advocate for protected weight bearing during early stages until reossification is complete. **Physical therapy or brace/cast.** NSAIDs for pain management.
- Surgical: pelvic osteotomy may be indicated in some children > 8 years of age, more advanced disease (eg, lateral pillar B and B/C).

LEGG-CALVÉ-PERTHES DISEASE

- Idiopathic avascular necrosis of the femoral head in children due to ischemia of the femoral epiphysis.

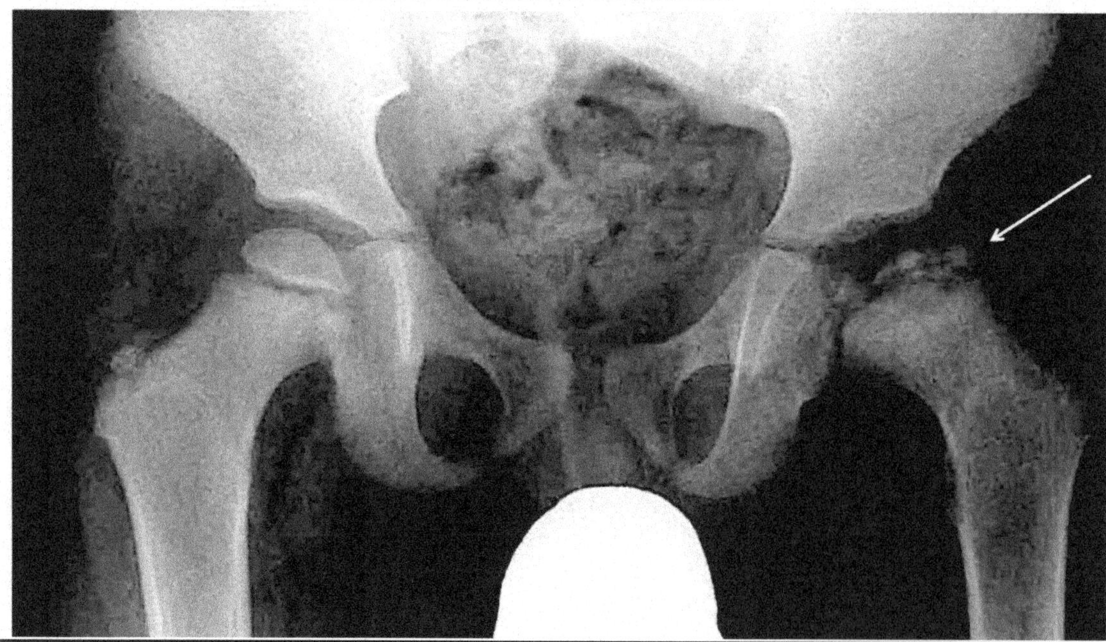

SLIPPED CAPITAL FEMORAL EPIPHYSIS

- Displacement of the femoral head (epiphysis) from the femoral neck through the growth plate.

RISK FACTORS

- Children 8-16y, **obese, African-Americans, males** during **adolescent growth spurt** (due to weakness of the growth plate & hormonal changes at puberty).
- **If seen in children before puberty, suspect hormonal or systemic disorders** (eg, **hypothyroidism,** hypopituitarism).

CLINICAL MANIFESTATIONS

- Ipsilateral dull, achy **hip, groin thigh or knee pain with a painful limp** worse with activity.
- Physical examination: **externally rotated leg** on the affected side (limited internal rotation abduction, and flexion on ROM of the hip), altered gait.

DIAGNOSIS

- Radiographs: **posterior displacement of femoral epiphysis,** similar to ice cream slipping off a cone. Best seen on frog-leg lateral pelvis or lateral hip view.

MANAGEMENT

- Non-weight bearing with crutches followed by internal fixation with pinning.

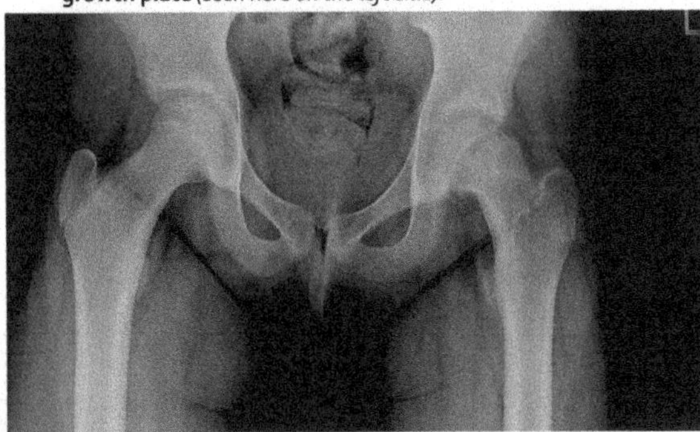

SLIPPED CAPITAL FEMORAL EPIPHYSIS
• Femoral head epiphysis slips POSTERIOR & INFERIOR @ growth plate (seen here on the left side).

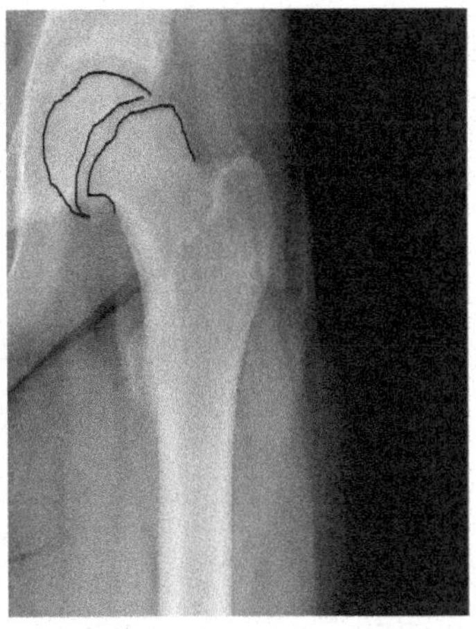

POPLITEAL (BAKER'S) CYST

- Popliteal synovial fluid (effusion) is displaced with subsequent cyst formation.
- Mechanism: degenerative or inflammatory joint disease.

CLINICAL MANIFESTATIONS

- Most are asymptomatic.
- Symptomatic: posterior knee pain and stiffness, mass behind the knee, knee effusion.
- **Ruptured cysts** may present with pseudothrombophlebitis syndrome, **mimicking a DVT (tenderness, warmth and erythema of the calf).**

DIAGNOSIS: Doppler often performed to rule out DVT (also helpful to identify the cyst).

MANAGEMENT

- **Conservative: initial management of choice** (eg, **ice, assisted weight bearing, NSAIDs**).
- Intraarticular corticosteroid injection.
- Surgical excision often reserved for refractory cases.

KNEE INJURIES

MCL (Medial) & LCL (lateral) COLLATERAL LIGAMENT INJURIES

- Medial collateral ligament: resists valgus force on the knee (lateral trauma). MCL injury more common than LCL.
- Lateral collateral ligament: resists varus force on the knee (medial trauma).

CLINICAL MANIFESTATIONS

- Localized knee pain, swelling, ecchymosis, stiffness.
- **LCL:** pain & laxity with **varus stress**.
- **MCL:** pain & laxity with **valgus stress.**

MANAGEMENT

- Grades I (sprains) & II (incomplete tears): **conservative**: pain control, physical therapy to restore range of motion & muscle strength, RICE, NSAIDs, knee immobilizer.
- Grades III (complete tears): may require surgical repair.

ANTERIOR CRUCIATE LIGAMENT (ACL) INJURIES

- **Most common knee ligamental injury** (may be associated with meniscal tears).
- 70% sports-related. More common in female athletes.

MECHANISM

- **Noncontact pivoting injury**, deceleration, changing direction, hyperextension, internal rotation.

CLINICAL MANIFESTATIONS

- Associated with **"pop" & swelling** followed by **hemarthrosis.**
- May develop **knee buckling**, inability to bear weight.

PHYSICAL EXAMINATION

- **Lachman test: most sensitive –** the knee is placed at 15° in supine position. Forward anterior translational movement > 2 mm when the tibia is pulled forward is positive for ACL injury.
- **Pivot shift test** while maintaining internal rotation, valgus force is applied to knee while it is slowly flexed. Positive if the tibia's position on the femur is reduced or there is anterior subluxation with extension.
- **Anterior drawer test:** similar to Lachman but at 90° - least reliable (spasms may stabilize the knee).

DIAGNOSIS

- Radiographs: usually initial test to rule out fracture.
  ±Segond fracture: avulsion of the lateral tibial condyle with varus stress to the knee. If present, ligamental injuries are most likely present. Pathognomonic for ACL tear.
- MRI: best test to assess ACL tears.

MANAGEMENT

- Controversial (depends on activity level of the patient). Therapy vs. surgical.
- Conservative: rest, NSAIDs, ICE, compression, & physical therapy.
- Surgical reconstruction: significant knee instability with desired activities, young active patients <40y, those with high demand jobs or athletes. May be performed with allograft.

Unhappy (O'Donoghue's) triad: injury to ❶ ACL + ❷ medial collateral ligament + ❸ medial meniscus.

POSTERIOR CRUCIATE LIGAMENT (PCL) INJURIES

MECHANISM

- **Most commonly associated with dashboard injuries** (anterior force to proximal tibia with knees flexed), direct blow injury or fall on a flexed knee. Usually associated with other ligamentous injuries.

CLINICAL MANIFESTATIONS

- Posterior knee pain, anterior bruising (especially to the anteromedial aspect of proximal tibia). Large effusion.
- Physical examination: **posterior drawer test** – posterior translational movement of the tibia.

DIAGNOSIS

- MRI

MANAGEMENT

- Conservative: rest, ice, compression and elevation (RICE) therapy, NSAIDs & knee immobilization. May be done if isolated PCL injury.
- Surgical: may indicated if acute injury or if associated with multiple injuries.

MENISCAL TEARS

MECHANISM

- Degenerative or acute. Axial loading & rotation (eg, squatting, twisting, compression or trauma with femur rotation on the tibia).
- **Medial 3 times more common** than lateral.

CLINICAL MANIFESTATIONS

- **Popping, "giving way"** during ambulation or climbing or descending stairs, **effusion after activities.**
- **Locking** (inability to fully extend the knee).

PHYSICAL EXAMINATION

- **Positive McMurray sign:** pop or click when the knee is flexed and then externally rotated and extended.
- Apley test, joint line tenderness, **joint effusion, & swelling.**

DIAGNOSIS

- MRI

MANAGEMENT

- Conservative: ice, NSAIDs, orthopedic follow up, physical therapy.
- Surgical: arthroscopic repair or partial meniscectomy. Severe symptoms, persistent symptoms despite conservative management.

PATELLAR FRACTURE

- Mechanism: **direct blow most common** (eg, fall on a flexed knee, forceful quadriceps contraction).
- Most common in young patients.

CLINICAL MANIFESTATIONS
- Pain, swelling, deformity. Limited knee extension with pain.

DIAGNOSIS
- Radiographs: **sunrise** & cross table lateral views allow better visualization of the patella.

MANAGEMENT
- Nondisplaced: knee immobilizer, leg cast.
- Displaced: surgery.

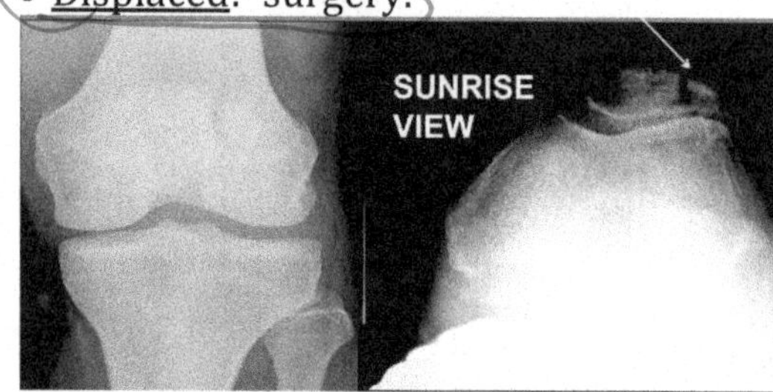

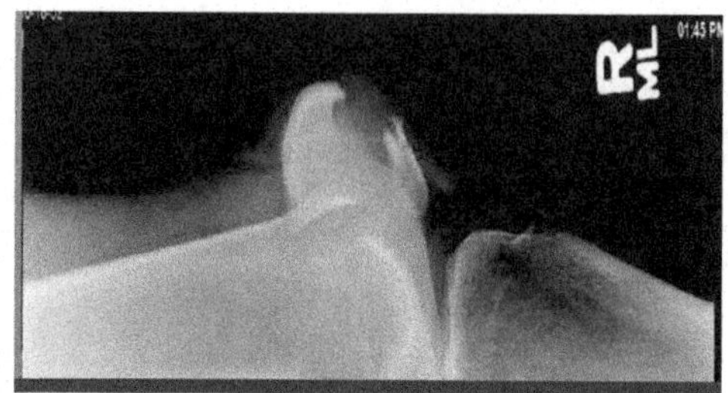

OSGOOD-SCHLATTER DISEASE

- Apophysitis of the tibial tuberosity (inflammation of the patellar tendon at the insertion of the tibial tubercle) due to **overuse** (repetitive stress microtrauma) or small avulsions from **repetitive knee extension & quadriceps contraction**.
- The apophysis is a muscle-tendon-bone attachment that is subject to injury from repetitive stress or an acute avulsion injury.

RISK FACTORS
- **Most common in males, 10-15 years, during growth spurts, athletes.**

CLINICAL MANIFESTATIONS
- **Activity-related anterior knee pain & swelling** (eg, running, jumping, kneeling) & relieved with rest.
- Prominence, **swelling & tenderness to the anterior tibial tubercle**.

DIAGNOSIS
- Imaging usually not necessary in classic presentations.
- Radiographs: elevation, heterotopic ossification, and/or bone fragmentation of the tibial tuberosity.

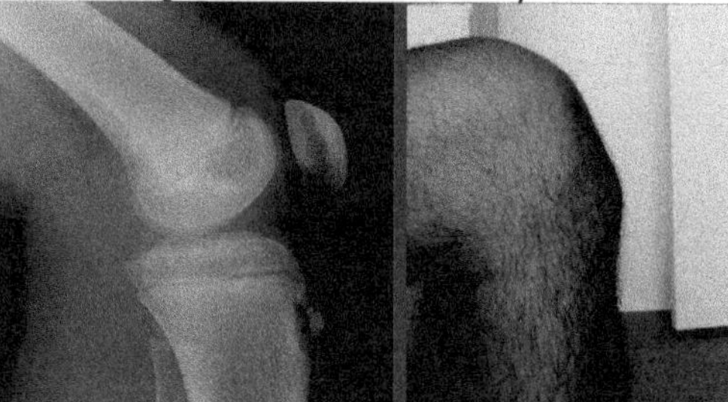

MANAGEMENT
- **Conservative: mainstay of treatment** - RICE (rest ice, elevation), NSAIDs, quadriceps stretching. Knee immobilization. Most symptoms resolve within 12 – 24 months.
- Surgery only in refractory cases (if done, usually performed after growth plate has closed).

PATELLAR & QUADRICEPS TENDON RUPTURES

MECHANISM
- **Forceful quadriceps contraction** (eg, fall on a flexed knee, walking up/down stairs).
- Quads > patellar. Quads rupture usually >40y; Patellar rupture usually <40y.

RISK FACTORS
- **Males >40y,** history of **systemic disease** (eg, DM, Gout, obesity, renal disease).

CLINICAL MANIFESTATIONS
- Sharp proximal knee pain with ambulation, **inability to extend knee & perform straight leg raise.**
- **Quadriceps tendon rupture:** palpable **defect above** the knee.
- **Patellar tendon rupture:** palpable **defect below** the knee.

DIAGNOSIS
- **Quadriceps tendon rupture: patella baja** (low-riding patella).
- **Patellar tendon rupture: patella alta** (high-riding patella).

MANAGEMENT
- Knee immobilizer, non or partial weight bearing, RICE.
- **Surgical repair** usually performed within 7-10 days.

NORMAL KNEE
Lateral View

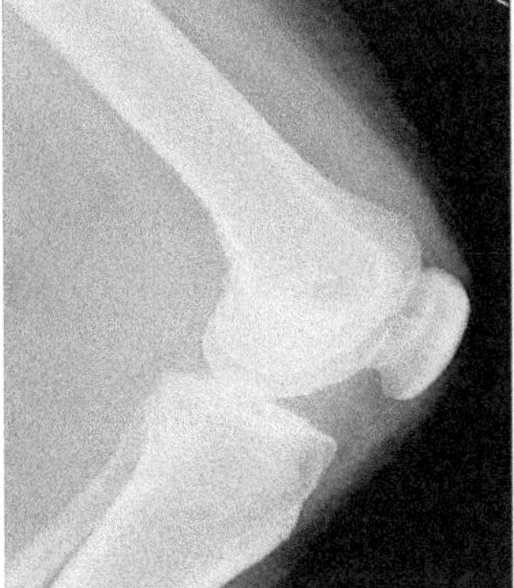

PATELLAR TENDON RUPTURE
"Patella Alta" Lateral View

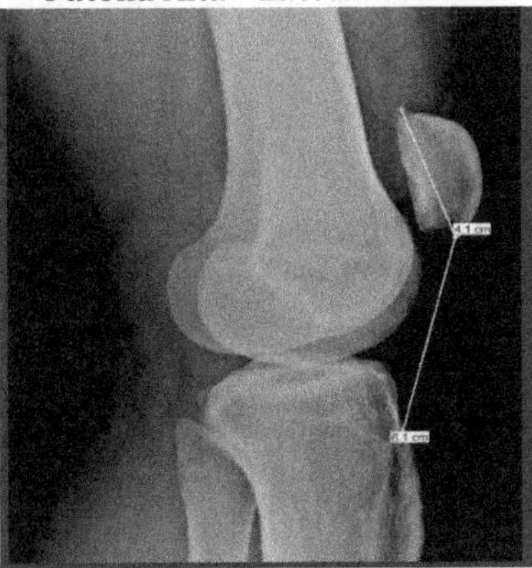

QUADRICEPS TENDON RUPTURE
"Patella Baja" - Lateral View

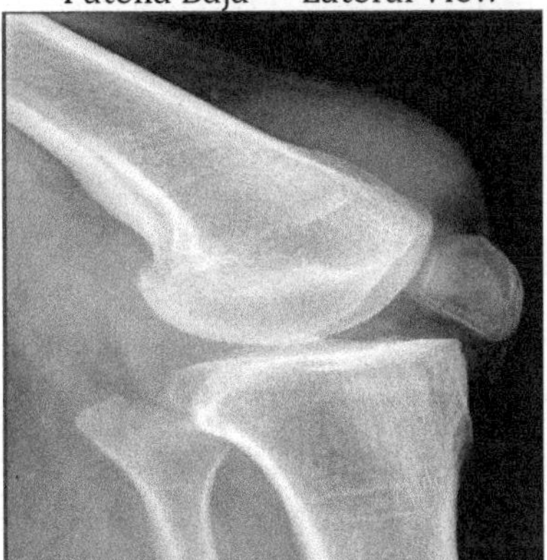

PATELLAR DISLOCATION

- MECHANISM: **valgus stress** after twisting injury, direct blow.
- **Lateral most common.**
- **Most common in females.**

DIAGNOSIS
- **Apprehension sign:** patient exhibits anxiety/forcefully contracts the quadriceps when the examiner pushes laterally. Only performed if patellar is already reduced. Radiographs.

MANAGEMENT
- **Closed reduction -** push anteromedially on the patella while gently extending the leg.
- Post reduction films. Knee immobilizer (full extension), quads strengthening.

KNEE (Tibial-femoral) DISLOCATIONS

- **Severe limb-threatening emergency.** Anterior most common, posterior (highest incidence of popliteal artery injury), lateral, rotational, medial.
- Mechanism: high velocity trauma, often associated with multiple trauma.
- Gross deformity. 50% spontaneously reduce before arriving to ER (so believe patients).

MANAGEMENT

- **Immediate orthopedic consult for prompt reduction** via longitudinal traction with vascular status check. If intact, place a splint. Most cases will need emergent surgical intervention.

COMPLICATIONS

- Vascular: **popliteal artery injury in 1/3 of patients – must perform arteriography or arterial duplex if pulses are diminished or absent**. Normal pulses do not rule out arterial injury. If pulses are normal, an ankle brachial index can be performed. If ABI > 0.9, serial examinations can be performed. If < 0.9, perform arteriography or arterial duplex.
- Neurological: peroneal or tibial nerve injuries (**peroneal injury most common**).

FEMORAL CONDYLE FRACTURES

MECHANISM

- **Axial loading** (fall from height); direct blow to the femur.

CLINICAL MANIFESTATIONS: pain, swelling, inability to bear weight.

COMPLICATIONS

- **Peroneal nerve injuries: foot drop** or decreased sensation to the posterior first web space of foot.
- **Popliteal artery injury.**

MANAGEMENT: **immediate orthopedic consult.** ORIF. Usually heals poorly.

TIBIAL PLATEAU FRACTURES

- Mechanism: axial loading, rotation, direct trauma (most commonly seen in children in MVAs).
- Location: **lateral plateau most common** > bicondylar > medial.

CLINICAL MANIFESTATIONS

- Pain, swelling, hemarthrosis. If displaced, **check for peroneal nerve injury (foot drop).**

DIAGNOSIS

- Radiographs: may be hard to see. CT scan: for further definition & pre-surgical planning.

MANAGEMENT

- Conservative: non-weight bearing initially with hinged knee brace + partial weight bearing & passive ROM + orthopedic follow up may be used if nondisplaced.
- Surgical: if displaced or severe.

COMPLICATIONS

- **Often associated with soft tissue injuries** - meniscal & ligamental tears **(lateral meniscal tears most common)**, compartment syndrome.
- Post degenerative arthritis (>50%), loss of joint congruity.

PATELLOFEMORAL SYDNROME (CHONDROMALACIA)

- Idiopathic softening or fissuring of the patellar articular cartilage from overuse.

RISK FACTORS

- **Most commonly in seen in runners or cyclists,** women.

CLINICAL MANIFESTATIONS

- **Anterior knee pain behind or around the patella** worsened with knee hyperflexion (eg, prolonged sitting, jumping or climbing).

- Physical examination: compression of the patella during knee extension will produce symptoms or a **positive apprehension sign** (anticipated pain).

MANAGEMENT

- **NSAIDs, rest, & rehabilitation initial management** of choice (strengthening the vastus medialis obliquus of the quadriceps, weight loss).

- Elastic knee sleeve for patellar stabilization.

ILIOTIBIAL BAND (ITB) SYNDROME

- Inflammation of the iliotibial band bursa due to lack of flexibility of the ITB bursa.
- Pathophysiology: excessive friction between the iliotibial band & the femoral condyle.

RISK FACTORS

- **Runners & cyclists.**

CLINICAL MANIFESTATIONS

- **Lateral knee pain** (especially where the ITB courses over the lateral femoral epicondyle). The pain is classically sharp or burning & **worse with changes in terrain** (eg, **climbing stairs or running downhill**), usually relieved with rest.

PHYSICAL EXAMINATION

- Positive **tenderness over the lateral condyle.** Pain reproduced with single leg squat.

- **Positive Noble compression test**: positive if pain over the distal ITB especially at 30 degrees of knee flexion with pressure applied to the ITB.

- **Positive Ober test:** pain or resistance to adduction of the leg parallel to the table in neutral position. Also tests the tensor fascia lata.

MANAGEMENT

- **Conservative: initial management** of choice (eg, NSAIDs, ice, avoid overuse, physical therapy, stretching of the iliotibial band).

- Corticosteroid injections.

- Surgical intervention may be indicated in refractory cases.

ANKLE & FOOT INJURIES

ANKLE SPRAINS

- **Lateral:** 85% of ankle sprains involve the lateral ligament complex: **Anterior talofibular (ATFL) most common,** Calcaneofibular (CFL) Posterior talofibular ligaments. **ATFL is the main stabilizer during inversion.**
- **Medial:** deltoid ligament sprains are usually due to eversion injuries. Talar tilt test

CLINICAL MANIFESTATIONS
- Patient may have felt a "pop" followed by swelling, pain, inability to bear weight. May be ecchymotic.

DIAGNOSIS
- Anterior drawer test can be performed to assess ATFL integrity.
- Talar tilt test assesses CFL stability.

OTTAWA ANKLE RULES	
ANKLE FILMS	**FOOT FILMS**
Pain along the **lateral malleolus**	**navicular** (midfoot) **pain**
Pain along the **medial malleolus**	**5th metatarsal pain**
Inability to walk >4 steps at the time of injury & in the ER.	

MANAGEMENT
- **Conservative: RICE** (rest, ice, compression & elevation); **NSAIDs,** crutches for the first 2-3 days. ACE wrap of brace for support.

ACHILLES TENDON RUPTURE

- Mechanism: mechanical overload from eccentric contraction of gastrocsoleus complex.

RISK FACTORS
- 75% occur as a sports-related injury, episodic athletes "weekend warrior".
- **Increased risk with Fluoroquinolone use,** corticosteroid injections. Common 30-50y.

CLINICAL MANIFESTATIONS
- **Sudden heel pain after push-off movement, "pop", sudden, sharp calf pain.**
- Inability to weight bear.
- **Positive Thompson test:** positive if **weak, absent plantar flexion** when the gastrocnemius is squeezed.

DIAGNOSIS
- Radiographs: usually initial test ordered to rule out ankle fracture or other causes of pain.
- **MRI best test.**

MANAGEMENT
- Nonoperative: splint initially in mild plantar flexion (resting equinus) with subsequent splinting employing gradual dorsiflexion towards neutral.

- Surgical repair allows for early range of motion.

WEBER ANKLE FRACTURE CLASSIFICATION

Way to classify ankle fractures on the basis of the lateral malleolus (fibular bone).

NORMAL

LEVEL OF FIBULAR FRACTURE RELATIVE TO THE SYNDESMOSIS

A- BELOW THE SYNDESMOSIS

B- LEVEL OF SYNDESMOSIS

C- ABOVE LEVEL OF SYNDESMOSIS

WEBER A

- **Fibular fx BELOW syndesmosis**
- **Tibiofibular syndesmosis intact**
- **Deltoid ligament intact**
- **Usually stable**
- ± medial malleolar fracture

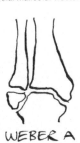

WEBER A

WEBER B

- **Fibular fx AT LEVEL of syndesmosis**
- Tibiofibular syndesmosis intact or mild tear (talofibular joint not widened).
- Deltoid ligament intact or may be torn
- Can be Stable or Unstable

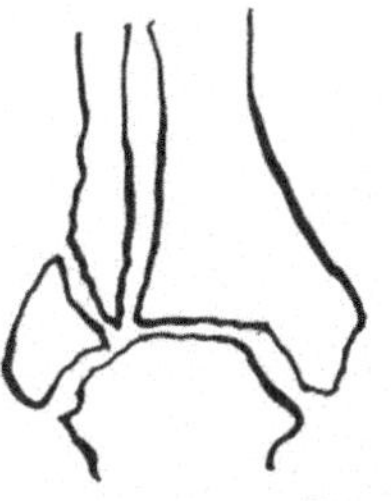

WEBER B

WEBER C

- **Fibular fx ABOVE Mortise**
- Tibiofibular syndesmosis torn widening of talofibular joint
- **Deltoid ligament damage or**
- **Medial malleolar fx**
- **Unstable – requires ORIF**

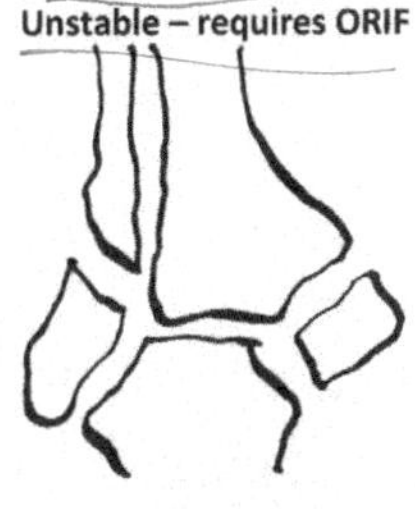

WEBER C

MAISONNEUVE FRACTURE

- **Spiral fracture of the proximal third of the fibula associated with a distal medial malleolar fracture or rupture of the deep deltoid ligament.**
- The proximal fibular fracture is a result of tearing of the distal talofibular syndesmosis and the interosseous membrane.
- Anyone with a distal ankle fracture should have proximal films performed to rule out Maisonneuve fracture.

MAISONNEUVE FRACTURE

PROXIMAL

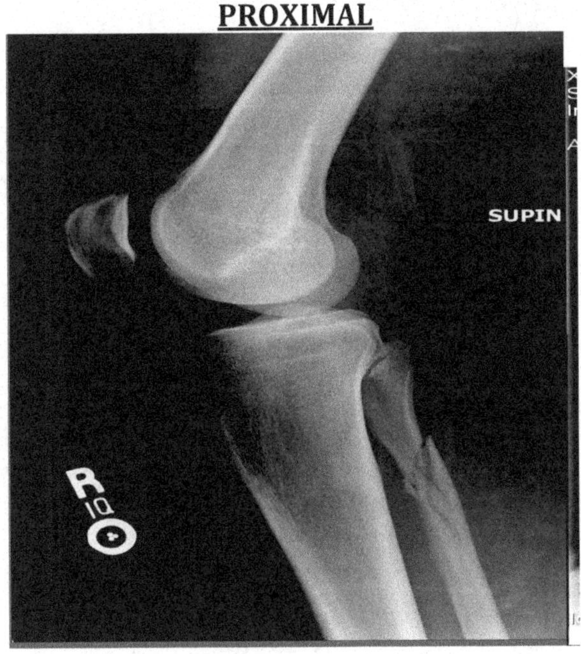

DISTAL

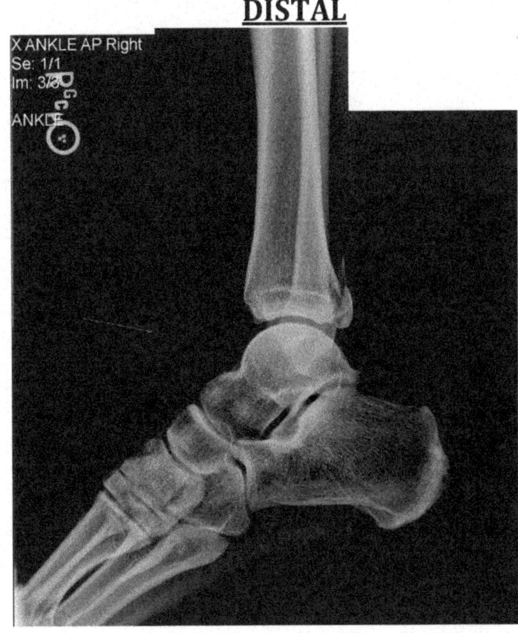

PILON (TIBIAL PLAFOND) FRACTURE

- Fracture of the distal tibia from impact with the talus (axial load), interrupting the ankle joint space eg, high-impact trauma. The fracture extends into the ankle joint.

CLINICAL MANIFESTATIONS

- Severe pain, swelling, deformity.

MANAGEMENT

- ORIF (open reduction internal fixation).

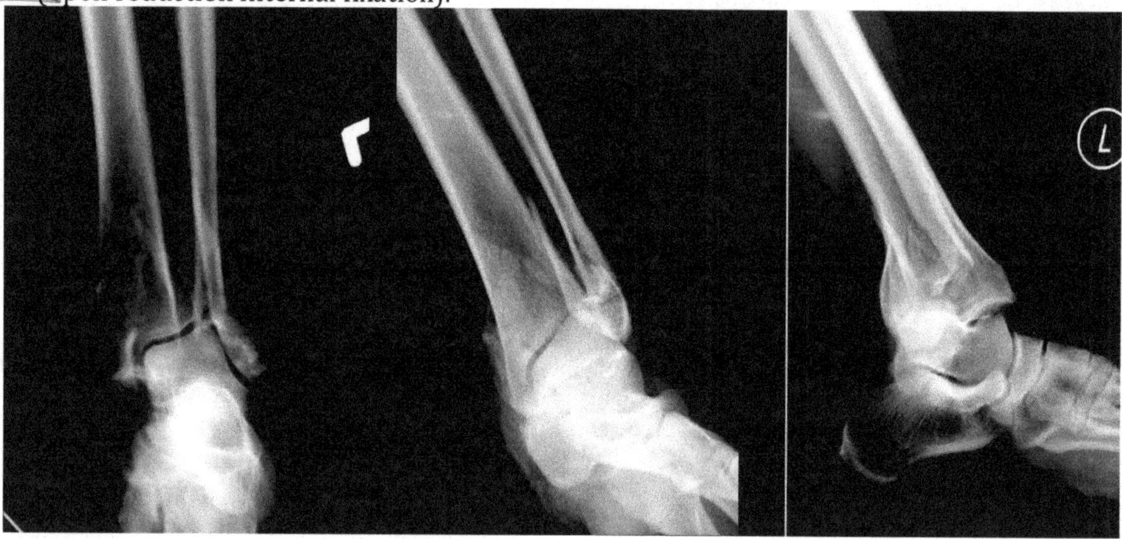

STRESS (MARCH) FRACTURE

- **Fracture due to overuse or high-impact activities** (eg, **athletes, military personnel**). Females at increased risk.
- Most common bones involved are the metatarsals **(third metatarsal most common)**, tibia, fibula, navicular bones.

CLINICAL MANIFESTATIONS

- Insidious onset of **localized aching pain, swelling & tenderness that increases with activity**. **Localized bone tenderness** at the fracture site.

- May develop pain with weight bearing as it progresses.

DIAGNOSIS

- Radiographs: 50% of radiographs will be negative initially (especially in the first 2 weeks) so it is mainly a clinical diagnosis. The radiographs may be positive with healing of the fracture (callous).

- MRI or bone scan usually only performed if radiographs are negative in high-risk areas (eg, proximal fourth or fifth metatarsal, navicular, talus or patella) or if symptoms persist.

MANAGEMENT

- **Conservative** - rest, avoidance of high-impact activities, ice, splint or post-op shoe, analgesia.

- Orthopedic surgery may be needed for high-risk fractures (eg, fifth metatarsal).

PLANTAR FASCIITIS

- Mechanism: inflammation & microscopic tears of the plantar fascia due to overuse (especially in patients with flat feet, high arches or heel spurs).
- Most common in females, 40-60y, older, & obese patients.

CLINICAL MANIFESTATIONS

- **Inferior heel pain** (often sharp), **usually worse after period of rest** (eg, **first few steps in the morning**). Pain usually decreases throughout the day with gradual increased activity, walking, massage, stretching, and rest. May worsen towards the end of the day after prolonged weight bearing with a return of the pain at night.

PHYSICAL EXAM

- **Local point tenderness** to the underside of the heel.
- **Pain increases with dorsiflexion of toes** (stretching of the plantar fascia).

DIAGNOSIS

- **Mainly a clinical diagnosis.**
- Radiographs not useful for the diagnosis. May show a flat foot deformity or a heel spur.

MANAGEMENT

- **Conservative:** rest, ice, NSAIDs, heel/arch support (orthotics), physical therapy (plantar stretching exercises).
- Corticosteroid injections (reserved for pain refractory to NSAIDs).
- Surgery in severe cases or refractory to conservative and corticosteroid injections.

TARSAL TUNNEL SYNDROME

MECHANISM

- **Posterior tibial nerve compression** as it travels through the tarsal tunnel. Compression may be a result of overuse, restrictive footwear or edematous states.

CLINICAL MANIFESTATIONS

- **Compression symptoms:** alternating **pain & numbness at the medial malleolus, heel, & sole.** Classically, the **pain increases throughout the day,** is worse at night, with dorsiflexion and **pain does not improve with rest**.

- **Positive Tinel sign:** tapping at the tarsal tunnel (posterior medial malleolus) reproduces symptoms.

DIAGNOSIS

- Clinical + Tinel sign at the tarsal tunnel.

- Electromyography: confirms the diagnosis.

MANAGEMENT

- **Conservative initial therapy of choice -** rest, NSAIDs, properly fitted shoes, & orthotics.

- Corticosteroids if refractory to initial treatment.

- Surgical: tunnel release in severe cases.

BUNION (HALLUX VALGUS)

- Hallux valgus deformity at the **first metatarsophalangeal joint** with **lateral deviation** of the proximal phalanx.
- **History of wearing poorly-fitted, tight or pointed shoes most common**, pes planus (flat feet), rheumatoid arthritis, women.

CLINICAL MANIFESTATIONS
- Pain over the great toe at the MTP joint with a lateral deformity.

MANAGEMENT
- **Conservative:** comfortable, wide-toed shoes.
- Surgical if no response to conservative treatment.

HAMMER TOE

- Deformity of PIP joint: **flexion of PIP joint & hyperextension of MTP & DIP joint.**
- Seen if 2nd, 3rd or 4th toe is longer than the first, people who wear tight fitting shoes, OA, RA.
- Clinical manifestations: **PIP pain** (due to contact with shoe). PIP deformity.

NEUROPATHIC (CHARCOT) ARTHROPATHY

MECHANISM
- **Joint damage & destruction as a result of peripheral neuropathy** from Diabetes mellitus, peripheral vascular disease, or other diseases.

PATHOPHYSIOLOGY
- Decreased sensation, autonomic dysfunction & repetitive microtrauma leads to bone resorption & weakening.
- Most commonly affects the midfoot & ankle. Neuropathic arthritis of the knee can be seen with Diabetes mellitus & tabes dorsalis (a form of tertiary Syphilis).

CLINICAL MANIFESTATIONS
- Acute: nontender, swollen, warm & erythematous joint.
- Chronic: **joint or foot deformity, alteration of the shape of the foot, ulcer or skin changes.**

DIAGNOSIS
- Radiographs: **obliteration of the joint space**, fragmentation of bone, increased bone density & **disorganization of the joint**.
- MRI or bone scintigraphy followed by indium scintigraphy may be needed in some cases to rule out Osteomyelitis.
- Labs: usually associated with normal WBC & inflammatory markers but may have an elevated ESR.

MANAGEMENT
- Conservative: rest, non-weight bearing. Accommodative footwear.
- Surgical rarely performed. May be indicated if severe deformity.

INTERDIGITAL (MORTON'S) NEUROMA

- **Compressive neuropathy of the interdigital nerve.**
- Most commonly involves the second or third interdigital nerve between the metatarsal heads.

MECHANISM

- Repetitive microtrauma leading to degeneration & proliferation of the interdigital nerve.

RISK FACTORS

- Most common in women 25-50y especially if they wear **tight-fitting shoes, high heels** (overpronation) or have **flat feet.**

CLINICAL MANIFESTATIONS

- **Lancinating or burning pain** especially with weight bearing. **Most common in the third intermetatarsal space (between third & fourth metatarsals).** Reproducible pain on palpation or squeezing the foot.
- May be associated with **numbness or paresthesia** of the toes or plantar aspect of the web space.

PHYSICAL EXAMINATION

- May have a palpable, painful mass near the tarsal heads.
- Mulder's sign: clicking sensation when palpating the involved interspace while simultaneously squeezing the metatarsal joints.

DIAGNOSIS

- Clinical diagnosis.
- Ultrasound is an inexpensive method for neuroma detection. MRI

MANAGEMENT

- **Conservative:** metatarsal support or pad, broad-toed shoes with firm soles are first line.
- Glucocorticoid injection may be used if refractory to initial management.
- Surgical resection: if failed conservative management. Complications of resection include permanent numbness or residual stump.

JONES FRACTURE

- **Transverse fracture through the diaphysis of the fifth metatarsal** at the **metaphyseal – diaphyseal junction**.

MECHANISM

- May occur with ankle sprains or when then heel is off the ground while the forefoot is planted.
- Complications: 15-50% **risk of nonunion or malunion** because it involves the vascular watershed area.

CLINICAL MANIFESTATIONS

- **Pain over the fifth metatarsal area** and lateral border of the midfoot especially with weight bearing.

DIAGNOSIS:

- Radiographs: transverse fracture involving the metaphyseal-diaphyseal junction.

MANAGEMENT

- **Non weight-bearing in short leg cast** x 6-8 weeks, followed by repeat radiographs as it is often complicated by nonunion or malunion.
- Frequently requires ORIF/pinning.

PSEUDOJONES FRACTURE

- Fracture through the **base (tuberosity) of the fifth metatarsal** due to plantar flexion with inversion.
- Much more common and less serious than a true Jones fracture.

MANAGEMENT

- **Walking cast** x 2-3 weeks; ORIF if displaced.

JONES FRACTURE

- JONES: Transverse fx through *DIAPHYSIS of* 5th *metatarsal*
- PSEUDO JONES: Transverse avulsion fx @ base (tuberosity) of 5th metatarsal

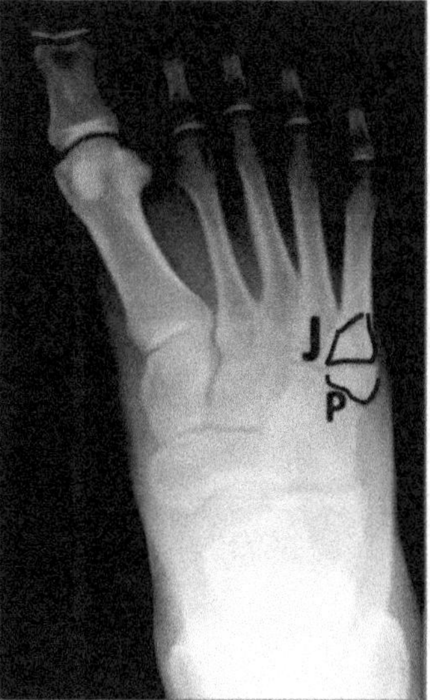

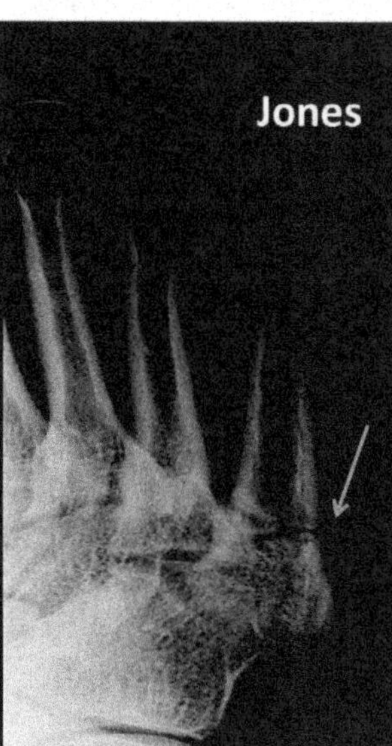

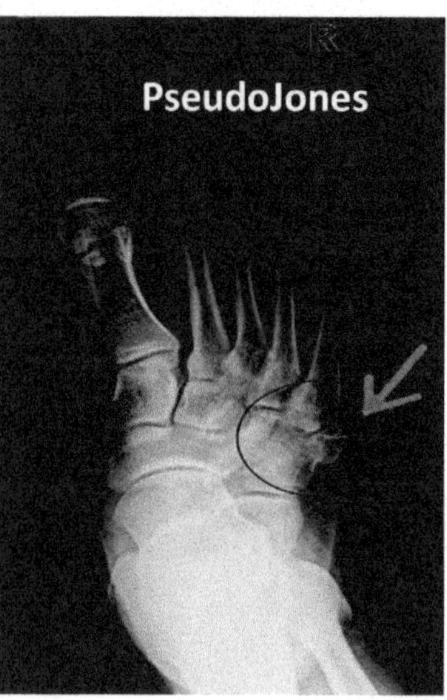

LISFRANC INJURY

- Lisfranc joint: bases of the first 3 metatarsal heads & their respective cuneiforms.
- Lisfranc Injury: injury where **one or more of the metatarsal bones are displaced from the tarsus.**

PATHOPHYSIOLOGY
- Disruption between the articulation of the medial cuneiform & the base of the second metatarsal, leading to ligamentous injury (dislocation) and or fracture **(tarsometatarsal fracture-dislocation)**.
- Mechanism: varied but includes rotational (midfoot) & severe axial load.

CLINICAL MANIFESTATIONS
- Severe pain, inability to bear weight.
- Physical exam: swelling, bruising, tenderness over the tarsometatarsal joint, instability (dorsal subluxation with dorsal force to the forefoot).

RADIOGRAPHS
- Most common variant is one metatarsal away from the other ones.
- **Fleck sign - fracture at the base of the second metatarsal pathognomonic** for disruption of the tarsometatarsal ligaments. May be associated with multiple fractures of the metatarsals.

MANAGEMENT
- **ORIF** (open reduction internal fixation) followed by non-weight bearing cast for 12 weeks.

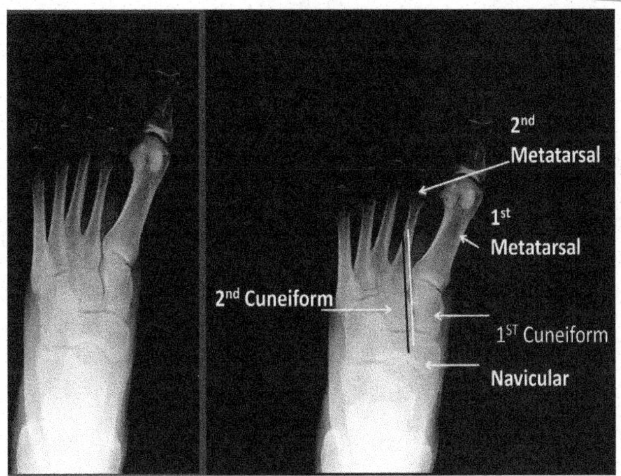

Normal radiographs

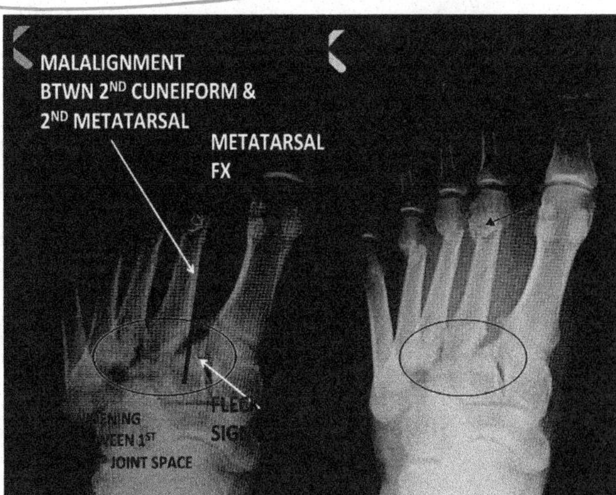

LISFRANC INJURY

\

PEDIATRIC FRACTURES

GREENSTICK FRACTURES

- Incomplete fracture with cortical disruption & periosteal tearing on the convex side of the fracture (intact periosteum on the concave side) **"bowing"**.

TORUS (BUCKLE) FRACTURES

- Incomplete fracture with **"wrinkling or bump"** of the metaphyseal-diaphyseal junction (where the dense bone meets the more porous bone) due to axial loading.

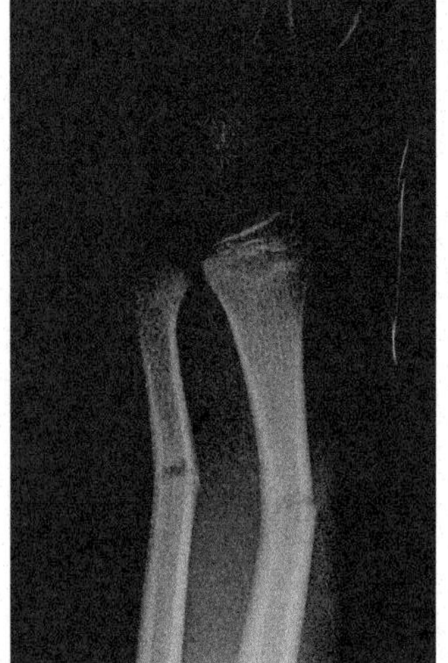

GREENSTICK FRACTURE

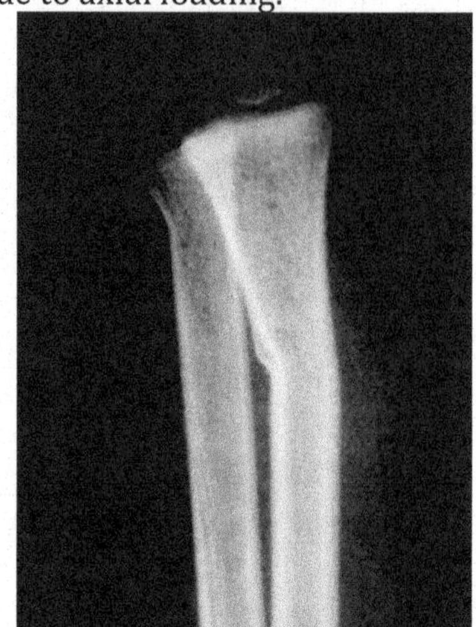

TORUS (BUCKLE) FRACTURE

SALTER- HARRIS CLASSIFICATION OF FRACTURES

- ***Growth (Epiphyseal) Plate Fractures. "SALTR"*** **useful mnemonic IN RELATION TO PLATE**

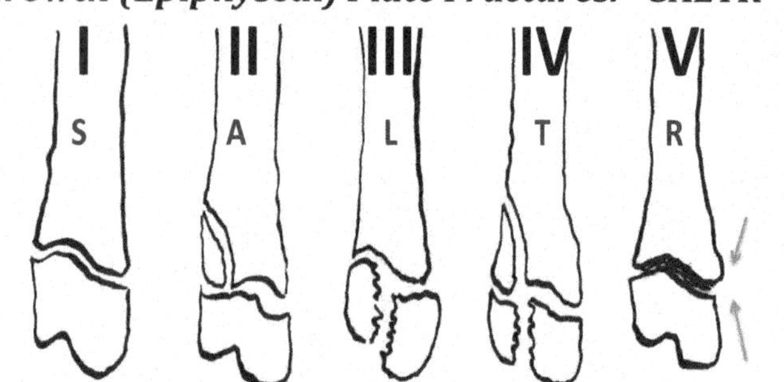

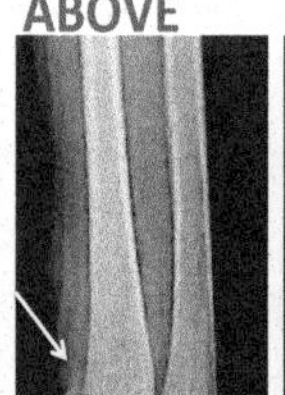

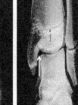

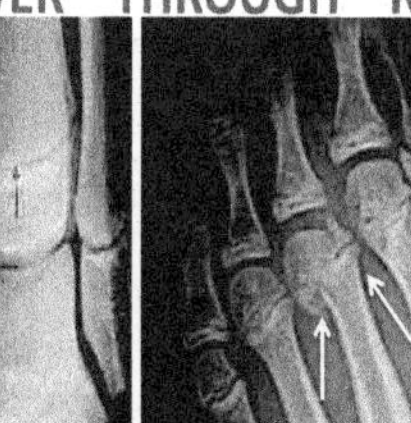

Type I: isolated growth plate fracture (may look normal). Best outcome.

Type II: growth plate fracture + **fracture of the metaphysis (good prognosis). MC of all Salter-Harris Fractures.**

Type III: growth plate fracture + **fracture of the epiphysis.** (good prognosis).

Type IV: fracture **extending across the metaphysis, growth plate & epiphysis (needs reduction).**

Type V: **Growth plate compression injury** (may arrest growth). **Worst type!**

MALIGNANT BONE TUMORS

OSTEOSARCOMA – Peds

- Malignant tumor of osteoblastic proliferation.
- **Most common primary bone malignancy in children and young adults.**
- 90% occur in the metaphysis of the long bones **(distal femur most common)**, proximal tibia, & proximal humerus. **Most common METS to the lungs** (most common cause of death).

BIMODAL
- **Most common in adolescents** (80% occur <20y).
- Second peak 50-60y especially if history of Paget disease of the bone or radiation therapy.

CLINICAL MANIFESTATIONS
- Localized **bone pain** (may occur after injury) and can be **worse at night.**
- Joint swelling without systemic symptoms.
- Physical exam: palpable soft tissue mass (may be tender to palpation).

DIAGNOSIS
- Radiographs: **"hair on end"** or **"sunburst" appearance** due to tumor spicules of calcified bone radiating in right angles is classic (not specific). Other findings: mixed sclerotic & lytic lesions. Codman's triangle: ossification of raised periosteum (can also be seen in Ewing sarcoma). MRI.
- **Biopsy: definitive diagnosis** - malignant osteoid within the tumor & malignant sarcomatous stroma.

MANAGEMENT
- Chemotherapy + surgical removal, with amputation (if neovascular) or limb-sparing resection (if not neovascular).

Hair On End

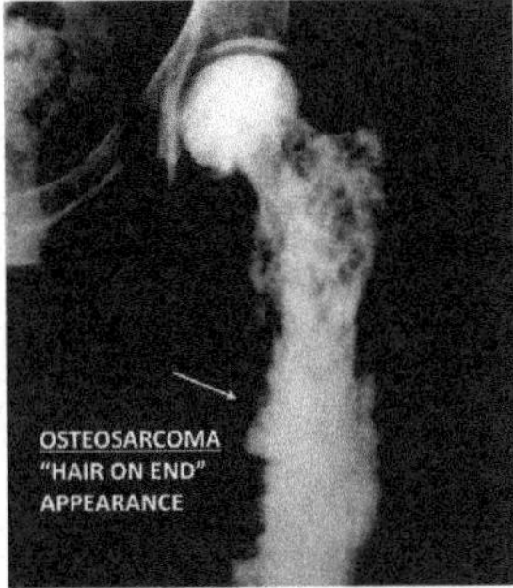

Codman's Triangle

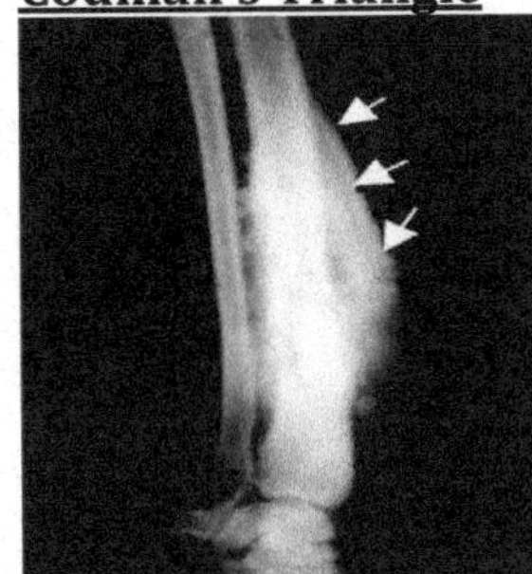

CHONDROSARCOMA – Adults

- **Cancer of the cartilage.** Most commonly seen in adults 40-75y.
- Location: proximal femur, pelvic bones and proximal humerus most common sites.
- CLINICAL MANIFESTATIONS: localized pain and swelling. Pathologic fractures.

DIAGNOSIS
- Radiographs: mineralized chondroid matrix with **punctate or ring & arc appearance** calcification.
- CT or MRI provide more details. Histology: increased malignant cartilage matrix production.

MANAGEMENT
- Surgical resection: nonmetastatic Chondrosarcoma.
- Chemotherapy may be used in select cases of advanced disease.

EWING SARCOMA

- **Second most common primary bone malignancy in children and young adults (after Osteosarcoma).**
- Due to translocation between chromosomes 11 & 22
- Most common in Caucasian males 5-25y.
- Bone, bone marrow, & lung are common sites for metastasis. Lung METS is a common cause of death.

Location:

- 50% found in the diaphysis of the long bones - **Femur most common; pelvis,** tibia, fibula, & pelvis are common sites.

CLINICAL MANIFESTATIONS

- Localized bone pain & swelling that may be accompanied by systemic symptoms (eg, fever, malaise, weight loss).
- Physical exam: may have a palpable mass, local tenderness, or joint swelling.

DIAGNOSIS

- Radiographs: layered **periosteal reaction "onion skin"** appearance, lytic lesions with a **"moth-eaten" appearance**.
  Codman's triangle: ossification of raised periosteum (can also be seen in Osteosarcoma).
- Labs: increased ESR, leukocytosis.
- Histology: sheets of monotonous small round blue cells. May have pseudo-rosettes (circle of cells with central necrosis).

MANAGEMENT

- Chemotherapy followed by limb-sparing resection when possible.
- Radiation therapy when complete excision is not possible.

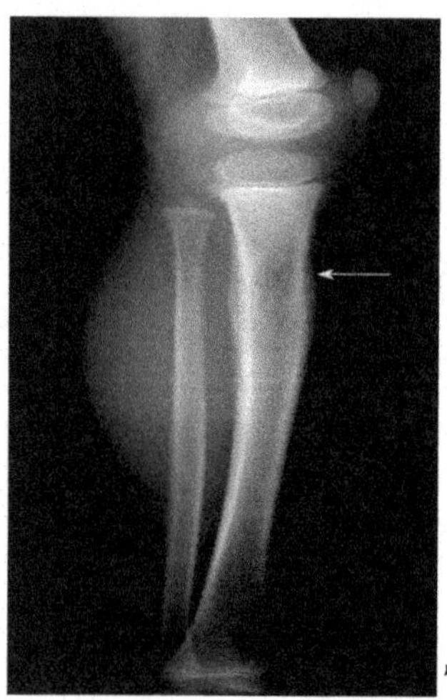

"Onion" peel appearance (periosteal reaction)

BENIGN BONE TUMORS

OSTEOCHONDROMA

- Cartilage-capped bony overgrowth arising on the external surface of a bone & areas of tendon insertion (eg, proximal tibia, femur, & proximal humerus).
- **Most common benign bone tumor.** 10% may become chondrosarcomas.
- Most commonly seen in between **10-20 years of age & in males.**
- Begins in childhood & grows until skeletal maturity.

CLINICAL MANIFESTATIONS
- Painless, palpable mass. May develop symptoms of neurovascular compression.

DIAGNOSIS
- Radiographs: often **pedunculated** (narrow stalk) that **grows away from the growth plate** & involves the medullary tissue. Biopsy: definitive.

MANAGEMENT
- Observation if asymptomatic.
- Marginal resection including cartilage cap if it becomes painful or if located in the pelvis (pelvis most common site of malignant transformation). Usually delayed until skeletal maturity.

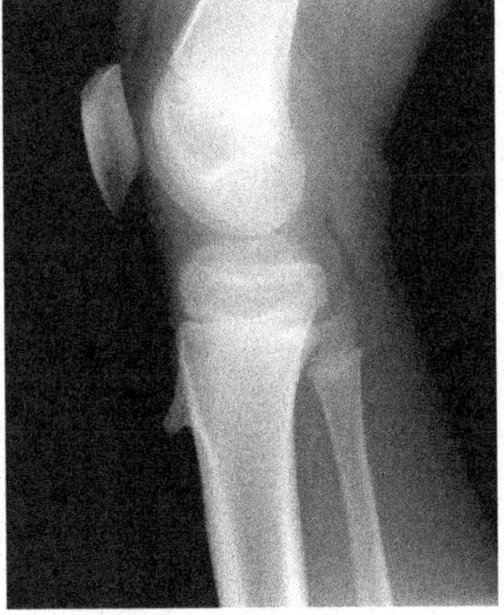

OSTEOID OSTEOMA

- **Benign bone tumor characterized by a small radiolucent nidus** (usually < 1 to 1.5 cm in diameter).
- Most commonly presents in the second decade. More common in males.
- Locations: proximal femur most common, tibia, the remainder of the femur, and spine.
- Pathophysiology: the nidus **produces high levels of prostaglandins.**

CLINICAL MANIFESTATIONS
- Progressively increasing pain that is worse at night and unrelated to activity. **The pain in relieved within 20-25 minutes of administration of NSAIDs** (prostaglandin inhibition).
- May develop a limp, localized tenderness, and limitation of range of motion.

DIAGNOSIS
- Radiographs: small round lucency (nidus) with a sclerotic margin. CT or MRI more sensitive.

MANAGEMENT
- NSAIDs with serial examinations or radiographs every 6 months. Untreated osteoid osteoma often spontaneously resolve over several years.
- Surgical resection for symptomatic lesions not responsive to conservative treatment.

RHEUMATOLOGIC DISORDERS

FIBROMYALGIA → TCAs (Amitriptyline)

- A disorder characterized by abnormal pain perception of unknown etiology.
- Most common in **women** 20-55y.

CLINICAL MANIFESTATIONS

- **Chronic, widespread musculoskeletal pain, extreme fatigue,** stiffness; Sleep & cognitive disturbances (fibro fog), headache, neurologic symptoms (eg, numbness).

DIAGNOSIS

- Primarily a clinical diagnosis. Associated with normal laboratory tests.
- **Tenderness in at least 11 out of 18 trigger points** + chronic pain > 3 months.
- Sleep studies show no REM cycle.

MANAGEMENT

- **Conservative measures:** initial treatment involves a multidisciplinary approach: patient education, sleep hygiene, **low-impact aerobic exercise** (eg, **swimming & water aerobics,** walking, & biking).
- Medical: **Tricyclic antidepressants (Amitriptyline) first-line medical agent in patients not responsive to conservative measures**. SSNRI: Duloxetine, Milnacipran. Cyclobenzaprine an alternative if mild to moderate symptoms.
- **Pregabalin** is FDA approved for Fibromyalgia (especially helpful for sleep symptoms).

POLYMYALGIA RHEUMATICA

- Idiopathic **inflammation of the joints, bursae, and tendons**.
- **Closely associated with Giant cell arteritis.**
- Most common **>50y,** women.

CLINICAL MANIFESTATIONS

- **Pain & stiffness in the proximal joints and muscles** - shoulder, neck, hips and pelvic girdle (worse in the morning) > 2 weeks. May have difficulty combing hair & rising from a chair.
- Constitutional symptoms: low-grade fever, fatigue, weight loss

PHYSICAL EXAMINATION

- **Normal muscle strength** (no muscle inflammation or objective weakness).
- May have decreased active and passive ROM.

DIAGNOSIS

- **Increased ESR & CRP.** Normocytic normochromic anemia.
- Normal muscle enzymes (creatine kinase & aldolase) distinguishes PMR from Polymyositis.

MANAGEMENT

- **Low-dose corticosteroids** initial treatment of choice (associated with rapid response).
- Methotrexate an option if no response to corticosteroids or if corticosteroids are contraindicated.

RHABDOMYOLYSIS

- Acute breakdown & necrosis of skeletal muscle.

ETIOLOGIES
- Trauma, strenuous activity, prolonged immobility, crush injuries, seizures, cocaine, **statin therapy**, viral infections, snake bites.

PATHOPHYSIOLOGY
- Myoglobin from muscle breakdown is extremely toxic to the renal tubular cells, leading to **Acute tubular necrosis** (acute kidney injury).

CLINICAL MANIFESTATIONS
- Classic triad: **muscle pain + muscle weakness** or swelling + **dark (tea-colored) urine** (myoglobinuria).

DIAGNOSTIC WORKUP
- **ECG: most important initial test** to look for signs of life threatening hyperkalemia.

- Urine dipstick & UA: **first lab tests ordered** - **dipstick positive for heme but negative for RBCs on microscopic examination** of the urine (indicates myoglobin is spilling into the urine). Urine myoglobin most specific test.

- Muscle enzymes: **increased creatinine phosphokinase** >20,000, increased LDH, ALT, & AST.

- Electrolytes: **hyperkalemia, hyperuricemia, hypocalcemia,** hypophosphatemia, & increased creatinine classic.

MANAGEMENT
- **IV fluids first line & mainstay of treatment** (with a target urine output 0.5 – 1.0 mL/kg/h). Treat the underlying cause.

- Osmotic diuretic (Mannitol) or Sodium bicarbonate (alkalinization of the urine) may be added in some patients.

- ECG changes of hyperkalemia: calcium gluconate (stabilize cardiac membranes). Insulin with glucose (shifts K+ intracellularly).

POLYMYOSITIS

- Idiopathic autoimmune disorder leading to **muscle inflammation,** primarily involving the proximal limbs, neck, and pharynx. May affect the heart, lungs, & GI tract.
- Most common in women, 30-50 years of age.

PATHOPHYSIOLOGY
- Inflammatory myopathy due to CD8+ lymphocyte infiltration of the endomysium.

CLINICAL MANIFESTATIONS
- **Progressive symmetric proximal muscle weakness (shoulders, hips)** - may have difficulty combing hair, raising arms, rising from a chair, and climbing stairs due to weakness.

- Systemic symptoms: dysphagia, polyarthralgias,
- Constitutional symptoms: low-grade fever, fatigue, weight loss

PHYSICAL EXAMINATION
- **Decreased muscle strength** – especially the proximal muscles, often symmetrical (due to muscle inflammation). Muscle atrophy may be present.

- Not usually associated with rash (helpful to distinguish from Dermatomyositis).

DIAGNOSIS
- **Increased muscle enzymes (CK & aldolase) – best initial test.**

- Autoantibodies:
  - **Anti Jo-1** (myositis-specific antibody often associated with interstitial lung fibrosis and "mechanic hands" – hyperkeratotic palms with a dirty appearance)
  - **Anti-signal recognition protein** (most specific for PM), ANA.

- Increased ESR & CRP, Rheumatoid factor. Normocytic normochromic anemia.
- Abnormal electromyography.

- **Muscle biopsy: definitive diagnosis** (most accurate) - endomysial inflammation.

MANAGEMENT
- **High-dose glucocorticoids first-line.**

- Methotrexate, Azathioprine, IVIG, Mycophenolate can be used if no response to corticosteroids or if corticosteroids are contraindicated.

- **EXAM TIP**
- Polymyalgia rheumatica vs. Polymyositis
- Both can have hip and shoulder pain, difficulty rising from chair and combing their hair.
- **Polymyositis: decreased muscle strength on physical examination,** symmetrical proximal muscle weakness reproducible on physical exam (decreased muscle strength), elevated muscle enzymes (creatinine kinase & aldolase), abnormal EMG.
- **Polymyalgia rheumatica normal muscle strength** (no objective weakness). Normal muscle enzymes.

DERMATOMYOSITIS

- Idiopathic autoimmune disorder leading to **dermatologic manifestations + muscle inflammation,** primarily involving the proximal limbs, neck and pharynx.
- May affect the heart, lungs & GI tract.
- **Associated with cancer in 25% of cases** (eg, lung, ovarian, GI).

PATHOPHYSIOLOGY
- Inflammatory myopathy due to CD4+ lymphocyte infiltration of the perimysium (perivascular involvement).

CLINICAL MANIFESTATIONS
- **Progressive symmetric proximal muscle weakness (shoulders, hips)** - may have difficulty combing hair, raising arms, rising from a chair, and climbing stairs due to weakness.
- Systemic symptoms: dysphagia, polyarthralgia, low-grade fever, fatigue, weight loss.

PHYSICAL EXAMINATION
- **Decreased muscle strength** – especially the proximal muscles, often symmetrical (due to muscle inflammation). Muscle atrophy may be present.
- **Gottron's papules**: raised violaceous scaly patches (eg, dorsum of the PIP & MCP joints).
- **Heliotrope rash**: edema & blue or purple discoloration of the upper eyelids.
- Malar rash, Photosensitive poikiloderma: **shawl sign** (erythema of the shoulder, upper chest and back) or V sign (erythema of the neck & upper chest).

DIAGNOSIS
- **Increased muscle enzymes (CK & aldolase) – best initial test**.
- Autoantibodies: **Anti Jo-1** (myositis-specific antibody often associated with interstitial lung fibrosis and "mechanic hands" – hyperkeratotic palms with a dirty appearance), **Anti-Mi-2** (most specific for DM), ANA.
- Increased ESR & CRP, Rheumatoid factor. Normocytic normochromic anemia.
- Abnormal electromyography.
- **Muscle biopsy: definitive diagnosis** (most accurate) – perifascicular and perivascular inflammation.

MANAGEMENT
- **High-dose glucocorticoids first-line**.
- **Hydroxychloroquine useful for skin lesions.**
- Methotrexate, Azathioprine, IVIG, Mycophenolate can be used if no response to corticosteroids or if corticosteroids are contraindicated.

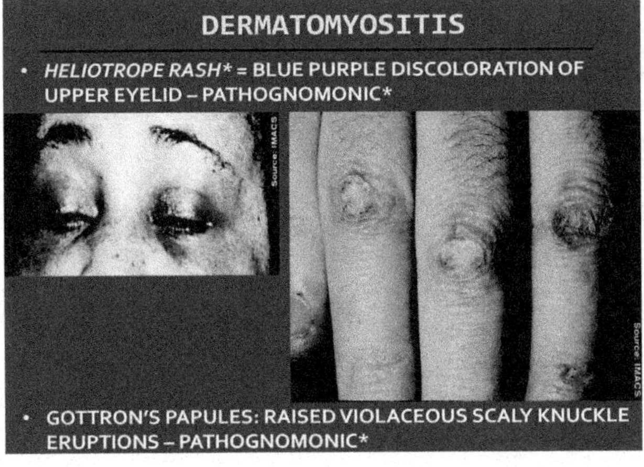

DERMATOMYOSITIS
• HELIOTROPE RASH* = BLUE PURPLE DISCOLORATION OF UPPER EYELID – PATHOGNOMONIC*
Source: IMACS
Source: IMACS
• GOTTRON'S PAPULES: RAISED VIOLACEOUS SCALY KNUCKLE ERUPTIONS – PATHOGNOMONIC*

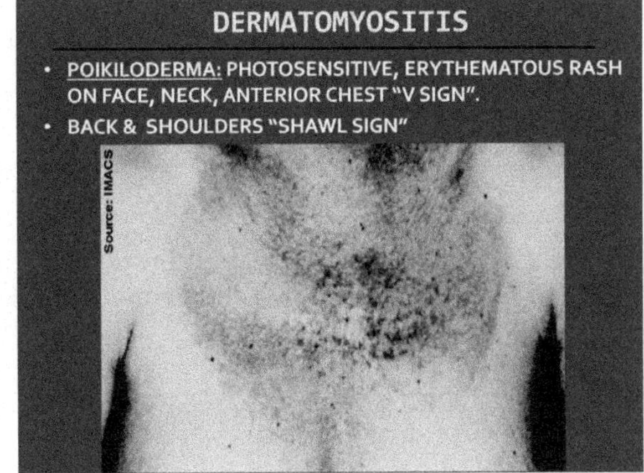

DERMATOMYOSITIS
• POIKILODERMA: PHOTOSENSITIVE, ERYTHEMATOUS RASH ON FACE, NECK, ANTERIOR CHEST "V SIGN".
• BACK & SHOULDERS "SHAWL SIGN"
Source: IMACS

SYSTEMIC LUPUS ERYTHEMATOSUS (SLE)

- Chronic systemic, multi-organ autoimmune disorder of connective tissues.
- Primarily a Type III hypersensitivity reaction (Ag-Ab immune complexes).

RISK FACTORS

- **Young females** (onset 20-40s), **African-American,** Hispanic, & Native American women. Genetic, environmental, **sun exposure,** infections, **estrogen** (eg, oral contraceptives).

CLINICAL MANIFESTATIONS

- Triad: **joint pain + fever + malar "butterfly" rash** - fixed erythematous rash on the cheeks or bridge of the nose sparing the nasolabial folds.
- Constitutional symptoms: fever, chills, fatigue, night sweats.
- **Discoid lupus: annular,** erythematous patches on the face & scalp that **heal with scarring.**
- Systemic: CNS (headache, stroke seizures), cardiovascular, glomerulonephritis, retinitis, oral ulcers, alopecia; Serositis (pericarditis, pleuritis).

DIAGNOSIS

- **Anti-nuclear antibodies (ANA): screening test of choice** (most sensitive but not specific).
- **Anti-double-stranded DNA & Anti-Smith: pathognomonic & specific for SLE** (not sensitive). During flares, dsDNA antibodies rise & complement (C3, C4) decrease (dsDNA used in monitoring).
- **Antiphospholipid antibodies: increased risk of arterial & venous thrombosis** (eg, atherosclerosis & DVTs). Includes Anti-cardiolipin antibodies & lupus anticoagulant.
- Pancytopenia: anemia of chronic disease (more common), hemolytic anemia, leukopenia, lymphopenia & thrombocytopenia.
- **Decreased complement levels** (eg, **C3, C4**).

MANAGEMENT

- Management choice depends on the level of organ involvement:
- Sunscreen and avoidance of prolonged sun exposure in all patients.
- **Mild lupus:** (skin, joint, mucosal). **Hydroxychloroquine with or without NSAIDs,** and/or short-term use of low-dose glucocorticoids. In mild cases, NSAIDs may be used alone.
- **Moderate** (significant but non-organ threatening): Hydroxychloroquine or Chloroquine plus short-term glucocorticoid therapy.
- **Severe** (life or organ-threatening): **high-dose glucocorticoids or intermittent IV "pulses" of Methylprednisolone** with other immunosuppressive agents (eg, Cyclophosphamide, Mycophenolate, Rituximab).
- Belimumab - monoclonal antibody that inhibits B-lymphocyte stimulator binding to B cells, which inhibits B-cell survival. It was designed for SLE & is usually reserved for active cutaneous or musculoskeletal disease unresponsive to glucocorticoids or other immunosuppressive agents.

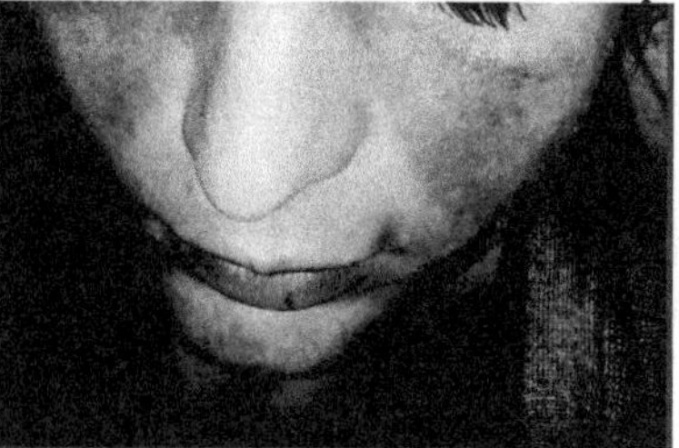

Butterfly malar rash

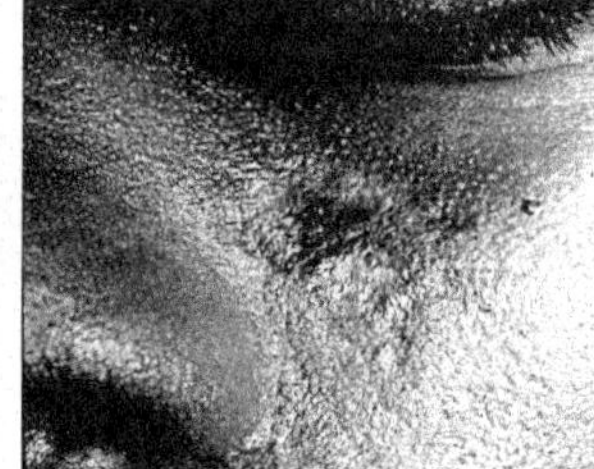

Discoid lupus

DIAGNOSTIC CRITERIA for SYSTEMIC LUPUS ERYTHEMATOSUS

At least 4 of the 11 needed

ANA SMITH was stranded on an island & developed a **RASH** when the **RAIN** made way for the **sun**

- Rash: Malar, Discoid, Oral ulcers, **Photosensitivity** (each count as 1)
- Arthritis
- Serositis: pericarditis, pleuritis, peritonitis
- Hematologic: hemolytic anemia, leukopenia, leukocytosis, thrombocytopenia

@pance_prep_pearls

- Renal disease: glomerulonephritis, proteinuria
- Anti-nuclear antibody (ANA)
- Immunologic disorders: anti-double stranded DNA, anti-Smith, false-positive tests for syphilis (RPR, VDRL) with a negative FTA.
- Neurologic: seizures or psychosis in absence of any other causes.

DRUG-INDUCED LUPUS

Autoimmune disorder similar to SLE caused by the use of certain drugs:

- **Hydralazine, Procainamide, Isoniazid, Quinidine** (high yield on exams). Methyldopa, Minocycline, Chlorpromazine, Pyrazinamide, D-penicillamine, Carbamazepine, Phenytoin & Minoxidil.

CLINICAL MANIFESTATIONS

- SLE-type symptoms: rash, fever, arthralgias, arthritis, & serositis (pleuritis, pericarditis).
- Unlike SLE, it is not usually associated with alopecia, hematologic, kidney injury, or CNS symptoms.

DIAGNOSIS

- **Anti-histone antibodies are hallmark.** Positive ANA.
- Hypocomplementemia & anti-double-stranded DNA antibodies are not usually seen.

MANAGEMENT

- **Discontinuation of the offending agent.**
- NSAIDs may be used for arthralgias & serositis. Topical corticosteroids for cutaneous symptoms.

ANTIPHOSPHOLIPID SYNDROME

- Idiopathic disorder characterized by venous or arterial thromboses due to antibodies against negatively-charged phospholipids.
- Can occur as a primary disease or in the setting of other diseases, such as **Systemic lupus erythematosus.**
- Pathophysiology: the autoantibodies activate complement-mediated thrombosis.
- Triggers: smoking, prolonged immobilization, estrogen (eg, oral contraceptive use, pregnancy, postpartum period, hormone replacement therapy), malignancy, hyperlipidemia, and Hypertension.

CLINICAL MANIFESTATIONS

- **Increased risk of arterial & venous thromboses** (eg, atherosclerosis, **recurrent DVT or PE, recurrent miscarriages**).
- Livedo reticularis, valvular heart disease, neurologic symptoms (eg, stroke, TIA, cognitive defects).

DIAGNOSIS

- **Anticardiolipin antibodies:** associated with **false-positive testing for Syphilis** - **positive RPR** or VDRL with a negative confirmatory FTA-ABS because the screening tests contain cardiolipin. May have normal or slightly prolonged prothrombin time (PT).
- **Lupus anticoagulant: increased partial thromboplastin time (PTT)** but associated with thrombosis. Despite its name, lupus anticoagulant positivity is associated with hypercoagulability.
- Beta-2 glycoprotein I autoantibodies.
- **Mixing studies: failure to correct PTT after mixing** the patient's blood with normal plasma due to the presence of an inhibitor (unlike clotting deficiency disorders where the mixing study will correct the aPTT).
- Prolonged Russell viper venom test: most specific for lupus anticoagulant. Official diagnosis requires two positive results with samples taken at least 12 weeks apart.

MANAGEMENT

- Asymptomatic patients do not need to be treated.
- Recurrent thrombosis may require lifelong Warfarin or novel oral anticoagulants (**Warfarin more effective**).
- Low molecular weight Heparin may be used in pregnant patients to prevent fetal loss.

SJÖGREN SYNDROME

- Autoimmune disease primarily affecting the **exocrine glands** (eg, salivary & lacrimal glands).

- Primary: occurs alone.
- Secondary: associated with other autoimmune disorders (eg, Hashimoto, SLE, Rheumatoid arthritis).
- Sjögren syndrome most common in females (90%), 40-60y. HLA-DR52.

CLINICAL MANIFESTATIONS
- Dry mucous membranes: **dry mouth** (xerostomia), **dry eyes** (keratoconjunctivitis sicca), **vaginal dryness** (may present as **dyspareunia**), bilateral **parotid gland enlargement**, dental caries (complication of xerostomia).

DIAGNOSIS
- **Screening labs:** Anti-nuclear antibodies (ANA), especially **antiSS-A (Ro)** & **antiSS-B (La)** best initial laboratory test.

- **Positive Schirmer test:** decreased tear production (wetting of <5 mm of the filter paper placed in the lower eyelid for 5 minutes).

- Rose Bengal stain: abnormal corneal epithelium.

- Definitive diagnosis: lip or parotid gland biopsy - gland fibrosis & lymphocytic infiltration.

- Nonspecific labs: positive rheumatoid factor, anemia, leukopenia.

MANAGEMENT
- Lifestyle: increase mucosal secretions - **artificial tears** to prevent corneal ulcers, **increase fluid intake**, sugar-free gum, artificial saliva and fluoride treatments.

- **Cholinergic drugs Pilocarpine or Cevimeline** lead to increased secretions.

COMPLICATIONS
- **Increased risk of Non-Hodgkin lymphoma,** pneumonitis, interstitial nephritis.

- Increased risk of congenital heart block if the mother has high antibody titers while pregnant.

PILOCARPINE

Mechanism:
- **Cholinergic (muscarinic)** drug that **increases lacrimation and salivation.**

Indications:
- **Sjögren syndrome** - improves dry mouth and dry eyes.
- Topical - **Acute angle-closure glaucoma** - causes pupillary constriction, opening the angle.

Adverse effects:
- **Diaphoresis, flushing, sweating, bradycardia, diarrhea, nausea, vomiting, incontinence, blurred vision.**
- Think SLUDD-C (**S**alivation, **L**acrimation, **U**rination, **D**efecation, **D**igestion, **C**onstriction of pupil).

SCLERODERMA (SYSTEMIC SCLEROSIS)

- Systemic autoimmune connective tissue disorder where collagen deposition leads to fibrosis of the skin and internal organs (lung, heart, kidney, & GI tract).
- Most common in women 30 – 50 years of age.

TYPES
- **Limited (CREST syndrome):** 80%. Characterized by **tight, shiny, thickened skin** involving the face, neck, as well as **distal to the elbows & knees.** Spares the trunk. Pulmonary hypertension with advanced disease. **C**alcinosis cutis, **R**aynaud's phenomenon: red-white-blue vasospastic changes of the digits, **E**sophageal motility disorder, **S**clerodactyly (claw hand), **T**elangiectasias.

- **Diffuse:** (20%). **Tight, shiny, thickened skin** involving the **trunk & proximal extremities.** Associated with greater internal organ involvement (eg, restrictive lung disease due pulmonary fibrosis, myocardial fibrosis).

DIAGNOSIS
- **Anti-centromere antibodies:** associated with **Limited (CREST) - specific.**
- **Anti-SCL-70 antibodies (anti-topoisomerase):** associated with **diffuse disease** & multiple organ involvement. Poorer prognosis than limited.
- ANA: nonspecific but positive in 90% in patients with Scleroderma.

MANAGEMENT
Treatment is organ specific:
- GERD: PPIs
- Hypertensive renal disease: ACE inhibitors
- Raynaud: vasodilators - calcium channel blockers, prostacyclin (prostaglandin).
- Severe: DMARDs: Methotrexate, Mycophenolate. Cyclophosphamide usually reserved for refractory cases.
- Pulmonary fibrosis: Cyclophosphamide
- Pulmonary hypertension: Bosentan, Sildenafil, Prostacyclin analogues

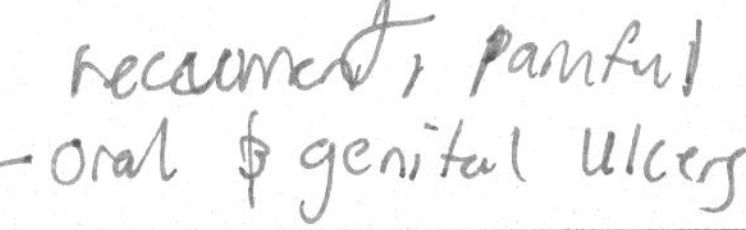

BEHÇET'S SYNDROME

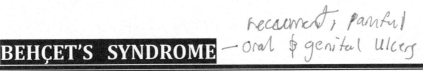

- Multisystemic autoimmune disorder characterized by **recurrent, painful oral & genital ulcers** (aphthous), **erythema nodosum**, eye (**uveitis**, conjunctivitis), arthritis, & CNS involvement (may mimic Multiple sclerosis).
- Increased incidence in **Asian or Middle Eastern** or **Mediterranean** persons.
- Initial presentation usually 20-40 years.

DIAGNOSIS
- **Primarily a clinical diagnosis.**
- Biopsy for definitive diagnosis (leukocytoclastic vasculitis or lymphocytic vasculitis). Increased ESR, CRP, and leukocytes.
- **Pathergy** = sterile skin papules or pustules from minor trauma (eg, needle stick) – less common in patients from N. America or N. Europe.

MANAGEMENT
- **Corticosteroids** during flares.
- Other treatment options include Colchicine, Cyclophosphamide, Azathioprine.

TAKAYASU ARTERITIS

- Chronic large-vessel vasculitis that affects the **aorta & its primary branches** (aortic arch & pulmonary arteries).
- Risk factors: **women** (80-90%), age of onset **10-40 years, Asians**.

CLINICAL MANIFESTATIONS

- Constitutional symptoms: flu-like, weight loss, low-grade fever, fatigue, arthralgias.
- **Vessel ischemia:** coronary arteries, carotid arteries (TIA, stroke), renal artery (HTN crisis), subclavian artery (arm claudication), **lower extremity claudication,** aneurysm rupture.

PHYSICAL EXAMINATION

- Bruits (carotid, subclavian or abdominal), **diminished pulses, asymmetric blood pressure measurements between arms** (>10 mmHg), hypertension, symptoms of peripheral arterial disease.

DIAGNOSIS

- **Angiography (MRA or CTA) necessary to confirm diagnosis** and extent of the disease.
- Nonspecific: may have increased ESR, CRP, normochromic, normocytic anemia, leukocytosis.

MANAGEMENT

- **High-dose corticosteroids first-line treatment.**
- Cytotoxic drugs: Methotrexate, Azathioprine.
- Revascularization in some.

KAWASAKI SYNDROME

- Medium & small vessel necrotizing vasculitis including the **coronary arteries.**
- AKA Mucocutaneous lymph node syndrome.

PATHOPHYSIOLOGY

- Thought to be an unidentified respiratory agent or viral pathogen with a propensity towards vascular tissue.

RISK FACTORS

- **Children (especially <5y), boys, & Asians** (highest risk).

DIAGNOSIS

Warm + CREAM = fever > 5 DAYS + 4 of the following 5:

- Conjunctivitis, Rash (erythematous or morbiliform or macular), Extremity changes: edema, erythema, or desquamation of palms & soles, Beau's lines (transverse nail grooves), arthritis. Adenopathy (cervical) & Mucositis: **strawberry tongue,** lip swelling, fissures, pharyngeal erythema.
- Labs: nonspecific - elevated WBC and platelet count, anemia, increased ESR & CRP; Sterile pyuria.
- Echocardiogram and ECG are recommended to look for complications.
- Complications: **coronary vessel arteritis: coronary artery aneurysm,** myocardial infarction, pericarditis, myocarditis.

MANAGEMENT

- **IV Immunoglobulin + Aspirin** for fever, joint pain, & prevention of coronary complications.

POLYARTERITIS NODOSA (PAN)

- Systemic vasculitis primarily of medium-sized vessels.
- Most commonly affects the renal, CNS, & GI vessels.
- **Pulmonary vessels (lung) not involved** (distinguishes PAN from the other vasculitides).

PATHOPHYSIOLOGY
- Type III hypersensitivity reaction leads to ischemia & microaneurysms of the affected vessels.
- Most common in men 40-60 years of age.
- **Increased association with chronic Hepatitis B & C.**

CLINICAL MANIFESTATIONS
- Renal: **Hypertension** (renal artery stenosis), renal ischemia. PAN is not usually associated with glomerulonephritis.
- GI: abdominal pain worse with eating (intestinal angina), nausea, vomiting.
- Constitutional: fever, arthralgia, myalgias.
- CNS: neuropathy, stroke, **Mononeuritis multiplex**. Multiple peripheral neuropathies - peroneal nerve (foot drop) most common, ulnar nerve, etc.
- Dermatologic: ulcers, **livedo reticularis,** purpura, Raynaud phenomenon.

DIAGNOSIS
- Labs: increased ESR, proteinuria.
- **Classic PAN is ANCA negative** (P-ANCA positive in <20% of cases).
- **Renal or Mesenteric angiography: microaneurysms** with abrupt cut-off of small arteries **(beading).**
- Biopsy: definitive - necrotizing medium vessel vasculitis & *no granulomas.*

MANAGEMENT
- **Glucocorticoids.** Cyclophosphamide added if severe or refractory.
- Hepatitis B-positive patients may treatment for HBV and possibly plasmapheresis.

EOSINOPHILIC GRANULOMATOSIS WITH POLYANGIITIS (EGPA- CHURG-STRAUSS)

- Systemic small- and medium-sized granulomatous necrotizing vasculitis.
- Can be a rare side effect of Montelukast and Zafirlukast.
- Lung most common organ involved, followed by the skin.

CLINICAL MANIFESTATIONS
- Triad: **Asthma + eosinophilia +** chronic **rhinosinusitis**.
- Prodromal phase: atopic disease, allergic rhinitis, Asthma (>90%)
- Eosinophilic phase: peripheral blood eosinophilia and infiltration of organs (eg, skin, lung, GI tract) – subcutaneous nodules, pulmonary opacities, abdominal pain, GI bleed, colitis.
- Vasculitic phase: constitutional symptoms (eg, fever, weight loss, malaise).

DIAGNOSIS
- Labs: **eosinophilia & P-ANCA positivity hallmark.** Increased ESR, CRP, IgE, rheumatoid factor.
- Biopsy: most accurate test – granulomatous necrotizing vasculitis.

MANAGEMENT
- **Glucocorticoids** (may add **Cyclophosphamide** if severe).

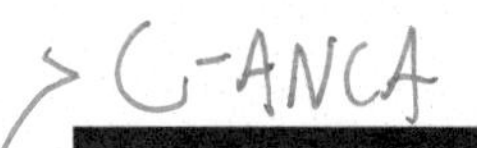

GRANULOMATOSIS WITH POLYANGIITIS (GPA - WEGENER'S)

- Small vessel vasculitis with granulomatous inflammation & necrosis of the **nose, lungs, & kidney.**

CLINICAL MANIFESTATIONS

- **Triad:** involvement of the **upper respiratory tract + lower respiratory tract + Glomerulonephritis.**
- Upper respiratory tract & nose: nasal congestion, **saddle nose deformity,** nasal perforation, mastoiditis, **otitis media**, stridor, **refractory sinusitis**.
- Lower respiratory tract: cough, dyspnea, hemoptysis, wheezing, pulmonary infiltrates, or cavitation (usually does not improve with antibiotics).
- **Glomerulonephritis: rapidly progressive** (**crescents** seen on biopsy). Hematuria, **RBC casts,** proteinuria.

DIAGNOSIS

- Chest radiograph: nonspecific abnormalities (eg, nodules, cavitations).
- **C-ANCA positivity: best initial lab test.**
  Cytoplasmic anti-nuclear cytoplasmic antibodies (anti-proteinase-3 antibodies) = C-ANCA.
- Biopsy definitive (lung preferred over sinus or kidney biopsy) - large **necrotizing granulomas.**

MANAGEMENT

- **Glucocorticoids PLUS Cyclophosphamide.**
- Methotrexate is an alternative to Cyclophosphamide.

MICROSCOPIC POLYANGIITIS (MPA)

- Small & medium-vessel vasculitis.
- Not associated with nasopharyngeal symptoms, necrosis, or granulomatous inflammation (as seen with GPA). Affects the capillaries (capillary involvement not seen with PAN).

CLINICAL MANIFESTATIONS

- Constitutional: fever, arthralgias, malaise, weight loss, **palpable purpura**. Mononeuritis multiplex.
- **Lung:** cough, dyspnea, hemoptysis.
- **Renal: acute glomerulonephritis - rapidly progressive (crescentic).**

DIAGNOSIS

- **+P-ANCA** (anti-neutrophil myeloperoxidase)
- CXR: nonspecific abnormalities.
- Biopsy: definitive – non-granulomatous inflammation.

MANAGEMENT

- **Glucocorticoids plus Cyclophosphamide.**

> - **EXAM TIP**
> - **Glucocorticoids plus Cyclophosphamide are used in the following diseases:**
> - Microscopic polyangiitis, Granulomatosis with polyangiitis (Wegener's), Eosinophilic granulomatosis with polyangiitis (Churg-Strauss), Systemic lupus nephritis, severe cases of Polyarteritis nodosa, & Rapidly-progressive glomerulonephritis.

	INCIDENCE	PATHOPHYSIOLOGY	CLINICAL	DIAGNOSIS	MANAGEMENT
LARGE VESSEL					
GIANT CELL (TEMPORAL) ARTERITIS	***Older women >50y****	• ***Cranial arteries*** - *Temporal & Ophthalmic artery**	• ***Headache, visual loss,* jaw claudication*** • Temporal artery sx	• ***Temporal Artery Bx*** • ***Clinical Dx****	***High-dose corticosteroids***
TAKAYASU ARTERITIS	***MC in young, Asian women <40y****	• ***Aorta & aortic arch**** • ***Pulmonary artery***	• ***Vessel aneurysm, occlusion (TIA, CVA, MYOCARDIAL INFARCTION**** • ***Lower extremity claudication, ↓pulses****	***Angiography***	***High-dose steroids*** Methotrexate (MTX) Azathioprine (AZA)
MEDIUM VESSEL	**Affects ARTERIOLES**				
KAWASAKI'S DISEASE	***MC in Asian children <5y****	Necrotizing vasculitis	***"warm + CREAM"*** ***Coronary aneurysms****	• ↑ESR/CRP, anemia • ***Clinical dx***	***IVIG + Aspirin****
POLYARTERITIS NODOSA (PAN)	Males ~45y ↑***Assoc c Hep B Virus****	Necrotizing vasculitis of arterioles. ***Capillaries not involved***	CNS, GI, derm, renal ***Lungs usually spared.*** ***Renovascular HTN****	• ***Angiogram*** • ***ANCA negative**** (⊕P-ANCA <20%) • ***No granulomas***	***Corticosteroids*** ± MTX, AZA
SMALL VESSEL	***Affects ARTERIOLES, CAPILLARIES & VENULES***				
GRANULOMATOUS **EOSINOPHILIC GPA (CHURG STRAUSS)**	Males >40y	Necrotizing ***granulomatous***	***Upper airway: allergic**** ***ASTHMA**** Skin, Lung MC involved	• ↑***EOSINOPHILS*, asthma*** • ***⊕P-ANCA****	***Corticosteroids*** Cyclophosphamide (Cyc), AZA
GPA (WEGENERS)	Men = Women Peaks 30-40y	Necrotizing ***granulomatous***	**TRIAD** ***1. Upper airway: necrotic**** ***2. Lower airway dz*** ***3. Acute Glomerulonephritis***	• ↑ESR/CRP, anemia • ***⊕ C-ANCA****	***Corticosteroids + Cyclophosphamide*** MTX
NONGRANULOMATOUS **MICROSCOPIC POLYANGIITIS (MPA)**	Males ~50y	***NON granulomatous capillaries, arteries, veins (unlike PAN)***	***Upp airway: unaffected*** ***Lung sx.*** ***Acute Glomerulonephritis***	***⊕P-ANCA****	***Steroids + Cyclophosphamide*** MTX
HENOCH-SCHÖNLEIN PURPURA (HSP)	***Children 3-15y*** ***Males MC***	• ***Ig-A deposition*** vasculitis • ***MC after URI****	❶ ***Purpura*** ❷ ***Arthritis*** ❸ ***Abdominal pain*** ❹ ***Hematuria***	• ↑***Ig-A**** • ***Normal coags, plts.*** • UA: RBC, proteinuria	***Self-limiting – supportive mgmt.*** ± Prednisone

IMMUNOGLOBULIN A VASCULITIS (HENOCH-SCHÖNLEIN-PURPURA)

- Acute systemic IgA-mediated small-vessel vasculitis.
- **90% occur in children** (especially 3-15 years of age).

PATHOPHYSIOLOGY
- Often occurs **after infection** (eg, **URI**, GABHS, Parvovirus B-19).

CLINICAL MANIFESTATIONS
4 cardinal symptoms: **HSP** affects Ig**A:**
- **H**ematuria. Azotemia (↑BUN/Creatinine), proteinuria.
- **S**ynovial (arthritis or arthralgia) – knees and ankles most common.
- **P**alpable purpura (especially on the lower extremities).
- **A**bdominal pain (may present with GI bleeding).

DIAGNOSIS
- Usually a clinical diagnosis.
- **Normal PT, PTT, & platelets** (the purpura is due to vasculitis, not due to thrombocytopenia or coagulopathy).
- Kidney biopsy: definitive diagnosis - **mesangial IgA deposits** & *leukocytoclastic vasculitis.*

MANAGEMENT
- **Supportive treatment mainstay** - bed rest, **hydration, & NSAIDs** for pain. Self-limited.
- Severe symptoms or progressive renal insufficiency may require hospitalization & glucocorticoids.

ANTI-GBM ANTIBODY (GOODPASTURE'S) DISEASE

- Type II hypersensitivity reaction: **IgG antibodies** against **type IV collagen of the alveoli & glomerular basement membrane** of the kidney.

CLINICAL MANIFESTATIONS
- **Symptoms limited to the lung & the kidney**
- Lung: **hemoptysis,** dyspnea, dry cough.
- Kidney: **hematuria,** oliguria.
- Systemic symptoms of vasculitides are usually absent (usually no fever weight loss, arthralgias, etc.)

DIAGNOSIS
- Glomerulonephritis: increased BUN/creatinine, UA: hematuria, proteinuria, dysmorphic RBCs, **RBC casts.**
- **⊕ anti-glomerular basement membrane antibodies** – **best initial test after UA**.
- May have anemia. Chest radiographs are usually abnormal but nonspecific.
- Biopsy of glomerulus or alveoli: definitive
  - **Linear IgG deposits** on immunofluorescence.
  - **Crescentic** (rapidly progressive) **glomerulonephritis.**

MANAGEMENT
- **Glucocorticoids PLUS Cyclophosphamide + Plasmapheresis**

Think **G**ood**P**astures ⇒ ❶ **G**lomerulonephritis (rapidly progressing) + ❷ **P**ulmonary hemorrhage (hemoptysis).

SERONEGATIVE SPONDYLOARTHROPATHIES

- Joint diseases affecting the vertebral column, associated with **rheumatoid factor & ANA negativity.**

RISK FACTORS
- Most common in **young males, <40 years of age** at initial presentation, **HLA-B27 positivity**.
- Characterized by **vertebral column involvement, sacroiliitis, uveitis, & enthesitis** (inflammation at the site of attachment of a tendon or ligament to the bone).

DISEASES: **PEAR - P**soriatic arthritis, **E**nteropathic arthritis (associated with Crohn or Ulcerative colitis), **A**nkylosing spondylitis, **R**eactive arthritis

PSORIATIC ARTHRITIS

- Inflammatory arthritis in patients with Psoriasis.

INCIDENCE
- 15-20% of patients with Psoriasis develop Psoriatic arthritis.
- 80% will have Psoriasis preceding the arthritis by months to years.

CLINICAL MANIFESTATIONS
- **Arthritis**: joint stiffness. May be asymmetric, symmetric, or clinically indistinguishable from Rheumatoid arthritis but unlike RA, may **involve the DIP joint**.
- **Dactylitis** (sausage digits hands > feet), **sacroiliitis,** & chronic uveitis.
- **Psoriasis:** erythematous plaques with **thick silvery-white scales & nail pitting.**

DIAGNOSIS
- Radiographs: **best initial test - "pencil in a cup" deformities** (description of the appearance of the periarticular bony erosions & bone resorption). The bony erosions look like the thin end of one bone is being inserted into a thicker bone, similar to a pencil in a cup.

MANAGEMENT
- **Mild: NSAIDs first-line initial therapy.**
- **Severe: Methotrexate is the drug of choice for severe disease** (eg, > 5 joints, severe damage on radiographs), or no response to NSAIDs. Leflunomide alternative.
- TNF inhibitors used if Methotrexate is unsuccessful (eg, Adalimumab, Infliximab).
- Interleukin antagonists (eg, Ustekinumab or Secukinumab) if refractory to anti-TNF agents.

PSORIATIC ARTHRITIS
- SAUSAGE DIGITS*
- X RAYS: PENCIL IN CUP DEFORMITY*

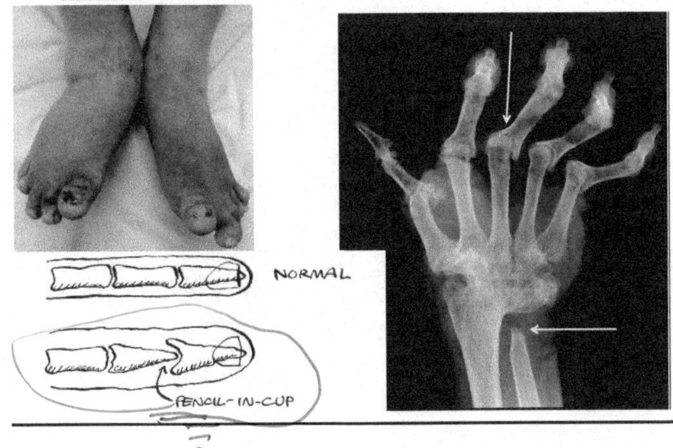

ENTEROPATHIC ARTHRITIS: associated with IBD: **Crohn, Ulcerative Colitis.**

ANKYLOSING SPONDYLITIS

- Chronic inflammatory arthropathy of the axial skeleton - spine & sacroiliac joints with progressive spine stiffness (ankylosis = stiffness of joints due to fusion of the joints).

RISK FACTORS

- **Young males 15-30y, HLA-B27 positivity**.

CLINICAL MANIFESTATIONS

- **Back pain, stiffness & decreased ROM** that is worse in the morning, with rest & **decreases with exercise & activity.** Kyphosis, **Sacroiliitis,** & large joint arthritis
- Extraarticular: Achilles tendon enthesitis, dactylitis, **uveitis,** cardiac (eg, AV cardiac blocks, aortic regurgitation), pulmonary fibrosis (decreased chest expansion).

DIAGNOSIS

- Labs: Increased ESR. Negative Rheumatoid factor & ANA.

- Radiographs:
  - Radiograph of the SI joint often initial test ordered - **sacroiliitis (narrowing of the joint)** early finding.
  - **Bamboo spine = straightening of the spine** (loss of normal lumbar curvature) + **squaring & fusion of the vertebrae** by bridging syndesmophytes is a classic but late finding.

- MRI: most accurate test.

MANAGEMENT

- **NSAIDs first-line**, exercise program & physical therapy.
- Anti-TNF drugs if no response to NSAIDs (eg, Etanercept, Adalimumab, Infliximab).

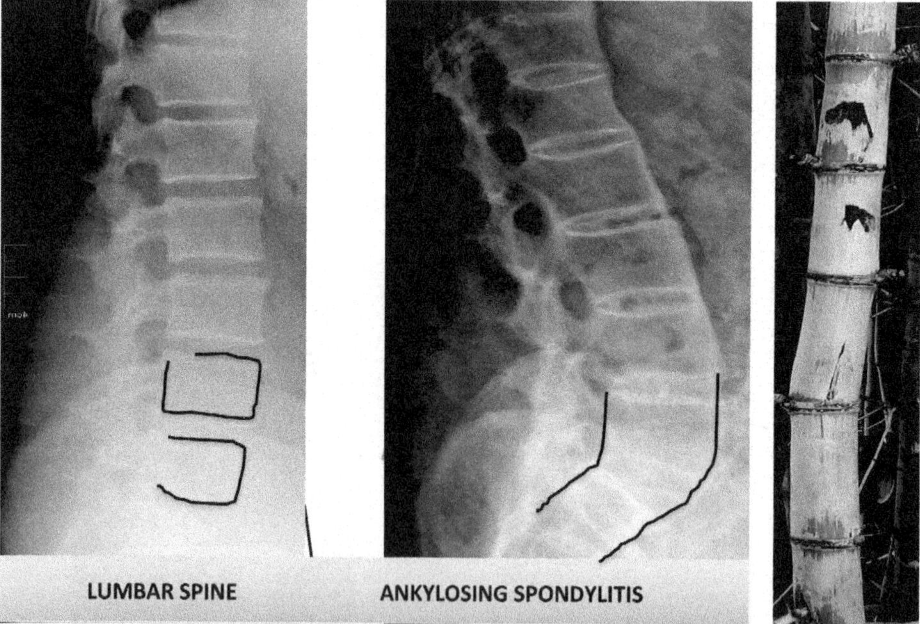

REACTIVE ARTHRITIS

- Inflammatory arthritis in response to an infection or inflammation in another part of the body. Formerly Reiter syndrome.
- May be seen 1-4 weeks after ***Chlamydia trachomatis*** or **GI infection** (eg, *Salmonella, Shigella, Campylobacter & Yersinia*).
- **HLA-B27** associated with increased incidence.

CLINICAL MANIFESTATIONS
- **Triad: arthritis + ocular (conjunctivitis,** uveitis) + **genital (urethritis,** cervicitis, balanitis).
- Lower extremity joints most commonly affected (especially the knees).
- **Keratoderma blennorrhagicum** - hyperkeratotic lesions on the palms & soles.

DIAGNOSIS
- **Arthrocentesis to rule out septic arthritis -** findings of Reactive arthritis are similar to other inflammatory arthritides - increased WBC count but <50,000, predominantly neutrophils with negative cultures (no evidence of Septic arthritis).
- Nonspecific: increased ESR & IgG, normochromic anemia.

MANAGEMENT
- **NSAIDs first-line treatment.**
- Sulfasalazine or Methotrexate second-line treatment if no response to NSAIDs. Intraarticular glucocorticoid injections may also be used as second-line agent.
- Antibiotics do not reverse reactive arthritis once the joint pain has begun but may be indicated to treat the underlying cause (eg, *Chlamydia trachomatis*).

TUMOR MARKERS

TUMOR MARKER	MAIN ASSOCIATIONS
ALPHA FETOPROTEIN	• **Hepatocellular carcinoma** • **Nonseminomatous germ cell testicular cancer** • Decreased in Down syndrome "AFP is down in Down syndrome"
Beta-hCG	• **Nonseminomatous germ cell testicular cancer** • **Choriocarcinoma,** Teratomas • **Trophoblastic tumors** (eg, Hydatidiform molar pregnancy)
CA-125	• **Ovarian cancer**
CA 19-9	• **Pancreatic cancer** • GI – colorectal, esophageal, & hepatocellular cancers
CALCITONIN	• **Medullary thyroid cancer**
CEA	• **Colorectal cancer** • Medullary thyroid, pancreatic, gastric, lung, & breast cancers
PROSTATE SPECIFIC ANTIGEN	• **Prostate cancer** • Can also be elevated in BPH & Prostatitis

ARTHRITIS SYNDROMES

GOUT

- **Uric acid deposition** in the soft tissues, joints, & bones.
- **90% occur in men.**

ETIOLOGIES

- Renal uric acid underexcretion (90%) – can be worsened with renal insufficiency, Thiazides, Aspirin; Uric acid overproduction - increased cell turnover (eg, cancer, chemotherapy, hemolysis).

TRIGGERS

- Attacks associated with **purine-rich foods** (alcohol, liver, seafood, yeasts) causing rapid changes in uric acid concentrations. Meds: **Thiazide & loop diuretics, ACEI, Pyrazinamide, Ethambutol, Aspirin,** & ARBs (notable **exception is Losartan**, which decreases uric acid levels).

CLINICAL MANIFESTATIONS

- Acute gouty arthritis: **first MTP joint of the great toe most common (podagra)** & lower extremity (knees, feet, & ankles). Severe **joint pain, erythema, warmth, swelling, & tenderness,** fever.

DIAGNOSIS

- **Arthrocentesis diagnostic test of choice - negatively birefringent, needle-shaped crystals.** Increased WBC count (but < 50,000), predominantly neutrophils.

- Radiographs: **mouse or rat bite lesions (punched out erosions with sclerotic & overhanging margins)**. Tophi may be seen in longstanding disease.

- Increased ESR & WBC.

ACUTE MANAGEMENT (ATTACKS)

- **NSAIDs initial treatment of choice.** Avoid Aspirin.

- Corticosteroids reserved if refractory to NSAIDs or if NSAIDs are contraindicated (eg, renal disease). Can be injected into a single joint or given as oral therapy.

- Colchicine usually reserved if unable to use NSAIDs or Corticosteroids. Adverse effects include diarrhea and bone marrow suppression (neutropenia).

CHRONIC MANAGEMENT (PROPHYLAXIS)

- Lifestyle: decrease alcohol consumption (especially beer), weight loss, decrease high-purine intake (eg, meats, seafood).

- **Allopurinol (first line)** & Febuxostat are xanthine oxidase inhibitors (decreases uric acid production). Not started during acute attacks. Allopurinol safe in renal insufficiency.

- Uricosuric drugs: Probenecid & Sulfinpyrazone. Both are contraindicated in renal insufficiency.

- Colchicine.

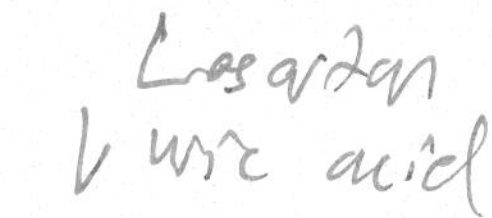

ACUTE GOUT MANAGEMENT

NSAIDs (eg, Naproxen, Indomethacin)

- Mechanism: anti-inflammatory (superior to Colchicine).
- Indications: **initial management of choice for acute Gout**, especially in patients < 60 years of age without significant cardiovascular, renal or active GI disease. Avoid Aspirin.
- Contraindications: **renal insufficiency.**

Glucocorticoids

- Mechanism: anti-inflammatory. Can be administered intraarticular or orally
- Indications: **acute Gout refractory to NSAIDS or if NSAIDs are contraindicated** (eg, **severe renal disease**).
- Cautions: used with caution in patients with glucose intolerance, Heart failure, or poorly controlled Hypertension.

Colchicine

- Mechanism: anti-inflammatory.
- Indications: **patients who cannot use either NSAIDs or Corticosteroids**. Safe in mild renal injury. The only medication that can be used in both acute and chronic Gout.

CHRONIC GOUT MANAGEMENT

Allopurinol

- Mechanism: **xanthine oxidase inhibition** leads to decrease uric acid production
- Indications: **first-line prophylaxis for Gout** (not used for acute attacks). Prevents urate nephropathy from tumor lysis syndrome. Allopurinol safe in patients with renal insufficiency.
- Adverse reactions: hypersensitivity (eg, rash hemolysis, Stevens-Johnson syndrome), allergic interstitial nephritis.
- Febuxostat is another xanthine oxidase inhibitor.

Colchicine

- Mechanism: anti-inflammatory (impairs neutrophil chemotaxis).
- Indications: **patients who cannot use either NSAIDs or Corticosteroids**. Safe in mild renal injury. The only medication that can be used in both acute and chronic Gout.
- Adverse reaction: **neutropenia,** GI irritation.

Uricosuric drugs

Probenecid, Sulfinpyrazone

- Mechanism: increase urinary uric acid excretion (uricosurics).
- Indications: prophylaxis for Gout. Used in uric acid underexcreters.
- Adverse effects: uric acid calculi, can cause prolonged Penicillin levels.
- Contraindications: renal insufficiency, prior history of uric acid renal calculi.

Pegloticase

- Mechanism: **dissolves uric acid -** recombinant uricase (catalyzes metabolism pf uric acid to allantoin, which is more water soluble).
- Indications: prophylaxis for Gout.
- Adverse effects: increased risk of new gout flare (not used in acute attacks).

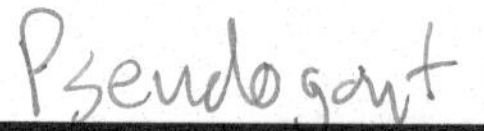

CALCIUM PYROPHOSPHATE DIHYDRATE DEPOSITION DISEASE

- **Calcium pyrophosphate dihydrate deposition in the joints & soft tissue**, leading to inflammation & bone destruction.
- Risk factors: Hemochromatosis, Hyperparathyroidism, & Hypomagnesemia.
- Joints involved: **knee most common. Elbow, wrist, & MCP joint** also common.

CLINICAL MANIFESTATIONS
- Asymptomatic: (majority). Incidental finding of chondrocalcinosis on radiographs.
- **Acute CPP crystal arthritis (Pseudogout):** clinically indistinguishable from Gout - **severe joint pain, erythema, warmth, swelling, & tenderness**.
- Pseudo-RA: mimics RA (inflammation, joint pain, and morning stiffness).
- Pyrophosphate arthropathy: resembles Osteoarthritis.

DIAGNOSIS OF PSEUDOGOUT
- **Arthrocentesis: diagnostic test of choice - positively birefringent, rhomboid-shaped calcium pyrophosphate** crystals & increased WBC 2,000 – 50,000, primarily neutrophils.
- Radiographs: linear **calcification of the cartilage (chondrocalcinosis**).

PSEUDOGOUT MANAGEMENT
- **Corticosteroids: intraarticular corticosteroids if 1 or 2 joints**. Oral if > 2 joints.
- **NSAIDs:** first-line option if > 2 joints. Contraindications include renal insufficiency, active PUD, GI bleed, cardiovascular (eg, Heart failure, uncontrolled Hypertension), or anticoagulant use.
- **Colchicine:** first-line option that can be used in acute & chronic CPP disease (can be used as prophylaxis between acute attacks).

PROPHYLAXIS
- Colchicine can be used in patients with 3 or more attacks of Pseudogout annually.

JUVENILE IDIOPATHIC (RHEUMATOID) ARTHRITIS

- Autoimmune mono or polyarthritis in **children <16y** for **>6 weeks**.

THREE TYPES
- **Systemic (Still's disease): daily or diurnal high fever,** daily arthritis. **Salmon-colored pink migratory rash.** No iridocyclitis but associated with systemic symptoms (hepatosplenomegaly, lymphadenopathy). 20% of all cases.
- Pauci (oligo) articular: <5 **joints involved**. Most commonly affects medium to large joints (eg, knees, ankle). **Iridocyclitis (anterior uveitis).** 50% of all cases.
- Polyarticular: **5 or more small joints** (usually symmetric). **Most similar to adult RA** (including morning stiffness). **Iridocyclitis** (anterior uveitis). Worse prognosis if RF positive.

DIAGNOSIS
- Primarily a **clinical diagnosis.**
- Increased ESR & CRP. Positive ANA in oligoarticular. Increased ferritin. Rheumatoid factor positive in only 15%. Systemic (Still's) usually associated with negative RF & ANA.

MANAGEMENT
- **NSAIDs first-line therapy.** Glucocorticoids if no response to NSAIDS. Physical therapy.
- Second line or severe disease: Anakinra (intereukin-1 receptor inhibitor), Methotrexate, Leflunomide.
- ANA positivity associated with increased risk of Iridocyclitis so routine eye exam every 3 months is recommended.

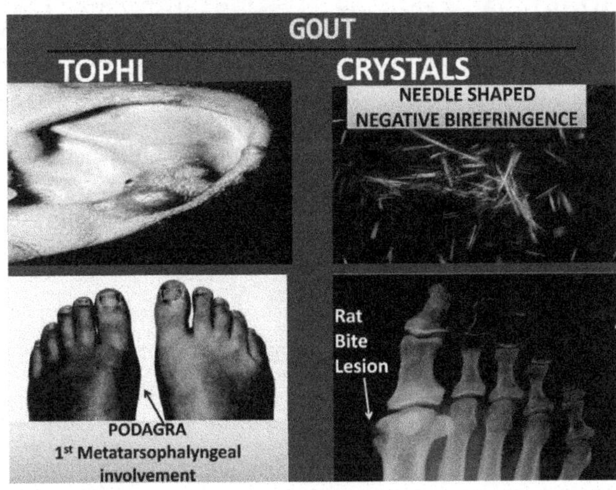

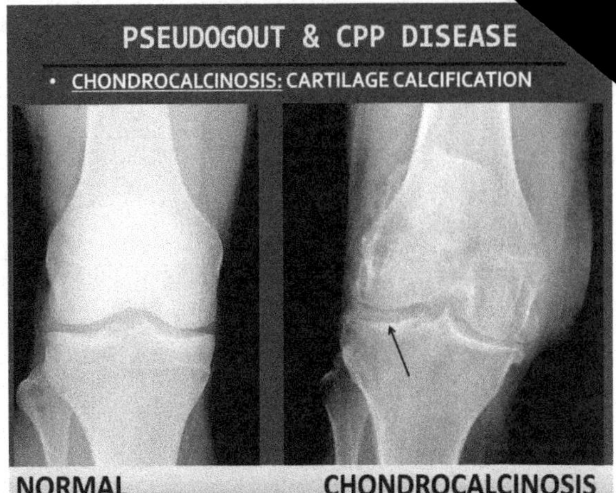

	GOUT	PSEUDOGOUT
PREVALENCE	• 17-20 per 1,000 individuals. • **Mostly adult men** Postmenopausal women.	• <1 per 1,000 individuals. • **Female predominance, elderly**
CRYSTAL CHEMISTRY	**Monosodium urate**	**Calcium pyrophosphate dihydrate**
SYNOVIAL FLUID CRYSTALS	NEGATIVELY BIREFRINGENT; NEEDLE-SHAPED.	WEAKLY POSITIVE; RHOMBOID-SHAPED.
MOST FREQUENTLY AFFECTED JOINTS	• **First MTP joint MC (Podagra)** 50% initially; 90% eventually. • **80% monoarticular typically lower extremities** (ankle, knees, foot)	• Knees, wrists, MCP joints, elbows, MTP.
RADIOGRAPH FINDINGS	• **"MOUSE BITE" (PUNCHED OUT) EROSIONS**	• **CHONDROCALCINOSIS** - calcification of the cartilage
THERAPEUTIC OPTIONS	**ACUTE ATTACKS:** • **NSAIDs 1st line, Colchicine** • Corticosteroids **CHRONIC MANAGEMENT:** • **Uric acid-lowering agents** Allopurinol, Febuxostat, Probenecid • Colchicine	**ACUTE ATTACKS:** • **Intraarticular steroids 1st line.** • **NSAIDs, Colchicine** **CHRONIC MANAGEMENT:** • **NSAIDs** • ± Colchicine

Note that the **medications used in the chronic management of gout are NOT initiated during an acute attack** (because it may precipitate an attack). Colchicine can be used for acute & chronic. Any acute increase OR decrease in serum uric acid levels can cause an acute attack. Note that measuring serum uric acid levels are generally not helpful to determine if the attack is due to gout.

ARTHOCENTESIS ANALYSIS OF FLUID

[illegible]	WBCs (/μL)	MICROSCOPIC	CULTURES
[illegible]	200		
[illegible]MATORY ARTHRITIS			
• GOUT	<50, 000 (mostly PMN)	• **Needle shaped crystals - negatively birefringent** • **Uric Acid Crystals**	Negative
• PSEUDOGOUT	<50, 000 (mostly PMN)	• **Rhomboid-shaped crystals- positively birefringent** • **Calcium Pyrophosphate crystals**	Negative
• REACTIVE ARTHRITIS & OTHER INFLAMMATORY ARTHRITIS	<50, 000 (mostly PMN) PMN = Polymorphonuclear neutrophils		Negative
SEPTIC ARTHRITIS	**≥50,000 (>90% PMNs)**	**Bacteria, Cloudy**	**Positive**

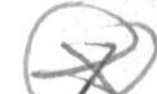

ANTIBODIES/AUTO ANTIBODIES	CLASSIC DISEASE ASSOCIATION
ACETYLCHOLINE RECEPTOR	Myasthenia Gravis
β-2 GLYCOPROTEIN 1	Antiphospholipid Antibody Syndrome (SLE)
CARDIOLIPIN	Antiphospholipid Antibody Syndrome (SLE)
CENTROMERE	CREST syndrome (Limited Systemic Sclerosis)
CYCLIC CITRULLINATED PEPTIDE (PROTEIN) – CCP	Specific for Rheumatoid Arthritis. Rheumatoid Factor used for screening but is not specific.
DOUBLE-STRANDED DNA	Systemic Lupus Erythematosus (*specific*, not sensitive)
ENDOMYSIAL	Celiac disease
GLOMERULAR BASEMENT MEMBRANE	Goodpasture's syndrome
HISTONE	Drug-induced Lupus
JO-1	Polymyositis, Dermatomyositis
LA (SS-B)	Sjögren syndrome
LUPUS ANTICOAGULANT	Antiphospholipid Antibody Syndrome (SLE)
Mi-2	Dermatomyositis
MITOCHONDRIAL	Primary Biliary Cirrhosis
MUSK (Muscle specific receptor tyrosine kinase)	Myasthenia Gravis - may be positive in AChR-negative patients with MG.
P-ANCA	Microscopic Polyangiitis (MPA), Churg Strauss Ulcerative Colitis, Primary Sclerosing Cholangitis
RHEUMATOID FACTOR	Rheumatoid Arthritis
RIBONUCLEOPROTEIN (RNP)	Mixed Connective Tissue disease, SLE
RO (SS-A)	Sjögren syndrome, Systemic Lupus Erythematosus
SACCHAROMYCES CEREVISIAE	Crohn disease
SCL-70 (TOPOISOMERASE)	Diffuse Systemic Sclerosis (Scleroderma)
SIGNAL RECOGNITION PROTEIN (SRP)	Polymyositis
SMITH	Systemic Lupus Erythematosus (*specific,* not sensitive)
SMOOTH MUSCLE	Autoimmune hepatitis
THYROGLOBULIN	Hashimoto's thyroiditis, Autoimmune thyroiditis
THYROID PEROXIDASE (TPO)	Hashimoto's thyroiditis, Autoimmune thyroiditis
TOPOISOMERASE (SCL-70)	Diffuse Systemic Sclerosis (Scleroderma)
TRANSGLUTAMINASE	Celiac disease, Dermatitis Herpetiformis
TSH (THYROTROPIN) RECEPTOR	Graves' disease
VOLTAGE-GATED CALCIUM CHANNEL	Lambert-Eaton Syndrome

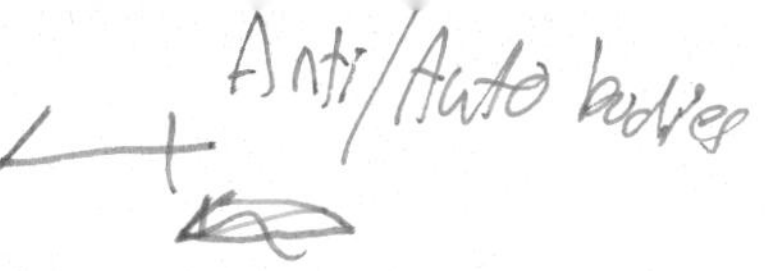

OSTEOPOROSIS

- **Loss of bone density (both mineral & matrix)** over time due to imbalance of increased bone resorption > formation of new bone (decreased). Osteopenia is a precursor to Osteoporosis.

PRIMARY
- **Postmenopausal & senile.**
- Risk factors: **Caucasians** > Asians > African-Americans, low BMI (**thin body habitus**), corticosteroid use, smoking, chronic kidney disease, alcohol, low calcium & vitamin D intake, physical inactivity.

SECONDARY
- Due to chronic disease or medications – hypogonadism, high cortisol states (eg, **Glucocorticoid use, Cushing's syndrome)**, Hyperthyroid states, Diabetes mellitus, low estrogen, malignancy, **Heparin, Phenytoin, Lithium, & Levothyroxine.**

CLINICAL MANIFESTATIONS
- Usually asymptomatic.
- Bone fractures: may develop pathologic fractures, back pain or deformity. **Pathologic fractures – vertebrae most common**, hip, distal radius.
- **Spine compression** - lumbar & thoracic. **Loss of vertebral height** (shortening of stature), kyphosis ("hunchback" bowing forward curvature of spine with forward thrust of head). **Back pain.**

DIAGNOSIS

DEXA scan (bone densitometry) **best diagnostic test.**

Normal = 1.0 or greater. T score compares bone density with the bone density of a young woman.

Osteopenia: T score -1.0 to -2.5

Osteoporosis: bone density T score -2.5 or less

Ancillary
- **Normal** serum calcium, phosphate, PTH, & alkaline phosphatase. Slight elevations of alkaline phosphatase may occur after acute fractures. Decreased Vitamin D; screen for thyroid, celiac disease.

MANAGEMENT
- Lifestyle modification: **Vitamin D** (eg, Ergocalciferol 800mg/IU) + **calcium supplementation initial therapy** (1500 mg/IU) & weightbearing exercise (weightlifting, high impact, resistance training, jogging, jumping, walking), smoking cessation, fall prevention. Periodic height & bone mass measurements.
- **Bisphosphonates: first-line medical management & prevention of Osteoporosis.** They inhibit osteoclast-mediated bone resorption & turnover. [See page 218 for details of Bisphosphonate therapy].
- Denosumab: option for initial therapy in certain patients with high risk for fracture intolerant or unresponsive to other therapies (including IV bisphosphonates). RANKL inhibitor.
- Teriparatide: anabolic recombinant human PTH analog that is an option in men or postmenopausal women with **severe** osteoporosis (T-score -3.5 or less even in the absence of fractures, or T-score of -2.5 or less + a fragility fracture).
- Raloxifene: SERM (selective estrogen receptor modifier) that inhibits bone resorption and reduces the risk of vertebral fractures in postmenopausal women. It has an additional benefit of breast cancer prophylaxis. May also be used to prevent Osteoporosis.
- Calcitonin usually used as last-line therapy because of its relatively weak effect on bone density, poor antifracture effects, and increased risk of cancer.

Screening:
- **DEXA scan in patients 65 years or older** (or anyone with the risk = that of a 65y Caucasian female).

DISORDERS OF THE BACK/SPINE

HERNIATED DISC (NUCLEUS PULPOSUS)

- **Most common at L5-S1** (because it is the junction between the mobile & non-mobile spine); L4-L5.

CLINICAL MANIFESTATIONS

- **Radicular back pain:** usually **unilateral,** may radiate down the leg with paresthesias or numbness in a **dermatomal pattern.** Pain may increase with coughing, straining, bending, sitting, & Valsalva.

PHYSICAL EXAMINATION

- **Positive straight leg raise**, crossover test.

	L4	L5	S1
Sensory "ALP"	• **ANTERIOR** thigh pain. • Sensory loss to the medial ankle.	• **LATERAL thigh/leg, hip groin** paresthesias & pain. • **Dorsum of the foot:** especially between 1st & 2nd toes.	• **POSTERIOR leg/calf,** gluteus. • **Plantar surface of the foot.**
Weakness	• **ANKLE DORSIFLEXION**	• **BIG TOE EXTENSION (big toe dorsiflexion).** • Walking on heels more difficult than on toes.	• **PLANTAR FLEXION** • Walking on toes more difficult than on heels.
Reflex Diminished	• **LOSS OF KNEE JERK.** • Weak knee extension – quads).	Reflexes usually normal. ± loss of ankle jerk.	• **LOSS OF ANKLE JERK.**

DIAGNOSIS

- Radiographs: loss of disc height, loss of lordosis due to spasm, degenerative changes.

- **MRI:** diagnostic test of choice for suspected herniation, persistent pain or refractory pain.

MANAGEMENT

- **Conservative: preferred initial management - NSAIDs + continuation of ordinary activities as tolerated**. If bed rest is advised, it should be brief. Physical therapy. Muscle relaxers or oral steroid taper in select patients.

- Corticosteroid injection: second line if refractory to first-line therapy (eg, epidural). Usually performed after MRI confirmation of disc disease.

- Operative: laminectomy & discectomy if persistent disabling pain >6 weeks not responding to nonoperative options or evidence of cauda equina syndrome.

CAUDA EQUINA SYNDROME

- Constellation of symptoms as a result of terminal spinal nerve compression in the lumbosacral region.
- Massive central herniation compresses several nerve roots of the cauda equina.
- **Considered a neurosurgical emergency.**

ETIOLOGIES
- **Lumbar disc herniation most common.**
- Spinal stenosis, trauma, tumors, epidural abscess, epidural hematoma, & vertebral fractures.

CLINICAL MANIFESTATIONS

Back pain plus any one of the following:
- Radiculopathy: **bilateral leg radiation of pain** and weakness in multiple root distributions (L3-S1). May be unilateral.

Involvement of S2-S4 spinal nerve roots
- **Saddle anesthesia** - decreased sensation to the buttocks, perineum, and inner surfaces of the thigh. Erectile dysfunction.
- New onset of **urinary or bowel retention or incontinence.**
- **Decreased anal sphincter tone** on physical examination (decreased anal wink test).

DIAGNOSIS
- **MRI: study of choice**.
- CT myelography if unable to perform MRI (eg, pacemaker).

MANAGEMENT
- **Emergent decompression** (considered a neurosurgical emergency).
- Corticosteroids to reduce inflammation.

VERTEBRAL COMPRESSION FRACTURE

- "Burst" fractures occur in children from jumping/fall from height.
- Pathologic lumbar compression fractures may occur in the **elderly** (eg, osteoporosis), **malignancy** (eg, Multiple myeloma, Prostate cancer), or systemic illness.

CLINICAL MANIFESTATIONS
- **Localized back pain with focal midline tenderness** at the level of fracture.
- Nerve root deficits may be present in the presence of retropulsed bone fragments in the spinal canal.

DIAGNOSIS
- Radiographs: loss of vertebral height.
- MRI or CT usually not necessary but may provide additional information. Imaging indicated if neurologic deficits are present.

MANAGEMENT
- Orthopedic & neurosurgery consult to determine appropriate workup & management.
- Conservative: observation, analgesics, bracing with gradual return to activity.
- Surgical: kyphoplasty may be used if symptoms are severe or persistent.

LUMBAR SPINAL STENOSIS (Pseudoclaudication) (Neurogenic)

- **Narrowing of the spinal canal** with impingement of the nerve roots.

- Etiologies: **degenerative arthritis or Spondylolysis most common - especially >60y,** post-surgical, congenital, traumatic, inflammatory.

CLINICAL MANIFESTATIONS

- **Back pain, numbness & paresthesias** that may radiate to buttocks & thighs bilaterally. The symptoms are:
  - **worsened with extension:** prolonged standing, walking upright, walking downhill.
  - **relieved with flexion: sitting, leaning over a shopping cart, walking uphill, cycling** (unlike claudication). Lumbar flexion increases the canal volume.

- Not worsened with Valsalva (as is the case with a herniated disc).

DIAGNOSIS

- **MRI: test of choice**

- Radiographs: nonspecific degenerative changes. CT myelogram

MANAGEMENT

- **Conservative:** pain control, physical therapy (ex. cycling, swimming), **lumbar corticosteroid injections** (epidural or foraminal) may reduce the need for surgical intervention.

- Surgical management for severe or refractory cases (eg, decompression laminectomy).

LUMBOSACRAL SPRAIN OR STRAIN

- Acute strain or tear of the paraspinal muscles, especially after twisting or lifting injuries.
- Most common cause of lower back pain.

CLINICAL MANIFESTATIONS

- **Back pain & muscle spasms** that is activity-related, **does not radiate to the leg and is not associated with neurological symptoms**. May develop stiffness & difficulty bending.

- Physical examination: decreased ROM, **paraspinal muscle tenderness** may be present, **no neurological changes.**

DIAGNOSIS

- Clinical. Radiographs are not needed unless symptoms are persistent or alarm symptoms are present.

MANAGEMENT

- **Analgesics** (eg, **NSAIDs**) **& resumption of ordinary activity is preferred**.

- BRIEF bed rest (maximum 2 days) may be indicated if moderate pain.

- Muscle relaxers may help with spasm in some cases.

SPINAL EPIDURAL ABSCESS

- Pus-filled collection often associated with Osteomyelitis & Discitis. The abscess can expand, compressing the brain or the spinal cord.
- Posterior most common type.

ETIOLOGIES
- ***Staphylococcus aureus* most common** (60%), gram-negatives (eg, *E. coli*), *Streptococci,* coagulase-negative *Staphylococci*. *Mycobacterium tuberculosis* in the developing world.

RISK FACTORS
- >50y, **IV drug abuse, immunodeficiency** (eg, diabetes, HIV, immunosuppressive medications – corticosteroids), recent spinal procedure, epidural catheter placement.

CLINICAL MANIFESTATIONS
- The classic triad for epidural abscess is **fever + spinal pain + neurologic deficits**.
- Back pain: usually **focal & severe** (most common symptom).
- **Radiculopathy** (nerve root pain).
- **Myelopathy (neurologic deficits)** - motor, sensory, bowel or bladder dysfunction. Paralysis is associated with increased risk of irreversibility.

DIAGNOSIS
- **MRI with gadolinium: test of choice** – will reveal a ring-enhancing lesion. Radiographs are usually normal. CT scan may be used if MRI is contraindicated.
- Inflammatory markers: increased ESR, CRP. May have an elevated WBC count.

MANAGEMENT
- Primary goals are elimination or reduction of the inflammatory mass & treatment of the organism.
- **Aspiration, drainage, & antibiotics:** eg, decompression laminectomy & drainage usually indicated if neurologic deficits, large abscess, or spinal instability.
- **Antibiotics: Vancomycin PLUS either Cefotaxime or Ceftriaxone**. Cefepime or Ceftazidime if *Pseudomonas aeruginosa* is suspected.
- IV Corticosteroids may be used in some cases to control the acute neurologic deficits.
- Conservative (nonsurgical): systemic antibiotics alone may be used in selected patients (eg, no neurologic deficits, patient not a surgical candidate due to medical comorbidities).

SPINAL CORD COMPRESSION

- External compression of the spinal cord (eg, due to **malignancy or infection).**
- A neurologic emergency.

CLINICAL MANIFESTATIONS
- **Sudden onset of focal neurologic deficits** (eg, at a sensory level), hyperreflexia below the level of compression.

DIAGNOSIS: MRI test of choice

MANAGEMENT
- Systemic glucocorticoids for acute neurologic symptoms, management of the underlying cause.
- Surgical decompression if not responsive to initial management.

SCOLIOSIS

- **Lateral curvature of the spine**.
- May be associated with **kyphosis** (humpback) **or lordosis** (sway back).
- Most common in girls & positive family history.
- Adolescent idiopathic: Cobb angle ≥ 10 degrees, age of onset at least 10 years, & no underlying etiology (eg, neuromuscular, congenital).

SCREENING
- **Adams forward bend test: most sensitive physical finding.** Thoracic or lumbar prominence on one side is seen with Scoliosis.
- Scoliometer: a 7-degree curve is considered abnormal.
- Forward bending sitting test.
- Assessment includes leg length, waistline asymmetry, midline skin defects, cafe-au-lait spots, foot deformities, and abdominal reflex asymmetry.

CONFIRMATORY
- **Radiographs - Cobb's angle ≥ 10 degrees** measured on AP & lateral films.
- MRI: not part of the initial evaluation without red flags or abnormal curve types. MRI may be indicated if rapid curve progression, left thoracic curve, abnormal reflexes, excessive kyphosis, or foot abnormalities.

MANAGEMENT
Based on skeletal maturity of the patient, severity of the deformity, & curve progression.
- **Observation:** Cobb angle <25 degrees: & Risser grade 0 to 2 at time of presentation. Regular follow up to monitor progression every 6-9 months. Bracing may be recommended if the Cobb angle increases 5 degrees or more over a 3 to 6-month period.
- **Bracing** may be needed **to stop progression** in patients with a flexible deformity & still skeletally immature: 1) if the Cobb angle increases 5 degrees or more over a 3 to 6-month period or 2) some patients with Cobb angle of 30 – 39 degrees.
- Bracing is contraindicated if skeletally mature, little growth remaining, Cobb angle ≥ 50 degrees or < 20 degrees.
- Surgical correction may be an alternative to bracing if > 40 degrees & Risser grade 0 to 2 (skeletally immature).

THORACIC OUTLET SYNDROME

- **Idiopathic compression of the brachial plexus** (most common)**, subclavian vein, or subclavian artery** as they exit the narrowed space between shoulder girdle & first rib.
- Most common in women 20-50y.

CLINICAL MANIFESTATIONS
- Nerve compression: **ulnar neuropathy,** pain or paresthesia to the forearm or arm.
- Vascular compression: swelling and/or discoloration of the arm **especially with abduction of the arm** (erythema, edema or cyanosis of affected arm)**.**

PHYSICAL EXAMINATION
- **Positive Adson sign - loss of the radial pulse with head rotated to affected side.** Confirmed with MRI.

MANAGEMENT
- Controversial. Physical therapy first line, avoid strenuous activity. Orthopedic consult, surgery.

SPONDYLOLYSIS

- **Pars interarticularis defect** due to **failure of fusion or stress fracture**. Most common at **L5-S1.**

MECHANISM
- Often from repetitive hyperextension trauma (eg, football players, gymnasts, weight lifters).
- Often the first step to Spondylolisthesis (forward slipping of a vertebra on another).

CLINICAL MANIFESTATIONS
- Most cases are asymptomatic.
- **Low back pain with activity.** Most common form of back pain in children & adolescents. May develop hamstring tightness, sciatica.

DIAGNOSIS
- Lateral radiographs: lateral view - **radiolucent defect in pars**.
- Oblique radiographs: the normal appearance of the lumbar spine has been described to resemble a **scotty dog**. If spondylolysis is present, the pars interarticularis (neck of the scotty dog) will have a defect or break (looks like a collar around the neck). CT scan. Bone scan.

MANAGEMENT
- Low-grade or asymptomatic: observation with no activity limitations if asymptomatic & low grade.
- Symptomatic: physical therapy & activity restriction in some patients.
- Bracing may be helpful for acute pars stress reaction or if failed physical therapy.

SPONDYLOLISTHESIS

- **Forward slipping of a vertebra on another** - bilateral fracture or defect of the pars interarticularis.
- Mechanism: usually a **complication of Spondylolysis**.

CLINICAL MANIFESTATIONS
- Most cases are asymptomatic. **Lower back pain most common symptom**.
- Nerve compression: sciatica. Bowel or bladder dysfunction and neurologic deficits if severe.

DIAGNOSIS
- Radiographs: **forward slipping of a vertebra.** Lateral views used to measure slip angle and grade. Flexion & extension views can help to evaluate stability.
- MRI: indicated if neurologic symptoms are present to assess for stenosis or complications.

MANAGEMENT
- Mild: treated like spondylolysis - physical therapy & activity restriction in some symptomatic patients.
- Severe cases may need surgical intervention

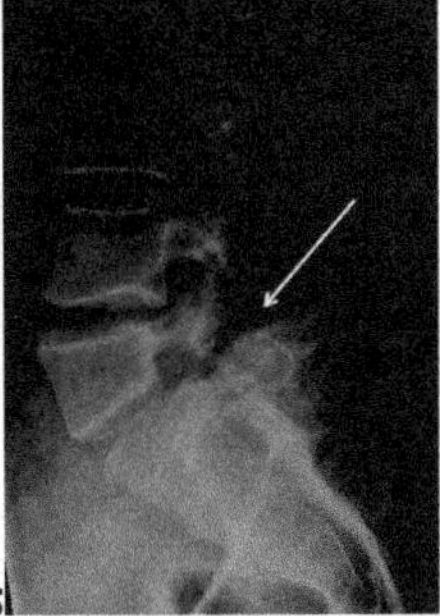
Spondylolysis

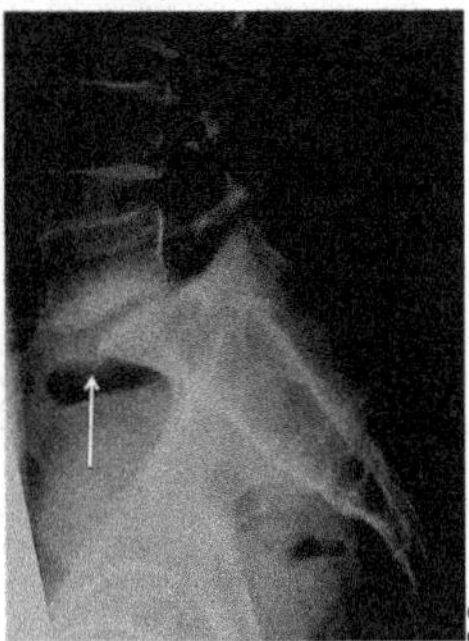
Spondylolisthesis

SHOULDER INJURIES

ANTERIOR GLENOHUMERAL DISLOCATION

- Mechanism: most common after a blow to an abducted, externally rotated, and extended extremity; fall on an outstretched hand (FOOSH), or posterior humeral force.
- Anterior is the most common type of shoulder dislocation.

PHYSICAL EXAMINATION
- Arm held in **abduction & external rotation** (elbow pointing outward).
- Humeral head is often palpable inferiorly with loss of the deltoid contour or **"squared off shoulder".**

DIAGNOSIS
- Shoulder radiographs: usually the initial test of choice. Axillary & scapular "Y" views most helpful in distinguishing anterior from posterior dislocations.
  - Hill sach lesion: groove fracture of the humerus. Bankart lesion: glenoid rim fracture.
- CT or MRI: gives more details about associated soft tissue injuries.

MANAGEMENT
- Reduction & immobilization. **Check deltoid pinprick sensation for axillary nerve injury** pre- and post-reduction. Physical therapy.
- Complications include injuries to the **axillary nerve (most common),** axillary artery, brachial plexus, suprascapular nerve & radial nerve. Neurovascular examination done pre and post reduction.

POSTERIOR GLENOHUMERAL SHOULDER DISLOCATION

- Mechanism: forced adduction, internal rotation.
- **Most commonly associated with seizures, electric shock,** or trauma.

PHYSICAL EXAMINATION
- Arm is usually **adducted & internally rotated.**
- The anterior shoulder appears flat with a prominent humeral head.

DIAGNOSIS
- Shoulder radiographs: **initial test. Scapular "Y" & Axillary lateral views best to distinguish anterior vs. posterior.** AP films may show the "**light bulb" sign** (the appearance of the humeral head looks like a light bulb or ice cream cone).
- CT or MRI may be used to assess for complications.

MANAGEMENT
- Reduction & immobilization. Neurovascular compromise is uncommon.
- Glenolabral and capsular injuries may lead to posterior shoulder instability.

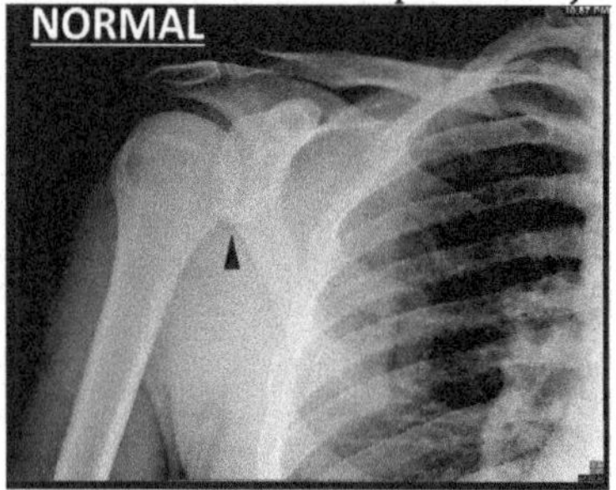

NORMAL AP: humeral head articulates with glenoid (arrowhead). Appears overlapped.

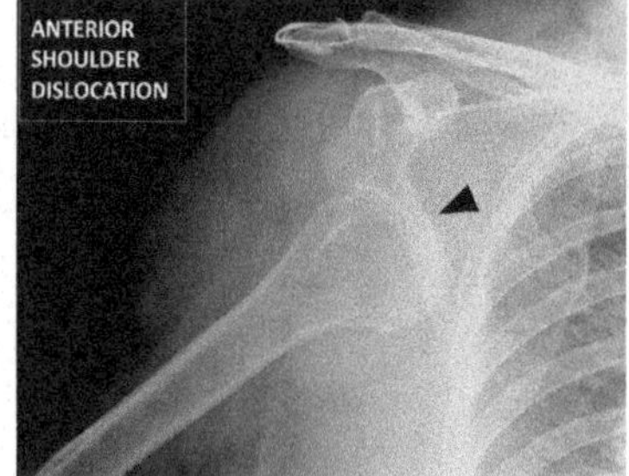

ANTERIOR DISLOCATION: Humeral head **anterior & inferior to glenoid**

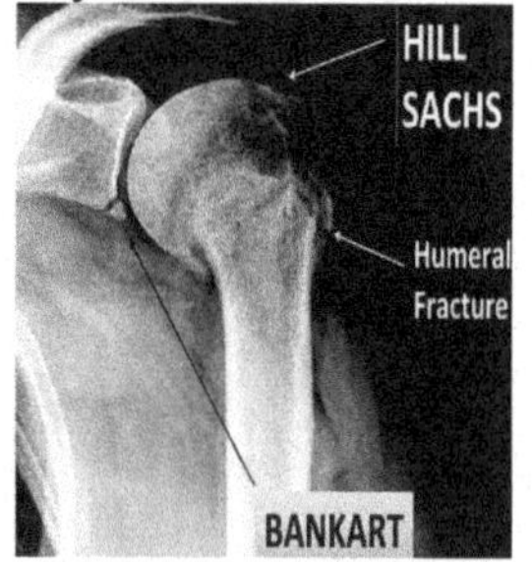

HILL-SACHS: Humeral head groove
BANKART: fracture of glenoid rim

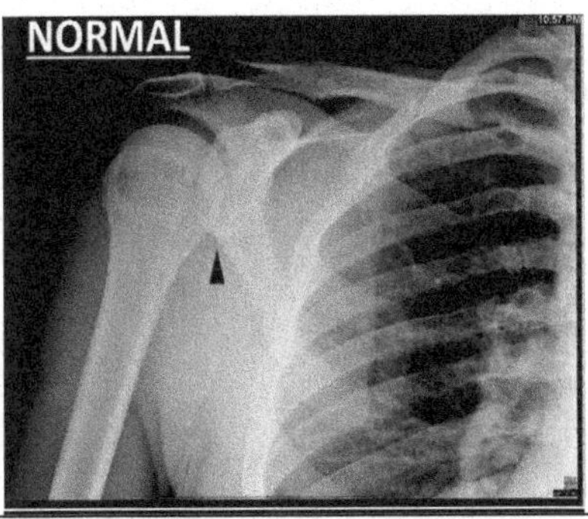

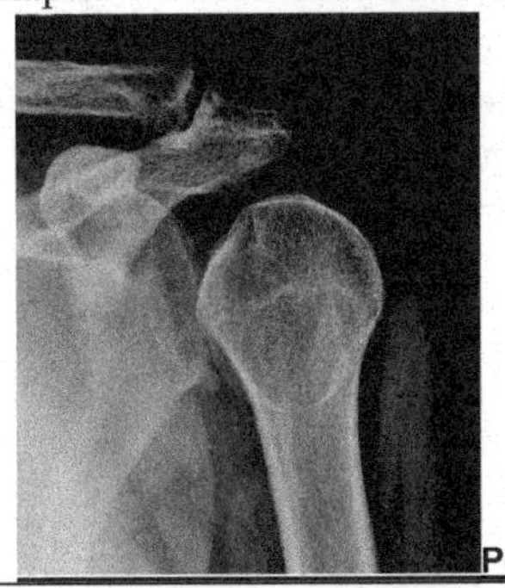
Posterior

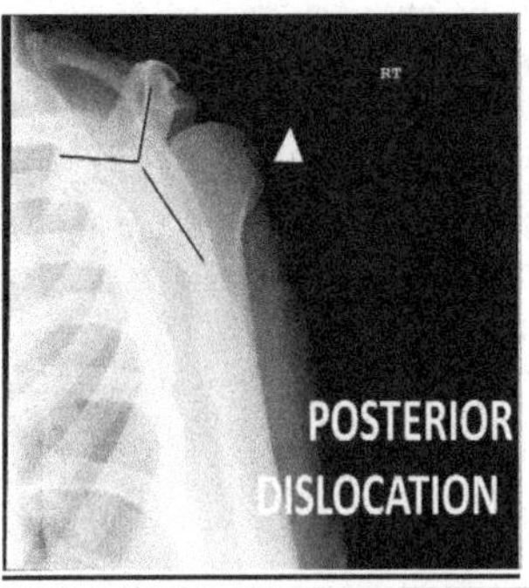

The humeral head may be rotated (ice cream on cone/light bulb appearance) and isn't centered on the glenoid. May look normal on AP view, or may show increased distance from the glenoid rim (normally there is overlap between glenoid rim & the humeral head).

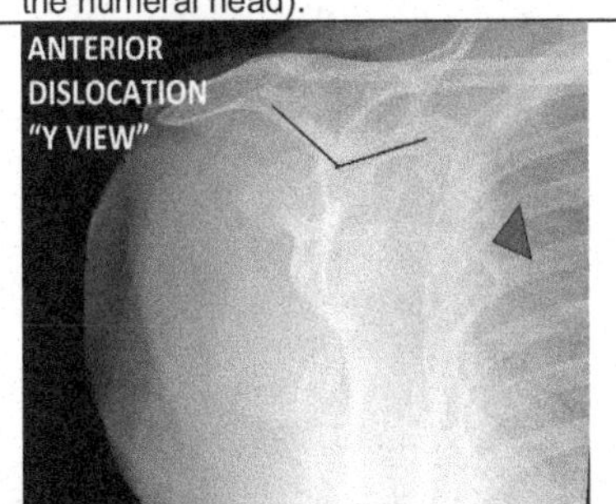

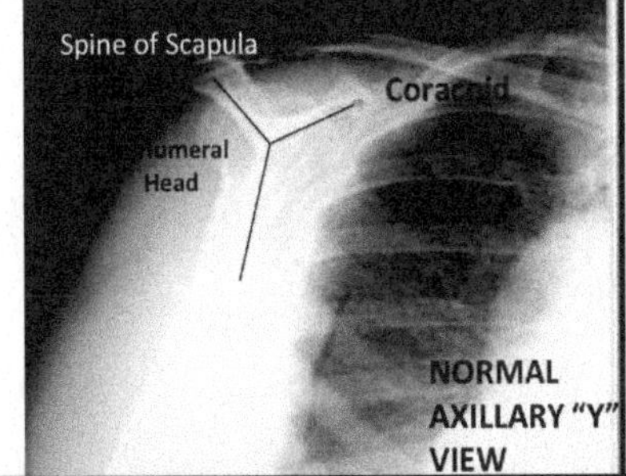

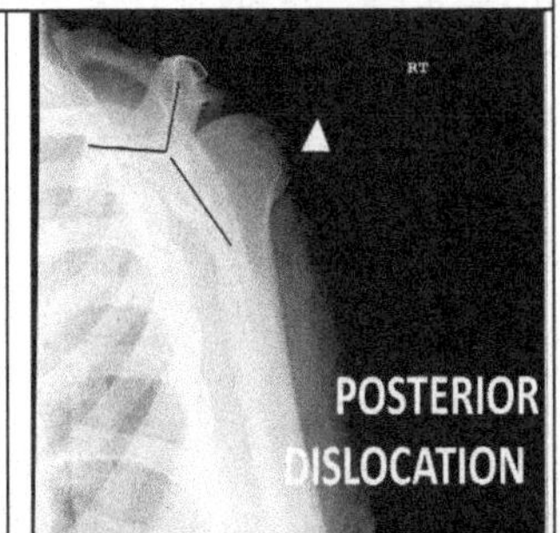

ACROMIOCLAVICULAR JOINT DISLOCATION "shoulder separation"

- Mechanism: Direct blow to an adducted shoulder.
- Physiology: the acromioclavicular ligament provides horizontal stability. The coracoclavicular ligament provides vertical stability.

CLINICAL MANIFESTATIONS

- Pain with lifting arm, unable to lift the arm at the shoulder.
- There may be a deformity (step-off) at the AC joint.

DIAGNOSIS

- Radiographs taken without weights or with weights to reveal mild separations. Both shoulders may be visualized to compare the separation.

MANAGEMENT

- Nonoperative: in most Type I, type II, & most type III. Conservative management includes ice, brief sling immobilization, & rest. Early rehabilitation for ROM preservation.
- Surgical: Type IV and above with < 2cm clavicular displacement & some patients with Type III (eg, athletes, cosmetic concerns).

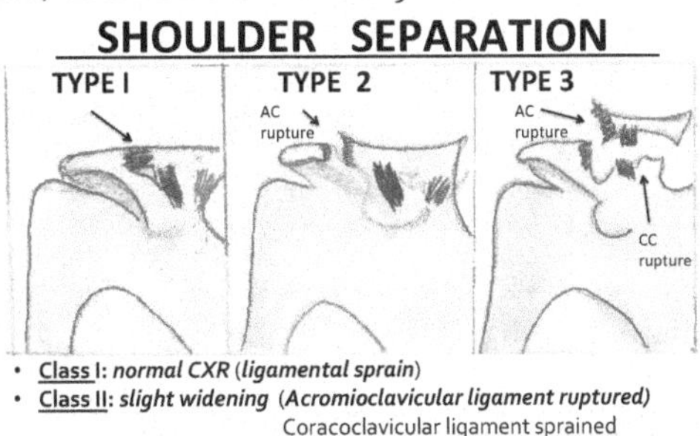

- Class I: *normal CXR (ligamental sprain)*
- Class II: *slight widening (Acromioclavicular ligament ruptured)* Coracoclavicular ligament sprained
- Class III: *significant widening: rupture of both AC & CC ligaments*
- Class IV: AC & CC rupture + displacement of clavicle into/through trapezius
- Class V: Class IV + disruption of the clavicular attachments

GRADE 2 SHOULDER SEPARATION

- Acromioclavicular (AC) ligament RUPTURED
- Coracoclavicular (CC) ligament sprained

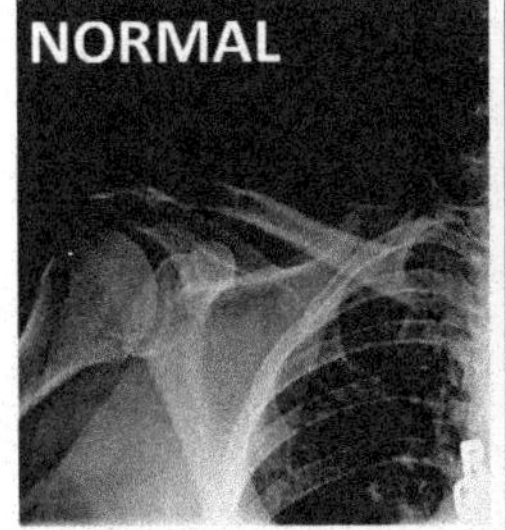

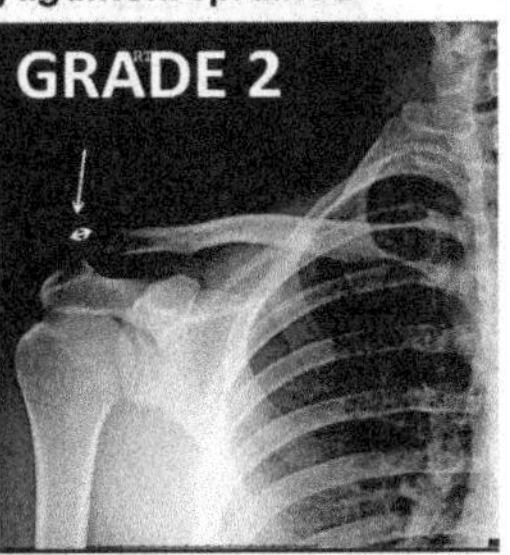

ROTATOR CUFF INJURIES

- Mechanism: chronic erosion, trauma. Impingement of the supraspinatus tendon.
- Common in athletes or laborers performing **repetitive overhead movements**, older age, smoking.
- **SITS (supraspinatus,** infraspinatus, teres minor, subscapularis).
  Supraspinatus is the most commonly injured muscle.

TENDONITIS
- Inflammation usually associated with subacromial bursitis: Most common in adolescents & <40 years.

ROTATOR CUFF TEAR
- Most common cause of shoulder pain **>40 years of age.** Trauma (50%) or chronic overuse.

CLINICAL MANIFESTATIONS:
- **Anterolateral shoulder (deltoid) pain** with decreased range of motion (ROM).
- **Decreased ROM especially with overhead activities, external rotation or abduction** (combing hair, reaching for wallet), inability to sleep on the affected side (especially with tears).
- Passive ROM greater than active.
- Weakness, atrophy, & continuous pain most commonly seen with tears.

PHYSICAL EXAMINATION:
- **Supraspinatus strength test:** the "empty can" test has **90% specificity for assessing supraspinatus involvement.**
- Impingement tests: positive Hawkins test, Drop arm test and Neer test.
  - ⊕ **Hawkins test**: Elbow/shoulder flexed @90° with **sharp anterior shoulder pain with internal rotation.**
  - ⊕ **Drop arm test:** pain with inability to lift arm above shoulder level or hold it or severe pain when slowly lowering the arm after the shoulder is abducted to 90°.
  - ⊕ **Neer test:** arm fully pronated (thumbs down) with pain during forward flexion (while shoulder is held down to prevent shrugging).
  - Supraspinatus test: pain with abduction against resistance.
- Subacromial lidocaine test: may help to distinguish tendinopathy from tears. Normal strength with pain relief = tendinopathy. Persistent weakness classically seen with large tears.

MANAGEMENT OF TEARS
- **Conservative:** physical therapy for rehab & NSAIDs for pain management. Intraarticular corticosteroids usually reserved for patients who fail NSAID management of pain.
- Surgery: patients who fail conservative management within 6 months or patients with complete tears.

MANAGEMENT OF TENDINITIS
- **Shoulder pendulum or wall climbing exercises**, ice, NSAIDs, stop offending activity.

ROTATOR CUFF INJURIES

PHYSICAL EXAMINATION

Impingement of subscapular nerve/supraspinatus between acromial process & humeral head:

- *⊕Hawkins test**: Elbow/shoulder flexed @90° c sharp anterior shoulder pain on passive internal rotation of humerus

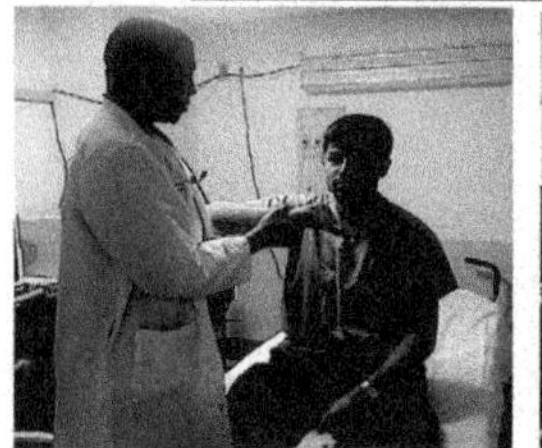
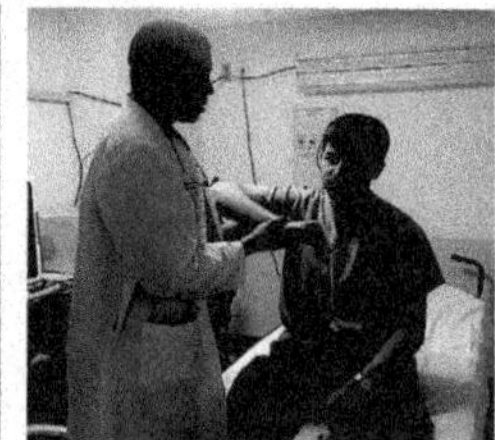

ROTATOR CUFF INJURIES

PHYSICAL EXAMINATION

Impingement of subscapular nerve/supraspinatus between acromial process & humeral head:

- *⊕ Neer test: arm fully pronated (thumb's down) c pain during forward flexion* (shoulder is held down to prevent shrugging)

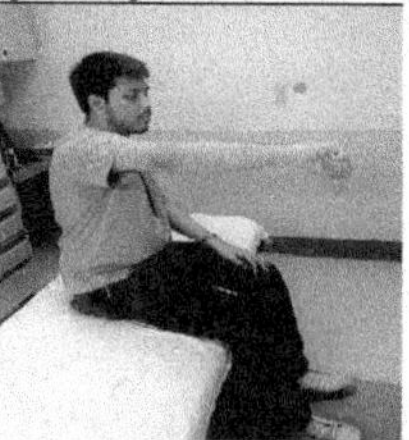
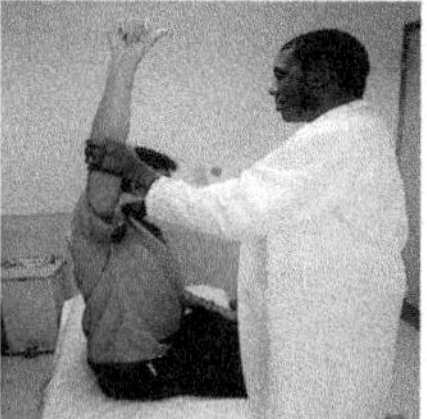

PROXIMAL HUMERUS/HUMERAL HEAD FRACTURES

- Mechanism: FOOSH, direct blow. Common site for pathologic fractures in metastatic breast cancer.
- Physical examination: arm held in adducted position. Decreased ROM, pain, swelling, & ecchymosis.

DIAGNOSIS
- Shoulder radiographs usually the initial test.
- CT scan: may be used to further evaluate (eg, preoperative planning). MRI

MANAGEMENT
- Sling immobilization, analgesics, & physical therapy for rehab for most fractures. Surgical for some.

HUMERAL SHAFT FRACTURES

MECHANISM
- Fall on an outstretched hand (FOOSH), direct trauma.

PHYSICAL EXAMINATION
- Pain & swelling to the arm, ecchymosis, decreased ROM. Must **rule out radial nerve injury.**

MANAGEMENT
- Nonoperative: coaptation splint or sling & swathe with prompt orthopedic follow up.
- Operative: ORIF for open fractures, vascular or brachial plexus injuries with pain and weakness.

PROXIMAL HUMERUS FRACTURE

arm usually held in adducted position.

Check deltoid sensation*, brachial plexus injury

± crepitus/ecchymosis

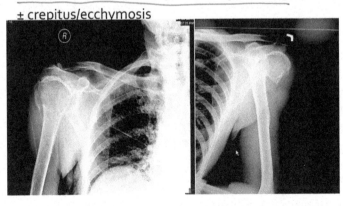

HUMERAL SHAFT FRACTURE

- MOI: FOOSH, direct trauma.
- *R/o radial nerve injury (may develop a wrist drop)**

NORMAL PATH OF RADIAL NERVE

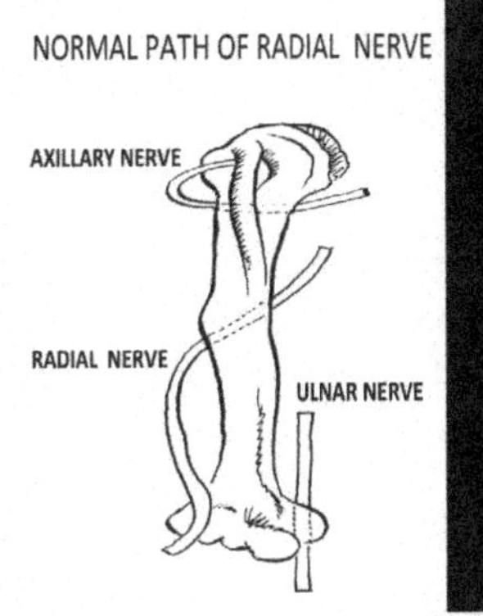

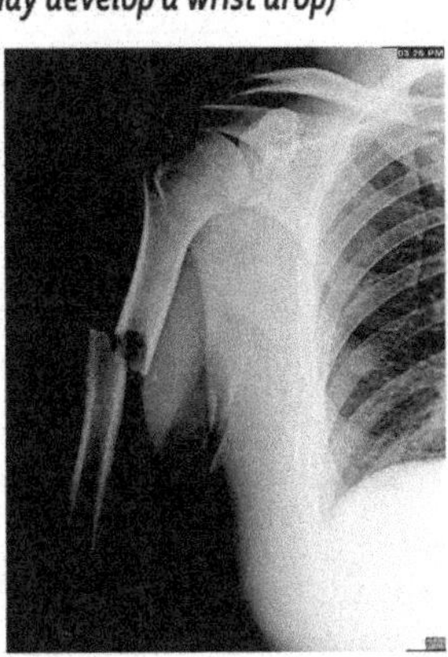

ADHESIVE CAPSULITIS (FROZEN SHOULDER)

- **Shoulder stiffness** due to inflammation (especially with **Diabetes mellitus & Hypothyroidism**). Also known as **"frozen shoulder".** Most common in 40s – 60s.

CLINICAL MANIFESTATIONS
- **Shoulder pain/stiffness**, decreased **ROM (especially with external rotation).** Stiff-pain cycle. Pain is usually worse at night.
- Associated with a gradual return of range of motion (may last 18-24 months).
- Physical Examination: resistance on passive range of motion (ROM) only on the affected side.

MANAGEMENT
- Rehab ROM therapy is the mainstay of treatment.
- Anti-inflammatories, intraarticular steroid injection & heat may be helpful.

CLAVICLE FRACTURES

- **Most commonly fractured bone in children, adolescents, & newborns during birth.**
- Most commonly seen in males.

CLASSIFICATION:
- **Group I (midshaft) middle 1/3 (most common).**
- Group II: lateral (distal) third.
- Group III: proximal (medial) third.

MECHANISM
- Mid-high energy impact to the area or fall on an outstretched hand (FOOSH).
- If no history of trauma, think malignancy, rickets, or child abuse (especially in children < 2 years of age).

PHYSICAL EXAMINATION
- Pain with ROM, deformity at the site, may have tenting of the skin (impending open fracture), & crepitus. May hold arm against the chest to protect against motion.

MANAGEMENT
- Mid 1/3: **Nonoperative: sling immobilization** in most adults. Sling or figure-of-eight splint in children. Operative: indicated for open fractures, displaced fractures with skin tenting, subclavian artery of vein injuries, severe displacement, or shortening.
- Proximal 1/3: orthopedic consult.

COMPLICATIONS
- Pneumothorax, hemothorax, coracoclavicular ligament disruption (distal), brachial plexus injuries.

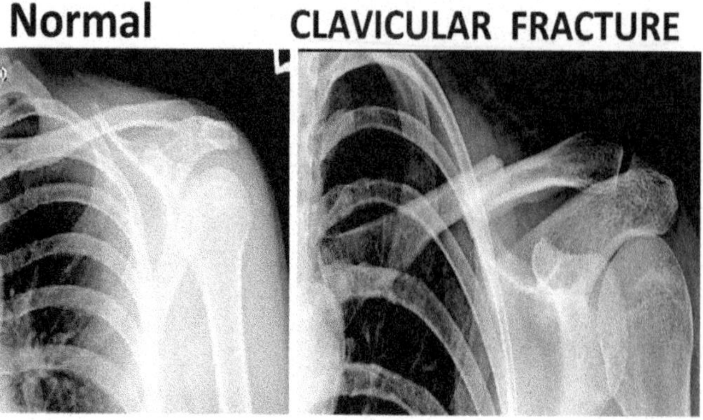

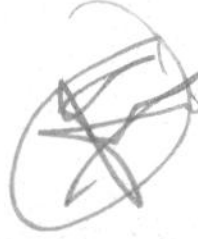

ELBOW & FOREARM INJURIES

SUPRACONDYLAR HUMERUS FRACTURES

- Mechanism: fall on outstretched hand (FOOSH) with hyperextended elbow.
- Most common in children 5-10y.
- Clinical manifestations: swelling & tenderness at the elbow, decreased ROM.

DIAGNOSIS
- Displaced: abnormal anterior humeral line may be seen on the lateral radiographs.
- Nondisplaced: **displaced anterior fat pad sign or posterior fat pad sign** (hemarthrosis) is suggestive of fracture.

COMPLICATIONS
- **Median nerve & brachial artery injury may lead to Volkmann ischemic contracture** (claw-like deformity from ischemia with flexion/contracture of wrist).
- **Radial nerve injury.**

MANAGEMENT
- Nondisplaced: long arm posterior splint followed by long arm casting.
- Displaced: closed reduction & pinning. All displaced fractures or severe swelling should be admitted for observation (immediate orthopedic consult).

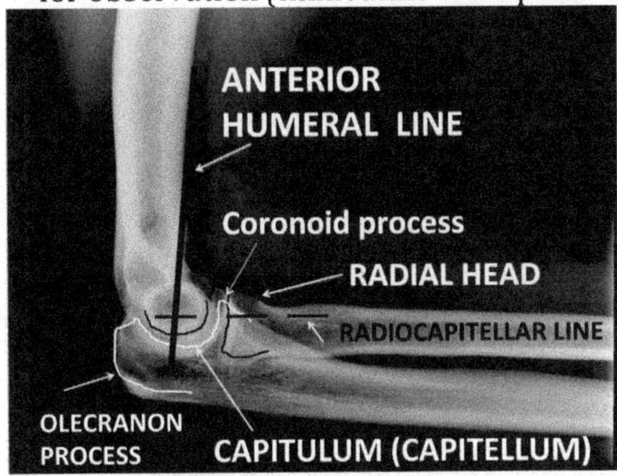

NORMAL LATERAL VIEW: the radial head dissects the capitellum. A line drawn from the anterior humerus should also dissect the capitellum.

SUPRACONDYLAR FRACTURE

DIAGNOSIS

• *Abnormal anterior humeral line on lateral view*

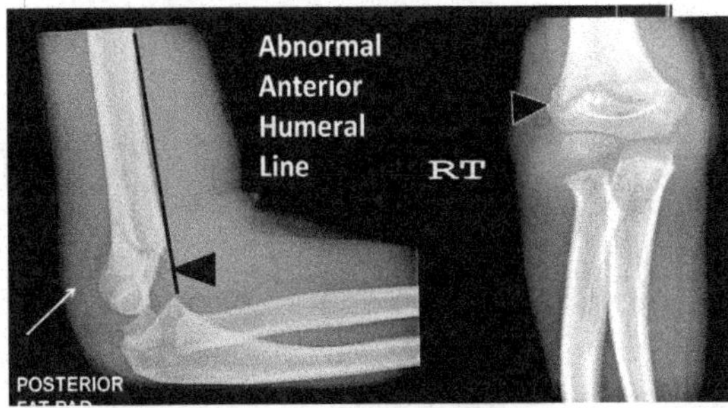

SUPRACONDYLAR FRACTURE: abnormal anterior humeral line (does not dissect the capitellum). Note the posterior fat pad sign. The fracture site is easily visible on the AP film (arrowhead)

SUPRACONDYLAR FRACTURE

DIAGNOSIS

• ⊕ Anterior or Posterior fat pad sign (hemarthrosis)

Normal SUPRACONDYLAR FRACTURE

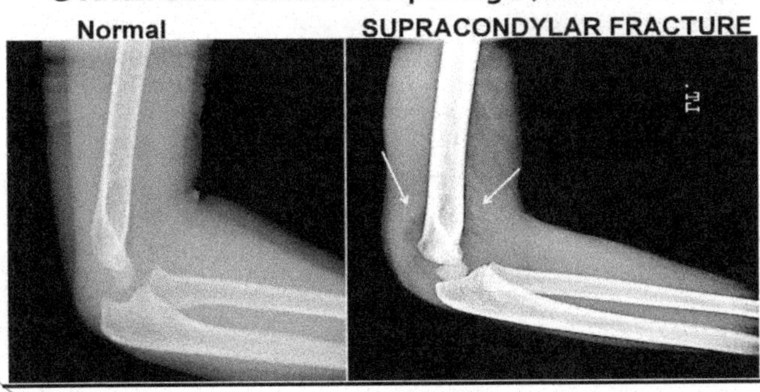

SUPRACONDYLAR FRACTURE:

Sometimes there is a normal anterior humeral line and the only clue is an abnormal anterior or ⊕ posterior fat pad (joint effusion).

Posterior fat pads are always abnormal.

Anterior fat pads may be seen as a normal variant if they are small and almost parallel to the humerus.

Anterior/posterior fad pad = supracondylar fracture in children (= radial head fracture in adults).

RADIAL HEAD FRACTURES

- Mechanism: fall on outstretched hand (FOOSH). Usually intraarticular.
- Physical examination: lateral (radial) elbow pain, **inability to fully extend the elbow.**

DIAGNOSIS
- Notoriously difficult to see.
- **Positive posterior or displaced anterior fat pad sign** (hemarthrosis) may be only radiologic evidence of occult fractures.

MANAGEMENT
- Nondisplaced: immobilization (eg, sling or long arm splint 90 degrees) with early ROM.
- Displaced: surgical (eg, ORIF).

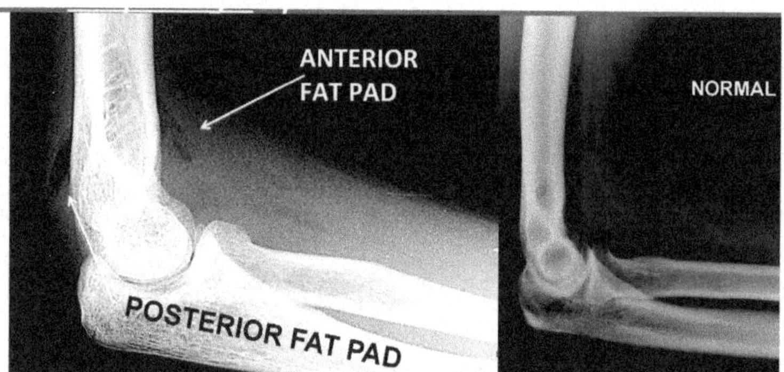

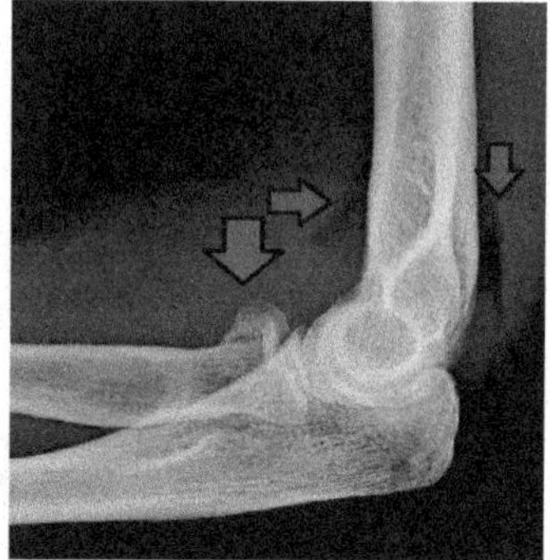

Photo credit: James Heilman, MD, *Wikimedia commons*

SUPPURATIVE FLEXOR TENOSYNOVITIS

- Infection of the flexor tendon synovial sheath of the finger.
- ***Staphylococcus aureus* most common**. *Staphylococcus epidermis*, group A *Streptococcus*; Others: Pseudomonas or mixed flora.
- Mechanism: often due to penetrating trauma or contiguous spread from adjacent tissues.

CLINICAL MANIFESTATIONS
- Pain & swelling especially to the palmar aspect of the affected finger.
- **Kanavel's signs (4): FLEX**or tenosynovitis
- **Finger held in flexion.**
- **Length of tendon sheath is tender** (tenderness along the tendon sheath).
- **Enlarged finger** (fusiform swelling of the finger).
- **Xtension of the finger causes pain** (**pain with passive extension**).

DIAGNOSIS
- Radiographs & MRI are often obtained but definitive diagnosis is via aspiration &/or biopsy.

MANAGEMENT
- Incision & drainage with irrigation of the tendon sheath, debridement & IV antibiotics.

OLECRANON FRACTURES

- Mechanism: direct blow (fall on a flexed elbow).

CLINICAL MANIFESTATIONS
- Pain, swelling, **inability to fully extend the elbow.**

COMPLICATIONS
- **Ulnar neuropathy**, posttraumatic arthritis, anterior interosseous nerve injury, & loss of extension strength.

MANAGEMENT
- Nondisplaced: reduction and posterior long arm splint (90 degrees flexion). All are considered intraarticular and need reduction.
- Displaced: ORIF.

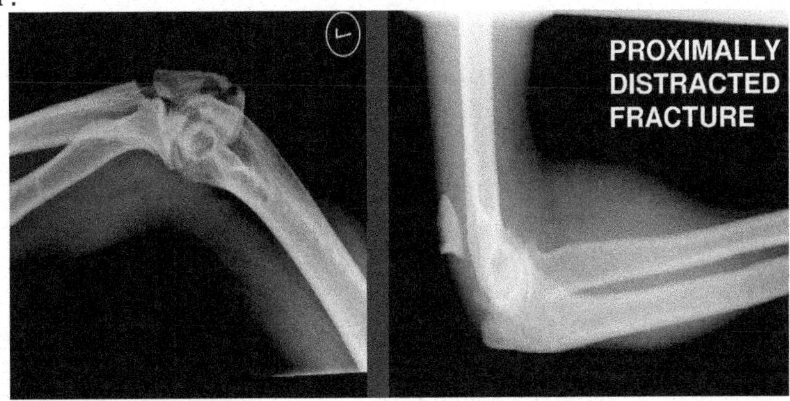

OLECRANON BURSITIS

ETIOLOGIES
- Direct trauma (repetitive microtrauma or pressure), Gout, inflammation.
- Infectious (septic bursitis) can occur after penetrating injury or break in the skin. *Staphylococcus aureus* is the most common organism.

CLINICAL MANIFESTATIONS
- **"Goose egg" boggy swelling to the posterior olecranon process area.**
- Repetitive trauma or chronic: usually painless or minimally tender. Often associated with full range of motion or mild discomfort with full flexion.
- Inflammatory or infectious: may have **erythema, warmth, tenderness with painful, limited ROM.** Evaluate for skin breaks or overlying cellulitis if suspected Septic bursitis.

DIAGNOSIS
- Clinical diagnosis in most patients.
- Aspiration of the bursa usually reserved for suspected Septic bursitis or if Gout is the suspected cause. WBC count <500/mm3 usually indicates noninfectious, non-crystalline bursitis. WBC count >2,000 cells/mm3 is often septic.

MANAGEMENT
- Olecranon bursitis: avoid further trauma, padding to the area, NSAIDs (if painful or inflammatory), ACE wrap for compression.
- Septic bursitis: drainage of infected bursal fluid and antibiotic therapy (eg, oral Dicloxacillin or Clindamycin).

ULNAR SHAFT (NIGHTSTICK) FRACTURE

- Mechanism: direct blow. May present with localized pain & swelling.
- Nightstick fracture: fracture of the middle portion of the ulnar shaft without any associated fractures.

MANAGEMENT
- Nondisplaced distal third: short arm cast.
- Nondisplaced mid-proximal third: long arm cast.
- Displaced >50%: open reduction & internal fixation.

MONTEGGIA FRACTURE

- **Fracture to the proximal 1/3 of the ulnar shaft + radial head dislocation.**
- Mechanism: direct blow to the forearm.

CLINICAL MANIFESTATIONS
- Elbow pain and swelling, thumb paresthesias.
- **Radial nerve injury** (17%) due to the radial head dislocation (may develop a **wrist drop**).

MANAGEMENT: unstable fractures require open reduction & internal fixation (ORIF).

GALEAZZI FRACTURE

- **Mid-distal radial shaft fracture with dislocation of the distal radioulnar joint**.
- Mechanism: FOOSH (fall on an outstretched hand) or direct blow.

CLINICAL MANIFESTATIONS
- Fracture & deformity on the radial side of the wrist. Additionally, the ulnar head will appear prominent at the wrist (because it is dorsally displaced).

MANAGEMENT
- Adults: **ORIF (it is an unstable fracture).** Long arm/sugar tong splint temporarily.

COMPLICATIONS
- Anterior interosseous nerve injury: loss of pinch between the thumb and index finger.
- Compartment syndrome.

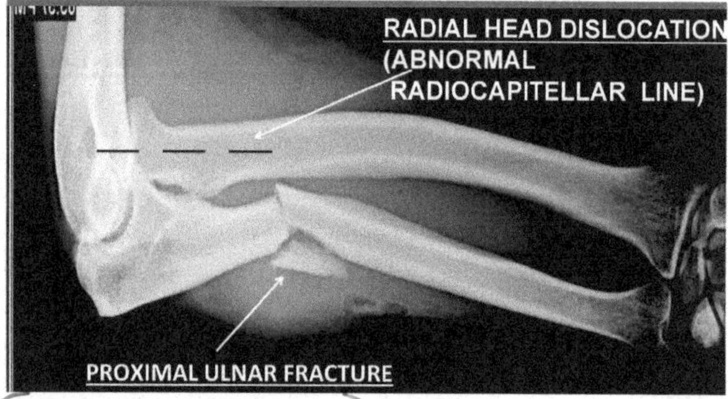

MONTEGGIA FRACTURE

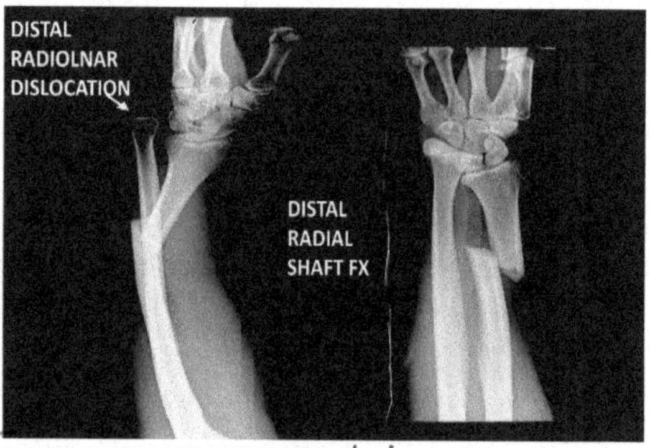

GALEAZZI FRACTURE

MU GR: **M**onteggia: proximal **U**lnar shaft fracture + radial head dislocation. **G**aleazzi: distal **R**adial fracture + dislocation of the distal radioulnar joint

RADIAL HEAD SUBLUXATION (NURSEMAID'S ELBOW)

- Radial head is wedged into the **stretched annular ligament.**
- **Most common in children 2-5 years of age.**

MECHANISM

- **Lifting, swinging or pulling a child** (longitudinal traction) while the forearm is pronated & extended.
- Physical examination: **arm slightly flexed & child refuses to use the arm** (usually no swelling). Tenderness to palpation of the radial head (lateral elbow).

DIAGNOSIS

- Clinical diagnosis (radiographs are normal).

MANAGEMENT

- **Closed reduction:** place **pressure on the radial head with supination of the elbow followed by flexion of the elbow**. Observe the child for normal function. If the child uses the arm after 15 minutes, no radiographs are needed. If no use after 15 minutes, consider radiographs to rule out fracture or reattempt reduction.

LATERAL EPICONDYLITIS (TENNIS ELBOW)

- Inflammation of the tendon insertion of the **extensor carpi radialis brevis muscle** due to repetitive pronation of the forearm & excessive wrist extension.

CLINICAL MANIFESTATIONS

- Lateral elbow pain especially with gripping, forearm pronation & **wrist extension against resistance.**
- May radiate down the forearm or worsen when lifting objects with the forearm prone.

MANAGEMENT

- Conservative: activity modification, RICE, NSAIDs, physiotherapy, counterbalance braces; Intraarticular steroid injections may provide short-term benefit.
- Surgery if refractory to conservative management.

MEDIAL EPICONDYLITIS (GOLFER'S ELBOW)

- Not as common as lateral epicondylitis. Common 40-60 years of age.
- Mechanism: Inflammation of the **pronator teres-flexor carpi radialis** muscles due to repetitive overuse & stress at the tendon insertion of flexor forearm muscle.
- Most common in golfers & patients who do household chores.

CLINICAL MANIFESTATIONS

- Tenderness over the medial epicondyle **worse with pulling activities.**
- Physical examination: pain reproduced by performing **wrist flexion against resistance** with the elbow fully extended.

MANAGEMENT

- Similar to lateral epicondylitis (however more difficult to treat).
- Activity modification, RICE, NSAIDs, physiotherapy, counter brace; Intraarticular steroid injections.
- Surgery if refractory to conservative management.

ELBOW DISLOCATION

- Mechanism: fall on outstretched hand (FOOSH) with hyperextension (high energy) & axial loading.
- **Posterior most common type.**

PHYSICAL EXAMINATION

- **Flexed elbow, marked olecranon prominence,** & inability to extend elbow.
- Often associated with radial head or coronoid process fracture.

MANAGEMENT

- Stable: **EMERGENT reduction with posterior splint** at 90 degrees with orthopedic follow up.
- Unstable: open reduction internal fixation (ORIF).

COMPLICATIONS

- Must rule out brachial artery; median, ulnar, or radial nerve injuries.
- Loss of terminal extension is the most common sequelae.
- Joint stiffness or contractures if the splint is left on > 3 weeks.
- Compartment syndrome.

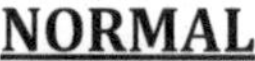
NORMAL

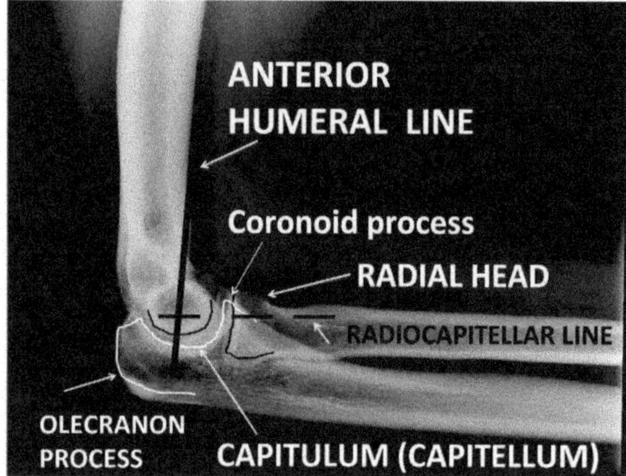

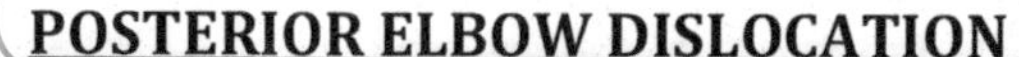
POSTERIOR ELBOW DISLOCATION

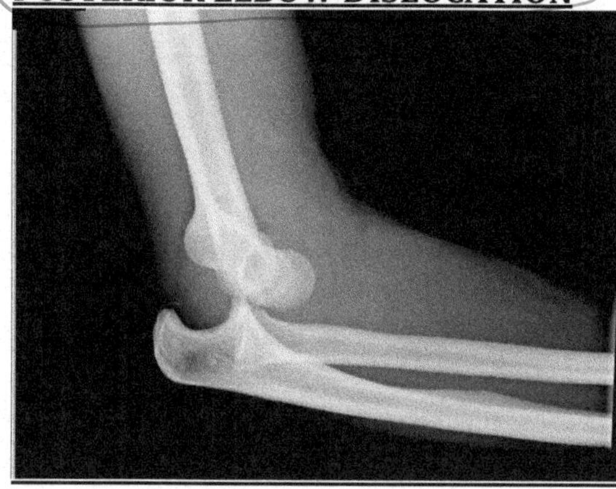

ulnar nerve

CUBITAL TUNNEL SYNDROME (ULNAR NEUROPATHY)

- **Ulnar nerve compression** at the cubital tunnel along the medial elbow.

CLINICAL MANIFESTATIONS

- **Paresthesia & pain along the ulnar nerve distribution** (worse with elbow flexion).

PHYSICAL EXAMINATION

- **Positive Tinel's sign at the elbow.**
- **Positive Froment sign** (ulnar nerve evaluation via adductor pollicis – holds paper & compensates with flexion of IP joint – pinching effect).
- Decreased sensation to the fifth and the ulnar side of the fourth finger.

MANAGEMENT

- Wrist immobilization especially with sleep, NSAIDs.
- Intraarticular steroids (chronic).

WRIST INJURIES

SCAPHOID (NAVICULAR) FRACTURE

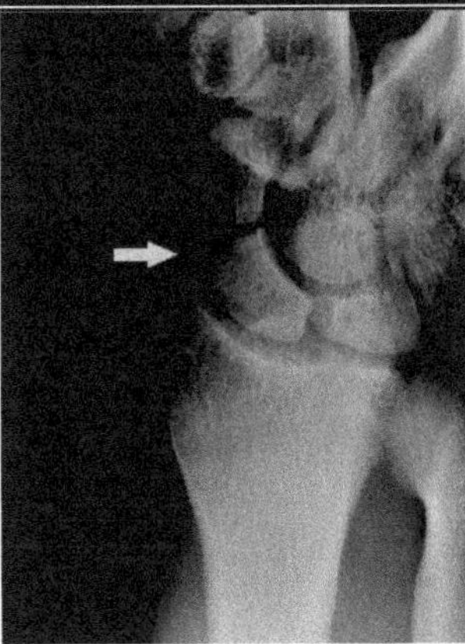

- Mechanism: fall on outstretched hand (FOOSH) on extended wrist.
- Most commonly fractured carpal bone. 65% occur at the waist.

CLINICAL MANIFESTATIONS:

- Pain along the radial surface of the wrist with **anatomical snuffbox tenderness.**

DIAGNOSIS

- Radiographs: the fracture may not be evident for up to 2 weeks. If **snuffbox tenderness is present, treat as fracture** because of the **high incidence of avascular necrosis** or **nonunion** (since the blood supply to scaphoid is distal to proximal).

MANAGEMENT

- **Nondisplaced fracture or snuffbox tenderness: thumb spica splint.**
- Displaced > 1mm: ORIF or percutaneous pin placement.

SCAPHOLUNATE DISSOCIATION

- Widened space between the scaphoid and lunate bones.
- Mechanism: fall on outstretched hand (FOOSH).

CLINICAL MANIFESTATIONS

- Pain on the dorsal radial side of the wrist with minimal swelling. Pain is increased with dorsiflexion. May have a click with wrist movement.
- Diagnosis: **widened scapholunate spaces >3mm** (aka Terry Thomas sign).

MANAGEMENT

- Initial: radial gutter splint.
- Surgical repair of the scapholunate ligament usually required to prevent SLAC of the wrist.

OSTEOGENESIS IMPERFECTA

- Autosomal dominant disease leading to defects in the gene that encodes for type I collagen.
- Associated with fetal or perinatal death & intrauterine growth retardation in its most severe form.

CLINICAL MANIFESTATIONS

- **Severe premature osteoporosis** – **multiple recurrent spontaneous fractures** with minimal or no trauma in childhood leading to limb deformities & shortening.
- **Presenile deafness**.

PHYSICAL EXAMINATION: **blue-tinted sclerae** hallmark. Brown teeth.

DIAGNOSIS: Clinical and radiologic findings. Confirmed with DNA or protein testing.

MANAGEMENT: Combination of bisphosphonates, physical therapy, & surgical interventions.

COLLES FRACTURE

- Distal radius fracture with dorsal angulation. Ulnar styloid fracture also seen in 60%.
- Mechanism: fall on outstretched hand **(FOOSH) with wrist extension**.
- Clinical manifestations: wrist pain worse with passive motion.
- Physical examination: **dinner fork deformity** appearance to the wrist.

DIAGNOSIS

- Radiographs: lateral view shows **dorsally displaced or angulated** extraarticular **fracture of the distal radius**. Lateral view needed to distinguish Colles vs Smith.

MANAGEMENT

- Stable: **closed reduction followed by sugar tong splint or cast** is the initial management.
- ORIF if comminuted or unstable (>20 degrees angulation, intraarticular, >1cm shortening).

COMPLICATIONS

- **Extensor pollicis longus tendon rupture most common.**
- Malunion or nonunion, joint stiffness, median nerve compression, residual radius shortening, & complex regional pain syndrome.

SMITH FRACTURE

- Extra-articular distal radius fracture with ventral angulation of the distal fragment.
- Mechanism: fall on outstretched hand **(FOOSH) with the wrist flexed.**
- Clinical manifestations: wrist pain worse with passive motion.
- Physical examination: **garden spade deformity** appearance of the wrist.

DIAGNOSIS

- Radiographs: lateral view shows **ventrally displaced or angulated** extraarticular **fracture of the distal radius**. Lateral view needed to distinguish Colles vs Smith.

MANAGEMENT

- Stable: **closed reduction followed by sugar tong splint or cast** is the initial management.
- ORIF if comminuted or unstable.

COLLES FRACTURE
DORSAL angulation.

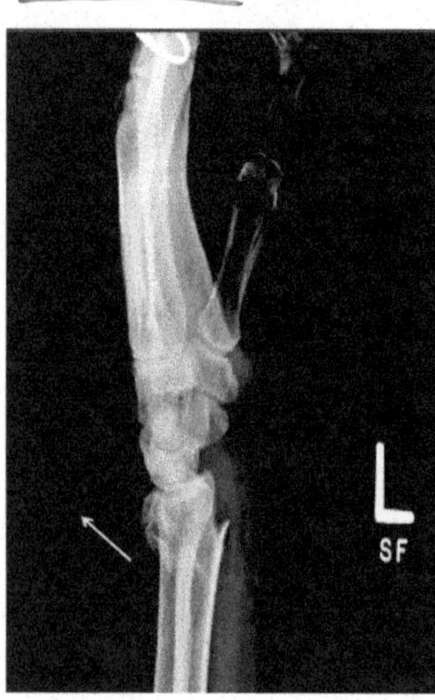

SMITH FRACTURE
VENTRAL angulation.

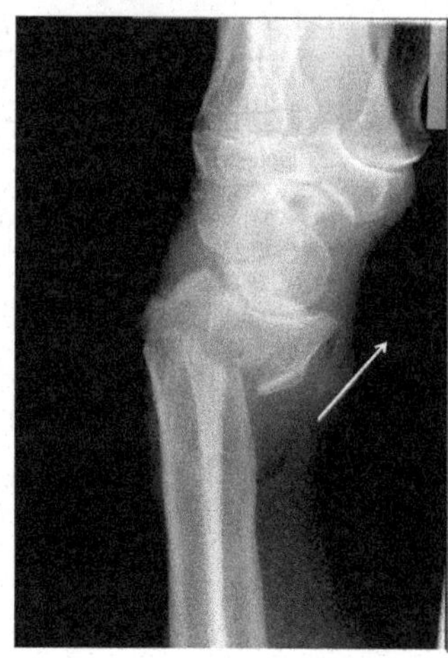

BARTON FRACTURE
Intra-articular distal radius fracture with **carpal displacement.**

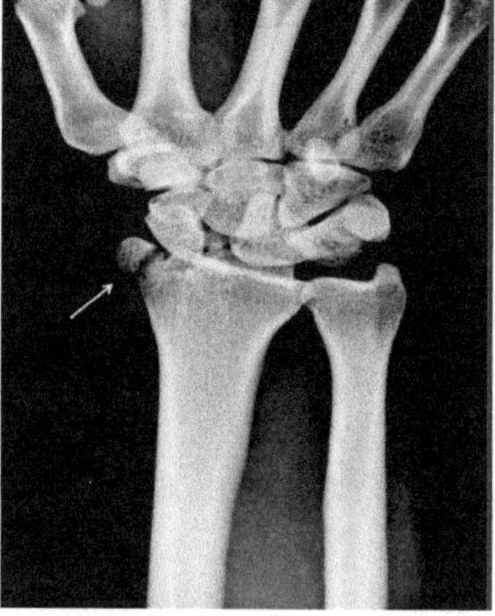

LUNATE DISLOCATION

- The lunate does not articulate with both the capitate and the radius.
- Mechanism: high energy injuries while the wrist is extended & ulnarly deviated.

CLINICAL MANIFESTATION
- Acute wrist swelling & pain. May develop median nerve symptoms.

DIAGNOSIS
- AP view: lunate appears triangular **"piece of pie" sign.**
- Lateral view: volar displacement & tilt of the lunate **"spilled teacup" sign.**

MANAGEMENT
- Emergent closed reduction & splint followed by ORIF (open reduction internal fixation). Orthopedic emergency.

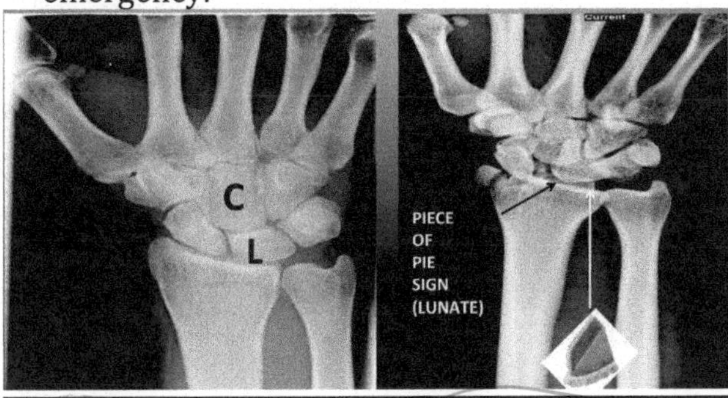

Normal Lunate dislocation
"Piece of pie sign" seen on the AP view.

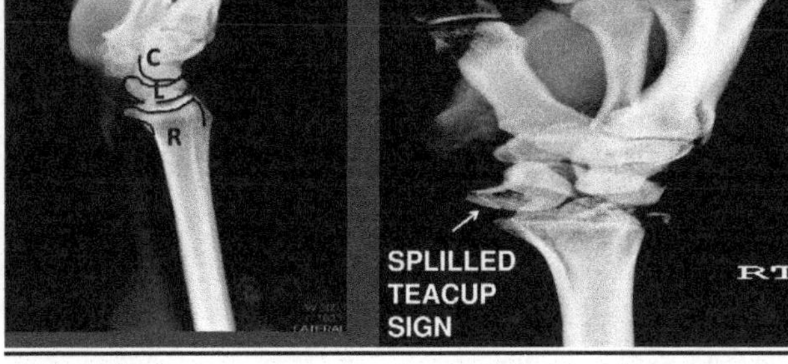

Normal Lunate dislocation
" Spilled teacup" sign" seen on the lateral view.

PERILUNATE VS LUNATE DISLOCATION

PERILUNATE: the lunate does not articulate with the capitate but still articulates with the radius.
LUNATE: the lunate doesn't articulate with the capitate OR radius "spilled teacup" sign on the lateral view.

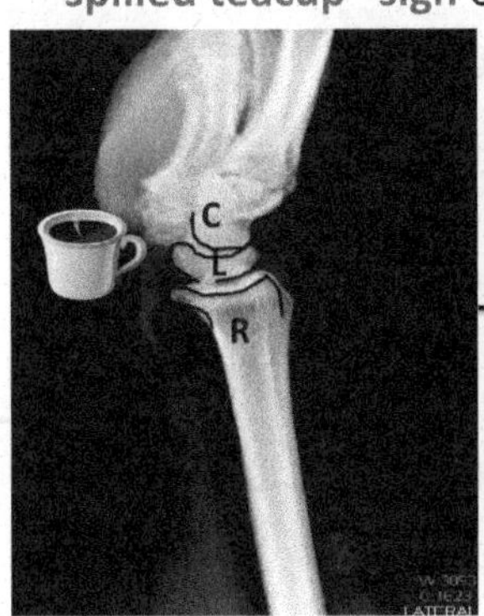

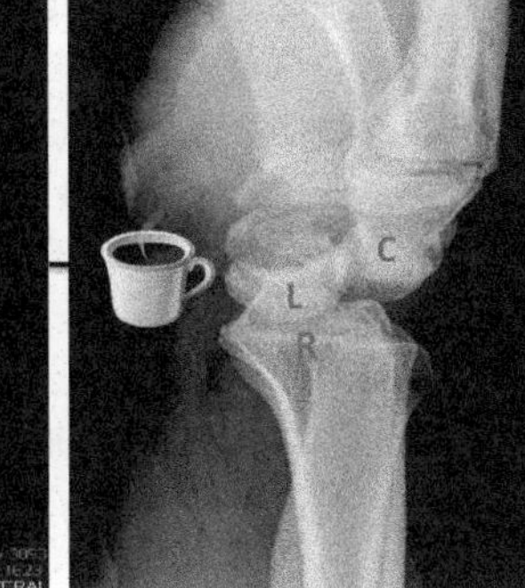

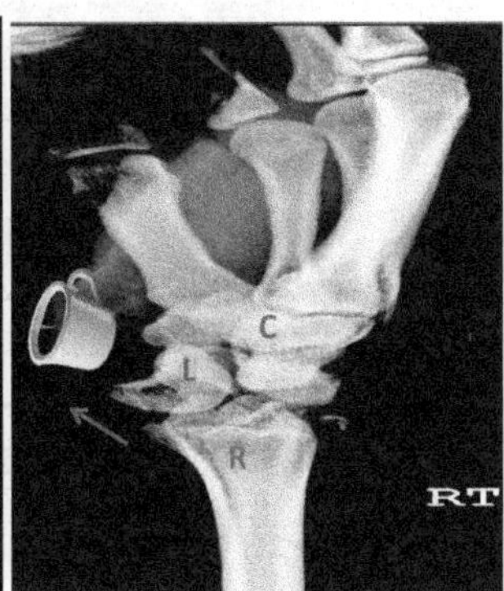

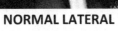

NORMAL LATERAL PERILUNATE LUNATE

LUNATE FRACTURE

- **Most serious carpal fracture** since the lunate occupies two-thirds of the radial articular surface. Radiographs are often negative.
- Complications: **avascular necrosis of the lunate bone (Kienböck's disease).**

MANAGEMENT
- Immobilization with orthopedic follow up.

COMPLEX REGIONAL PAIN SYNDROME (CRPS)

- Formerly known as reflex sympathetic dystrophy (RSD).
- **Autonomic dysfunction following bone or soft tissue injuries** (eg, wrist fracture or post-surgery). 30% have no history of injury.
- Most commonly affects the upper extremities, women & >30 years.

CLINICAL MANIFESTATIONS

- Characterized by 4 main symptoms after an initiating event:
- **Sensory – pain, hyperalgesia** often out of proportion to the initial injury.
- **Motor/trophic changes**: decreased range of motion & motor dysfunction with trophic changes (increased hair & nail growth initially followed by decreased growth).
- **Edema** or sweating changes
- **Vasomotor:** temperature & skin color asymmetry with **autonomic dysfunction**.

DIAGNOSIS:

- **Mainly a clinical diagnosis**
- Radiographs: may show patchy osteoporosis. Bone scintigraphy: increased uptake/activity.

Diagnostic criteria:

- An initiating event, or immobilization
- Persistent pain, allodynia, or hyperalgesia out of proportion to the initiating event
- Symptoms of edema, changes in skin blood flow, or abnormal sudomotor activity
- No other obvious diagnosis that could explain the symptoms

MANAGEMENT

- NSAIDs initial treatment. Physical & occupational therapy. Anesthetic blocks, oral corticosteroids, tricyclic antidepressants, transcutaneous electric nerve stimulation, etc.
- **Vitamin C prophylaxis after fractures may reduce the incidence of CRPS.**

DE QUERVAIN (TENDINOPATHY) TENOSYNOVITIS

- Stenosing inflammation of the tendons (**entrapment tendinitis**) of the first dorsal compartment: APL & EBP **abductor pollicis longus & extensor pollicis brevis.**
- Mechanism: excessive thumb use with repetitive action (thumb abduction & extension). Seen in golfers, clerical workers, **women postpartum (from lifting the newborn), diabetics**, posttraumatic etc.

CLINICAL MANIFESTATIONS

- **Pain along the radial aspect of the wrist & base of the thumb radiating to the forearm** especially with thumb extension or gripping.
- Pain & tenderness at the radial styloid.
- Swelling & thickness over the tendon sheath may be present.

DIAGNOSIS

- **Finkelstein test:** positivity = first dorsal compartment **pain with ulnar deviation** while the thumb is flexed in the palm or pain with thumb extension.

MANAGEMENT

- **Thumb spica splint initial management**, NSAID, physical therapy.
- Corticosteroid injection may be used if initial treatment is unsuccessful.
- Surgical release usually reserved for cases refractory to nonoperative management.

Mallet
Boutoniere
Swan neck

MALLET (BASEBALL) FINGER

- Mechanism *avulsion of the extensor tendon* after sudden blow to tip of the finger causing forced flexion of an extended finger.
- Physical exam: *unable to actively extend the DIP joint.*
- Radiographs: normal or avulsion fracture of the distal phalanx at the tendon insertion site.

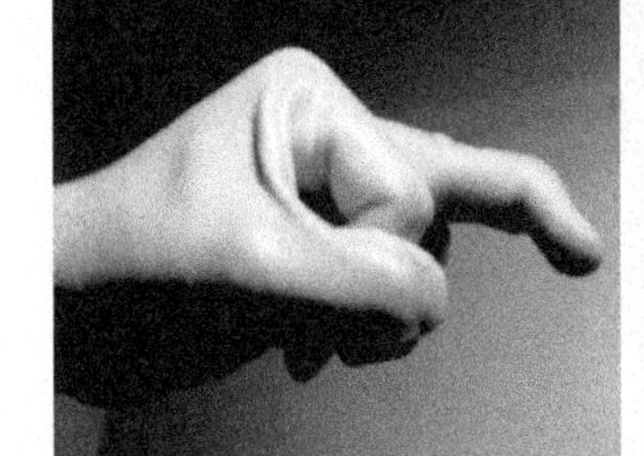
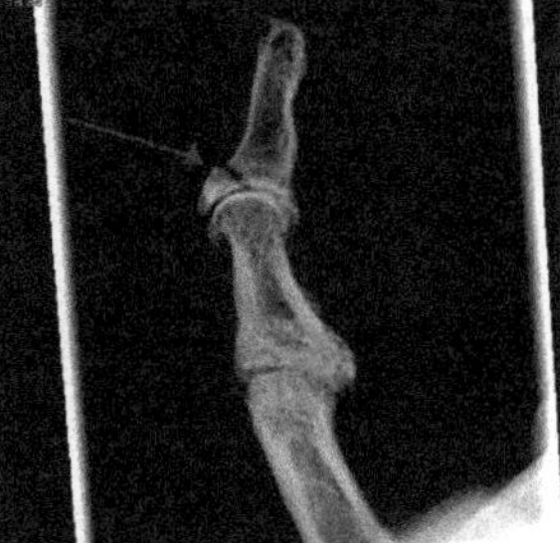

@pance_prep_pearls

MANAGEMENT

- Nonoperative: *uninterrupted extension splint of DIP joint x 6-8 weeks*
- Closed reduction & percutaneous pinning if displaced mallet finger with subluxation.
- Operative: ORIF (if CR & PP cannot be done), tendon reconstruction.

BOUTONNIERE DEFORMITY

- Mechanism: sharp force against the tip of a partially extended digit ⇨ hyperflexion at the PIP joint with hyperextension at the DIP. Disruption of extensor tendon at the base of the middle phalanx.

Management:

- Splint PIP in extension x 4-6weeks with hand surgeon follow up.

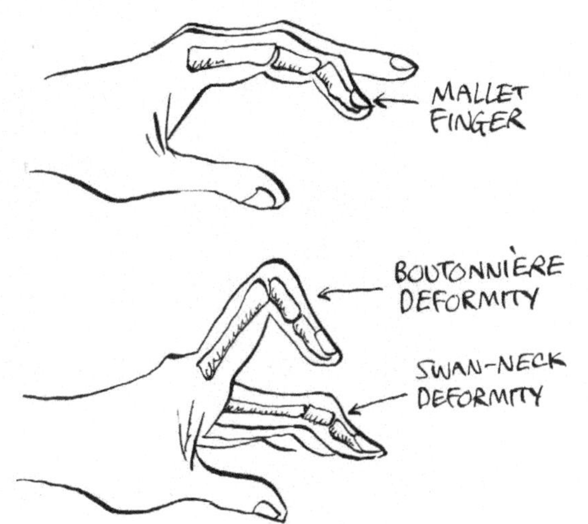

MALLET FINGER

Finger flexed at the DIP joint
unable to extend at the DIP joint

BOUTONNIERE DEFORMITY

Finger flexed @ PIP joint &
hyperextended @ DIP joint

SWAN NECK DEFORMITY

Finger hyperextended @ PIP joint &
flexed @ DIP joint

GAMEKEEPER'S (SKIER'S) THUMB

- Sprain or tear of the **ulnar collateral ligament of the thumb** ⇨ instability of MCP joint.
- Skier's thumb: acute condition (eg, after fall); Gamekeeper's: chronic hyperabduction injury.
- Mechanism: Forced abduction of the thumb (UCL functions to resist against valgus forces).

CLINICAL MANIFESTATIONS

- Thumb far away from the other digits (especially with **valgus stress** - pulling thumb away from the hand), MCP tenderness, weakness in pinch strength.
- **± Fracture at the base of the proximal phalanx** (if UCL ruptures, it may pull off piece of bone).

MANAGEMENT

- **Thumb spica splint** & referral to hand surgeon (because it affects pincer function).
- Complete rupture: surgical repair.

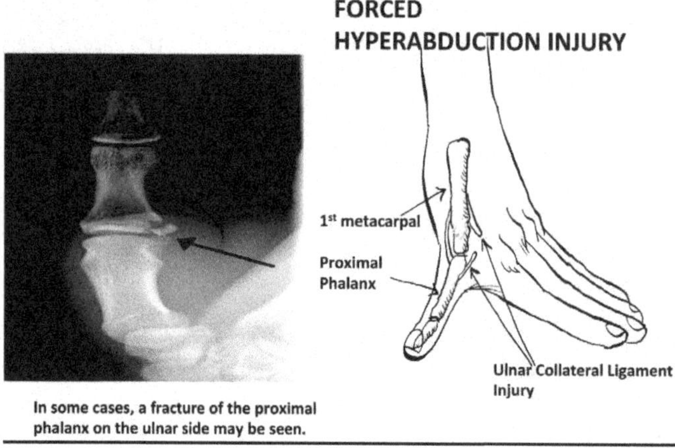

In some cases, a fracture of the proximal phalanx on the ulnar side may be seen.

BOXER'S FRACTURE

- **Fracture through the fifth metacarpal neck** (maybe the fourth).
- Mechanism: direct trauma to a closed fist against a hard surface (eg, wall).

CLINICAL MANIFESTATIONS

- Pain along the dorsum of the fifth metacarpal of the hand with swelling, ecchymosis (may have loss of the appearance of the fifth knuckle if angulated). May have rotational deformity.

DIAGNOSIS

- Radiographs

MANAGEMENT

- Initial: **ulnar gutter splint** with joints in at least 60 degrees flexion. Reduction required prior to splinting of any fracture > 25-30 degrees angulation.
- Open reduction internal fixation if the fifth remains > 40 degrees angulated (30 degrees for the ring finger).
- **Always check for bite wounds.** If present, treat with the appropriate antibiotics (eg, Amoxicillin-clavulanate).

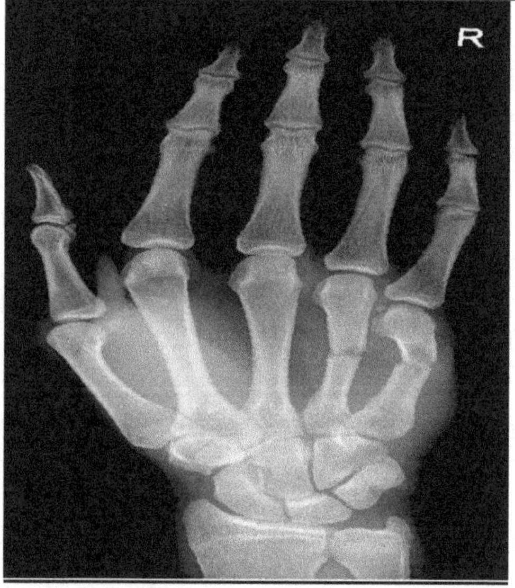

Boxer's fracture of the 5th.
4th metacarpal fracture also seen here.

BENNETT FRACTURE – DISLOCATION/ROLANDO FRACTURE

- **Metacarpal fractures involving the base of the thumb.**
- Mechanism: axial force applied to the thumb in flexion.
- **Bennett fracture: non-comminuted** partial intra-articular fracture.
- **Rolando fracture: comminuted** complete intra-articular fracture.

CLINICAL MANIFESTATIONS
- Pain, swelling, ecchymosis, and tenderness to the CMC joint (base of thumb).

DIAGNOSIS
- Bennett: small fragment of first metacarpal base articulating with the trapezium.
- Rolando: **Y sign** – splitting of the first metacarpal base into dorsal and volar fragments.

MANAGEMENT
- Immediate: **thumb spica splint** for temporary stabilization.
- Bennett: immobilization. Closed reduction & percutaneous pinning, ORIF if large fragment and joint displacement.
- Rolando: unstable often need ORIF, external fixation or closed reduction & percutaneous pinning.

BENNETT & ROLANDO FX

- **Bennett's Fracture:** ***intraarticular fracture through base of the 1st metacarpal (MCP)***
- **Rolando's fracture:** ***COMMINUTED Bennett's fracture.***

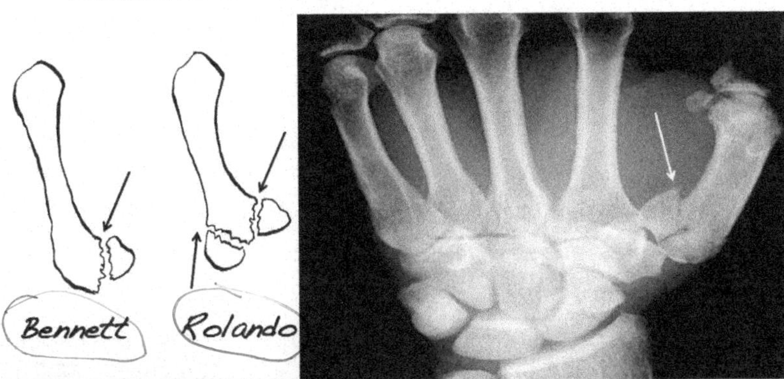

PRONATOR TERES SYNDROME

- Proximal forearm **median nerve compression** where the nerve traverses the pronator teres muscle.
- Usually due to entrapment of the median nerve between the 2 heads of the pronator teres muscle.

CLINICAL MANIFESTATIONS
- **Paresthesia or pain** of the lateral palmar aspect of the **first 3 (& radial half of the fourth) digits.** May have sensory loss over the thenar eminence.
- Symptoms are not worse at night (compared to Carpal tunnel syndrome).
- **Tenderness over the proximal median nerve aggravated by pronation** of the forearm.

MANAGEMENT
- Initial management: reduction in the symptom-inducing activity. NSAIDs for pain.
- Steroid injections if no relief with NSAIDs.
- Surgical decompression in refractory cases.

CARPAL TUNNEL SYNDROME

- **Median nerve entrapment & compression** at the carpal tunnel.
- Increased incidence in women, **Diabetes Mellitus, pregnancy,** hypothyroidism, rheumatoid arthritis, occupations with repetitive extension & flexion of the wrists (eg, typing).

CLINICAL MANIFESTATIONS

- **Paresthesias or pain** of the palmar aspect of the **first 3 (& radial half of the fourth) digits especially at night.** Clumsiness & weakness.
- Thenar muscle wasting may be seen in advanced cases.

DIAGNOSIS

- Workup may include electromyography & nerve conduction velocity studies.
- **Tinel test:** positive if percussion of the median nerve produces symptoms.
- **Phalen test:** positive if flexion of both wrists for 30-60 seconds reproduces the symptoms.

MANAGEMENT

- **Conservative: volar splint initial management,** NSAIDs, avoiding repetitive wrist movements.
- Corticosteroid injections.
- Carpal tunnel surgery in refractory or severe cases.

DIFFERENTIAL DIAGNOSIS:

PRONATOR TERES SYNDROME median nerve compression in the proximal forearm. May develop paresthesias in the same distribution as carpal tunnel. However, **pronator syndrome** associated more with **proximal forearm pain** than wrist/hand pain & **not associated with pain at night** (like seen in carpal tunnel).

DUPUYTREN CONTRACTURE

- Progressive fibrosis of the palmar fascia leading to contractures as a result of nodules or longitudinal bands (cords) in the palm.

RISK FACTORS

- **Men > 40 years of age, Northern Europeans,** ETOH abuse, Cirrhosis, Diabetes mellitus, cigarette smoking.

CLINICAL MANIFESTATIONS

- Visible or palpable **nodules over the distal palmar crease** or proximal phalanx (especially ring, little finger) along the course of the flexor tendons.
- May have thickened skin or bands in the palmar fascia. The nodules may be tender, the cords & contractures are usually painless.
- **Fixed flexion deformity at the MCP joint** with limited extension of the MCP or PIP joint.

MANAGEMENT

- Intralesional collagenase &/or corticosteroid injections, Physical therapy. High recurrence rate after injections.
- Surgical correction (fasciotomy or fasciectomy) for advanced stages, refractory cases or impaired function.

PHOTO CREDITS

Bankart Lesion By RSatUSZ (Own work) [CC-BY-SA-3.0 (http://creativecommons.org/licenses/by-sa/3.0)], via Wikimedia Commons
Thoracic Outlet Syndrome By English: Nicholas Zaorsky, M.D. (English: Nicholas Zaorsky, M.D.) [CC-BY-SA-3.0 (http://creativecommons.org/licenses/by-sa/3.0)], via Wikimedia Commons
Mallet Finger By Howcheng (Own work) [CC-BY-SA-3.0 (http://creativecommons.org/licenses/by-sa/3.0) or GFDL (http://www.gnu.org/copyleft/fdl.html)], via Wikimedia Commons
Mallet Finger By James Heilman, MD (Own work) [CC-BY-SA-3.0 (http://creativecommons.org/licenses/by-sa/3.0) or GFDL (http://www.gnu.org/copyleft/fdl.html)], via Wikimedia Commons
Galeazzi Fracture By Th. Zimmermann THWZ) (Own work) [CC-BY-SA-3.0-de (http://creativecommons.org/licenses/by-sa/3.0/de/deed.en)], via Wikimedia Commons. SPECIAL THANKS to Mr. Zimmerman. Photo Edited from original
Scaphoid Fracture
By Gilo1969 (Own work) [CC-BY-SA-3.0 (http://creativecommons.org/licenses/by-sa/3.0) or GFDL (http://www.gnu.org/copyleft/fdl.html)], via Wikimedia Commons
Lunate Fracture By Vanalstm at en.wikipedia [Public domain], from Wikimedia Commons
Triquetrum Fracture
By Hellerhoff (Own work) [CC-BY-SA-3.0 (http://creativecommons.org/licenses/by-sa/3.0)], via Wikimedia Commons
Gamekeeper's thumb
By James Heilman, MD (Own work) [CC-BY-SA-3.0 (http://creativecommons.org/licenses/by-sa/3.0) or GFDL (http://www.gnu.org/copyleft/fdl.html)], via Wikimedia Commons
Rolando Fracture
By Gilo1969 (Own work) [CC-BY-SA-3.0 (http://creativecommons.org/licenses/by-sa/3.0) or GFDL (http://www.gnu.org/copyleft/fdl.html)], via Wikimedia Commons
Legg Calves Perthes Disease
By J. Lengerke (Praxis Dr. Lengerke) [Public domain], via Wikimedia Commons
Buckle Fracture
© Nevit Dilmen [CC-BY-SA-3.0 (http://creativecommons.org/licenses/by-sa/3.0) or GFDL (http://www.gnu.org/copyleft/fdl.html)], via Wikimedia Commons
Patella Alta
By Hellerhoff (Own work) [CC-BY-SA-3.0 (http://creativecommons.org/licenses/by-sa/3.0)], via Wikimedia Commons
Patella Baja
By Hellerhoff (Own work) [CC-BY-SA-3.0 (http://creativecommons.org/licenses/by-sa/3.0)], via Wikimedia Commons
Osgood Schlatter
By Lucien Monfils (Own work) [GFDL (http://www.gnu.org/copyleft/fdl.html) or CC-BY-SA-3.0-2.5-2.0-1.0 (http://creativecommons.org/licenses/by-sa/3.0)], via Wikimedia Commons
Osgood
By D3aj86 (Own work) [CC-BY-3.0 (http://creativecommons.org/licenses/by/3.0)], via Wikimedia Commons
Hallux Valgus
By Michael Nebel http://de.wikipedia.org/wiki/Benutzer:Jakker [CC-BY-SA-2.0-de (http://creativecommons.org/licenses/by-sa/2.0/de/deed.en)], via Wikimedia Commons
Hallux Valgus
By Cyberprout at fr.wikipedia [CC-BY-SA-1.0 (http://creativecommons.org/licenses/by-sa/1.0)], from Wikimedia Commons
Lisfranc Injury
By James Heilman, MD (Own work) [CC-BY-3.0 (http://creativecommons.org/licenses/by/3.0)], via Wikimedia Commons
Jones Fracture
By Lucien Monfils (Own work) [GFDL (http://www.gnu.org/copyleft/fdl.html) or CC-BY-SA-3.0-2.5-2.0-1.0 (http://creativecommons.org/licenses/by-sa/3.0)], via Wikimedia Commons
Spondylolysis &other films
By Hellerhoff (Own work) [CC-BY-SA-3.0 (http://creativecommons.org/licenses/by-sa/3.0)], via Wikimedia Commons

Hammertoe
By Richard Huber (Own work) [CC-BY-SA-3.0 (http://creativecommons.org/licenses/by-sa/3.0)], via Wikimedia Commons

Normal Foot X ray
By Andrew Magill (Flickr) [CC-BY-2.0 (http://creativecommons.org/licenses/by/2.0)], via Wikimedia Commons

Spondylolisthesis
By Lucien Monfils (Own work) [GFDL (http://www.gnu.org/copyleft/fdl.html) or CC-BY-SA-3.0-2.5-2.0-1.0 (http://creativecommons.org/licenses/by-sa/3.0)], via Wikimedia Commons

Ostoechondroma
By Dr Frank Gaillard. Used With Permission.
http://images.radiopaedia.org/images/137159/aa2551e220f734fece9b37fd38f00e_big_gallery.jpg

Osteomyelitis
Case by Dr. Hani Salam. Copyrighted by radiopaedia.org. Used with permission.

Osteomyelitis
Sarindam7 at the English language Wikipedia [GFDL (http://www.gnu.org/copyleft/fdl.html) or CC-BY-SA-3.0 (http://creativecommons.org/licenses/by-sa/3.0/)], from Wikimedia Commons

Codman's triangle
By User:Ajimsha619 (Own work) [CC-BY-SA-3.0 (http://creativecommons.org/licenses/by-sa/3.0)], via Wikimedia Commons

Osteochondroma
By J Bovee (Orphanet J Rare Dis. 2008 Feb 13;3:3.) [CC-BY-SA-3.0-nl (http://creativecommons.org/licenses/by-sa/3.0/nl/deed.en)], via Wikimedia Commons
Ewing's Sarcoma
By Michael Richardson, M.D. on Oct 25th, 2004; Upload by Christaras A (EN:Wikipedia. IMG EwingSarcomaTibia.jpg) [GFDL (www.gnu.org/copyleft/fdl.html) or CC-BY-SA-3.0 (http://creativecommons.org/licenses/by-sa/3.0/)], via Wikimedia Commons
Dermatomyositis
By Elizabeth M. Dugan, Adam M. Huber, Frederick W. Miller, Lisa G. Rider [CC-BY-SA-3.0 (http://creativecommons.org/licenses/by-sa/3.0)], via Wikimedia Commons
Dermatomyositis
By Elizabeth M. Dugan, Adam M. Huber, Frederick W. Miller, Lisa G. Rider [CC-BY-SA-3.0 (http://creativecommons.org/licenses/by-sa/3.0)], via Wikimedia Commons
Dermatomyositis
By Elizabeth M. Dugan, Adam M. Huber, Frederick W. Miller, Lisa G. Rider [CC-BY-SA-3.0 (http://creativecommons.org/licenses/by-sa/3.0)], via Wikimedia Commons
Pagets disease of skull
By dr Laughlin Dawes (radpod.org) [CC-BY-3.0 (http://creativecommons.org/licenses/by/3.0)], via Wikimedia Commons
Paget's disease CT scan
By Hellerhoff (Own work) [CC-BY-SA-3.0 (http://creativecommons.org/licenses/by-sa/3.0)], via Wikimedia Commons
Osteosarcoma in Paget's disease
From Radiopaedia.org. Used with permission
Scleroderma
By AVM (talk) 02:54, 9 January 2009 (UTC) (Own work) [GFDL (http://www.gnu.org/copyleft/fdl.html) or CC-BY-3.0 (http://creativecommons.org/licenses/by/3.0)], via Wikimedia Commons
Systemic Lupus Erythematosus
By Sarella (Own work) [CC-BY-SA-3.0 (http://creativecommons.org/licenses/by-sa/3.0)], via Wikimedia Commons
Discoid Lupus
By Leonard C. Sperling, M.D., COL, MC, USA, Department of Dermatology, Uniformed Services University [Public domain], via Wikimedia Commons
Uric Acid crystals
By Bobjgalindo (Own work) [GFDL (http://www.gnu.org/copyleft/fdl.html) or CC-BY-SA-3.0-2.5-2.0-1.0 (http://creativecommons.org/licenses/by-sa/3.0)], via Wikimedia Commons
Tophi
By Herbert L. Fred, MD and Hendrik A. van Dijk (http://cnx.org/content/m14895/latest/) [Attribution], via Wikimedia Commons
Podagra
By Gonzosft (Own work) [CC-BY-3.0-de (http://creativecommons.org/licenses/by/3.0/de/deed.en)], via Wikimedia Commons
Rheumatoid Arthritis
By James Heilman, MD (Own work) [CC-BY-SA-3.0 (http://creativecommons.org/licenses/by-sa/3.0) or GFDL (http://www.gnu.org/copyleft/fdl.html)], via Wikimedia Commons
Ankylosing Spondylitis
By http://en.wikipedia.org/wiki/User:Glitzy_queen00 [Public domain], via Wikimedia Commons
Lspine X ray
© Nevit Dilmen [CC-BY-SA-3.0 (http://creativecommons.org/licenses/by-sa/3.0) or GFDL (http://www.gnu.org/copyleft/fdl.html)], via Wikimedia Commons
Bamboo
By Scott Sandars from Melbourne, Australia (Flickr) [CC-BY-2.0 (http://creativecommons.org/licenses/by/2.0)], via Wikimedia Commons
Maisonneuve fracture
By RotorMotor2 (Own work) [CC-BY-SA-3.0 (http://creativecommons.org/licenses/by-sa/3.0)], via Wikimedia Commons
Maisonneuve fracture
By RotorMotor2 (Own work) [CC-BY-SA-3.0 (http://creativecommons.org/licenses/by-sa/3.0)], via Wikimedia Commons
Boxer fracture and
By Hellerhoff (Own work) [CC BY-SA 3.0 (http://creativecommons.org/licenses/by-sa/3.0)], via Wikimedia Commons
Greenstick & Torus
By Hellerhoff (Own work) [CC BY-SA 3.0 (http://creativecommons.org/licenses/by-sa/3.0)], via Wikimedia Commons
By Hellerhoff (Own work) [CC BY-SA 3.0 (http://creativecommons.org/licenses/by-sa/3.0)], via Wikimedia Commons

CHAPTER 5 - ENT (EARS, NOSE, & THROAT DISORDERS)

ECTROPION

- **Eyelid & lashes are turned outward (everted)** due to relaxation of the orbicularis oculi muscle.
- Risk factors: most commonly seen in the elderly (tends to be bilateral) but can be congenital, infectious, or part of a cranial nerve 7 palsy.
- Clinical manifestations: irritation, ocular dryness, tearing, sagging of the eyelid, increased sensitivity.

MANAGEMENT
- Lubricating eye drops & moisture shields for symptom relief.
- Surgical correction if needed.

ENTROPION

- **Eyelid & lashes are turned inward (inverted).** Most commonly seen in the elderly.
- Pathophysiology: may be caused by spasms of the orbicularis oculi muscle.
- Clinical manifestations: eyelashes may cause corneal abrasion or ulcerations, erythema, tearing, increased sensitivity.

MANAGEMENT
- Lubricating eye drops & moisture shields for symptom relief. Surgical correction if needed.

DACRYOCYSTITIS

-Clindamycin

- **Infection of the lacrimal sac** due to obstruction of the nasolacrimal duct.
- Etiologies: *Staph epidermis, Staph aureus, GABHS, Pseudomonas, GABHS.*

CLINICAL MANIFESTATIONS
- Acute: **tearing** and **signs of infection** - tenderness, edema, erythema & warmth **to the medial canthal (nasal) side of the lower lid area.** May have purulent discharge.
- Chronic: mucupurulent drainage from the puncta without other signs of infection.

MANAGEMENT
- Acute: warm compresses + **antibiotics** (eg, Clindamycin, Vancomycin + Ceftriaxone).
- Chronic or severe acute: **Dacryocystorhinostomy**. Topical antibiotics may be used prior to surgery.

BLEPHARITIS

- **Inflammation of the eyelid margin.**
- Risk factors: Down syndrome, Atopic dermatitis, Rosacea, Seborrheic dermatitis.
- Posterior: Meibomian gland dysfunction. Most common type.
- Anterior: involves the skin & base of the eyelashes. 2 types: **Infectious** (***Staphylococcus aureus*** or *Staphylococcus epidermis*), viruses; **Seborrheic.**

CLINICAL MANIFESTATIONS
- Eyelid: burning, erythema, **crusting, scaling & red-rimming of the eyelid** (pink or erythematous eyelid edges) & **flaking on the lashes or lid margins.** May have entropion or ectropion.

MANAGEMENT
- **Eyelid hygiene mainstay of treatment** - warm compresses, eyelid scrubbing & lid washing with baby shampoo, artificial tears.
- Severe or refractory: topical antibiotics (eg, Azithromycin solution or ointment, Erythromycin or Bacitracin); oral antibiotics, topical glucocorticoids, topical Cyclosporine.

HORDEOLUM (STYE)

- Localized abscess of the eyelid margin.
- Etiologies: ***Staphylococcus aureus*** **most common cause** (>90%).
- Increased risk with Seborrheic dermatitis & Rosacea.

TYPES:
- External: infection of eyelash follicle or external sebaceous glands near the lid margin with production of pus (gland of Moll or gland of Zeis).
- Internal: inflammation or infection of a Meibomian gland. They are found deep from the palpebral margin under the eyelid.

CLINICAL MANIFESTATIONS
- Focal abscess: **erythematous, painful, warm, nodule or pustule on the eyelid.**

MANAGEMENT
- **Warm compresses mainstay of treatment** (most eventually point & drain spontaneously).
- Incision & drainage may be needed if no spontaneous drainage after 48 hours.
- May add topical antibiotic ointment (eg, Erythromycin, Bacitracin) if actively draining in some.

CHALAZION

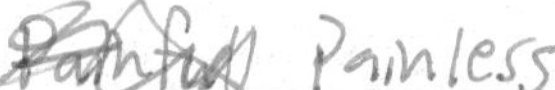

- **Painless indurated granuloma of the internal Meibomian sebaceous gland** away from the eyelid margin.
- Pathophysiology: obstruction of the Zeis or Meibomian glands.

CLINICAL MANIFESTATIONS
- **Non-tender localized, eyelid swelling** (nodule) on the conjunctival surface of the eyelid.
- May cause erythema of the affected eyelid.
- Chalazions are often larger, firmer, slower growing & less painful than Hordeola.

MANAGEMENT
- **Conservative:** eyelid hygiene & warm compresses. Small chalazia will often resolve without intervention in days to weeks.
- Refractory: ophthalmologist referral for injection of glucocorticoid or incision + curettage may be necessary if no resolution by an ophthalmologist.

PINGUECULA

- Slow growing thickening of the bulbar conjunctiva.
- **Yellow, slightly elevated nodule** most common on the nasal side of the sclera near the limbal conjunctiva – **does not grow** onto the cornea.
- Consists of fat, protein & calcium.

RISK FACTORS
- Often develop when the eye is irritated (eg, dry, windy and sunny conditions, ocular trauma).

MANAGEMENT
- **No treatment is needed**.
- May be resected if chronically inflamed or for cosmetic reasons.

PTERYGIUM

- Slow growing thickening of the bulbar conjunctiva.

RISK FACTORS

- Associated with **ultraviolet exposure in sunny climates (tropics)**
- **Sand, wind, & dust exposure**.

CLINICAL MANIFESTATIONS

- Elevated, superficial fleshy, **triangular-shaped growing fibrovascular mass** that usually starts **medially (nasal side of the eye**) & extends laterally.
- May cause irritation, erythema, or foreign body sensation.

MANAGEMENT

- **Observation for most.** Artificial tears may help irritation & erythema.
- **Removal only needed if the growth affects vision** (if it advances over the cornea or causes astigmatism) or significant cosmetic impact.

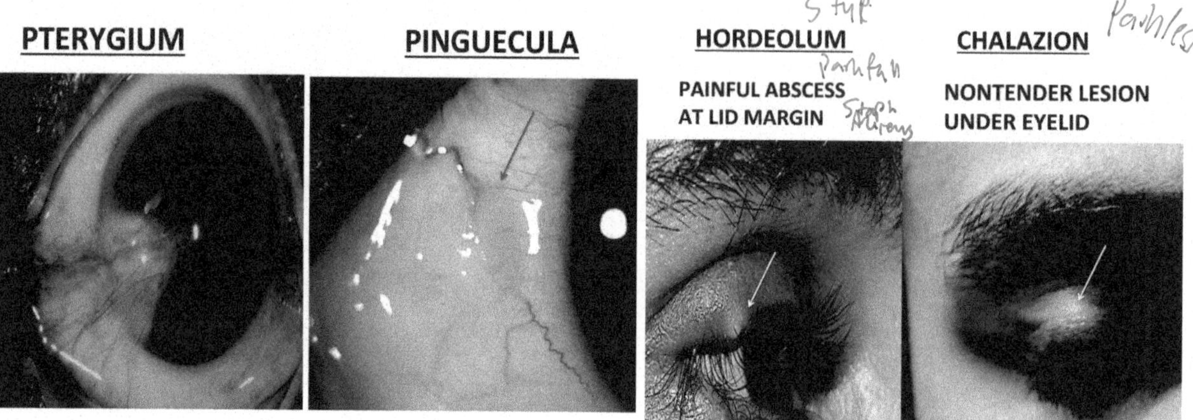

GLOBE RUPTURE

- The outer membranes of the eye are disrupted by blunt or penetrating trauma.
- **Ophthalmologic emergency – immediate ophthalmologist consult.**

PHYSICAL EXAMINATION

- Visual acuity: markedly reduced (may be light perception only), diplopia. Examination for a relative afferent pupillary defect.
- Orbits: **enophthalmos** or exophthalmos. Foreign bodies may be present. **Severe conjunctival hemorrhage (360 degrees bulbar).**
- Corneal/Sclera: misshapen pupil with prolapse of ocular tissue from the sclera or corneal opening. Prolapse of the iris through the cornea, **positive Seidel's test** = parting of fluorescein dye by a clear stream of aqueous humor from the anterior chamber. Obscured red-reflex, **teardrop or irregularly-shaped pupil,** hyphema (blood in anterior eye chamber).

MANAGEMENT

- **Rigid eye shield** protects the eye from applied pressure. **Impaled objects should be left undisturbed.** IV Antibiotics. Tetanus prophylaxis (if needed).
- **Emergent ophthalmology consult.** May need CT scan of the eye without contrast.
- In cases of suspected globe rupture, avoid topical eye solutions and avoid any procedure that may apply pressure to the eyeball (eg, tonometry, eyelid retraction, etc.).

ORBITAL FLOOR "BLOWOUT" FRACTURES

- Fractures to the orbital floor as a result of blunt trauma. May lead to trapping of eye structures.
- The orbital floor consists of the zygomatic, palatine, and maxillary bones.

TYPES

- **Inferior (floor, blowout) fractures are the most common type**. Orbital fat and/or the inferior rectus muscle may prolapse into the maxillary sinus.
- Medial (lamina papyracea): orbital fat and the medial rectal muscle may prolapse into the ethmoid air cells.
- Superior (roof) and lateral wall are uncommon.

CLINICAL MANIFESTATIONS

- Eyes: decreased visual acuity, **diplopia especially with upward gaze (inferior rectus muscle entrapment), orbital emphysema** from air from the maxillary sinus - eyelid swelling especially after blowing the nose.
- Facial: epistaxis. Dysesthesias, hyperalgesia or **anesthesia to the anteromedial cheek** (due to stretching of the **infraorbital nerve**).

DIAGNOSIS

- CT scan: test of choice – localizes the fracture. **"Teardrop" sign** (inferior herniation of the orbital fat inferiorly) may also be seen.

MANAGEMENT

- **Nasal decongestants** (decreases pain), **avoid blowing nose or sneezing,** corticosteroids (to reduce edema)
- **Antibiotics** (eg, Ampicillin-Sulbactam or Clindamycin).
- Surgical repair: severe cases, patients with enophthalmos or for persistent diplopia.

RETINOBLASTOMA

- Most common primary intraocular malignancy in childhood.
- **Most are diagnosed before 3 years of age** (almost exclusively found in children).

TYPES:

- Non heritable: due to somatic mutations in the RB1 gene in the tumor (RB1 is a tumor suppressor gene on chromosome 13).
- Heritable: due to germline mutations in the RB1 gene. May develop bilateral Retinoblastoma.

CLINICAL PRESENTATION

- **Leukocoria (presence of an abnormal white reflex** instead of the normal red reflex).
- May develop Strabismus or Nystagmus.

DIAGNOSIS

- Dilated ophthalmologic examination.
- Ocular ultrasound – intraocular calcified mass. MRI or CT.

MANAGEMENT

- Radiation therapy, chemotherapy, and/or enucleation. Retinoblastoma can be associated with bone neoplasms (eg, Osteosarcoma).
- Fatal if untreated but survival > 95% if treated promptly

MACULAR DEGENERATION

- **Most common cause of permanent legal blindness & vision loss in older adults** (especially > 75 years of age).

TYPES:

- Dry (atrophic): most common type. Dry is progressive (over decades).
- Wet (neovascular or exudative): not as common but more aggressive (within months).

CLINICAL MANIFESTATIONS

- **Bilateral, progressive central vision loss (including detailed & colored vision).** Central scotomas. **Metamorphopsia** (straight lines appear bent). Micropsia (object seems smaller in the affected eye).
- Wet macular degeneration may occur more rapidly and is more severe (responsible for most cases of blindness due to Macular degeneration).

FUNDUSCOPIC EXAMINATION

- **Dry (atrophic): Drusen bodies** - small, round, yellow-white spots on the outer retina. They represent localized deposits of extracellular material.
- **Wet (neovascular or exudative): new, abnormal vessels** that can cause retinal hemorrhaging & scarring.

DIAGNOSIS

- Funduscopy, fluorescein angiography, Amsler grid

MANAGEMENT OF DRY

- **Zinc & antioxidant vitamins (C & E) may slow progression** in patients with extensive intermediate-size Drusen but do not reverse changes.
- Amsler grid at home to monitor stability.

MANAGEMENT OF WET

- **Intravitreal VEGF inhibitors** (eg, **Bevacizumab,** Ranibizumab, Aflibercept) decrease new, abnormal vessel formation.
- Laser photocoagulation.

MACULAR DEGENERATION

Loss of central & detail vision

AMSLER GRID
Metamorphopsia =
Straight lines appear bent in central vision

Age-related Macular Degeneration

MACULAR DEGENERATION

DRUSEN (diffuse)

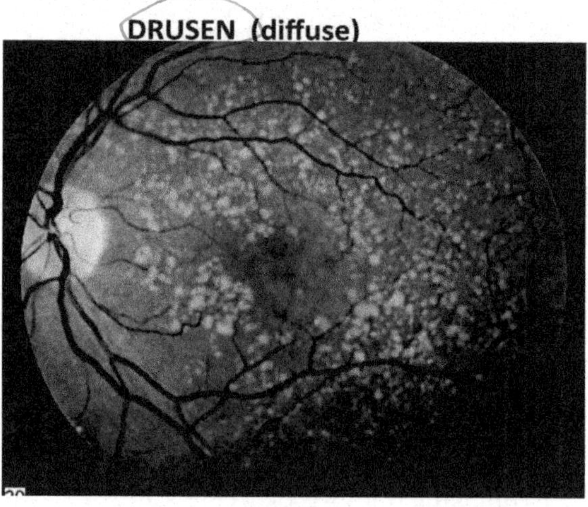

DIABETIC RETINOPATHY

- **Most common cause of new, permanent vision loss in 20-74 years** (usually due to maculopathy).

TYPES

- Nonproliferative (background): **microaneurysms,** cotton wool spots (soft exudates that resemble fluffy gray-white spots due to nerve layer microinfarctions), **hard exudates:** yellow spots with sharp margins often **circinate** (due to lipid or lipoprotein deposits from leaky blood vessels), **blot & dot hemorrhages** (bleeding into the deep retinal layer); **Flame-shaped hemorrhages** (nerve fiber layer hemorrhage).
- Proliferative: **neovascularization** – growth of **new abnormal blood vessels** that can lead to **vitreous hemorrhage**.
- Maculopathy: macular edema or exudates, blurred or decreased central vision loss. Can occur at any stage. Vision loss in nonproliferative often occurs due to macular edema.

MANAGEMENT

- Nonproliferative: strict glucose control, laser treatment.
- **Proliferative: VEGF inhibitors** (eg, Bevacizumab), laser photocoagulation treatment, strict glucose control.
- Prevention: annual eye exams are performed in diabetics to detect diabetic retinopathy.

HYPERTENSIVE RETINOPATHY

- Damage to the retinal blood vessels from longstanding high blood pressure.

MILD

- Arteriolar narrowing due to vasospasm. Shows up as abnormal light reflexes on dilated tortuous arteriole. Copper wiring describes moderate narrowing. Silver wiring = severe narrowing. **AV nicking** – venous compression at the arterial-venous junction.

MODERATE

- Hemorrhages (flame or dot-shaped), cotton-wool spots (soft exudates), hard exudates, and microaneurysms.

SEVERE (GRADE IV)

- All of the above + **papilledema (blurring of the optic disc).**
- Considered an **ophthalmologic emergency.**

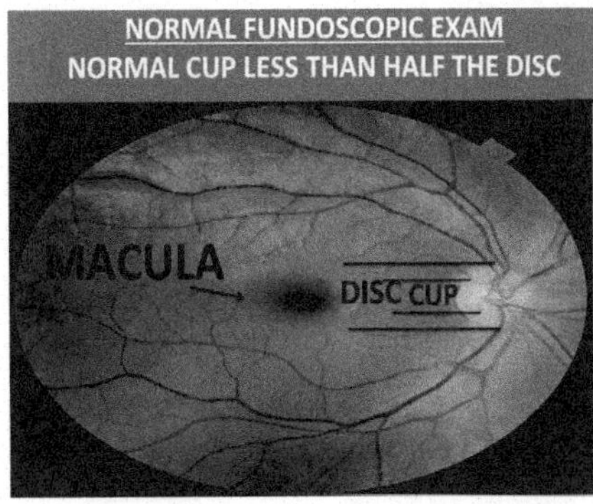

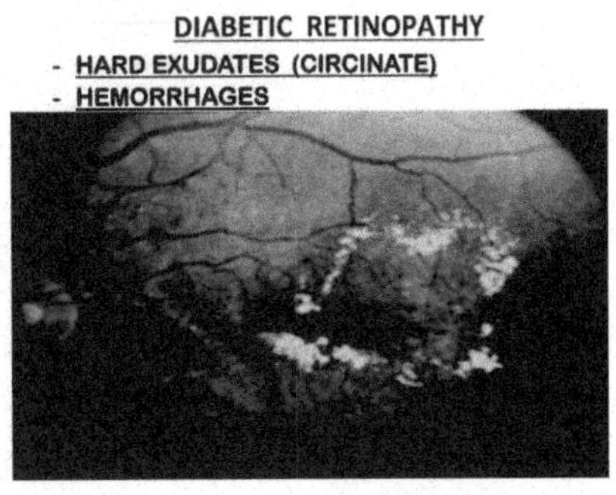

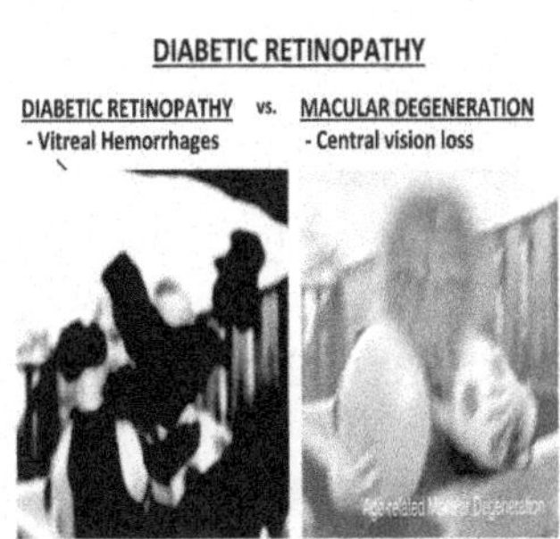

RETINAL DETACHMENT

- Separation of the retina from the underlying retinal pigment epithelium.
- RISK FACTORS: **myopia, previous cataract surgery**, advancing age, trauma.

3 TYPES
- **Rhegmatogenous: most common type** - full-thickness retinal tear causes the retinal inner sensory layer detachment from the choroid plexus.
- Tractional: adhesions separate the retina from its base (eg, proliferative diabetic retinopathy, Sickle cell disease, trauma).
- Exudative (serous): fluid accumulates beneath the retina causing detachment (eg, HTN, CRVO, papilledema).

CLINICAL MANIFESTATIONS
- **Photopsia (flashing lights)** with detachment followed by **floaters** (spots in the visual fields) followed by **progressive unilateral peripheral vision loss: shadow or "curtain coming down"** in the periphery initially followed by loss of central visual field.
- No ocular pain or redness.

DIAGNOSIS
- Funduscopy: retinal tear (detached tissue "flapping" in the vitreous humor). **Positive Shafer's sign** = clumping of brown-colored pigment vitreous cells in the anterior vitreous humor resembling "tobacco dust".

MANAGEMENT
- **Ophthalmologic emergency - keep patient supine** while awaiting consult with the **head turned toward the side of the detachment**. Do not use miotic drops.
- Laser, cryotherapy, or ocular surgery.

OPHTHALMIA NEONATORUM (NEONATAL CONJUNCTIVITIS)

Neonatal conjunctival infection contracted by newborns during delivery.

Day 1:
- **Chemical conjunctivitis** due to silver nitrate. Artificial tears may be helpful once it occurs.

Days 2-5:
- **Gonococcal** most likely cause. Presents with purulent conjunctivitis with exudate and swelling of the eyelids.
- Management: **IM or IV Ceftriaxone needed once infection has occurred.**
- Prophylaxis: **Topical Erythromycin used prophylactically** to prevent infection.

Days 5-7:
- **Chlamydia trachomatis** most likely cause. May occur up to 23 days after birth.
- Management: **Oral erythromycin once infection has occurred.**

Prevention (Prophylaxis):
- Standard neonatal **prophylaxis against gonococcal conjunctivitis** given immediately after birth is **Erythromycin ointment 0.5%**.
- Other options include: topical Tetracycline 1.0%, Silver nitrate, or Povidone-iodine 2.5%.
- Neonatal ocular **prophylaxis is not effective in preventing neonatal chlamydial conjunctivitis.**

OCULAR FOREIGN BODY & CORNEAL ABRASION

CLINICAL MANIFESTATIONS
- Foreign body sensation, tearing, red & painful eye, photophobia, blepharospasms (hard to open the eye).

DIAGNOSIS
- Check visual acuity first.
- Fluorescein staining: **corneal abrasion = "ice rink"/linear abrasions** seen especially if the foreign body is underneath the eyelid (so evert the eyelid to look for it). Pain often relieved with instillation of ophthalmic analgesic drops.

MANAGEMENT

Antibiotic drops for both corneal abrasions & foreign bodies:
- Non-contact lens wearers: **Erythromycin ointment,** Polymyxin-Trimethoprim, Sulfacetamide.
- **Contact lens wearers: Pseudomonal coverage** (eg, **topical Ciprofloxacin or Ofloxacin**). Topical Tobramycin or Gentamicin are alternatives.
- Foreign body removal: remove with sterile irrigation or moistened sterile cotton swab (needle via slit lamp if experienced).
- Corneal abrasions: patching not indicated for small abrasions. May patch the eye in some patients with large abrasions (>5 mm) but do not patch longer than 24 hours. Do not send home with topical anesthetics (may delay healing and cause corneal toxicity).
- 24-hour ophthalmology follow up.
- Rust ring: remove rust ring at 24 hours usually with rotating burr by an ophthalmologist.

CONTRAINDICATIONS
- **Do not patch if *Pseudomonas aeruginosa* is suspected.**
- Antibiotics containing Corticosteroids are NOT used as they can prolong healing and increase susceptibility to superinfection.

BACTERIAL CONJUNCTIVITIS

- Most commonly due to *Staphylococcus aureus* in adults, *Streptococcus pneumoniae, H. influenzae, M. catarrhalis.*
- *N. gonorrhoeae, Chlamydia trachomatis.*
- Transmitted by direct contact and autoinoculation.

CLINICAL MANIFESTATIONS
- **Purulent discharge, lid crusting (eye "stuck shut"** in the morning**),** conjunctival erythema with no ciliary injection (limbal flush), usually no significant visual changes.

DIAGNOSIS
- Usually clinical. Fluorescein staining to look for keratitis or corneal abrasions.
- Culture & gram stain of the discharge.

MANAGEMENT
- **Topical antibiotics: Erythromycin ointment**, Trimethoprim-Polymyxin B, Fluoroquinolones (eg, Moxifloxacin, Ofloxacin).
- **Contact lens wearer: cover Pseudomonas** (eg, **topical Ciprofloxacin or Ofloxacin**). Topical aminoglycosides (eg, Tobramycin or Gentamicin) alternatives.

VIRAL CONJUNCTIVITIS

- Inflammation of the conjunctiva. **Adenovirus is the most common cause**.

TRANSMISSION:
- Highly contagious from **direct contact.**
- **Swimming pool most common source during outbreaks**. Most common in children.

CLINICAL MANIFESTATIONS
- Foreign body or gritty sensation, ocular erythema, & itching. Normal vision.
- Often starts unilateral and progresses to bilateral involvement in 1-2 days.
- May have accompanying viral symptoms.

PHYSICAL EXAMINATION
- Ipsilateral **preauricular lymphadenopathy,** copious **watery tearing** (may have mucoid discharge).
- The tarsal conjunctiva may have a bumpy appearance with lid eversion.
- **Punctate staining** on slit lamp examination may be seen.

MANAGEMENT
- **Supportive mainstay of treatment (self-limited)** – warm to cool compresses, artificial tears. Antihistamines for itching & redness (eg, Olopatadine). Antihistamines with decongestants (eg, Pheniramine-Naphazoline).

ALLERGIC CONJUNCTIVITIS

- Inflammation of the conjunctiva in response to an allergen.
- Contact of the allergen with the eye causes mast cell degranulation and release of histamine.

CLINICAL MANIFESTATIONS
- Conjunctival erythema (red eyes) with normal vision.
- May have other **allergic symptoms** (eg, nasal congestion, sneezing, **marked pruritus (hallmark)** distinguishes allergic from viral. Often bilateral.
- May have an atopic history (eg, Hay fever).

PHYSICAL EXAMINATION
- **Cobblestone mucosa** appearance to the inner upper eyelid, erythema, **watery or mucoid discharge, chemosis** (conjunctival edema). No visual deficits.

MANAGEMENT

Symptomatic treatment mainstay:
- **Topical Antihistamines (H$_1$ blockers): Olopatadine** (antihistamine/mast cell stabilizer), **Pheniramine-Naphazoline** (antihistamine & decongestant), Emedastine.

- Topical NSAIDs: Ketorolac.

OCULAR CHEMICAL BURNS

- Ophthalmologic emergency
- **Alkali burns: worse than acids –** causes **liquefactive necrosis,** denatures proteins & collagen, causes thrombosis of vessels.
- **Acid Burns: coagulative necrosis** (H+ precipitates protein barrier) - cleaners, batteries.

CLINICAL PRESENTATION

- Ocular pain, decreased vision, blepharospasm (inability to open the eyelids), photophobia.

MANAGEMENT

- **Immediate irrigation until a neutral pH (7.0 – 7.4) is achieved** with **lactated ringers or normal saline** (LR ideal because it is closer to a normal pH & is less irritating). Unless there is a strong suspicion for globe rupture, do not delay irrigation. Often irrigated for at least 30 minutes. Once the pH is normal, the eye can safely be examined.
- **Topical antibiotic**: Polymyxin-Trimethoprim, Erythromycin ointment or Moxifloxacin.

STRABISMUS

- **Misalignment of one or both eyes**.
- Stable ocular alignment is not usually present until age 2-3 months.
- **Referral needed for intermittent manifest strabismus needed if it persists >4-6 months of age** to reduce incidence of amblyopia.

MAJOR TYPES:

- **Esotropia:** convergent strabismus - **deviated inward (nasally)** "crossed eyed".
- **Exotropia:** divergent strabismus – **deviated outward (temporally).**

CLINICAL MANIFESTATIONS

- Diplopia, scotomas or amblyopia.

PHYSICAL EXAMINATION

- Asymmetric corneal reflex.

DIAGNOSIS

- **Hirschberg corneal light reflex testing** often used as **initial screening** – asymmetric deflection of the corneal light reflex in one eye is seen in strabismus.
- Cover test refixation of the uncovered eye consistent with manifest strabismus (tropia).
- **Cover-uncover test** looks for latent strabismus (phoria) – the misaligned will appear to deviate inward or outward. Convergence testing.

MANAGEMENT OF REFRACTIVE ERROR

- **Patch (occlusive) therapy first-line** - normal eye is covered to stimulate & strengthen the affected eye.
- Eyeglasses.
- Corrective surgery if severe or unresponsive to conservative therapy.

ORBITAL (SEPTAL) CELLULITIS

- Infection of the orbit (fat & ocular muscles) posterior to the orbital septum.
- Often polymicrobial: *S. aureus, streptococci, GABHS, H. influenzae.*
- Most common in children especially 7-12 years of age.

ETIOLOGIES

- **Most common secondary to sinus infections** (eg, **Ethmoid**).
- Less common: untreated blepharitis, facial trauma, ophthalmic surgery, facial or dental infections.

CLINICAL MANIFESTATIONS

- **Ocular pain especially with eye movements, ophthalmoplegia** (extraocular muscle weakness) with diplopia, **proptosis** (bulging) & visual changes.
- Eyelid edema & erythema.

DIAGNOSIS

- Clinical diagnosis. Can be confirmed by CT scan.
- **High resolution CT scan** – infection of the fat & ocular muscles behind the septum. MRI.

MANAGEMENT

- **Admission + IV antibiotics**: **Vancomycin PLUS** one of the following – **Ceftriaxone or Cefotaxime**, Ampicillin-Sulbactam, Piperacillin-Tazobactam, Clindamycin.

PRESEPTAL (PERIORBITAL) CELLULITIS

- Infection of the eyelid and periocular tissue anterior to the orbital septum.
- Most commonly due to sinusitis or contiguous infection of the soft tissues of the eyelids and face (eg, insect or animal bites).
- Most common causes include *Staphylococcus aureus* (including MRSA), *Streptococci,* & anaerobes.

CLINICAL MANIFESTATIONS

- Unilateral ocular pain, eyelid erythema and edema.
- **The absence of proptosis, ophthalmoplegia, and ocular pain with extraocular movements clinically distinguishes preseptal from postseptal cellulitis.**

DIAGNOSIS

- Often clinical.
- CT scan best test to distinguish between preseptal and postseptal cellulitis if the diagnosis is uncertain.

MANAGEMENT

Outpatient management if > 1 year of age & mild.

- **MRSA coverage:** Oral Clindamycin monotherapy.
- Other options include: Trimethoprim-sulfamethoxazole PLUS either Amoxicillin, Amoxicillin-clavulanic acid or Cefpodoxime.

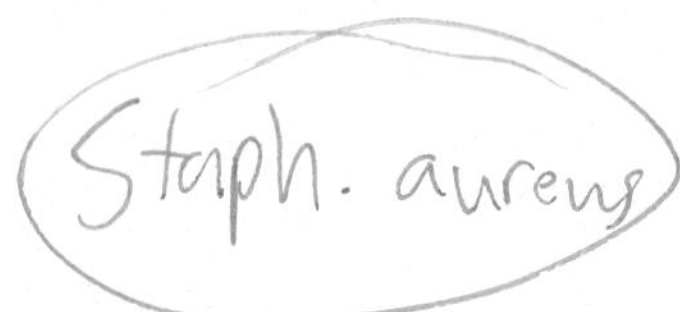

KERATITIS (CORNEAL ULCER/INFLAMMATION)

BACTERIAL KERATITIS

- **Cornea ulceration** & or inflammation. May rapidly progress & be sight-threatening.

PATHOGENS

- Include *S. aureus, Streptococci*. ***Pseudomonas aeruginosa*** **increased in contact lens wearers.**

RISK FACTORS

- **Improper contact lens wear greatest risk factor.**
- Dry ocular surfaces (eg, inability to fully close eyes with Bell palsy).
- Topical corticosteroid use and immunosuppression.

CLINICAL MANIFESTATIONS

- **Ocular pain, photophobia, eye redness, vision changes,** ocular discharge, tearing, foreign body sensation, difficulty keeping the affected eye open.

PHYSICAL EXAM

- Conjunctival erythema, **ciliary injection (limbal flush), hazy cornea (corneal opacification** & ulceration). Hypopyon in severe cases.
- Slit lamp: **increased fluorescein uptake** (deeper than an abrasion).

MANAGEMENT

- **Fluoroquinolone topical** (Moxifloxacin, Gatifloxacin) after obtaining corneal cultures if possible + same-day ophthalmology follow-up.
- **Do not patch the eye.**
- Use of topical corticosteroids controversial (at the discretion of the ophthalmologist).

HERPES KERATITIS

- Corneal infection and inflammation usually due to reactivation of herpes simplex virus in the **trigeminal ganglion**. Major cause of blindness in the US.

CLINICAL MANIFESTATIONS

- Acute onset of unilateral **ocular pain, photophobia, eye redness,** watery discharge, **blurred vision**.

PHYSICAL EXAMINATION

- Conjunctival erythema, **limbic injection (ciliary flush),** hazy cornea. Preauricular lymphadenopathy.

Diagnosis

- **Dendritic (branching) corneal ulceration with fluorescein staining hallmark.**

MANAGEMENT

- **Topical antivirals**: *Trifluridine*, Ganciclovir ointment. **PO Acyclovir.**
- Corneal transplantation may be needed in severe cases.

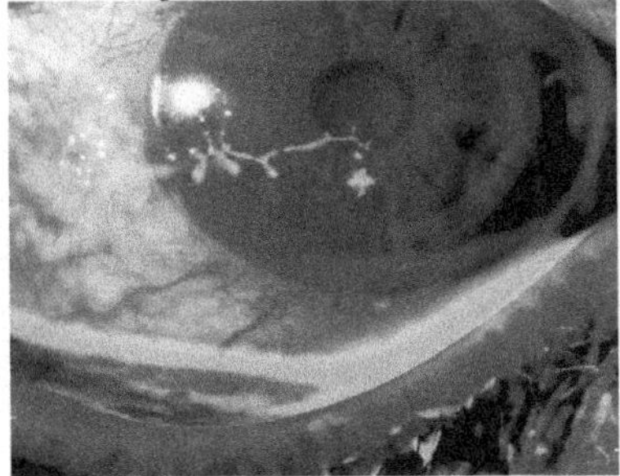

Dendritic (branching) lesion of HSV keratitis
Photo credit: Shutterstock (used with permission)

UVEITIS (IRITIS)

- Anterior: inflammation of iris (iritis) or ciliary body (cyclitis).
- Posterior: choroid inflammation.

ETIOLOGIES

- **Systemic inflammatory & autoimmune diseases:** eg, HLA-B27 spondyloarthropathies, Sarcoidosis, Inflammatory bowel disease.
- Infectious: CMV, Toxoplasmosis, Syphilis, Tuberculosis.
- Trauma.

CLINICAL MANIFESTATIONS

- Anterior: **unilateral severe ocular pain & photophobia, eye redness,** tearing, **blurred or decreased vision**.
- Posterior: **blurred or decreased vision,** floaters. May not be painful.

PHYSICAL EXAMINATION

- Conjunctival erythema, **ciliary injection (limbal flush), consensual photophobia.**
- **Constricted pupil (miosis)**. Hypopyon in severe cases.

DIAGNOSIS

- Slit lamp: **inflammatory "cells & flare"** (cells = WBCs & flare = proteins in the vitreous humor).

MANAGEMENT

- Anterior: **topical glucocorticoids.** Relief of spasm with Scopolamine or topical cycloplegics (eg, Cyclopentolate or Homatropine).
- Posterior: systemic glucocorticoids.
- Infectious: treat as appropriate (viral, bacterial, etc.)

CATARACT

- **Lens opacification (thickening).** Usually bilateral.
- Most common cause of blindness in the world.

RISK FACTORS

- **Aging** (most common >60y).
- **Cigarette smoking, glucocorticoid use, Diabetes mellitus,** UV light, malnutrition, trauma.
- Neonatal cataracts: congenital ToRCH syndrome (Toxoplasmosis, Rubella, CMV HSV)

CLINICAL MANIFESTATIONS

- Painless, slow, progressive blurred or vision loss over months to years (difficulty with night driving, reading signs).

PHYSICAL EXAMINATION

- **Absent red reflex, opaque lens**.

MANAGEMENT

- Observation if mild
- Surgery indicated if the visual changes affect activities of daily living.

PAPILLEDEMA

- **Optic nerve (disc) swelling** secondary to **increased intracranial pressure** (usually bilateral).
- Etiologies: Idiopathic intracranial hypertension, space-occupying lesion (eg, cerebral tumor, abscess), increased CSF production, cerebral edema, severe hypertension (Grade IV).

CLINICAL MANIFESTATIONS

- Headache, nausea, vomiting. Vision is often preserved.

DIAGNOSIS

- Funduscopy: swollen optic disc with blurred margins.
- MRI or CT scan of the head first to rule out mass effect, followed by lumbar puncture (increased CSF pressure).

MANAGEMENT

- Acetazolamide – decreases production of aqueous humor and CSF production).
- Treat the underlying cause.

	PAPILLEDEMA	PAPILLITIS	RETROBULBAR NEURITIS	GLAUCOMA
DEFINITION	Edema of the optic nerve head due to **↑CSF pressure**	Edema of optic nerve head in the orbit (eye) - **Optic Neuritis**	Edema of optic nerve behind the eye - **Optic Neuritis**	Edema of the optic nerve from **↑intraocular pressure**
LATERALITY	Bilateral	Unilateral	Unilateral	Acute: Unilateral Chronic: Bilateral
VISUAL DEFICIT	Enlarged blind spot	Range from central scotoma to complete loss of vision	Range from central scotoma - complete loss of vision	Halos around light to blindness
FUNDUSCOPIC	Blurred disc-cup	Blurred disc-cup	Normal	Blurred disc-cup
MARCUS GUNN	Negative	**POSITIVE**	**POSITIVE**	Negative
MANAGEMENT	Reduce ICP	Corticosteroids	Corticosteroids	Reduce IOP

OPTIC NEURITIS (OPTIC NERVE/CN II INFLAMMATION)

- **Acute inflammatory demyelination of the optic nerve.**
- Risk factors: most common in women and young patients 20-40y.

ETIOLOGIES

- Multiple sclerosis. Autoimmune. Medications: **Ethambutol,** Chloramphenicol, PDE5 inhibitors.

CLINICAL MANIFESTATIONS

- **Painful loss of vision, decrease in color vision (desaturation),** visual field defects: **central scotoma** (blind spot) over hours to a few days. Usually **unilateral.**

PHYSICAL EXAMINATION

- **Ocular pain worse with eye movement.**
- **Marcus-Gunn pupil** (relative afferent pupillary defect) – during swinging-flashlight test **from the unaffected eye into the affected eye, the pupils appear to dilate.**
- Funduscopy: 2/3 normal disc/cup (retrobulbar) or 1/3 **optic disc swelling/blurring (papillitis).**
- MRI confirms the diagnosis when Multiple sclerosis is suspected.

MANAGEMENT

- **IV Methylprednisolone initial management** followed by oral corticosteroids.
- Vision usually returns with treatment.

MARCUS GUNN PUPIL (RELATIVE AFFERENT PUPILLARY DEFECT)

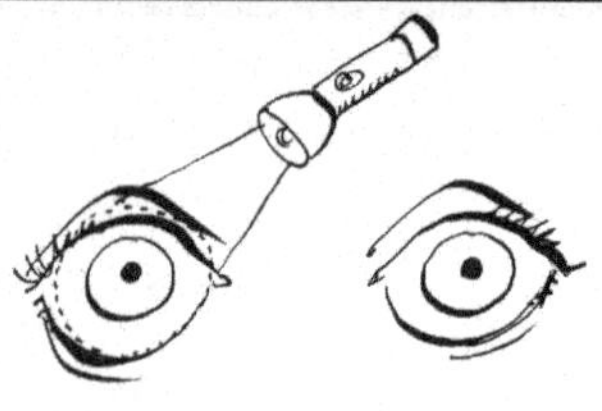

1. **Optic neuritis MC cause.**
2. Severe retinal disease (eg, CRVO, CRAO, significant retinal detachment).

- During swinging-flashlight test into the unaffected eye, both pupils constrict.

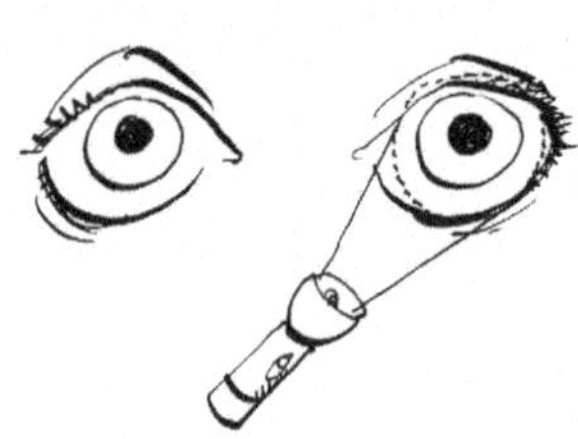

- **MARCUS GUNN:** during swinging-flashlight test **from the unaffected eye into the affected eye, the pupils appear to dilate** (due to less than normal constriction).
- **R**elative **A**fferent **P**upillary **D**efect mnemonic = when you shine a **R**ay in the **A**ffected **P**upil it **D**ilates

ARGYLL-ROBERTSON PUPIL

- Near-light dissociation. Pupil **constricts on accommodation but does not react to bright light.**

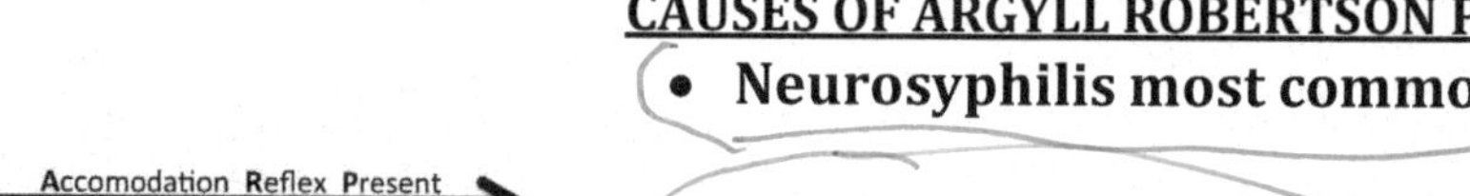

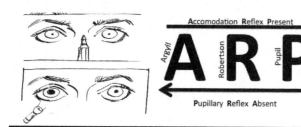

Accomodation Reflex Present

Argyll **A** Robertson **R** Pupil **P**

Pupillary Reflex Absent

CAUSES OF ARGYLL ROBERTSON PUPIL

- **Neurosyphilis most common**
- Midbrain lesions (eg, Parinaud syndrome)
- Diabetic neuropathy

VISUAL PATHWAY DEFECTS

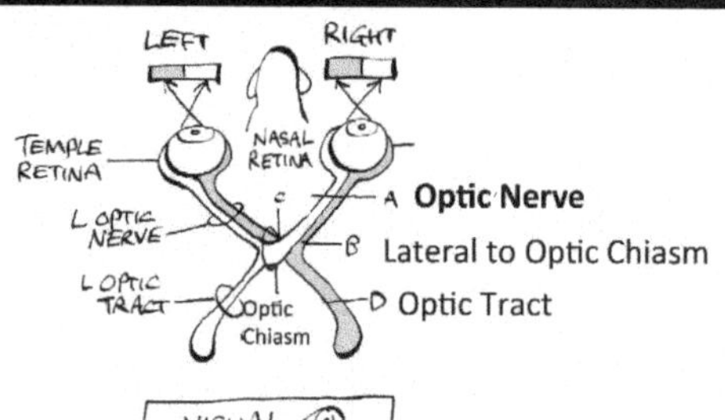

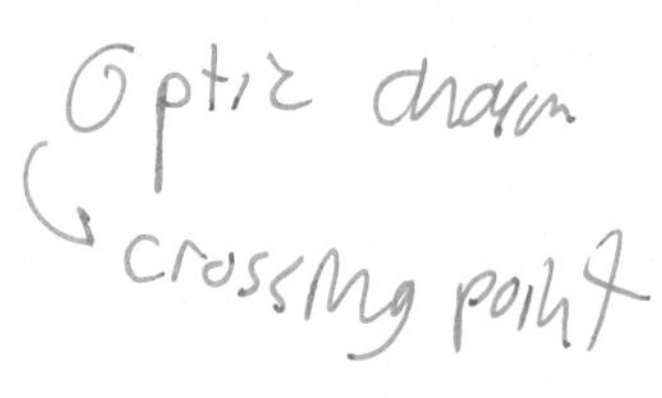

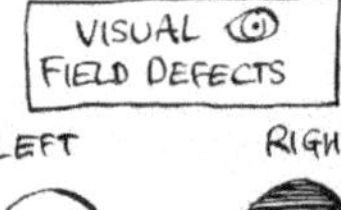

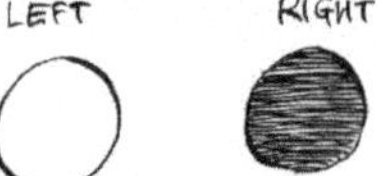

A. **TOTAL BLINDNESS OF IPSILATERAL EYE**
If lesion is on ***Optic Nerve or Retina****

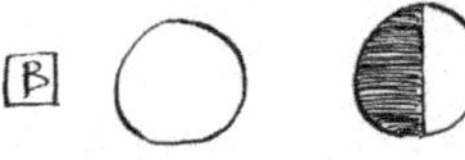

B. IPSILATERAL NASAL HEMIANOPSIA
If lesion is **lateral** to the optic chiasm.

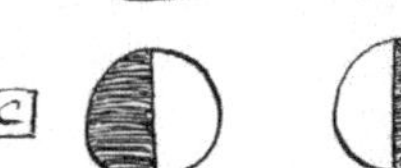

C. **BITEMPORAL HETERONYMOUS HEMIANOPSIA**
If ***midline optic chiasm lesion (ex. pituitary adenoma)****

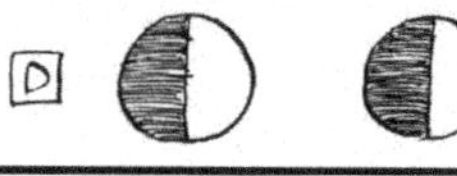

D. **CONTRALATERAL HOMONYMOUS HEMIANOPSIA**
If lesion at ***optic tract*** or in ***occipital lobe stroke***

ACUTE NARROW ANGLE-CLOSURE GLAUCOMA

- Increased intraocular pressure leading to damage of the optic nerve.
- Ophthalmologic emergency. Leading cause of preventable blindness in US.
- Risk factors: patients with preexisting narrow angle or large lens – age > 60 years, hyperopes (far-sighted), females & Asians.

PATHOPHYSIOLOGY
- Decreased drainage of aqueous humor via trabecular meshwork & canal of Schlemm.
- Precipitants: **mydriasis** (pupillary dilation) further closes the angle (eg, **dim lights, sympathomimetics, anticholinergics**).

CLINICAL MANIFESTATIONS
- **Sudden** onset of **severe, unilateral ocular pain.**
- Vision changes include **halos around lights & loss of peripheral vision** (tunnel vision).
- Nausea, vomiting, headache.

PHYSICAL EXAMINATION
- **Conjunctival erythema, cloudy "steamy" cornea**, **mid-dilated fixed pupil** (reacts poorly to light), eye hard on palpation.

DIAGNOSIS
- Tonometry: **increased intraocular pressure** (>21 mmHg).
- Funduscopy: **optic disc blurring** or "cupping" of optic nerve (thinning of the outer rim of the optic nerve head).

MANAGEMENT

Combination of topical agents (eg, **Timolol, Apraclonidine, Pilocarpine**) with a systemic agent to lower intraocular pressure (eg, **PO or IV Acetazolamide** or IV Mannitol).
- Topical Beta-blockers: (eg, Timolol) **does not affect visual acuity.**
- Alpha-2 agonists: Apraclonidine, Brimonidine
- Miotics/cholinergics: Pilocarpine or Carbachol
- Prostaglandins: Latanoprost

Definitive:
- **Iridotomy** – laser (preferred) or surgical.

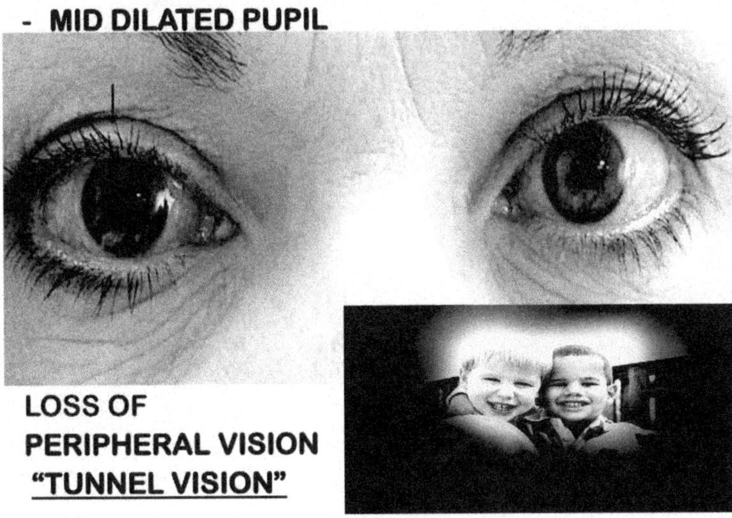

CHRONIC (OPEN ANGLE) GLAUCOMA

- **Slow, progressive painless bilateral peripheral vision loss** (compared to rapid painful unilateral vision in acute glaucoma).
- Risk factors: African-Americans, age >40y, family history, Diabetes Mellitus.
- Pathophysiology: open angle: normal anterior chamber. The increased intraocular pressure in chronic open angle glaucoma is due to reduced aqueous drainage through the trabeculum, which eventually damages the optic nerve.

CLINICAL MANIFESTATIONS

- Usually **asymptomatic** until late in the disease course & vision loss is usually the presenting symptom.
- **Slow, progressive painless bilateral peripheral vision loss (tunnel vision)** progressing to central loss.

PHYSICAL EXAM

- **Cupping of optic discs**, increased cup to disc ratio, notching of the disc rim.

MANAGEMENT

- Reduce intraocular pressure: **Prostaglandin analogs first-line** (eg, **Latanoprost** – greater reduction of IOP), beta-blockers (Timolol), alpha-2 adrenergic agonists (Brimonidine), Acetazolamide (carbonic anhydrase inhibitor).
- Laser therapy (trabeculoplasty) if medical therapy fails. Increases aqueous outflow by improving drainage of aqueous humor via the trabecular meshwork.
- Surgery last-line treatment.

AMAUROSIS FUGAX

- **Transient monocular vision loss** (lasting minutes) with complete recovery (may be binocular).

ETIOLOGIES

- Disorders affecting the eye or the optic nerve: **retinal emboli or ischemia.**
- Can be seen with transient ischemic attack (carotid artery disease), Giant cell arteritis, central retinal artery occlusion, migraine (visual aura), systemic lupus erythematosus & other vasculitis disorders.

CLINICAL MANIFESTATIONS

- **Vision loss descending over the visual field** described as a **temporary "curtain or shade" comes down and resolves ("lifts up")** usually **within 1 hour**. TIA usually lasts 1-15 minutes. Migraine aura usually 10-30 minutes.

DIAGNOSIS

- Determined by likely cause based on history and physical examination.
- Often includes carotid duplex ultrasound and ophthalmologic examination.
- MRI, EEG

CENTRAL RETINAL ARTERY OCCLUSION (CRAO)

- Retinal artery thrombus or embolus. Ophthalmologic emergency.
- Most common 50-80y, history of **atherosclerotic disease.**

ETIOLOGIES
- **Emboli from carotid artery atherosclerosis most common.**
- **Cardiogenic emboli** - second most common cause overall but most common cause in young patients & patients without atherosclerosis.
- Vasculitis.

CLINICAL MANIFESTATIONS
- **Acute, sudden painless monocular vision loss.** May be preceded by Amaurosis fugax.
- May have an ipsilateral carotid bruit.

DIAGNOSIS
- Funduscopy: retinal ischemia
  Pale retina with a cherry-red macula.
  Boxcar appearance of the retinal vessels (segmentation of blood flow).
  Emboli may be seen (20%).

MANAGEMENT
- No consensus on optimal treatment - initial treatment may include CO_2 rebreathing, 100% oxygen, ocular massage (to dilate vessels & attempt to dislodge the clot), decompression of the anterior chamber (Acetazolamide or chamber paracentesis), ophthalmology consult, and in-situ fibrinolysis.

PROGNOSIS
- Poor prognosis even with treatment.
- No treatment has been shown truly effective but should be attempted.

CENTRAL RETINAL VEIN OCCLUSION (CRVO)

- Thrombus in the central retinal vein that leads to fluid backup in the retina.

RISK FACTORS
- Hypertension, Diabetes mellitus, glaucoma, hypercoagulable states (eg, Polycythemia vera), Multiple myeloma, & smoking.

CLINICAL MANIFESTATIONS
- **Sudden onset of painless monocular vision loss.**

DIAGNOSIS
- Funduscopy:
  - **extensive retinal hemorrhages (blood & thunder appearance)**
  - retinal vein dilation, macular edema, optic disc swelling may be seen.
- May have relative afferent pupillary defect (Marcus-Gunn pupil).

MANAGEMENT
- No definitive treatment.

EAR DISORDERS

OTITIS EXTERNA

- Inflammation of the external auditory canal.

RISK FACTORS
- **Water immersion** aka **"swimmer's ear"** – excess moisture raises the pH from the normal acidic pH of the ear, facilitating bacterial overgrowth.
- **Local mechanical trauma** (eg, use of Q-tips), age 7-12 years, aberrant ear wax (too much or too little).

ETIOLOGIES
- ***Pseudomonas aeruginosa* most common** (50%).
- *Staphylococcus* (eg, aureus & epidermis), GABHS, Proteus, anaerobes; Aspergillus. Fungi.

CLINICAL MANIFESTATIONS
- **Ear pain, pruritus** in the ear canal (may have recent activity of swimming).
- Auricular discharge, ear pressure or fullness, hearing loss.
- Physical exam: **pain on traction of the ear canal or tragus, purulent auricular discharge.**

DIAGNOSIS
- Clinical + otoscopy: **edema of the external auditory canal** with erythema, debris, or discharge.

MANAGEMENT
- Protect the ear against moisture (drying agents include isopropyl alcohol & acetic acid) + removal of debris & cerumen + topical antibiotics with coverage against *Pseudomonas* & *Staphylococcus* (with or without glucocorticoids for inflammation).
- Topical antibiotics:
  - **Ciprofloxacin-dexamethasone, Ofloxacin.**
  - Aminoglycoside combination: Neomycin/Polymyxin-B/Hydrocortisone otic. **Not used if tympanic perforation suspected or if TM cannot be visualized - aminoglycosides are ototoxic**.

MALIGNANT (NECROTIZING) OTITIS EXTERNA

- **Invasive infection of the external auditory canal and skull base** (temporal bone, soft tissue, and cartilage). A complication of Acute otitis externa.
- ***Pseudomonas aeruginosa*** >95%.
- Risk factors: **immunocompromised states - elderly diabetics most common,** high-dose glucocorticoid therapy, chemotherapy, advanced HIV.

CLINICAL MANIFESTATIONS
- **Severe auricular pain, otorrhea. Cranial nerve palsies** (eg, CN VII) if Osteomyelitis occurs.
- May radiate to temporomandibular joint (pain with chewing).
- Physical examination: **severe auricular pain on traction of the ear canal or tragus.**

DIAGNOSIS
- Otoscopy: edema of the external auditory canal with erythema, discharge, **granulation tissue at the bony cartilaginous junction of the ear canal floor,** frank necrosis of the ear canal skin.
- **CT or MRI** to confirm the diagnosis. Biopsy is the most accurate test.

MANAGEMENT
- **Admission + IV Antipseudomonal antibiotics – IV Ciprofloxacin first-line.**
- Alternatives include Piperacillin-tazobactam, Ceftazidime, Cefepime.

MASTOIDITIS

Infection of the mastoid air cells of the temporal bone. Largely a disease of childhood (esp. < 2 years).

- Etiologies: usually a **complication of Acute otitis media.**
- Clinical manifestations: **deep ear pain** (usually worse at night), fever, lethargy, malaise.

PHYSICAL EXAMINATION
- Otalgia, **fever,** signs of Otitis media (bulging & erythematous tympanic membrane).
- **Mastoid (postauricular) tenderness, edema, & erythema**.
- **Protrusion of the auricle.** May develop cutaneous abscess (fluctuance). Narrowed auditory canal.

DIAGNOSIS
- **CT scan with contrast first-line diagnostic test**. MRI.

MANAGEMENT
- **IV antibiotics + middle ear or mastoid drainage (myringotomy)** with or without **tympanostomy tube placement.** IV Vancomycin PLUS either Ceftazidime or Cefepime or Piperacillin-tazobactam.
- Tympanocentesis can be performed to get cultures. Refractory or complicated: **mastoidectomy**

CHRONIC OTITIS MEDIA

- **Recurrent or persistent infection of the middle ear** &/or mastoid cell system **in the presence of tympanic membrane perforation** > 6 weeks.
- Complication of Acute otitis media, trauma, or cholesteatoma.

ETIOLOGIES
- ***Pseudomonas* most common,** *S. aureus*, gram-negative rods (eg, *Proteus*), anaerobes, *Mycoplasma*.
- Can become worse after a URI or after water enters the ear.

CLINICAL MANIFESTATIONS
- **Perforated tympanic membrane + persistent or recurrent purulent otorrhea (often painless),** ear fullness, varying degrees of **conductive hearing loss**.
- May have a primary or secondary Cholesteatoma.

MANAGEMENT
- Removal of infected debris + **topical antibiotic drops first-line (Ofloxacin or Ciprofloxacin)**.
- Systemic antibiotics reserved for severe cases.
- **In patients with a tympanic membrane rupture, avoid water, moisture, & topical aminoglycosides in the ear whenever there is a tympanic membrane rupture.**
- Surgical: tympanic membrane repair or reconstruction.

EXAM TIP

Acute otitis media: effusion + signs or symptoms of inflammation (fever, ear pain with bulging, & marked erythema of the tympanic membrane).

Chronic otitis media: perforated tympanic membrane + persistent or recurrent purulent otorrhea, otalgia (ear pain), ear fullness, & varying degrees of conductive hearing loss.

Serous otitis media (otitis media with effusion): asymptomatic effusion + no signs or symptoms of inflammation (no fever, no ear pain & no marked erythema or bulging of the TM).

ACUTE OTITIS MEDIA (AOM)

- Infection of middle ear, temporal bone, & mastoid air cells.
- Acute otitis media: rapid onset + signs or symptoms of inflammation.
- Risk factors: peak age 6 – 18 months (Eustachian tube in children is shorter, narrower, & more horizontal), day care, pacifier or bottle use, second-hand smoke, not being breastfed.

4 MOST COMMON ORGANISMS:
- ***Streptococcus pneumoniae* most common,** *H. influenzae, Moraxella catarrhalis,* Group A *Streptococcus* (same organisms seen in Acute sinusitis).

PATHOPHYSIOLOGY
- **Most commonly preceded by viral URI,** leading to blockage of the Eustachian tube.

CLINICAL MANIFESTATIONS
- Fever, **otalgia** (ear pain), **ear tugging in infants**, stuffiness, conductive hearing loss.
- Tympanic membrane rupture: rapid relief of pain + otorrhea (usually heals in 1-2 days).

PHYSICAL EXAMINATION
- **Bulging & erythematous tympanic membrane (TM) with effusion,** loss of landmarks.
- Pneumatic otoscopy: **decreased TM mobility (most sensitive).**

DIAGNOSIS
- Clinical.
- Tympanocentesis for a sample of fluid for culture definitive (eg, in recurrent cases).

MANAGEMENT
- Observation can be done depending on age and severity. Children over age of 2 should receive antibiotics if the diagnosis is certain and the infection is severe.
- **Amoxicillin initial antibiotic of choice.**
- Second-line: Amoxicillin-Clavulanic acid, Cefuroxime, Cefdinir, Cefpodoxime.
- Penicillin allergy: Azithromycin, Clarithromycin, Erythromycin-Sulfisoxazole, Trimethoprim–sulfamethoxazole.
- Severe or recurrent cases: myringotomy (surgical drainage) with tympanostomy tube insertion.
- In children with recurrent otitis media, may need an Iron deficiency anemia workup & CT scan.

SEROUS OTITIS MEDIA WITH EFFUSION

- Middle ear fluid **+ no signs or symptoms of acute inflammation** (no fever, no ear pain, & no marked erythema or bulging of the TM).
- May be seen after resolution of Acute otitis media or in patients with Eustachian tube dysfunction

DIAGNOSIS
- Otoscopy: effusion with **tympanic membrane that is retracted or flat.** Hypomobility with insufflation.

MANAGEMENT
- **Observation in most cases** (usually spontaneously resolves).
- Persistent or complicated: Tympanostomy tube for drainage (eg, children with hearing impairment, developmental delays, or specific conditions).

EUSTACHIAN TUBE DYSFUNCTION

- Eustachian tube (ET) swelling inhibits the ET ability to autoinsufflate, causing negative pressure.
- **Often follows viral URI or allergic rhinitis;** sinusitis, tumors.

CLINICAL MANIFESTATIONS
- Obstructive dysfunction: ear fullness or pressure, **popping of the ears, underwater feeling,** disequilibrium, fluctuating conductive hearing loss, tinnitus.

DIAGNOSIS
- Clinical. Otoscopic findings usually normal. May have fluid behind the TM (serous otitis media).

MANAGEMENT
- Treating the underlying cause & symptom management is the mainstay of treatment.
- **Autoinsufflation** (eg, swallowing, yawning, blowing against a slightly-pinched nostril).
- Intranasal corticosteroids if sinonasal inflammation present.
- **Decongestants for congestive symptoms**: Pseudoephedrine, Phenylephrine, Oxymetazoline nasal.

BAROTRAUMA

- Damage to the tympanic membrane can occur with sudden pressure changes (eg, flying, diving, decompression, hyperbaric oxygen).

CLINICAL MANIFESTATIONS
- **Ear pain, fullness, & hearing loss that persists after the etiologic event.**

PHYSICAL EXAMINATION
- May have bloody auricular discharge if traumatic.
- Visualization of the tympanic membrane may reveal rupture or petechiae.

MANAGEMENT
Avoidance is the best treatment:
- Avoidance of flying with a cold.
- **Autoinsufflation** (eg, swallowing, yawning, chewing gum).

AUDITORY EXAMINATION FINDINGS

AC = air conduction. BC = bone conduction.

Assessed with a tuning fork	**WEBER:** place on top head	**RINNE:** place on mastoid by ear
NORMAL	No lateralization	Normal (Positive) AC > BC
SENSORINEURAL LOSS (INNER EAR):	Lateralizes to **NORMAL ear**	**Normal: AC > BC.** Difficulty hearing their own voice & deciphering words.
CONDUCTIVE LOSS (EXT/MIDDLE):	Lateralizes to **AFFECTED ear**	**BC ≥ AC (Negative)**

sensoriNeural lateralizes to Normal ear + Normal Rinne (think of the N for sensoriNeural).

CONDUCTIVE HEARING LOSS:	SENSORINEURAL HEARING LOSS:
External or middle ear disorders: defect in sound conduction (ex. obstruction from a foreign body or cerumen impaction), damage to ossicles (otosclerosis, cholesteatoma), mastoiditis, otitis media. **Cerumen impaction most common cause**	**Inner ear disorders:** ex presbycusis, chronic loud noise exposure, CNS lesions (eg, acoustic neuroma), Labyrinthitis, Meniere syndrome. **Presbycusis most common cause**

CERUMEN IMPACTION

- External auditory canal wax impaction.

CLINICAL MANIFESTATIONS
- May lead to **conductive hearing loss** & ear fullness.

PHYSICAL EXAMINATION
- Otoscopy: direct visualization of the impacted cerumen
- Conductive hearing loss pattern: **lateralization to the affected ear** on Weber testing. Bone conduction > air conduction.

MANAGEMENT
Cerumen softening:
- **Hydrogen Peroxide** 3%
- **Carbamide peroxide**

Aural toilet:
- Irrigation, curette removal of cerumen, suction.
- Irrigation (if no evidence of tympanic membrane perforation & water must be at body temperature to prevent vertigo).

TYMPANIC MEMBRANE PERFORATION

- Rupture of the tympanic membrane
- May lead to Cholesteatoma development.

ETIOLOGIES
- Most commonly occurs due to penetrating or noise trauma (most commonly occurs at the pars tensa) or Otitis media.

CLINICAL MANIFESTATIONS
- Acute ear pain, hearing loss.
- Patients with otalgia prior to rupture may develop **sudden pain relief with bloody otorrhea.**
- Tinnitus & vertigo.

DIAGNOSIS
- Otoscopic examination: perforated TM. Do not perform pneumatic otoscopy.
- May have conductive hearing loss (Weber: lateralization to the affected ear, Rinne: bone conduction greater than air conduction.

MANAGEMENT
- Most perforated TMs heal spontaneously. Follow up to ensure resolution.
- Topical antibiotics (eg, Ofloxacin in some).
- **Avoid water & topical aminoglycosides in the ear whenever there is a TM rupture.**

(Neomycin ect)

CHOLESTEATOMA

- Abnormal keratinized collection of desquamated squamous epithelium in the middle ear that can lead to bony erosion of the mastoid.
- Etiologies: most commonly due to **chronic middle ear disease or Eustachian tube dysfunction.**

CLINICAL MANIFESTATIONS
- **Painless otorrhea (brown or yellow discharge with a strong odor).**
- May develop peripheral vertigo, tinnitus, dizziness, or cranial nerve palsies.

DIAGNOSIS
- Otoscopy: **granulation tissue (cellular debris).** May have perforation of the tympanic membrane.
- **Conductive hearing loss** – lateralization to the affected ear on Weber testing and bone conduction > air conduction in the affected ear on Rinne.

MANAGEMENT
- Surgical excision of the debris & Cholesteatoma with reconstruction of the ossicles.

OTOSCLEROSIS

- Abnormal bony overgrowth of the footplate of the stapes bone leading to **conductive hearing loss.**
- Autosomal dominant disorder (may have **family history** of conductive hearing loss)

CLINICAL MANIFESTATIONS
- Slowly progressive **conductive hearing loss,** especially **low-frequencies**, tinnitus.
- Vertigo uncommon.

DIAGNOSIS
- **Conductive hearing loss** – lateralization to the affected ear on Weber testing and bone conduction > air conduction in the affected ear on Rinne.
- Tone audiometry (most useful)

MANAGEMENT
- Stapedectomy with prosthesis or hearing amplification (eg, hearing aid).
- Cochlear implantation if severe.

VERTIGO

- **False sense of motion** (or exaggerated sense of motion). 2 types:

	PERIPHERAL VERTIGO		CENTRAL VERTIGO
LOCATION OF PROBLEM	**Labyrinth or Vestibular nerve** (which is part of CN VIII/8).		**Brainstem or cerebellar**
ETIOLOGIES	1. BENIGN POSITIONAL VERTIGO (MC) 2. MENIERE: 3. VESTIBULAR NEURITIS 4. LABYRINTHITIS: 5. Cholesteatoma	**episodic vertigo, no hearing loss** **episodic vertigo + hearing loss** **continuous vertigo, no hearing loss** **continuous vertigo + hearing loss**	Cerebellopontine tumors Migraine Cerebral vascular disease Multiple sclerosis Vestibular Neuroma
CLINICAL	• **HORIZONTAL nystagmus** (usually beats away from affected side). **Fatigable.** • Sudden onset of tinnitus & hearing loss usually associated with peripheral compared to central causes.		• **VERTICAL nystagmus. Nonfatigable** (continuous) • Gait issues more severe. • Gradual onset. • **Positive CNS signs.**

MANAGEMENT OF NAUSEA/VOMITING IN PATIENTS WITH VERTIGO:

Nausea & vomiting is caused by sensory conflict **mediated by the neurotransmitters GABA, acetylcholine, histamine, dopamine, & serotonin.**

Therefore, antiemetics work primarily by blocking these transmitters.

ANTIHISTAMINES/ ANTICHOLINERGICS **Meclizine** **Scopolamine** - anticholinergic **Dimenhydrinate** **Diphenhydramine**	MOA: acts on the brain's control center for nausea, vomiting & dizziness. Ind: **first-line for vertigo** (nausea/vomiting), **motion sickness.** S/E: **anticholinergic** - dry mouth, blurred vision (dilated pupils), urinary retention, constipation, dry skin, flushing, tachycardia, fever, delirium. CI/Caution: **acute narrow angle glaucoma, BPH with urinary retention.**
DOPAMINE BLOCKERS **Prochlorperazine** **Promethazine** **Metoclopramide**	MOA: **blocks CNS dopamine receptors (D_1 D_2)** in the brain's vomiting center. Ind: nausea/vomiting, motion sickness. S/E: **QT prolongation, sedation,** constipation. **Extrapyramidal Sx (EPS): rigidity, bradykinesia, tremor, akathisia (restlessness).** 3 EPS syndromes include: 1. **Dystonic Reactions (Dyskinesia):** reversible EPS **hours-days after initiation** ⇨ intermittent, spasmodic, sustained involuntary contractions **(trismus, protrusions of tongue, forced jaw opening, difficulty speaking, facial grimacing, torticollis).** **Mgmt: Diphenhydramine IV** or add **anticholinergic agent** (eg, Benztropine). 2. **Tardive Dyskinesia:** repetitive involuntary movements mostly involving extremities & face – lip smacking, teeth grinding, rolling of tongue.* Seen with long-term use.* 3. **Parkinsonism:** (due to ↓dopamine in nigrostriatal pathways) – rigidity, tremor. **Neuroleptic Malignant Syndrome (NMS):** life threatening disorder due to D_2 inhibition in basal ganglia: **mental status changes, extreme muscle rigidity, tremor, fever, autonomic instability (tachycardia,** blood pressure changes, tachypnea, profuse diaphoresis, incontinence, dyspnea). Ice to axilla/groin, ventilatory support. **Dopamine Agonists: Bromocriptine,** Amantadine, Levodopa/Carbidopa.
BENZODIAZEPINES	Lorazepam, Diazepam used in refractory patients (potentiates GABA).
SEROTONIN ANTAGONISTS **Ondansetron** **Granisetron** **Dolasetron**	MOA: **blocks serotonin receptors** (5-HT3) both peripherally & centrally in the chemoreceptor trigger zone of the medulla (suppressing the vomiting center). S/E: neurologic: headache, fatigue. GI sx: nausea, constipation. Cardiac: prolonged QT interval & cardiac arrhythmias.

BENIGN PAROXYSMAL POSITIONAL VERTIGO

- A type of peripheral vertigo most commonly due to **displaced otolith particles** (calcium crystals) within the semicircular canals of the inner ear (canalithiasis).
- Most common cause of peripheral vertigo.

CLINICAL MANIFESTATIONS

- Recurrent episodes of **sudden, episodic peripheral vertigo (lasting 60 seconds or less) & provoked with specific head movements** (eg, rolling over in bed, lying down, getting up from bed, looking up).
- May be accompanied by nausea or vomiting.
- **Not associated with hearing loss,** tinnitus, or ataxia.

DIAGNOSIS

- **Dix Hallpike (Nylen Barany) test** - produces fatigable nystagmus.

MANAGEMENT

- **Canalith repositioning treatment of choice - Epley maneuver** or Semont maneuver.
- Because the episodes are so brief, medical therapy is not usually needed.

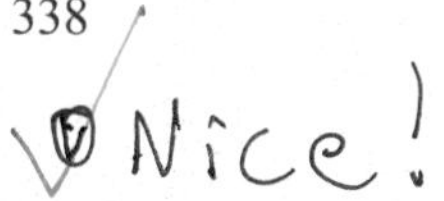

VESTIBULAR NEURITIS & LABYRINTHITIS

DEFINITIONS

- Vestibular neuritis: inflammation of the vestibular portion of cranial nerve VIII.
- Labyrinthitis: inflammation of the vestibular and cochlear portion of CN VIII.

ETIOLOGIES

- Idiopathic. May be associated with **viral or postviral inflammation.**

CLINICAL MANIFESTATIONS

- **Vestibular symptoms (both): continuous peripheral vertigo,** dizziness, nausea, vomiting, & gait disturbances. **Nystagmus is usually horizontal and rotary** (away from the affected side in the fast phase).
- **Cochlear symptoms (Labyrinthitis only):** unilateral **hearing loss, tinnitus.**

DIAGNOSIS

- Primary clinical (imaging not usually needed).
- Neuroimaging (MRI preferred > CT) to rule out alternative causes if the symptoms are not fully consistent with a peripheral lesion.

MANAGEMENT

- **Glucocorticoids first-line management.**
- **Symptomatic relief:** antihistamines (eg, **Meclizine**) or anticholinergics. Benzodiazepines.
- Both are self-limited - symptoms usually resolve in weeks even without treatment.

MÉNIÈRE'S DISEASE (IDIOPATHIC ENDOLYMPHATIC HYDROPS)

- **Idiopathic distention of the endolymphatic compartment of the inner ear due to excess fluid.**
- Meniere SYNDROME is due to an identifiable cause. Meniere DISEASE is idiopathic.

CLINICAL MANIFESTATIONS

- Characterized by 4 findings - **episodic peripheral vertigo** (lasting minutes – hours) + fluctuating **sensorineural hearing loss** (low-tones initially), **tinnitus**, & **ear fullness.**
- **Horizontal nystagmus,** nausea, vomiting.

DIAGNOSIS

- Diagnosis of exclusion (no specific test).
- Transtympanic electrocochleography, loss of nystagmus with caloric testing seen with Meniere.

MANAGEMENT

- **Initial: dietary modifications: avoidance of salt, caffeine, nicotine, chocolate, & alcohol** (because they increase endolymphatic pressure).
- Medical: if no relief with dietary modifications. Antihistamines (**Meclizine,** Dimenhydrinate); Prochlorperazine or Promethazine, benzodiazepines (Diazepam), anticholinergics (Scopolamine), & **Diuretics** (eg, **Hydrochlorothiazide**) to reduce endolymphatic pressure are all options.
- Refractory: surgical decompression (eg, tympanostomy tube), labyrinthectomy, or intraaural Gentamicin.

ACOUSTIC (VESTIBULAR) CN VIII NEUROMA

- **Vestibular Schwannoma** – benign tumor involving Schwann cells, which produce myelin sheath.
- Arises in the **cerebellopontine angle** & can compress structures (eg, **Cranial nerves VIII, VII, & V**).

CLINICAL MANIFESTATIONS
- **Unilateral sensorineural hearing loss is an Acoustic neuroma until proven otherwise.**
- **Tinnitus,** vertigo, ataxia, headache, **facial numbness** (CN V), **or facial paresis** (CN VII).

DIAGNOSIS
- **MRI imaging test of choice**. CT scan.
- **Audiometry** is the laboratory test of choice: asymmetric sensorineural hearing loss most common.

MANAGEMENT
- Surgery or focused radiation therapy (depending on age, tumor location, size, etc.).

NOSE/SINUS DISORDERS

ACUTE RHINOSINUSITIS

- Symptomatic inflammation of the nasal cavity and paranasal sinuses.
- Acute = 1 - 4 weeks. Subacute: 4-12 weeks. Chronic >12 weeks.

ETIOLOGIES
- Viral: most cases are viral in etiology - rhinovirus, influenza & parainfluenza.
- Bacterial: same organisms associated with Acute otitis media - ***Streptococcus pneumoniae*** **(most common),** *Haemophilus influenzae, Moraxella catarrhalis,* & group A *Streptococcus.*

RISK FACTORS
- **Most common in the setting of a viral URI,** dental infections, smoking, allergies, Cystic fibrosis,

CLINICAL MANIFESTATIONS
- **Facial pain or pressure worse with bending down & leaning forward, headache,** malaise, **purulent nasal discharge, fever**, nasal congestion.
- Often, patients develop **worsening symptoms after a period of improvement.**

DIAGNOSIS
- Primarily a clinical diagnosis.
- **Imaging is not indicated if classic presentation & uncomplicated.**
- **CT scan is the imaging test of choice** if imaging is needed. Sinus radiographs not usually needed (if ordered, Water's view most helpful).
- Biopsy or aspirate: definitive diagnosis. Usually not needed in most uncomplicated cases.

MANAGEMENT
- Symptomatic management: **decongestants (promote sinus drainage)**, analgesics, antihistamines, mucolytics, intranasal glucocorticoids, analgesics, nasal lavage.

Antibiotics:
- **Indications: symptoms should be present for >10-14 days** with worsening of symptoms or earlier if severe.
- **Amoxicillin-clavulanic acid is often the antibiotic of choice.**
- Second-line: **Doxycycline.** Respiratory fluoroquinolones (Levofloxacin, Moxifloxacin) usually reserved to prevent resistance.

CHRONIC SINUSITIS

- Inflammation of the nasal cavity and paranasal sinuses for **at least 12 consecutive weeks.**

ETIOLOGIES
- Bacterial: *S. aureus* most common bacterial cause, *Pseudomonas,* anaerobes.
- Wegener's granulomatosis (necrotic).
- Fungal: **Aspergillus most common fungal cause, Mucormycosis** second most common fungal cause.

CLINICAL MANIFESTATIONS
- Same as Acute sinusitis - facial pain or pressure worse with bending down & leaning forward, headache, malaise, purulent nasal discharge, fever, nasal congestion.

DIAGNOSIS
- **Biopsy or histology diagnostic test of choice** (allows for identification of the organism and determination of the appropriate management).

MANAGEMENT
- Depends on etiology.
- The goal of therapy is to promote sinus drainage, reduce edema, & eliminate infections. This is usually achieved with a combination of nasal irrigation, topical or oral glucocorticoids, ENT follow-up.
- Antibiotics (if bacterial) with ENT follow up.

MUCORMYCOSIS (ZYGOMYCOSIS)

- Invasive fungal infection that infiltrates the sinuses, lungs & central nervous system.
- The fungus rapidly dissects the nasal canals and eye into the brain. High mortality.

ETIOLOGIES
- **Mucor, Rhizopus, Absidia, & Cunninghamella** fungal species.

RISK FACTORS
- **Most commonly seen with Diabetes mellitus (especially in DKA)** & other **immunocompromised** states (eg, post-transplant, chemotherapy, HIV).

CLINICAL MANIFESTATIONS
- **Rhino-orbital-cerebral infections: Sinusitis** (facial pain or pressure worse with bending down & leaning forward, headache, malaise, purulent nasal discharge, fever & nasal congestion) progressing to orbit & brain involvement.
- Physical examination: may develop erythema, swelling necrosis or **black eschar on the palate, nasal mucosa, or face.**

DIAGNOSIS
- Biopsy and histopathologic examination of involved tissue – **non-septate broad hyphae with irregular right-angle (90 degree) branching.**

MANAGEMENT
- **IV Amphotericin B first-line + surgical debridement** of necrotic areas.
- Posaconazole or Isavuconazole.

RHINITIS

3 types: allergic, infectious, & vasomotor.

- **Allergic: most common type overall - IgE-mediated** mast cell histamine release due to allergens (eg, pollen, mold, dust etc.).
- **Infectious: Rhinovirus most common infectious cause** (common cold). *Streptococcal* species less commonly seen.
- Vasomotor: nonallergic & noninfectious dilation of the blood vessels (eg, temperature change, strong smells, humidity etc.).

CLINICAL MANIFESTATIONS

- Sneezing, nasal congestion, itching, **clear, watery rhinorrhea**.
- Eyes, ears, nose & throat may be involved.
- Bluish discoloration around the eyes may be seen in allergic.

PHYSICAL EXAMINATION:

- **Allergic: pale or violaceous boggy turbinates, nasal polyps** with **cobblestone mucosa** of the conjunctiva. May develop an "allergic shiner" purple discoloration around the eyes or a nasal bridge crease from constant rubbing.
- **Viral: erythematous turbinates.**

MANAGEMENT OF ALLERGIC:

- **Intranasal corticosteroids first-line if allergic or nasal polyps.**
- Antihistamines, mast cell stabilizers & short-term decongestants may also be used. Anticholinergics can be used for rhinorrhea.
- Avoidance and environmental control, exposure reduction. **Intranasal corticosteroids if allergic.**

Intranasal glucocorticoids:

Mometasone, Fluticasone.

- Indications: **most effective medication for Allergic rhinitis** (moderate to severe or persistent) **especially with nasal polyps.**

Decongestants:

- MOA: improve congestion (little effect on rhinorrhea, sneezing, pruritus).
- Intranasal: Oxymetazoline, Phenylephrine, Naphazoline. Oral: Pseudoephedrine.
- **Intranasal decongestants used >3-5 days may cause rhinitis medicamentosa** (rebound congestion).

NASAL POLYPS

- **Allergic rhinitis most common cause.** May be seen with Cystic Fibrosis.

CLINICAL MANIFESTATIONS

- Most are incidental findings but if large, they can cause obstruction or anosmia (decreased smell).

DIAGNOSIS

- Direct visualization: **pale boggy mass on the nasal mucosa**. May have findings associated Allergic rhinitis (eg, pale or violaceous, boggy turbinates & cobblestone mucosa of the conjunctiva).

MANAGEMENT

- **Intranasal glucocorticoids initial treatment of choice.**
- Surgical removal may be needed in some cases that are large and if medical therapy is unsuccessful.

EPISTAXIS

ANTERIOR EPISTAXIS

- Source: **Kiesselbach venous plexus most common site.**
- Etiologies: most commonly associated with nasal trauma (eg, *nose picking most common in children*, blowing nose forcefully etc.), low humidity, hot environments (dried nasal mucosa), rhinitis, alcohol, cocaine use, antiplatelet meds, foreign body. Hypertension doesn't cause it but may prolong it.

POSTERIOR EPISTAXIS

- Source: **sphenopalatine artery branches & Woodruff's plexus most common site** (may cause bleeding in both nares & the posterior pharynx).
- Risk factors: Hypertension, older patients, nasal neoplasms.

MANAGEMENT OF ANTERIOR

- **Direct pressure first-line therapy in most cases.** Pressure applied at least 5-15 minutes with the patient in the seated position, **leaning forward** (to reduce vessel pressure). Untreated septal hematomas can lead to septum destruction if not evacuated.
- Adjunct medications: **topical vasoconstrictors** may be adjunctive therapy with direct pressure (eg, **Oxymetazoline** nasal, lidocaine with epinephrine, 4% cocaine) - cautious use in patients with hypertension.
- Cauterization: electrocautery or silver nitrate if the above measures fail & the bleeding site can be visualized.
- **Nasal packing: if direct pressure, vasoconstrictors, & cautery are unsuccessful or in severe bleeding.** May consider antibiotic (Cephalexin or Clindamycin) to prevent toxic shock syndrome if packed (controversial).
- Septal hematomas are associated with loss of cartilage if the hematoma is not removed.
- Post treatment care: avoid exercise for a few days, avoid spicy foods (they cause vasodilation). Bacitracin, petroleum gauze & humidifiers helpful to moisten the nasal mucosa.

MANAGEMENT OF POSTERIOR

- **Balloon catheters most common initial management.**
- Foley catheter
- Cotton packing

NASAL FOREIGN BODY

- Most commonly seen in children.
- Many are asymptomatic.
- Classically presents with **epistaxis associated with a mucopurulent discharge, foul odor,** & nasal obstruction (**mouth breathing**).

DIAGNOSIS

- Direct visualization (head light & otoscope).
- Rigid or flexible fiberoptic endoscopy.
- Radiographs not usually needed (may be helpful if button batteries are suspected & not visualized).

MANAGEMENT

- Removal via positive pressure technique or instrument.
- Positive pressure technique: involves having the patient blow his or her nose while occluding the nostril opposite of the foreign body.
- Oral positive pressure: parent blows into the mouth while occluding the unaffected nostril (used in smaller children).

ACUTE PHARYNGITIS/TONSILLITIS

ETIOLOGIES

- **Viral most common overall cause of pharyngitis** - Adenovirus, Rhinovirus, Enterovirus, Epstein-Barr virus, Respiratory syncytial virus, Influenza A & B, Herpes zoster virus.
- Bacterial: **Group A *Streptococcus* (*S. pyogenes*) most common bacterial cause.**

CLINICAL MANIFESTATIONS

- Sore throat, pain or swallowing or with phonation. Other symptoms based on the etiology.
- Viral often associated with cough, hoarseness, coryza, conjunctivitis, diarrhea.

DIAGNOSIS

- Usually clinical.
- Rapid strep or throat culture may be performed to rule out bacterial cause if suspected.

MANAGEMENT

- **Symptomatic mainstay of treatment** - fluids, warm saline gargles, topical anesthetics, lozenges, NSAIDs.

STREPTOCOCCAL PHARYNGITIS ("STREP THROAT")

- Group A *Streptococcus* (*Streptococcus pyogenes*).
- Rare in children < 3 years of age.
- Highest incidence of Rheumatic fever if untreated in children 5-15 years of age.

CLINICAL MANIFESTATIONS

- Dysphagia (pain on swallowing), fever.
- Not usually associated with symptoms of viral infections (eg, cough, hoarseness, coryza, conjunctivitis, diarrhea).

PHYSICAL EXAMINATION

- Pharyngeal edema or exudate, tonsillar exudate and/or petechiae
- **Anterior cervical lymphadenopathy.**

DIAGNOSIS

- **Rapid antigen detection test: best initial test.** 95% specific but only 55-90% sensitive (most useful if positive, but **if negative, throat cultures should be obtained** especially **in children 5-15y**).
- **Throat culture: definitive diagnosis** (gold standard).

MANAGEMENT

- **Penicillin first-line treatment** (eg, PCN G or VK, Amoxicillin).
- Penicillin allergy: **Macrolides,** Clindamycin, Cephalosporins.

COMPLICATIONS

- **Rheumatic fever (preventable with antibiotics)**
- Acute glomerulonephritis (not preventable with antibiotics)
- Peritonsillar abscess

LARYNGITIS

- Acute inflammation of the mucosa of the larynx.

ETIOLOGIES
- **Viral upper respiratory tract infection most common** - Adenovirus, Rhinovirus, Influenza, Respiratory Syncytial virus (RSV), Parainfluenza.
- Bacterial causes include *M. catarrhalis* & *Mycoplasma pneumoniae*.
- Vocal strain (eg, screaming or singing), irritants (eg, acid - GERD), polyps, & laryngeal cancer.

CLINICAL MANIFESTATIONS
- **Hoarseness hallmark, aphonia.** Dry or scratchy throat.
- May have viral (URI) symptoms (eg, rhinorrhea, cough, sore throat).

DIAGNOSIS: **usually a clinical diagnosis.**

MANAGEMENT
- **Supportive care mainstay** - hydration, humidification, vocal rest, warm saline gargles, anesthetics, lozenges, and reassurance that it is usually self-limited.
- ENT follow-up if workup needed.

PERITONSILLAR ABSCESS (QUINSY)

- Abscess between the palatine tonsil & the pharyngeal muscles resulting from a complication of tonsillitis or pharyngitis. Most common in adolescents & young adults 15-30y.

ETIOLOGIES
- Often polymicrobial - the predominant species include **Group A *Streptococcus* (*S. pyogenes*)**, *Staphylococcus aureus,* and respiratory anaerobes.

CLINICAL MANIFESTATIONS
- Dysphagia, severe unilateral pharyngitis, high fever.
- **Muffled "hot potato" voice, difficulty handling oral secretions (drooling), trismus** (lockjaw).

PHYSICAL EXAMINATION
- **Swollen or fluctuant tonsil** causing **uvula deviation to the contralateral side**, bulging of the posterior soft palate, anterior cervical lymphadenopathy.

DIAGNOSIS
- Primarily a clinical diagnosis without the need for imaging or labs if classic. Ultrasound.
- **CT scan imaging test of choice if imaging is needed** to differentiate Cellulitis vs. Abscess.

MANAGEMENT

Drainage (aspiration or I & D) + antibiotics.
- Drainage: **needle aspiration (preferred) or incision & drainage.**
- Antibiotics: oral (Amoxicillin-clavulanic acid, Clindamycin); Parenteral (Ampicillin-sulbactam, Clindamycin).
- Tonsillectomy: usually reserved for patients who fail to respond to drainage, PTA with complications, prior episodes of PTA, or recurrent severe pharyngitis.

PREVENTION
- Prompt treatment of Streptococcal infections.

RETROPHARYNGEAL ABSCESS

- Deep neck space infection located behind the posterior pharyngeal wall.
- Most common in children 2 – 4 years. In adults, it is often a result of penetrating trauma (eg, chicken or fish bones, instrumentation, dental procedures).

ETIOLOGIES

- Similar to Peritonsillar abscess - often polymicrobial (eg, **Group A *Streptococcus*,** *Staphylococcus aureus* & respiratory anaerobes).

CLINICAL MANIFESTATIONS

- Neck: **torticollis** (unwilling to move the neck secondary to pain and spasms), **neck stiffness especially with neck extension**.
- Fever, drooling, dysphagia, odynophagia, chest pain, muffled "hot potato" voice, trismus.

PHYSICAL EXAMINATION

- **Midline or unilateral posterior pharyngeal wall edema (most common).**
- Anterior cervical lymphadenopathy, lateral neck mass or swelling.

DIAGNOSIS

- Lateral neck radiograph: **increased prevertebral space >50%** of the width of adjacent vertebral body (may be performed if low suspicion).
- **CT scan of neck with contrast preferred if suspicion is high.**
- In smaller children with respiratory distress, evaluation often done in the operating room.

MANAGEMENT

- Surgical incision & drainage with antibiotics for large & mature abscesses in the OR.
- Abscess <2.5cm^2 may be observed for 24-48 hours with antibiotic therapy.
- Antibiotics: IV Ampicillin-Sulbactam or Clindamycin (similar to Peritonsillar abscess).

COMPLICATIONS

- Airway obstruction, Mediastinitis (due to spread of the infection), sepsis, atlantoaxial dislocation.

ORAL LICHEN PLANUS

- Idiopathic cell-mediated autoimmune response affecting the skin & mucous membranes.
- Most common in middle-age range. **Increased incidence with hepatitis C infection.**

CLINICAL MANIFESTATIONS

- **Reticular: lacy reticular leukoplakia** of the oral mucosa most common **(Wickham striae).** Usually painless. **Most common type.**
- Erythematous: red patches (may accompany the reticular lesions). May be painful.
- Erosive: erosions or ulcers. Usually painful.

DIAGNOSIS

- Mainly clinical. Biopsy often performed in the erythematous & erosive types to rule out malignancy.

MANAGEMENT

- **Local glucocorticoids initial management of choice** (eg, Clobetasol, Betamethasone)
- Second-line: topical (Tacrolimus, Pimecrolimus, Cyclosporine), intralesional corticosteroid injections.
- Systemic glucocorticoids if no response to topical therapy.

LUDWIG'S ANGINA

- Rapidly spreading **cellulitis of the floor of the mouth** (bilateral infection of submandibular space).
- Risk factors: most commonly due to spread of oral flora **secondary to dental infections** (second or third mandibular molars). Increased incidence in Diabetes & HIV.
- Polymicrobial (oral flora).

CLINICAL MANIFESTATIONS
- Fever, chills, malaise, stiff neck, dysphagia, drooling, muffled voice.
- Respiratory difficulty if severe (eg, stridor).

PHYSICAL EXAMINATION
- **Tender, symmetric swelling, "woody" induration, & erythema of the upper neck & chin** (may have palpable crepitus). Pus on the floor of the mouth.
- Swelling of the tongue *can lead to airway compromise.* No lymphadenopathy or abscess formation.

DIAGNOSIS
- **CT scan initial test of choice**. MRI.

MANAGEMENT IF IMMUNOCOMPETENT
- IV antibiotics: **Ampicillin-sulbactam** OR Ceftriaxone plus Metronidazole OR Clindamycin plus Levofloxacin.
- Add Vancomycin if MRSA suspected.

MANAGEMENT IF IMMUNOCOMPROMISED
- IV antibiotics: Cefepime plus Metronidazole OR Imipenem OR Meropenem OR Piperacillin-tazobactam. Add Vancomycin if MRSA suspected.

OROPHARYNGEAL CANDIDIASIS (THRUSH)

- *Candida albicans* is part of the normal flora but can become pathogenic due to local or systemic immunosuppressed states.
- Risk factors: **immunocompromised states** (HIV, chemotherapy, diabetics), use of **inhaled Corticosteroids without a spacer**, antibiotic use, xerostomia, or denture use.

CLINICAL MANIFESTATIONS
- Asymptomatic. Loss of taste or cotton-like feel in the mouth, loss of taste, throat or mouth pain with eating or swallowing.

PHYSICAL EXAMINATION
- **White curd-like plaques** on the buccal mucosa, tongue, palate, &/or the oropharynx that are easily scraped off **(may leave behind erythema & friable mucosa if scraped).**
- The denture form may be associated with erythema only.

DIAGNOSIS
- Clinical.
- **Potassium Hydroxide: budding yeast, & pseudohyphae.** Smear performed on scrapings.
- Fungal culture (rarely done).

MANAGEMENT
- **Topical therapy: first-line therapy – Nystatin liquid** swish and swallow, **Clotrimazole troches** or Miconazole mucoadhesive buccal tablets.
- Oral Fluconazole usually reserved for refractory cases or patients with both oropharyngeal + esophageal Candidiasis.

APHTHOUS ULCERS (CANKER SORE, ULCERATIVE STOMATITIS)

- Unknown cause but may be associated with human herpes virus 6.
- Recurrent disease seen in patients with Inflammatory bowel disease, HIV, Celiac disease, SLE, Methotrexate, & neutropenia.

CLINICAL MANIFESTATIONS

- Small, **painful, shallow round or oval shallow ulcer (yellow, white or grey central exudate) with erythematous halo.** Most common on the buccal or labial mucosa (nonkeratinized mucosa).

MANAGEMENT

- **Topical oral glucocorticoids first-line management** (eg, Clobetasol gel or ointment, Dexamethasone elixir swish and spit, Triamcinolone in orabase).
- Topical analgesics: **2% viscous lidocaine**, Diphenhydramine liquid; aluminum hydroxide + magnesium hydroxide + simethicone

ORAL LEUKOPLAKIA

- Oral potentially malignant disorder characterized by hyperkeratosis due to chronic irritation.
- Up to 6% are dysplastic or **Squamous cell carcinoma**.
- Risk factors: chronic irritation due to tobacco, cigarette smoking, alcohol, dentures, HPV infections.

CLINICAL MANIFESTATIONS

- Most are asymptomatic.
- **Painless white patchy lesions that cannot be scraped off** (in comparison to Candida which is painful & can be scraped off).

DIAGNOSIS

- Biopsy to rule out Squamous cell carcinoma.

MANAGEMENT

- Cessation of irritants (eg alcohol, smoking).
- Cryotherapy, laser ablation and surgical excision are options if increased risk for malignancy or malignant.

ERYTHROPLAKIA

- Uncommon oral lesion with a high risk of malignant transformation.
- **90% of Erythroplakia is either dysplastic or shows evident of Squamous cell carcinoma.**
- Risk factors: chronic irritation due to tobacco, cigarette smoking, age > 65 years.

CLINICAL MANIFESTATIONS

- Most are asymptomatic.
- **Painless erythematous, soft, velvety, patch** in the oral cavity, most commonly on the mouth floor, soft palate, and ventral aspect of the tongue.

DIAGNOSIS: biopsy to rule out Squamous cell carcinoma.

MANAGEMENT

- Complete excision may be needed depending on the biopsy results.

SIALOLITHIASIS (SALIVARY GLAND STONES)

- Stones within the salivary glands or ducts (no inflammation).
- **Most common in Wharton's duct (submandibular gland duct); Stensen's duct** (parotid gland duct).

RISK FACTORS
- Decreased salivation (eg, dehydration, anticholinergic mediations, diuretics).

CLINICAL MANIFESTATIONS
- **Sudden onset of salivary gland pain & swelling with eating or in anticipation of eating.**

PHYSICAL EXAMINATION
- Stone may be palpated in the salivary gland.
- If the gland is compressed and no saliva flows, the stone can be obstructive.

DIAGNOSIS
- Usually clinical.

MANAGEMENT
- **Conservative management: first-line therapy - sialagogues** to increase salivary flow (eg, **tart, hard candies, lemon drops,** Xylitol-containing gum or candy), increase fluid intake, gland massage, moist heat to affected area. Avoid anticholinergic drugs if possible (anticholinergics decrease salivation).
- Minimally invasive therapy: includes sialoendoscopy, laser lithotripsy, extracorporeal lithotripsy.
- Surgery (eg, sialoadenectomy) reserved for recurrent stone or failure of less invasive techniques.

ACUTE BACTERIAL SIALADENITIS (SUPPURATIVE SIALADENITIS)

- **Bacterial infection of the parotid or submandibular salivary glands.**
- Etiologies: ***S. aureus* most common,** *S. pneumoniae, S. viridans, H. influenzae, Bacteroides.*
- Risk factors: salivary gland obstruction from a stone, dehydration, chronic illness.

CLINICAL MANIFESTATIONS
- Sudden onset of very firm and **tender gland swelling with purulent discharge** (may be able to express **pus if the duct is massaged), dysphagia, trismus** (reduced opening of the jaw due to spasms of the muscles of mastication).
- **Fever & chills** if severe.

DIAGNOSIS
- **CT Scan** to assess for associated abscess or extent of tissue involvement.

MANAGEMENT
- **Anti-staphylococcal antibiotics + sialagogues** to increase salivary flow (eg, tart or hard candies).
- Dicloxacillin or Nafcillin. Metronidazole can be added for anaerobic coverage.
- Clindamycin.

ACUTE HERPETIC GINGIVOSTOMATITIS

- Inflammation of the gums and the oral mucosa.
- **Primary manifestation of HSV-1 in children.**
- Most commonly occurs between 6 months – 5 years.

CLINICAL MANIFESTATIONS
- Prodrome: sudden onset of fever, anorexia, malaise and refusal to eat and/or drink followed by oral lesions.
- Gingivostomatitis: **ulcerative lesions of the gingiva (gum swelling with friability & bleeding)** & **vesicles** on the mucous membranes of the mouth, often with **perioral vesicular lesions clustered on an erythematous base** (dew drops on a rose petal).
- After rupture, the vesicles become **ulcerated**, yellow, and are surrounded by an erythematous halo. They may coalesce to form painful ulcers.
- Regional lymphadenopathy.

DIAGNOSIS: clinical

MANAGEMENT
- **Supportive care mainstay** – hydration, oral hygiene, barrier cream (eg, petroleum jelly) to the lips. Lesions usually heal within 1 week.
- **Oral Acyclovir** if within 72-96 hours of disease onset if they are unable to drink, have significant pain.
- IV Acyclovir if immunocompromised.

ACUTE HERPETIC PHARYNGOTONSILLITIS

- **Primary manifestation of herpes simplex virus-1 in adults.**

CLINICAL MANIFESTATIONS: fever, malaise, headache, sore throat.

PHYSICAL EXAMINATION: **vesicles** that rupture, leaving **ulcerative lesions with grayish exudates** in the posterior pharyngeal mucosa.

MANAGEMENT: oral hygiene - lesions usually resolve within 7-14 days.

ORAL HAIRY LEUKOPLAKIA

- Mucocutaneous manifestation of **Epstein-Barr virus** (Human herpesvirus-4).

RISK FACTORS
- **Almost exclusively seen with HIV infection.**
- Other immunocompromised states - post-transplant, chronic steroid, chemotherapy.

CLINICAL MANIFESTATIONS
- **Painless, white smooth or corrugated "hairy" plaque** along the **lateral tongue borders** or buccal mucosa **that cannot be scraped off**.

MANAGEMENT
- No specific treatment required (may spontaneously resolve & not considered a premalignant lesion).
- Antiretroviral treatment in patients with HIV.

OTOTOXIC MEDICATIONS

- Loop diuretics: Furosemide, Bumetanide, Ethacrynic acid (most ototoxic)
- Antibiotics: Vancomycin, Aminoglycosides (Gentamicin), Macrolides (Erythromycin), Tetracyclines.
- Anti-inflammatories: Aspirin, NSAIDs
- Anti-neoplastics: Cisplatin, Carboplatin, Cytarabine
- Anti-malarials: Chloroquine, Hydroxychloroquine, Quinine

PHOTO CREDITS

Pinguecula
By Red eye2008 (Own work) [CC-BY-SA-3.0 (http://creativecommons.org/licenses/by-sa/3.0) or GFDL (http://www.gnu.org/copyleft/fdl.html)], via Wikimedia Commons

Pterygium
By Jmvaras José Miguel Varas, MD (Own work) [GFDL (http://www.gnu.org/copyleft/fdl.html) or CC-BY-3.0 (http://creativecommons.org/licenses/by/3.0)], via Wikimedia Commons

Hypertensive retinopathy
By Frank Wood ([1]) [CC-BY-3.0 (http://creativecommons.org/licenses/by/3.0)], via Wikimedia Commons

Papilledema
By Jonathan Trobe, M.D. - University of Michigan Kellogg Eye Center (The Eyes Have It) [CC-BY-3.0 (http://creativecommons.org/licenses/by/3.0)], via Wikimedia Commons

Eye changes
By National Eye Institute, National Institutes of Health [Public domain], via Wikimedia Commons

Normal Funduscopic Exam
By Mikael Häggström (Own work) [CC0], via Wikimedia Commons

Glaucoma
By James Heilman, MD (Own work) [CC-BY-SA-3.0 (http://creativecommons.org/licenses/by-sa/3.0) or GFDL (http://www.gnu.org/copyleft/fdl.html)], via Wikimedia Commons

HordeolumBy Andre Riemann (Own work) [Public domain], via Wikimedia Commons

Chalazion

By Poupig (Own work) [CC-BY-SA-3.0 (http://creativecommons.org/licenses/by-sa/3.0)], via Wikimedia Commons

Orbital Fracture
By James Heilman, MD (Own work) [CC BY-SA 4.0 (http://creativecommons.org/licenses/by-sa/4.0)], via Wikimedia Commons

Macular degeneration By Credit to: National Eye Institute, National Institutes of Health - http://www.nei.nih.gov/health/maculardegen/webAMD.pdf page 14, Public Domain, https://commons.wikimedia.org/w/index.php?curid=862686

CHAPTER 6 - REPRODUCTIVE SYSTEM (MALE AND FEMALE)

ACUTE MASTITIS

- Infection of the breast **most common in lactating women** secondary to nipple trauma (especially **primigravida** in the first 6 weeks postpartum).
- Etiologies: ***Staphylococcus aureus* most common.** Streptococcus. *Candida albicans.*

CLINICAL MANIFESTATIONS
- **Unilateral localized breast pain**, tenderness, warmth, swelling, induration, & skin redness.
- **Cracked nipples or visible fissure.**
- May have purulent nipple discharge.
- Systemic symptoms may include fever, myalgias, chills.

DIAGNOSIS
- Clinical in most cases.
- Culture of breast milk in some cases for culture and sensitivities.
- Imaging usually reserved for cases not responding to empiric antibiotics within 48-72 hours.

MANAGEMENT
- **Supportive** - warm or cool compresses, breast pump, anti-inflammatory medications.
- **Anti-staphylococcal antibiotics - Dicloxacillin, Nafcillin**. Cephalosporin. Erythromycin can be used if penicillin-allergic. Fluconazole if fungal.
- **Mothers encouraged to continue breastfeeding** - milk drainage (either breastfeeding, pumping, or hand expression) is critical for resolution of infection and for relief of symptoms.

BREAST ABSCESS

- Rare complication of Acute mastitis.
- **Most common in lactating women** secondary to nipple trauma (especially **primigravida**).

ETIOLOGIES
- ***Staphylococcus aureus* most common.** Streptococcus. *Candida albicans.*

CLINICAL MANIFESTATIONS
- **Symptoms of acute mastitis** - unilateral breast pain (especially one quadrant) with tenderness, warmth, swelling.
- Cracked nipples or visible fissure **+ induration & fluctuance** (due to pus).
- May have purulent nipple discharge.

DIAGNOSIS
- Clinical (based physical examination).
- Ultrasound may be ordered if there is a question of cellulitis vs. abscess – ill-defined mass with septations if breast abscess.

MANAGEMENT
- **Drainage** via **needle aspiration (lactational abscess) or incision & drainage +** antibiotics.

- **Antibiotics: Dicloxacillin, Cephalexin**, Clindamycin. If MRSA suspected, Trimethoprim-sulfamethoxazole, or Clindamycin.

- Breast infection, including breast abscess, is not a contraindication to breastfeeding. Milk drainage (eg, breastfeeding, pumping, or hand expression) is important to facilitate resolution of infection.

CONGESTIVE MASTITIS

- Bilateral breast enlargement 2-3 days postpartum due to **milk stasis.**

CLINICAL MANIFESTATIONS

- **Bilateral** breast pain & swelling.

MANAGEMENT

- **Breast drainage mainstay of treatment (manually or breast pump).**
- If the woman does not want to breastfeed, treat with ice packs, tight-fitting bras, analgesics, and breast drainage.
- If breastfeeding is desired, manually empty the breasts completely after baby is done breastfeeding, local heat, analgesics, & continue nursing.

FIBROCYSTIC BREAST CHANGES

- Noncancerous, fluid-filled breast cysts due to exaggerated response to hormones.
- Also known as glandular hyperplasia – duct dilation, breast cysts, & stromal fibrosis.
- **Most common benign breast disorder in reproductive age women** (especially 30-50 years).
- Often regresses after menopause.

CLINICAL MANIFESTATIONS

- Multiple, painful or painless **breast masses that may increase or decrease in size with menstrual hormonal changes (often worse prior to menstruation).**

PHYSICAL EXAMINATION

- Usually **multiple, nodular, mobile, smooth round or ovoid lumps in both breasts** of varying sizes.
- Often bilateral and not usually associated with axillary lymph node involvement.
- Most commonly found in the upper outer sections of the breast.

DIAGNOSIS

- **Ultrasound initial test of choice.**
- Fine needle aspiration – straw-colored or green fluid (no blood). Not usually performed.
- A mammogram may be required if lesion is suspicious or persistent after drainage.

MANAGEMENT

- **Supportive management – observation**, supportive bra, warm or cool compresses, analgesics.
- Oral contraceptives can reduce symptoms.
- FNA removal of fluid is diagnostic & therapeutic in complex cases.

FIBROADENOMA OF THE BREAST

- **Benign solid tumor** composed of glandular & fibrous tissue.
- Second most common benign breast mass (after fibrocystic disease) & most common breast tumor in women < 30 years. Increased incidence in African-Americans.

CLINICAL MANIFESTATIONS
- Breast mass. Usually nontender but may become tender prior to menstruation.
- Gradually grows over time but **may enlarge in pregnancy.**
- **Does not change significantly in size with menstrual cycle.**

PHYSICAL EXAMINATION
- **Firm, nontender, solitary,** smooth, **well-circumscribed**, **freely mobile**, **rubbery lump in the breast.** Usually 2-3 cm & no axillary involvement.

DIAGNOSIS
- Clinical diagnosis. Ultrasound – solid, well-circumscribed, avascular mass.
- Fine needle aspiration: definitive diagnosis – fibrous tissue & **collagen arranged in a "swirl"**.

MANAGEMENT
- **Conservative: observation, reassurance and follow-up** - most small tumors resorb with time. Can repeat ultrasound in 3-6 months.
- Excision: may be needed if enlarging after repeat ultrasounds or for large masses.
- Cryoablation: alternative to surgery if < 4cm

GYNECOMASTIA

- Enlargement of glandular breast tissue & adipose tissue in males due to increased effective estrogen (increased production or reduced degradation) or due to decreased androgens.
- **Hormonal:** seen in 3 main groups: **Infants:** due to high maternal estrogen; **during puberty:** especially 10 – 14 years (classically may last between 6 months – 2 years) & **older males**.
- **Idiopathic**, persistent pubertal gynecomastia.
- Medications: **Spironolactone**, Ketoconazole, Cimetidine, 5-alpha reductase inhibitors, Digoxin, GnRH agonists (eg, Leuprolide), Thiazides, Phenothiazines, Verapamil, & Theophylline.
- Other: malignancies - large cell lung cancer, renal cell, hepatic, testicular and gastric cancers. Cirrhosis, hyperthyroidism, chronic renal disease, Klinefelter syndrome, & alcoholism.

CLINICAL MANIFESTATIONS
- **Palpable mass of tissue at least 0.5 cm in diameter**, centrally located (usually underlying the nipple), symmetrical, **classically bilateral** and often tender to palpation.

DIAGNOSIS: **clinical.** Check testosterone levels. Mammogram if breast cancer is suspected.

MANAGEMENT
- **Supportive:** stop offending medications, **observation if early in the disease course or physiologic**.
- If treatment is needed, initiate it within the first 6 months of onset (after 12 months, fibrosis may occur).

Medical:
- **Tamoxifen** is selective estrogen receptor modifier that is an **estrogen antagonist in the breast**. Often first-line medication if medical management indicated. Androgens used in hypogonadism.

Surgical:
- Reserved for severe disease refractory to medical therapy, large breasts, cosmetically unappealing, fibrosis etc.

BREAST CANCER

- Most common non-skin malignancy in women. 1 in 8 lifetime incidence.
- Second most common cause of cancer death in women (after lung).

RISK FACTORS

- Genetics: **BRCA 1 & BRCA 2** - genetic mutation associated 60-85% lifetime development of Breast cancer & 15-40% development of Ovarian cancer. BRCA positivity seen in 5 -10% of cases of Breast cancer. First-degree relative with Breast cancer.
- Increasing age: >50% occur >60y.
- Increased number of menstrual cycles: nulliparity, late first full-term pregnancy >35y, early onset of menarche (<12y), late menopause, never having breastfed.
- Increased estrogen exposure: postmenopausal hormonal replacement therapy, prolonged unopposed estrogen, obesity, alcohol use. Endometrial cancer increases the risk of Breast cancer and vice versa.

TYPES

- **Infiltrative ductal carcinoma: most common type of breast cancer** (75%). Associated with lymphatic metastases (especially axillary). **Ductal carcinoma in situ** – does not penetrate the basement membrane.

- Infiltrative lobular carcinoma (10%).
- Medullary, mucinoid, tubular, papillary, metastatic, inflammatory.

- **Paget disease of the breast**: ductal carcinoma presenting as an **eczematous nipple lesion**. May have bloody discharge from the nipple.

PREMALIGNANT LESIONS

- **Lobular carcinoma in situ** not considered cancer but is **associated with increased risk of invasive breast cancer in either breast.**
- Atypical ductal hyperplasia

CLINICAL MANIFESTATIONS

- **Painless, hard fixed immobile lump most common presentation** (may be mobile early on & may be painful in <10%). May complain of unilateral discharge (may be bloody).

PHYSICAL EXAMINATION

- Mass **most common in the upper outer quadrant** (65%), areola (18%).

- **Skin changes:** asymmetric erythema, discoloration, ulceration, skin retraction (dimpling if Cooper's ligament involvement), changes in breast size & contour, nipple inversion, & skin thickening.

- Locally advanced disease: **axillary lymphadenopathy.**
- Metastatic disease: most common sites are the **bone** (vertebrae, ribs, pelvis, & femur), **lungs** (eg, dyspnea or cough), liver (abdominal pain, nausea, jaundice) or brain. Think 2Bs and 2Ls.

- **Paget disease of the breast: chronic eczematous itchy scaly rash on the nipples & areola** (may ooze). <5%. A lump is often present.

- **Inflammatory breast cancer: red, swollen, warm, itchy breast**. Often with nipple retraction, **peau d'orange** = skin changes that looks like the peel of an orange due to **lymphatic obstruction** (associated with **poor prognosis**). Usually not associated with a lump.

BREAST MASS – DIAGNOSIS

A combination of physical exam, mammography, and fine needle aspiration or core biopsy is highly accurate. Ultrasound is sometimes used to see if the mass is cystic.

- **Mammography: initial modality to evaluate breast masses in women >40y - microcalcifications & spiculated** masses are **highly suspicious for malignancy**.

- **Ultrasound: recommended initial modality to evaluate breast masses in women <40y** (due to high density of breast tissue). May also be used to guide FNA with biopsy or determine if a mass seen on mammogram is cystic or solid.

- MRI: rapid uptake of contrast is characteristic of a malignant mass.

BIOPSY OPTIONS

- **Fine needle aspiration:** advantages: removes the least amount of tissue. Disadvantages: if positive, it **doesn't allow for receptor testing** (estrogen, progesterone and HER 2/neu) and associated with a false negative rate of 10%.

- **Large needle (core biopsy):** advantages: allows for receptor testing if positive (estrogen, progesterone and HER 2/neu). Disadvantages: can leave greater deformity with the procedure and the needle may miss the lesion.

- **Open biopsy:** advantages: **most accurate diagnostic test,** allows for frozen section to be done followed by immediate resection of the cancer followed by sentinel node biopsy.

BREAST CANCER MANAGEMENT

Treatment based on TNM staging. Metastatic workup recommended for stage III and above.

- **Early stage cancer: breast conservation therapy (lumpectomy) with sentinel node biopsy + follow-up radiation** usually preferred when possible. A negative sentinel node eliminates the need for axillary lymph node dissection.

- Modified radical mastectomy may be needed if diffuse, large tumor, prior radiation to the breast, or if radiation post-lumpectomy is contraindicated.

- **Radiation therapy: usually done after lumpectomy or post mastectomy to destroy residual tumor cells** (eg, external beam radiation or brachytherapy).

- Anti-estrogen Hormonal therapy: in **estrogen receptor positive tumors – Tamoxifen. Most useful in premenopausal patients**. Estrogen-receptor (ER) positivity associated with a better prognosis. Adverse effect of Tamoxifen: venous thrombosis & endometrial cancer.

- **Aromatase inhibitor Hormonal therapy: most useful in postmenopausal** ER-positive patients (eg, **Letrozole, Anastrozole, Exemestane**) AIs are slightly more effective than Tamoxifen.
  Adverse effects: Osteoporosis.

- **Anti-HER2/neu Hormonal therapy: Trastuzumab.** HER2/neu positivity is associated with more aggressive tumors. Adverse effects: cardiotoxicity.

- Adjuvant chemotherapy: used to treat any residual disease. Indications include lesions > 1 cm, positive axillary lymphadenopathy, breast cancers stage II-IV, & inoperable disease (especially estrogen receptor-negative disease).
  - Options include Doxorubicin, Cyclophosphamide, Fluorouracil, & Docetaxel.

BREAST CANCER SCREENING

- **Mammogram: best screening in women > 40 years of age**. Detects breast cancer as early as 2 years before a mass can be palpated clinically.
- Breast self-examination has not been shown to reduce long-term overall mortality.
- Average-risk: USPSTF guidelines recommends **Mammogram every 2 years beginning at 50 years until 74 years.** Women over the age of 74 can be offered screening if their life expectancy is at least 10 years (every 2 years).
- Moderate risk: (eg, most patients with first-degree relative with breast cancer) in some patients, screening at age 50y and every 2 years (or 10 years prior to the age the first-degree degree relative was diagnosed, whichever is earlier).
- Women with breast implants should undergo the same screening schedule as women without implants.

Clinical breast exam:

- At least every 3 years in women 20-39 years (annually after age 40).

BREAST CANCER PREVENTION

SERM:

- Tamoxifen & Raloxifene are selective estrogen receptor modulators that can be used for Breast cancer prevention in high-risk individuals.
- **Tamoxifen or Raloxifene can be used in postmenopausal or women >35y with high risk.**
- Treatment usually used for 5 years.
- Tamoxifen preferred (more effective but associated with Endometrial cancer. Tamoxifen also associated with increased risk of DVT compared to Raloxifene.

Aromatase inhibitors

- An alternative to the SERMs.

HPV VACCINATION

- **HPV types 16 and 18 cause ~70% of all Cervical cancers worldwide and nearly 90 percent of anal cancers**, as well as a significant proportion of oropharyngeal cancer, vulvar, vaginal cancer, and penile cancer.
- **HPV types 6 and 11 cause ~90% of genital warts.**

INDICATIONS:

- Females: **given in women age 11 up to 26 years of age.**
- Males: given age 11 up to 21 years of age. Men who have sex with men and individuals with weakened immune systems can be vaccinated until age 26.

VACCINES:

- **Gardasil 9 (preferred):** targets the same as Gardasil (**6, 11, 16, 18**) as well as HPV types 31, 33, 45, 52, & 58.
- Gardasil: quadrivalent HPV vaccine that targets **HPV 6, 11, 16, & 18.**

DOSING:

- $\leq$15y: 2 doses of HPV vaccine at least 6 months apart.
- 15y or older or immunocompromised: should receive *3 doses over a minimum of 6 months.* Classically administered at day 0, at 2 month & at 6 months. Minimum interval between first 2 doses is 4 weeks, minimum interval between the second & 3rd is 12 weeks.
- HPV vaccine is contraindicated if pregnant or lactating.

CERVICAL INSUFFICIENCY (INCOMPETENT CERVIX)

- Inability to maintain pregnancy secondary to **premature cervical dilation (especially in the 2nd trimester).**

RISK FACTORS
- Previous cervical trauma or procedure (eg, LEEP, cervical conization, etc.)
- Uterine defects, DES exposure in utero.

CLINICAL MANIFESTATIONS
- Usually asymptomatic.
- May develop pressure, Braxton-Hix-like contractions, bleeding or vaginal discharge especially in the 2nd trimester.

PHYSICAL EXAMINATION
- **Painless dilation & effacement of the cervix.**

DIAGNOSIS
- Clinical.
- **Transvaginal ultrasound most accurate & predictive** to measure cervical length. Findings include wide internal os, shortening of the cervical canal, hourglass appearance, bulging of the fetal membranes into the os. **Insufficiency is present if cervical length 25 mm or less before 24 weeks.**

MANAGEMENT
- **Cerclage** (suturing of cervical os) **and bed rest** especially if prior history. If not performed initially, cerclage can also be performed for women who develop a short cervix (25 mm or less) before 24 weeks as determined by ultrasound surveillance.
- May also use **weekly injection of 17 alpha-hydroxyprogesterone** in addition in some women with preterm birth history.

INFERTILITY

- **Failure to conceive after 1 year** of regular unprotected sexual intercourse.
- 60% of couples achieve pregnancy in the first 3 years in the absence of a cause for infertility.

- Etiologies in males: 40% of causes (eg, abnormal spermatogenesis).
- Etiologies in females: anovulatory cycles or ovarian dysfunction 30%, congenital or acquired disorders.

DIAGNOSIS
- **Hysterosalpingography** helps evaluate tubal patency or abnormalities.

MANAGEMENT
- **Clomiphene induces ovulation.**
- Amenorrhea or Oligomenorrhea: correct endocrine problems to improve fertility. Intrauterine insemination.
- In vitro fertilization (especially if fallopian tube defect is present).

CERVICAL CANCER SCREENING

PAP SMEAR RESULTS				
RESULT	**21-24 YEARS OLD**	**25 – 29 YEARS OLD**	**≥30 YEARS & HPV NEGATIVE**	**≥30 YEARS & HPV POSITIVE**
Normal	• **Pap every 3 years**	• **Pap every 3 years**	• **HPV and Pap cotest every 5 years** (preferred) OR • **Pap every 3 years** (acceptable)	• Co-testing in 1 year or • HPV Genotype testing
ASC-US Atypical squamous cells of undetermined significance	• **Pap test in 1 year (preferred)** OR • Reflex HPV test (acceptable)	• **Reflex HPV testing (preferred)** OR • Pap testing in 1 year (acceptable)	• Repeat co-testing in 3 years	• Colposcopy
LSIL Low-grade squamous intraepithelial lesion	• Repeat pap in 1 year	• Colposcopy	• Repeat pap in 1 year OR • Colposcopy	• Colposcopy
ASC-H Atypical cells can't exclude HSIL	• **Colposcopy**	• **Colposcopy**	• **Colposcopy**	• **Colposcopy**
HSIL High-grade squamous cell intraepithelial lesion	• Colposcopy	• Excisional treatment OR • Colposcopy	• Excisional treatment OR • Colposcopy	• Excisional treatment OR • Colposcopy

Excisional treatment options include:

- Loop electrosurgical excision procedure (LEEP)
- Cold-knife conization
- Laser conization

CERVICAL BIOPSY RESULTS			
PAP SMEAR RESULT	**BIOPSY (HISTOLOGY) RESULTS** **CIN = Cervical intraepithelial neoplasia**	**DESCRIPTION**	**MANAGEMENT**
LSIL Low-grade squamous intraepithelial lesion	• **CIN I**	• **Mild dysplasia** contained to basal 1/3 of epithelium. • Cellular changes seen with HPV (often transient in young women)	• For women with **CIN 1 + ASC-US, LSIL or normal cytology** in the presence HPV 16 or 18, **recommended follow-up is cotesting with cytology and an HPV test at one year.** For women with CIN 1 + HSIL or ASC-H either: • Excisional procedure or • Observation with contesting at 12 & 24 months are recommended.
HSIL High-grade squamous cell intraepithelial lesion	• **CIN II**	• **Moderate dysplasia** including 2/3 thickness of basal epithelium • Usually due to persistent HPV	**For HSIL lesions (CIN I or CIN II) excision or ablation is the mainstay of treatment** (high risk of progression). • **Excision:** LEEP (Loop electrical excisional procedure) or Cold knife conization. • **Ablation:** cryocautery, laser cautery or electrocautery
	• **CIN III**	• **Severe dysplasia** including > 2/3 up to full thickness of the basal epithelium. • **Full thickness = carcinoma in situ** (hasn't invaded basement membrane)	

- ASCUS = Atypical squamous cells of undetermined significance
- LSIL = Low-grade squamous cell intraepithelial lesion
- HSIL = High-grade squamous intraepithelial lesion
- ASC-H = Atypical squamous cells, cannot rule out HSIL

CERVICAL CANCER

- **3rd most common gynecologic cancer** (#1 = endometrial cancer; #2 = ovarian cancer).
- Most commonly metastasize to local areas: vagina, parametrium, & pelvic lymph nodes.

MAJOR TYPES
- **Squamous cell carcinoma is most common (90%).**
- Adenocarcinoma 10%.
- Clear cell carcinoma is a type linked with DES exposure.

SPREAD
- In order, primary node groups involved in the spread of cervical cancer include the **paracervical (most common),** parametrial, obturator, hypogastric, external iliac, and sacral nodes
- It takes on average 2-10 years for carcinoma to penetrate the basement membrane.

RISK FACTORS
- **Human papilloma virus associated with 99.7% - especially 16, 18** (70%), **31 & 33,** 45, 52, & 58.
- Early onset of sexual activity, increased number of sexual partners, smoking, DES exposure (Diethylstilbestrol was a synthetic estrogen used in OCPs), cervical intraepithelial neoplasia, immunosuppression, STIs.
- 40-50 years is the most common age range for diagnosis.

CLINICAL MANIFESTATIONS
- Cervical cancer is usually asymptomatic in the early stages.
- **Post coital bleeding or spotting most common symptom.**
- Irregular or heavy vaginal bleeding or watery vaginal discharge.
- Advanced disease may present with pelvic or back pain.
- Physical examination: may have cervical discharge or ulceration if invasive.

DIAGNOSIS
- **Colposcopy with biopsy.**

MANAGEMENT
- Carcinoma in situ (Stage 0): **Excision preferred** (Loop electrical excision procedure/LEEP, cold knife conization) or **ablation** (cryotherapy or laser). Total abdominal hysterectomy + bilateral salpingo-oophorectomy.

- Stage IA1: total hysterectomy, radical hysterectomy, conization.

- IA2, IB, IIA: combined external beam radiation with brachytherapy OR radical hysterectomy with bilateral pelvic lymphadenectomy.

- Locally advanced (IIB, III, IVA): radiation therapy + chemotherapy (Cisplatin-based).

- Advanced: radiation therapy, systemic chemotherapy.

SPONTANEOUS ABORTION

- A pregnancy that ends **before 20 weeks' gestation.** Almost 80% occur prior to 12 weeks.
- Includes threatened, inevitable, incomplete, complete, missed, & septic.
- **Threatened is the only one that is potentially viable.**

ETIOLOGIES
- **Chromosomal abnormalities most common** (60-80%).
- Maternal factors include STIs, antiphospholipid syndrome, trauma, Rh isoimmunization, malnutrition, and anatomic abnormalities.

CLINICAL MANIFESTATIONS
- Crampy abdominal pain & vaginal bleeding.

DIAGNOSIS
- Ultrasound, CBC, blood type and Rh screen, serial beta-hCG titers, & progesterone levels.

TYPE OF ABORTION	ULTRASOUND & CERVICAL FINDINGS	MANAGEMENT
THREATENED	• **Products of conception (POC) intact** • **Cervical os closed**	• **Supportive: observation at home**, bedrest and **close follow up** to see if either symptoms resolve or progress to abortion. • Serial beta-hCG to see if doubling to see if viable.
INEVITABLE	• **POC intact** • **Cervical os DILATED**	Options include: • **Surgical evacuation:** dilation & curettage <16 weeks or dilation & evacuation ≥ 16 weeks. • Medical: **Misoprostol** • Expectant management
INCOMPLETE	• **Some POC expelled from the uterus** • **Cervical os DILATED**	Options include: • **Expectant** – allow POC to fully pass with serial beta-hCG & transvaginal US to determine when complete. • **Surgical evacuation:** dilation & curettage <16 weeks or dilation & evacuation ≥ 16 weeks. • Medical: **Misoprostol**
COMPLETE	• **All POC expelled from the uterus** • Cervical os usually closed	• RhoGAM if indicated, follow up beta-hCG
MISSED	• **POC intact** • **Cervical os closed.**	• **Surgical evacuation:** dilation & curettage <16 weeks or dilation & evacuation ≥ 16 weeks. • Medical: **Misoprostol**
SEPTIC	• Some POC retained • Cervical os closed. **Cervical motion tenderness.** • Foul brown discharge, fever, chills	• **D & E to remove products of conception + broad spectrum antibiotics** (e.g., Levofloxacin + Metronidazole)

All women who are Rh-negative should also receive anti-D Rh immunoglobulin at this time for all abortions.

ELECTIVE (INDUCED) ABORTION

MEDICAL

- **Mifepristone followed by Misoprostol** 24 - 48 hours afterwards. Safe up to 10 weeks.
  - Mifepristone is a progesterone receptor antagonist (leads to dilation and softening of the cervix, and placental separation).
  - Misoprostol is a prostaglandin E1 analog (causes uterine contractions). Patient must return day 7-14 days after Mifepristone to confirm complete termination of pregnancy.

- **Methotrexate followed by Misoprostol** 3 - 7 days later (safe up to 7 weeks).
  - Methotrexate is a folic antagonist. This regimen is less effective.

SURGICAL

Can be performed up to 24 weeks from LMP

- Dilation and Curettage (D & C): includes usage of a curette or suction curettage (manual or electric vacuum aspiration) . Used during the first 4-12 weeks' gestation.

- Dilation and Evacuation: > 12 weeks' gestation.

PLACENTAL INSUFFICIENCY

- Impairment or inability of the placenta to provide oxygen & nutrients.
- Etiologies: placenta previa or abruption, post-term pregnancy, intrauterine growth restriction.

DIAGNOSIS

- Fetal heart monitoring – **late decelerations** (gradual decrease in fetal heart rate initiating at the peak of contraction and into the second half of the contraction) due to mechanical compression of maternal vessels traversing the uterine wall during uterine contractions. May be associated with gradual return of heart rate to baseline.

INITIAL MANAGEMENT

- Placing the mother on her side, administering oxygen by mask, and correcting hypotension.

MULTIPLE GESTATIONS

- Associated with rapid maternal weight gain and growth of the uterus.
- **Dizygotic (fraternal):** due to fertilization of 2 ova by 2 different sperm (66%).
- **Monozygotic (identical):** formed from the fertilization of 1 ovum that splits. Increased risk of fetal transfusion syndrome and discordant fetal growth.

DIAGNOSIS:

- Ultrasound to visualize the fetuses.
- **Elevated levels of beta-hCG & maternal serum alpha-fetoprotein** higher than normal.

MATERNAL COMPLICATIONS

- Preterm labor, spontaneous abortion, preeclampsia, anemia.

FETAL COMPLICATIONS

- Intrauterine growth restrictions, placental abnormalities, breech presentation, umbilical cord prolapse, preeclampsia.
- Multiple gestations considered a high-risk pregnancy.

UNCOMPLICATED PREGNANCY

DIAGNOSIS

- Serum β-hCG: serum quantitative can detect pregnancy as early as 5 days after conception.
- Urine β-hCG: can detect pregnancy 14 days after conception; ↑Serum progesterone.

PHYSICAL EXAMINATION

- **Uterus changes**
  - **Ladin's sign:** uterus softening after 6 weeks.
  - **Hegar's sign:** uterine isthmus softening after 6-8 weeks' gestation.
  - **Piskacek's sign:** palpable lateral bulge or softening of uterine cornus 7-8 weeks' gestation.
- **Cervix changes**
  - **Goodell's sign:** cervical softening due to increased vascularization ~4-5 weeks' gestation.
  - Chadwick's sign: bluish coloration of the cervix & vulva ~8-12 weeks.
- Fetal heart tones: 10-12 weeks (towards the end of the 1st trimester). Normal is 120-160 bpm.
- Pelvic ultrasound: detects fetus ~5-6 weeks.
- Fetal movement: 16-20 weeks (quickening).

GPA CLASSIFICATION

- **Gravida:** # of times pregnant (regardless if carried to term).
- **Para:** # of births (>20 weeks) including viable or nonviable births (ex. stillbirth). Multiple gestations (eg, twins) count as 1 for notation.
- **Abortus:** # of pregnancies lost for whatever reason (miscarriages, abortions).

Ex: G_3P_3 = 3 pregnancies 3 births. $G_4P_3A_1$ = 4 pregnancies, 3 births, 1 miscarriage (or abortion).

FUNDAL HEIGHT MEASUREMENT

12 weeks	above the pubic symphysis
16 weeks	midway between the pubis & umbilicus
20 weeks	**at the umbilicus**
38 weeks	2-3 cm below the xiphoid process

MEASURING FUNDAL HEIGHT

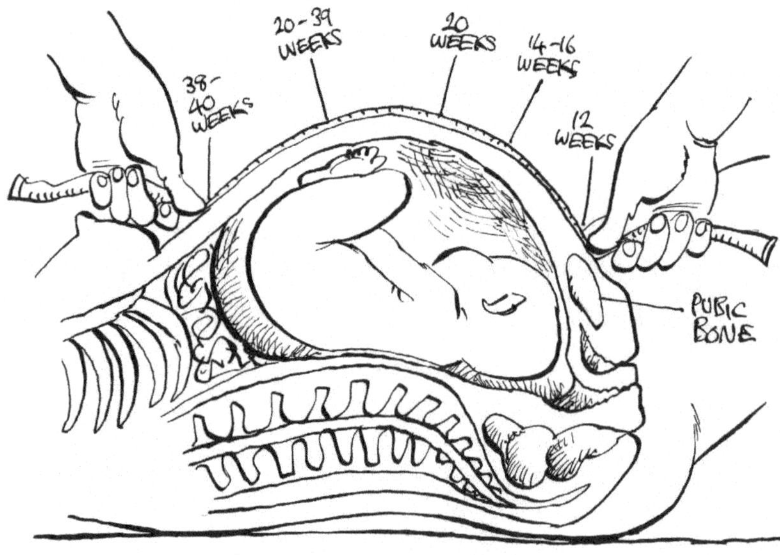

(1st day LMP + 7 − 3 months) Naegele's rule

PRENATAL CARE

ESTIMATED DATE OF DELIVERY (EDD) – NAEGELE'S RULE

- **1ST day of last menstrual period plus 7 days subtract 3 months**
  Example: LMP 8/7/16 EDD: 5/14/17

ROUTINE TESTS DURING FIRST PRENATAL VISIT

- Blood pressure, blood type & Rh, CBC, UA (glucose & protein), random glucose, HBsAg, HIV & syphilis, rubella titer, screening for sickle cell & cystic fibrosis. Pap smear.

FIRST TRIMESTER SCREENING/TESTS

Week 1 – 12 of pregnancy

Chromosomal screening tests:

- **Biochemical screening** may be performed:
  Free beta-hCG: abnormally high or low may be indicative of chromosomal abnormalities.
  PAPP-A: usually **low with fetal Down syndrome**
  (PAPP-A = serum pregnancy-associated plasma protein-A).
- **Nuchal translucency ultrasound** at 10-13 weeks. Screens for trisomies 13, 18, & 21 (Down syndrome). Increased thickness is abnormal. **If increased thickness, chorionic villous sampling or amniocentesis is offered.**

Other tests

- **Ultrasound:** fetal heart tones usually heard around 10-12 weeks by Doppler. **Transvaginal ultrasound can detect fetal heart activity as early as 5-6 weeks** after LMP.

- Uterine size & gestation: if abnormal, chorionic villus sampling (CVS) or amniocentesis can be offered at around 10-13 weeks.

- **Chorionic villus sampling:** may be performed ~10-13 weeks **(preferred technique before 15 weeks)**. **May be offered to women with increased risk of chromosomal abnormalities,** including those with a prior child with a chromosomal abnormality, maternal age >35y, abnormal 1st or 2nd trimester maternal screening tests, abnormal nuchal translucency & prior pregnancy losses.
  Advantage: allows for the option of early termination of the pregnancy if abnormalities are found.
  Disadvantages: performing it increases the risk of spontaneous abortion, increased infection, or fluid leak. Cannot be used in alpha-fetoprotein testing for neural tube defects.

SECOND TRIMESTER SCREENING/TESTS

Week 13 – 27 of pregnancy

- **Triple screening:** measures **alpha-fetoprotein, unconjugated estriol,** & **beta-hCG** usually at 15-20 weeks. Quadruple adds Inhibin A.

α-FP	β-hCG	Unconjugated Estriol (uE3)	Diagnosis
Low	**High**	Low	**Down Syndrome (Trisomy 21).**
High			**Open neural tube defects** eg, **Spina bifida** (or multiple gestation).
Low	Low	Low	Trisomy 18: often born stillborn or die within the 1st year of life.

High levels of inhibin A indicate chromosomal abnormalities

- **Gestational diabetes screening: 24 – 28 weeks.**

- **Amniocentesis:** may be offered to women including those with a prior child with a chromosomal abnormality, maternal age >35y, abnormal 1st or 2nd trimester maternal screening tests, abnormal ultrasound, prior pregnancy losses. Usually performed ~15-18 weeks.

NEURAL TUBE DEFECTS

- Birth defects of the brain, spine or spinal cord.
- **The two most common types are spina bifida and anencephaly.**
- **Increased incidence with maternal folate deficiency.**

PATHOPHYSIOLOGY

- Anencephaly: failure of closure of the portion of the neural tube that becomes the cerebrum.
- Spina bifida: incomplete closure of the embryonic neural tubule leads to non-fusion of some of the vertebrae overlying the spinal cords. This may lead to protrusion of the spinal cord through the opening. Most commonly seen at the lumbar and sacral areas of the spine.

TYPES OF SPINA BIFIDA

- **Spina bifida with myelomeningocele: most common type.** Meninges and spinal cord herniates thought the gap in the vertebrae. Often leads to disability.

- Spina bifida occulta: mildest form. No herniation of the spinal cord. The overlying skin may be normal or have some hair growing over it, dimpling of the skin or birthmark over the affected area.

- Spina bifida with meningocele: only the meninges herniate through the gap in the vertebrae

CLINICAL MANIFESTATIONS

- Sensory deficits, paralysis, hydrocephalus, hypotonia.

SCREENING

- Increased maternal serum alpha-fetoprotein followed by **amniocentesis showing increased alpha-fetoprotein & increased acetylcholinesterase.**

THIRD TRIMESTER SCREENING/TESTS Week 28 until birth

- **Gestational diabetes screening: 24 – 28 weeks.**

- Repeat antibody titers: **in Rh(D)-negative, antibody-negative (unsensitized) women:** **Anti-D Rh immunoglobulin** RhoGAM (300 micrograms) **given at 28 weeks' gestation**

- Hemoglobin & Hematocrit: 35 weeks.
- Group B *Streptococcus* screening: see below.
- Biophysical profile: looks at 5 variables including: fetal breathing, fetal tones, amniotic fluid levels, NST, & gross fetal movements. 2 points each (maximum score of 10 points).

- Non Stress Testing

NON STRESS Testing*:* baseline fetal heart rate is 120 – 160 bpm.

	DEFINITION	PROGNOSIS	MANAGEMENT
REACTIVE NST	• **≥2 accelerations of fetal heart rate ≥15 bpm** from baseline lasting at least 15 seconds over a 20-minute period. • Detection of two fetal movements	• **Fetal well being**	• Repeat weekly or biweekly
NONREACTIVE	• ***No fetal heart rate accelerations or*** ≤15bpm lasting ≤15 seconds	• Sleeping, immature or compromised fetus	• Vibratory stimulation to wake fetus up • May try contraction stress

CONTRACTION STRESS TEST (CST): measures fetal response to stress at times of uterine contraction.

	DEFINITION	PROGNOSIS	MANAGEMENT
NEGATIVE CST	• **No late decelerations** in the presence of 3 contractions in 10 minutes	• **Fetal well being**	• Repeat CST as needed
POSITIVE CST	• **Repetitive late decelerations** following ≥50% of contractions	• Worrisome especially if nonreactive NST	• **Hospitalize for prolonged fetal monitoring or delivery.**

GROUP B STREPTOCOCCUS SCREENING

- Group B *Streptococcus* (*S. agalactiae*) frequently colonizes the female reproductive tract and the upper respiratory tract of young infants.
- Vertical transmission of Group B *Streptococcus* infection during labor is the leading cause of neonatal infection and the major cause of sepsis in newborns.

COMPLICATIONS OF GBS INFECTION

- Maternal: chorioamnionitis, preterm labor, asymptomatic bacteriuria, cystitis, and pyelonephritis.
- **Neonates: early postpartum infection** (eg, meningitis, septic arthritis, osteomyelitis).

SCREENING

- **Rectovaginal screening culture:** new ACOG guidelines (August 2019) is now recommended at **36 0/7 to 37 6/7 weeks of gestation** (previously 35-37 weeks) with the following 2 exceptions:
- Exceptions to screening: 1. women with bacteriuria during the current pregnancy and 2. women who previously gave birth to an infant with invasive GBS disease. Women who fit either criteria should receive intrapartum antibiotic prophylaxis.

INTRAPARTUM PROPHYLAXIS

- If positive screening or one of the 2 exceptions, **prophylactic antibiotics given during labor** (most effective within 4 hours of delivery) - **IV Penicillin G first-line agent** (5 million units followed by 2.5 million units every 4 hours until delivery).
- Second-line: Ampicillin, extended-spectrum Penicillins, Cephalosporins (eg, Cefazolin), Clindamycin, and IV Vancomycin.

TOXIC SHOCK SYNDROME

- Exotoxins produced by ***Staphylococcus aureus.***

PATHOPHYSIOLOGY

- toxic shock syndrome toxin is a superantigen that activates a large number of T cells, which releases various inflammatory mediators (IL-2, IL-1, TNF). This causes capillary leakage, circulatory collapse, and multi-organ failure.

RISK FACTORS

- 50% associated with high absorbency **tampon use.**

- Nonmenstrual: surgical & postpartum wound infections, burns & contraceptive sponge use.

CLINICAL MANIFESTATIONS

- Sudden onset of **high fever** (≥39°C/102.2°F), tachycardia, nausea, vomiting, diarrhea, pharyngitis.

- **Skin: erythroderma = diffuse erythematous macular rash** (resembles sunburn – includes palms & soles), desquamation.

- Multisystemic involvement can manifest as **hypotension**, abdominal tenderness, headache, myalgias.

DIAGNOSIS

- Clinical, CBC, cultures, clinical.

MANAGEMENT

- **Supportive:** hospital admission, removal of offending object, **aggressive IV fluid replacement & antibiotics (eg, Clindamycin + Vancomycin** or Linezolid.

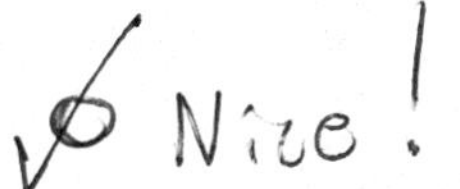

RH ALLOIMMUNIZATION

PATHOPHYSIOLOGY

- Occurs **when Rh(D)-negative women carry a Rh(D)-positive fetus** with exposure to fetal blood mixing of D-positive RBCs (eg, during C-section, abruptio placentae, placenta previa, amniocentesis, vaginal delivery etc.).

- The mixing causes maternal alloimmunization & maternal anti-Rh(D) IgG antibodies.

- **During subsequent pregnancies, if she carries another Rh(D)-positive fetus**, the antibodies may cross the placenta & attack the fetal RBCs, **leading to hemolysis of the fetal RBCs** (hemolytic disease of the fetus or newborn).

- If the mother of the fetus is Rh(D)-negative & father of the fetus is Rh(D)-positive, there's a 50% chance baby will be positive.

- At-risk pregnancy: **Rh(D)-negative mother + Rh(D)-positive father (or unknown).**

WORKUP

- Antibody screen: done at initial prenatal visit to see if mother is Rh(D)- or Rh(D)+. In D-negative women, the antibody screen may be repeated at 28 weeks of gestation and at delivery.

- Antibody titers: performed in Rh(D)-negative women. **Unsensitized = no Rh(D) antibodies present.** If sensitized (Rh antibodies present), titers should be performed via indirect antiglobulin test. The patient is considered sensitized if titer level is > 1:4. If titer is < 1:16 no further treatment is necessary.

If antibody titer 1:16 or greater, do initial amniocentesis at 16-20 weeks. If fetal cells are Rh(D)-negative, treat like normal pregnancy. If fetal cells are Rh(D)-positive and bilirubin is:

- low – repeat amniocentesis in 2-3 weeks.
- medium - repeat amniocentesis in 1-2 weeks.
- high - perform a percutaneous umbilical blood sample (fetal hematocrit). If fetal hematocrit is low, perform an intrauterine umbilical vein infusion.

PREVENTION

In Rh(D)-negative, antibody-negative women:

- **Anti-D Rh immunoglobulin** RhoGAM (300 micrograms) given in **3 instances:**
  1) **given at 28 weeks' gestation** AND
  2) **within 72h of delivery of a Rh(D)-positive baby** AND
  3) **after any potential mixing of blood** (spontaneous abortion, ectopic pregnancy, amniocentesis etc.).

PLACENTA PREVIA

- Abnormal placenta placement over or close to the internal cervical os.

Types:
- Complete: complete coverage of the cervical os by the placenta.
- Partial: partial coverage of the cervical os by the placenta.
- Marginal: adjacent to the internal os (leading edge of the placenta is < 2cm from the internal os).

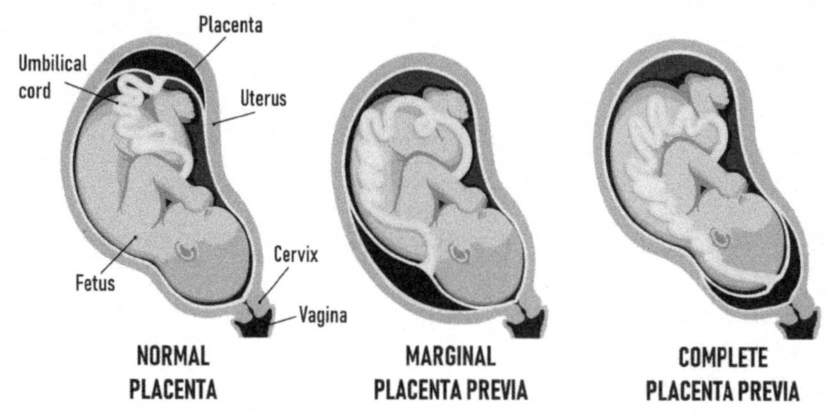

Photo credit: Shutterstock (used with permission)

RISK FACTORS
- Major: **previous placenta previa, previous C-section, and multiple gestations.**
- Increasing age & previous uterine surgery.

CLINICAL MANIFESTATIONS
- Sudden onset of **painless vaginal bleeding in the third trimester** (may be bright-red) usually after 28 weeks.
- **Absence of abdominal pain or uterine tenderness.**

PHYSICAL EXAMINATION
- **Soft, nontender uterus.**
- ***Do not perform digital vaginal or speculum exam*** if placenta previa is suspected (may cause increased separation, resulting in severe hemorrhage).

DIAGNOSIS
- **Transabdominal ultrasound often performed initially (screening)** with **confirmation by transvaginal ultrasound** (more sensitive and helps monitor placement of the placenta).

MANAGEMENT
- Stabilization with premature fetus: watchful waiting if the patient is stable. Pelvic rest (no vaginal intercourse).

- Delivery when stable: if L:S ratio > 2:1, > 36 weeks, blood loss > 500mL, coagulation defects, or persistent labor. **C-section usually preferred in complete, major degrees, & with fetal distress.** Vaginal delivery may be an option if the margins are at least 2cm away from internal os, mild degrees, & no fetal distress.

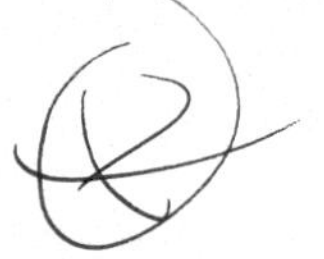

ABRUPTIO PLACENTAE

- Partial or complete premature separation of the placenta from the uterine wall (prior to delivery of the fetus).
- The blood may be concealed (within the uterine cavity) or external (blood drains through the cervix).

PATHOPHYSIOLOGY
- **Rupture of maternal blood vessels in the decidua basalis**, leading to bleeding into the separated space.
- The subsequent release of tissue factor, thrombin generation lead to the other findings.

RISK FACTORS
- **Maternal hypertension most common** (eg, chronic, preeclampsia, eclampsia).
- Prior abruption, smoking, alcohol use, **cocaine**, folate deficiency, advanced maternal age, abdominal trauma, multiple gestation, PPROM, & chorioamnionitis.
- More common in African-Americans.

CLINICAL MANIFESTATIONS
- Sudden onset of **painful third-trimester vaginal bleeding** (often dark red), **severe abdominal pain (uterine contractions).**
- May have back pain or signs of shock from blood loss.
- Premature delivery may occur.

PHYSICAL EXAMINATION
- **Tender rigid (hypertonic) uterus.**
- **Do not perform a pelvic exam.**
- Fetal distress may occur (eg, fetal bradycardia).

DIAGNOSIS
- **Primarily a clinical diagnosis.**
- Transabdominal ultrasound may show a retroplacental clot (but not reliable). May be helpful to distinguish between abruptio and previa.

- **EXAM TIP:**
- **Placenta previa vs. Abruptio placentae**
- Both are common causes of third trimester bleeding.

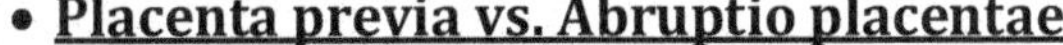

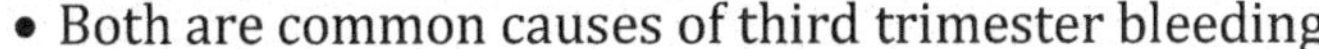

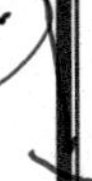

- Previa: painless vaginal bleeding + soft, nontender uterus
- Abruptio: painful vaginal bleeding + abdominal pain + firm tender uterus.
- Think **P**revia is **P**ainless whereas **Ab**ruptio is associated with **Ab**dominal pain.

VASA PREVIA

- Fetal vessels are present over the cervical os.
- Fetal mortality approaches 60% if not detected before delivery due to fetal exsanguination.

CLINICAL MANIFESTATIONS
- Triad of **rupture of membranes followed by painless, vaginal bleeding** + **fetal distress** (eg, **bradycardia).**

DIAGNOSIS: may be seen prior to delivery as the vessels crossing the os.

MANAGEMENT: **immediate Cesarean section.**

CHRONIC (PREEXISTING) HYPERTENSION

- Hypertension **(140/90 mmHg or greater)** occurring **BEFORE 20 weeks' gestation** or prior to pregnancy.
- Mild: 140/90 mmHg or greater.
- Moderate: 150/100 mmHg or greater.
- **Severe: 160/110 mmHg** or greater.

CLINICAL MANIFESTATIONS

- Usually asymptomatic but headache or visual symptoms may be seen if severe (> 160/110 mmHg).

MANAGEMENT OF MILD

- Monitor every 2-4 weeks, weekly between 34-36 weeks. Delivery may be recommended at 37 weeks or later.

MANAGEMENT OF MODERATE TO SEVERE

- **Medications – Labetalol,** long-acting calcium channel blockers (eg, **Nifedipine**) or **Methyldopa** are first-line agents. Hydralazine.
- Management of blood pressure helps to reduce maternal and fetal complications.
- **ACE inhibitors & Angiotensin receptor blockers are contraindicated in pregnancy.**

TRANSITIONAL HYPERTENSION

- AKA Gestational hypertension or Pregnancy-induced HTN.

- **New** onset of hypertension **140/90 mmHg or greater** occurring **after 20 weeks' gestation + no proteinuria, edema, or end-organ dysfunction.**

CLINICAL MANIFESTATIONS

- Asymptomatic.

DIAGNOSTIC WORKUP

- Primarily to distinguish gestational from preeclampsia – urine protein, platelets, LFTs, & assessment of fetal status.

MANAGEMENT

- **Supportive monitoring:** weekly blood pressure, urine protein, platelets & liver enzymes measurements. Ultrasound monthly to check for intrauterine growth restriction and weekly fetal nonstress testing in the third trimester.

- Severe hypertension (160/110 or greater): blood pressure medication only during pregnancy to reduce stroke risk - **Methyldopa, Labetalol, or Nifedipine**. Second-line – Clonidine, Hydralazine.

PREECLAMPSIA

- **New** onset of hypertension **(systolic >140/90 mmHg)** occurring **after 20 weeks' gestation** + **proteinuria or end-organ dysfunction** in a previously normotensive female.
- Blood pressure measurements done on at least 2 occasions at least 4 hours apart.

RISK FACTORS

- Preexisting hypertension, nulliparity, maternal age of < 20 years or >35 years, diabetes, chronic renal disease, or autoimmune disorders.

MILD PREECLAMPSIA

- Blood pressure 140/90 mmHg or greater + proteinuria of at least 300mg in a 24-hour urine specimen (or dipstick 1+ to 2+).

SEVERE FEATURES

- Blood pressure **160/110 mmHg** or greater + **proteinuria at least 5g** in a 24-hour urine specimen (or dipstick 3+ or greater).
- Symptoms of end-organ damage - **cerebral or visual symptoms** (eg, new-onset or persistent headaches, flashing lights, blurred vision, altered mental status changes), severe or persistent epigastric or right upper quadrant pain, DIC, pulmonary or peripheral edema.
- Progressive renal insufficiency: serum creatinine > 1.1 mg/dL or oliguria (<500ml of urine in 24 hours or 30cc/hour).
- Thrombocytopenia
- **HELLP syndrome:** Hemolytic anemia, Elevated Liver enzymes, and Low Platelets.

MANAGEMENT OF **MILD**:

- **37 weeks' gestation or greater is managed with delivery.**
- < 37 weeks' gestation: expectant management (eg, daily weights, weekly blood pressure and dipstick, bedrest, antenatal corticosteroids to mature lungs if elective delivery is planned) with delivery at 37 weeks' gestation.

MANAGEMENT OF **SEVERE FEATURES**:

- 37 weeks or greater: **prompt delivery definitive management** after hospitalization + **Magnesium sulfate** to prevent seizures + **blood pressure control** (eg, Labetalol, Nifedipine or Methyldopa). Hydralazine alternative.
- 34 - 37 weeks: **prompt delivery definitive management.**
- Viable to 33+6 weeks: If symptomatic, not controlled with antihypertensives – deliver. If asymptomatic or well-controlled with antihypertensives – expectant management followed by delivery at 34 weeks.

ECLAMPSIA

- Preeclampsia + **seizures or coma.**

CLINICAL MANIFESTATIONS

- Abrupt onset of **tonic-clonic seizures**.

MANAGEMENT

- **IV Magnesium sulfate for seizures & blood pressure stabilization followed by delivery of the fetus** (once the mother is stabilized).
- Lorazepam only used if refractory to Magnesium sulfate.
- Blood pressure control: **IV Labetalol or Hydralazine.** IV Nicardipine.

GESTATIONAL DIABETES MELLITUS

- **Glucose intolerance or Diabetes mellitus only present during pregnancy** (usually subsides postpartum).

RISK FACTORS

- Family or prior history of gestational diabetes, spontaneous abortion, history of infant >4,000g at birth, multiple gestations.
- **Obesity,** >25y of age.
- Non-Caucasians: African-American (highest), Hispanic, Asian or Pacific Islander, & Native American.

PATHOPHYSIOLOGY

- **Maternal insulin resistance in women with undiagnosed beta cell dysfunction** exacerbated by placental release diabetogenic hormones - **human placental lactogen** (human somatomammotropin), growth hormone, & corticotropin-releasing hormone.
- Maternal insulin resistance allows for increased glucose availability for the growing fetus.

Fetal complications:

- Fetal hyperinsulinemia leads **to fetal macrosomia (most common),** birth injuries from macrosomia (eg, shoulder dystocia), **preterm labor,** delayed fetal lung maturity, fetal hyperglycemia but **neonatal hypoglycemia** (high fetal insulin levels + abrupt removal of maternal glucose after delivery), **neonatal hypocalcemia,** hypomagnesemia, & hyperbilirubinemia.
- Congenital malformations (cardiac, musculoskeletal, and CNS) occur less because GDM occurs later in pregnancy.

Maternal complications:

- **>50% chance of developing type 2 Diabetes mellitus after pregnancy.**
- >50% chance of recurrence with subsequent pregnancies.
- Preeclampsia, Abruptio placentae.

SCREENING (two-step approach):

- Step 1: **50-gram 1-hour glucose challenge test, usually at 24 – 28 weeks' gestation.** Screen-positive patients (glucose > 130 – 140 mg/dL) go on to 3h-glucose tolerance test.
- Step 2: **100-gram 3-hour oral glucose tolerance test** (diagnostic gold standard). The threshold for glucose levels on a 3-hour glucose tolerance test are 2 of the 4: fasting >95 mg/dL, 1 hour >180 mg/dL, 2 hour >155 mg/dL, 3 hour >140 mg/dL.

SCREENING (alternative one-step approach):

- 75-gram 2-hour oral glucose tolerance test (may be more sensitive).

MANAGEMENT

- Lifestyle modifications: **diabetic diet and exercise** (eg, **walking**) **initial treatment of choice.** Note that *pregnant patients are not told to lose weight.* Daily fingersticks overnight and after each meal.

MEDICAL MANAGEMENT

- Indications: if fasting glucose > 95 mg/dL or greater and 1h-postprandial glucose > 130-140 mg/dL *after a trial of diet & exercise.*
- **Insulin first-line medical treatment of choice** (doesn't cross placenta). Goal of treatment is fasting glucose <95.
- Glyburide or Metformin also relatively safe in women who are unable to comply or refuse insulin therapy.
- Labor induction: at 38 weeks if uncontrolled/macrosomia. At 40 weeks if controlled/no macrosomia. C-section may be delivery method of choice if the child is macrosomic.

PREGESTATIONAL DIABETES MELLITUS

- Preexisting type I or type II Diabetes mellitus prior to pregnancy.

MATERNAL COMPLICATIONS
- Preeclampsia, spontaneous abortion, postpartum hemorrhage.

FETAL COMPLICATIONS
- **Congenital anomalies** (eg, cardiac and neural tube defects), macrosomia, and preterm labor.

SHOULDER DYSTOCIA

- Failure of the shoulders to spontaneously traverse the pelvis after delivery of the fetal head due to impaction (anterior shoulder is stuck behind the mother's pubic bone).
- Considered an obstetric emergency.

RISK FACTORS
- **Most commonly seen in macrosomic infants of diabetics,** post-term pregnancy, multiparity, prolonged second stage of labor, forceps delivery, maternal obesity, and advanced maternal age, epidural anesthesia.

FETAL COMPLICATIONS:
- **Brachial plexus injuries** due to traction during shoulder dystocia, Erb's palsy, Klumpke paralysis, Cerebral palsy.
- Erb-Duchenne palsy is a lesion in the upper trunk (root) injury (C5-C6 with or without C7) of the brachial plexus, leading to the characteristic "waiter's tip" deformity (arm in adduction with elbow extension, forearm pronation, and wrist flexion with the fingers curled up).
- **Clavicular fractures,** long bone fractures, fetal asphyxia, anoxic brain injury, death.

MATERNAL COMPLICATIONS:
- Perineal or vaginal tears, postpartum hemorrhage, uterine rupture.

CLINICAL MANIFESTATIONS
- During delivery, the turtle sign may occur (retraction of the baby's head, similar to a turtle retracting into its shell) or red, puffy face.

MANAGEMENT

Nonmanipulative:
- **McRoberts maneuver:** hyperflexion and abduction of the mother's hips towards the abdomen without and then with suprapubic pressure. An extending episiotomy may need to be performed.

Manipulative
- Delivery of the posterior arm to allow for a rotational maneuver (eg, Woods, Rubin I and II)
- **Woods corkscrew maneuver:** rotation of the fetal shoulders 180 degrees.

Others
- Gaskin all-fours maneuver.
- Zavanelli maneuver: pushing the fetal head back into the vaginal canal with immediate transport to cesarean section.

PREVENTION
- Cesarean delivery indicated if fetus us > 4,500g in weight in a diabetic mother or >5,000 in a nondiabetic mother.

BREECH PRESENTATION

- The fetus whose presenting part is the buttocks and/or feet.
- Occurs in 3-5% of fetuses at term (37-40 weeks).
- Risks of breech presentation include developmental dysplasia of the hip, torticollis, and mild deformations.
- Spontaneous version may occur at any time prior to delivery.

TYPES

- Frank: both hips are flexed and both knees are extended (the feet are adjacent to the fetal head). Most common type of breech presentation at term (50-70%).
- Complete: both hips and both knees are flexed (5-10% at term).
- Incomplete: one or both of the hips are not completely flexed (10-40%).

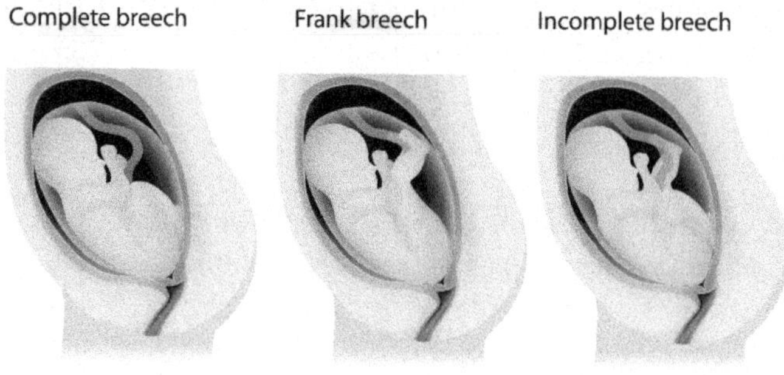

Photo credit:
Shutterstock (used with permission)

DIAGNOSIS

- Physical examination – a soft mass (eg, buttocks) instead of the normal hard surface of the skull. Leopold maneuvers are as set of 4 maneuvers that can determine the estimated fetal weight and presenting part of the fetus.
- Ultrasound can be used to confirm if the diagnosis is uncertain.

MANAGEMENT

Choice of delivery route includes patient preference, expertise of the provider, etc. Options include:

- External cephalic version before labor, followed by a trial of labor (if the version is successful) & cesarean delivery if version is unsuccessful is an option for women at or near term at a low risk of labor and delivery-related complications. Planned Cesarean delivery of the breech fetus if the breech persists reduces maternal and perinatal death.

- External cephalic version before labor, followed by a trial of labor if the version is successful. If the version is unsuccessful, a trial of labor and vaginal breech birth are offered to patients at low risk of labor and delivery-related complications. Cesarean delivery is offered to patients at increased risk or if patient does not want to attempt a vaginal breech birth.

- Planned cesarean delivery for breech presentation, without a trial of external cephalic version.

- A trial of labor and vaginal breech birth for patients thought to be at a low risk of labor and delivery-related complications, without a trial of external cephalic version.

UMBILICAL CORD PROLAPSE

- Occurs when the cord extends past the presenting part of the fetus and protrudes into the vagina.
- A prolapsed cord can lead to reduced fetal oxygenation as a result of umbilical artery vasospasm and/or umbilical vein occlusion.

RISK FACTORS

- Fetal and maternal factors include low birth weight, malpresentation, long umbilical cord, pelvic deformities, low-lying placentation, polyhydramnios, prematurity, etc.

CLINICAL MANIFESTATIONS

- **Sudden onset of severe, prolonged fetal bradycardia or variable decelerations** after a previously normal tracing.
- The cord may be palpable on vaginal examination.

MANAGEMENT

- **Emergent Cesarean section** to avoid fetal compromise or death.
  - Preoperative intrauterine resuscitation: aims at increasing oxygen delivery to the placenta and umbilical blood flow – eg, manual elevation of the fetal presenting part to prevent compression, placing the patient in Trendelenburg or knee-chest position, tocolytics, etc.
- Vaginal delivery is an option when delivery is impending and can be securely assisted.

CESAREAN DELIVERY

- The use of surgery for delivery of the fetus.

INDICATIONS

- Conditions where vaginal delivery would put the fetus or mother at risk – includes but not limited to **failure to progress during labor (most common), nonreassuring fetal status, fetal malpresentation**, problems with the placenta or the umbilical cord, multiple gestations, maternal hypertension, maternal infection with significant risk of perinatal transmission via vaginal birth, suspected macrosomia, uterine rupture.

TIMING

- Scheduled primary Cesarean deliveries at term is often performed in the 39th of 40th week of gestation.
- Obstetrically & medically indicated Cesarean deliveries are performed as deemed necessary.
- The timing of elective repeat Cesarean delivery is dependent on a multitude of factors.

ANTIBIOTIC PROPHYLAXIS

- Preoperative: up to 60 minutes prior to making the initial incision.
- **IV Cefazolin**. Azithromycin may be added if the Cesarean delivery is performed after rupture of membranes or intrapartum.
- Clindamycin and Gentamicin if penicillin-allergic.
- For women in labor &women with ruptured membranes, vaginal cleansing before cesarean delivery (eg, Povidone-iodine vaginal scrub for 30 seconds) reduces the frequency of postpartum Endometritis.

THROMBOPROPHYLAXIS

- For all women undergoing Cesarean delivery, mechanical thromboprophylaxis is suggested.
- Women at high risk of venous thromboembolism should receive mechanical thromboprophylaxis plus pharmacologic thromboprophylaxis. Pharmacologic prophylaxis is initiated 6 to 12 hours postoperatively, after concerns for hemorrhage have diminished and continued until the woman is fully ambulating.

MORNING SICKNESS & HYPEREMESIS GRAVIDARUM (HEG)

- Morning sickness: nausea &/or vomiting **up until 16 weeks (most common in the first trimester).**
- Hyperemesis gravidarum: **severe, excessive form of morning sickness** (nausea, vomiting) associated with **weight loss & electrolyte imbalance**. Develops during 1st or 2nd trimester (persists >16 weeks of gestation).
- Risk factors: primigravida, previous hyperemesis in past pregnancy, multiple gestations, molar pregnancy.
- Pathophysiology: vomiting center oversensitivity to hormones of pregnancy (eg, beta-hCG)

CLINICAL MANIFESTATIONS

- Nausea and or vomiting. **Hyperemesis gravidarum is associated with more severe symptoms, weight loss** of 5% of pre pregnant weight & acidosis (from starvation),

LABS IN HEG

- Electrolyte imbalance from vomiting – **hypokalemia, hypochloremic metabolic alkalosis,** ketones.

MANAGEMENT

- **Lifestyle modifications: initial management of choice - ginger**, dietary changes (eg, high protein foods, small & frequent meals, avoiding trigger foods, such as spicy or fatty foods), increase fluids.
- **Pyridoxine (vitamin B_6) with or without Doxylamine first-line medical management.**
- Second-line: if no relief, use antihistamines (eg, Doxylamine, Dimenhydrinate, Meclizine).
- Third-line: dopamine antagonists (eg, Metoclopramide or Promethazine).
- Fourth line: Ondansetron (serotonin antagonist).
- Hypovolemia: **IV rehydration, electrolyte repletion.** May need Dimenhydrinate, Meclizine, or Diphenhydramine. Ondansetron if severe vomiting. Total parenteral nutrition if severe.

UTERINE RUPTURE

- Complete transection of the uterus from the endometrium to the serosa. If the peritoneum remains intact, it is known as uterine dehiscence. Most occur during labor at the site of a prior C-section.
- **Life-threatening to the mother and fetus.**

RISK FACTORS

- **Previous uterine rupture, prior cesarean section** (eg, fundal or vertical), induction of labor, trauma (especially MVA), uterine myomectomy, uterine overdistention (eg, multiple gestation, polyhydramnios), placenta percreta, abdominal trauma.

DECREASED RISK

- A prior vaginal delivery either before or after the prior C-section significantly reduces rupture risk.

CLINICAL MANIFESTATIONS

- **Sudden onset of extreme abdominal pain, decreased or absent uterine contractions,** abnormal bump in the abdomen, & possible regression of the fetus.
- Vaginal hemorrhaging.
- The most common fetal heart rate pattern is fetal bradycardia. No FHR pattern is pathognomonic.
- High fetal mortality rate (50-75%) depending on if the placenta remains attached to the uterine wall.

MANAGEMENT

- **Immediate laparotomy & delivery of the fetus** to reduce fetal and maternal mortality followed by repair of the uterus or hysterectomy.
- If repair is performed, all subsequent pregnancies will be delivered via cesarean at 36 weeks'.

LABOR & DELIVERY

INTRA PARTUM

- **Braxton-Hicks contractions:** spontaneous uterine contractions late in pregnancy **not associated with cervical dilation.**
- **Lightening:** fetal head descending into the pelvis causing a change in the abdomen's shape and sensation that the baby has "become lighter".
- **Ruptured Membranes:** sudden gush of liquid or constant leakage of fluid.
- **Bloody show:** passage of blood-tinged cervical mucus late in pregnancy. Occurs when the cervix begins thinning (effacement).
- **True labor:** contractions of the uterine fundus with radiation to lower back & abdomen. Regular & painful contractions of the uterus causes cervical dilation & fetus expulsion.

CARDINAL MOVEMENTS OF LABOR

1. **Engagement:** when the fetal presenting part enters the pelvic inlet.
2. **Descent:** passage of the head into the pelvis (commonly called "lightening").
3. **Flexion:** flexion of the head to allow the smallest diameter to present to the pelvis.
4. **Internal Rotation:** fetal vertex moves from occiput transverse position to a position where the sagittal suture is parallel to the anteroposterior diameter of the pelvis.
5. **Extension:** vertex extends as it passes beneath the pubic symphysis.
6. **External rotation:** fetus externally rotates after the head is delivered so that the shoulder can be delivered.
7. Expulsion.

STAGES OF LABOR

3 STAGES OF LABOR.

STAGE I:	Onset of labor (true regular contractions) to **full dilation of cervix (10 cm).** - **Latent phase:** cervix effacement with gradual cervical dilation. - **Active phase:** rapid cervical dilation (usually beginning @ 3-4 cm).
STAGE II:	Time from full cervical dilation until **delivery of the fetus**. - **Passive phase:** complete cervical dilation to active maternal expulsive efforts. - **Active phase:** from active maternal expulsive efforts to delivery of the fetus.
STAGE III:	Postpartum until **delivery of the placenta**. 0-30 minutes usually (average 5). **3 signs of placental separation**: 1. **gush of blood** 2. **lengthening of the umbilical cord** 3. **anterior-cephalad movement** of the uterine **fundus (becomes globular and firmer)** after the placenta detaches. Placental expulsion: due to downward pressure of the retroplacental hematoma, uterine contractions

The period 1-2 hours after delivery where the mother is assessed for complications is sometimes called the 4th stage.

PRELABOR RUPTURE OF MEMBRANES (PROM)

- Rupture of the amniotic membranes before the onset of labor.
- If it occurs prior to 37 weeks' gestation, it is known as Preterm prelabor rupture of membranes (PPROM).

COMPLICATIONS
- **May lead to chorioamnionitis or endometritis if prolonged** (>24 hours).
- Cord prolapse, placental abruption.

RISK FACTORS
- STIs, smoking, prior preterm delivery, multiple gestations.

CLINICAL MANIFESTATIONS
- **Gush of fluid** or persistent leakage of fluid from the vagina or vaginal discharge.

DIAGNOSIS
- **Sterile speculum exam: pooling of secretions** in posterior fornix with inspection. Obtain fluid for cultures, nitrazine paper test or fern test. **Nitrazine paper test**: **turns blue if pH >6.5** (PROM is likely because normal amniotic fluid pH is ~7 compared to vaginal pH usually ~4). **Fern test**: amniotic fluid dries in a fern pattern (crystallization of estrogen & amniotic fluid).
- Ultrasound to check amniotic fluid index.
- Avoid digital vaginal examination unless delivery is imminent in most cases (to avoid introduction of infection).

MANAGEMENT
- Expectant: admit with fetal monitoring & await for spontaneous labor (90% will go into spontaneous labor within 24 hours after PROM). Monitor for infection (chorioamnionitis or endometritis).
- Labor induction: if chorioamnionitis or labor does not occur spontaneously within 18 hours or rupture. **Prostaglandin cervical gel or Oxytocin.**

PRETERM PRELABOR RUPTURE OF MEMBRANES (PPROM)

- Rupture of the amniotic membranes before the onset of labor occurring **prior to 37 weeks**.

COMPLICATIONS
- **May lead to chorioamnionitis or endometritis if prolonged** (>24 hours).
- Cord prolapse, placental abruption.

RISK FACTORS
- STIs, smoking, prior preterm delivery, multiple gestations.

MANAGEMENT
- Expectant management: **if no sign of maternal or fetal infection or distress.** Admit with fetal monitoring & await for spontaneous labor.
- **If under 34 weeks, administer corticosteroids** (eg, **Betamethasone**) to **enhance fetal lung maturity.** Amniocentesis can be done to assess fetal lung maturity.
- Tocolytics may be given to delay delivery 48 hours to allow Betamethasone to work if not in advanced labor (>4 cm dilation), no signs of chorioamnionitis, or if no signs of nonreassuring fetal testing.
- **Antibiotics** (Ampicillin + Azithromycin) often given to prevent infection.
- Prompt delivery: if **signs of maternal or fetal infection or distress.**

PRETERM PRELABOR

- **Labor = regular uterine contractions** >4-6/hour + **progressive cervical effacement & dilation** between 20-36 weeks' gestation.

CLINICAL MANIFESTATIONS
- **Contractions** (abdominal pain, pelvic pain, or lower back pain)

DIAGNOSIS
- **Preterm labor is cervical dilation <u>3 cm or greater</u> + >80% effacement or the presence of fetal fibronectin** between 20-34 weeks.
- PTL likely if cervical dilation 2-3 cm with <80% effacement or if >1cm cervical dilation between serial examinations.
- Signs of rupture of membrane include pooling of fluid in the vaginal fornix, positive ferning of vaginal fluid, and nitrate paper turning blue.
- <u>Workup:</u> rule out infections (eg, UTI, Group B streptococcus, STIs). Amniocentesis for L:S ratio **(L:S ratio < 2.0 suggests fetal lung immaturity).**

<u>Management 34 weeks or later</u> & fetal weight > 2,500g
- **Admit for delivery**. If after 4-6 hours, there is no progressive cervical dilation or effacement + fetal well-being is determined (reactive nonstress test), they are eligible for discharge home.

<u>Management < 34 weeks</u> + 600 – 2,500g:
- **Delay delivery with tocolytics + Betamethasone** to enhance fetal lung maturity.
- <u>Corticosteroids</u> decrease the incidence of infant respiratory distress syndrome and neonatal mortality.
- <u>Tocolytics</u> may be given to delay labor up to 48 hours to allow for Betamethasone to take full effect (effects begin at 24h, peak at 48h and last 7 days). **Magnesium sulfate** exposure in utero confers neuroprotection against sever motor dysfunction and cerebral palsy in preterm births.
- Antibiotic for GBS prophylaxis (eg, Ampicillin) may be used.

POSTPARTUM DEPRESSION

- **Major depression 2 weeks – 12 months postpartum**

	POSTPARTUM BLUES	POSTPARTUM DEPRESSION	POSTPARTUM PSYCHOSIS
ONSET	• 2-4 days postpartum	• 2 weeks – 2 months postpartum.	• Repeat weekly or biweekly
CLINICAL MANIFESTATIONS	• **Mild depression**: insomnia, anhedonia, fatigue, depressed mood, irritability. • **Concern if she is a good mother.** • **No thoughts of harming baby.**	• Irritability, sleep & mood disturbances, **loss of interest (anhedonia),** eating changes, anxiety, and **crying most days of the week.** • **May have thoughts of harming baby.**	• **Psychotic thoughts and delusions.** • **Thoughts of harming baby (baby is in danger).**
DURATION	• Resolves within 1-2 weeks	• Resolves within 3-14 months	
MANAGEMENT	• No treatment needed. • Cognitive behavioral therapy	• Antidepressants (SSRI) • Cognitive behavioral therapy	• **Admit patient & remove children to ensure their safety.** • Antidepressants (SSRI), antipsychotics • Cognitive behavioral therapy

INDUCTION OF LABOR

- Stimulation of uterine contractions to initiate labor prior to the onset of spontaneous labor.

INDICATIONS

- **Vaginal delivery when prolonged labor may lead to complications** for either the mother or the fetus and those risks are greater than continuing the pregnancy.

CONTRAINDICATIONS

- Situations in which the risks of induction of vaginal delivery is greater than cesarean delivery.
- **Absolute contraindications transmural myomectomy, placenta previa, prolapsed cord, active genital herpes, transverse fetal lie, uterine scar from classical C-section incision, & cephalopelvic disproportion.**
- Relative contraindications breech presentation, multiple gestation, prematurity, & previous C-section with transverse scar.

EARLY INDUCTION

- Used in women with unfavorable cervices to promote cervical ripening.
- **Prostaglandin gel** placed directly on the cervix. Promotes cervical ripening and may lead to uterine contractions.
- Balloon catheter or laminaria (dilates the cervix).

LATER INDUCTION

- Performed when the cervix is dilated <1cm with some effacement.
- **IV Oxytocin (Pitocin)** is a **uterotonic agent**. Monitor uterine activity & fetal heart rate.
- Amniotomy artificially rupturing the membranes with a small hook. May be performed if the cervix is partially dilated and there is effacement of the cervix.

APGAR SCORE

Usually done at 1 & 5 minutes after birth. Repeated at 10 minutes if abnormal.

Score from 1-10: ≥7 = normal; 4-6 fairly low ≤3 critically low

	0	1	2
Appearance Skin color changes	Blue-gray Pale all over	• **Acrocyanosis: body pink but blue extremities**	• **Pink baby (no cyanosis)**
Pulse	0	• *<100*	• ***≥100***
Grimace (Reflex irritability)	No response to stimulation	• Grimaces feebly	• Pulls away, sneezes or coughs
Activity (Muscle tone)	None	• Some flexion	• Flexes arm & legs • Resists extension
Respiration	Absent	• Weak, irregular	• Strong, crying (nml 30-60/min)

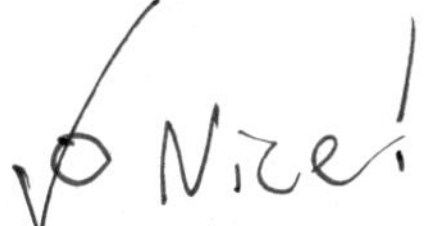

POSTPARTUM (PUERPERIUM) 6-week period after delivery

- **Uterus:** at the level of the umbilicus after delivery, involution (shrinks) after 2 days, descends into the pelvic cavity ~2 weeks. Normal size around 6 weeks postpartum.
- **Lochia serosa:** pinkish/brown vaginal bleeding especially postpartum days 4-10 (from the decidual tissue). Usually resolves by 3-4 weeks postpartum.
- **Breasts/menstruation:** breast milk in postpartum days 3-5 bluish-white. If lactating, mothers may remain anovulatory during that time. If not breastfeeding, menses may return 6-8 weeks postpartum.

POSTPARTUM HEMORRHAGE

- Bleeding >500 ml if vaginal delivery is performed or >1000 ml if C-section is performed. Loss requiring transfusion or a 10% decrease in hematocrit.
- Common cause of maternal death within 24 hours of delivery.
- Early: within 24 hours postpartum. Delayed > 24 hours up to 8 weeks postpartum.

ETIOLOGIES: **4 Ts:**
- **Tone uterine atony most common cause** (80%) - uterus unable to contract to stop the bleeding.
- **Tissue:** retained placental tissue
- **Trauma** to the cervix, perineum or vagina, uterine rupture, lacerations.
- **Thrombin:** coagulation abnormalities (Hemophilia A, von Willebrand diseases, ITP, or DIC).

RISK FACTORS FOR ATONY
- Rapid or prolonged labor, overdistended uterus, C-section, anesthesia, retained placenta.

CLINICAL MANIFESTATIONS
- Prolonged bleeding
- Hypovolemic shock - hypotension, tachycardia, pale or clammy skin, decreased capillary refill.

PHYSICAL EXAMINATION
- **Soft flaccid boggy uterus** (uterine atony) with dilated cervix.

WORKUP
- CBC to evaluate hemoglobin & hematocrit. IV access.
- Ultrasound may detect the bleeding source or retained products of conception.

MANAGEMENT OF ATONY
- **Bimanual uterine massage and compression first-line treatment.**
- Uterotonic Agents: **IV oxytocin first-line medical treatment** to increase uterine contractions. If Oxytocin ineffective, **Methylergonovine** (if no hypertension, coronary or cerebral artery disease) or Prostaglandin analogs: IM Carboprost tromethamine (if no asthma), Misoprostol.
- Refractory: Tamponade, surgical ligation of the uterine artery, arterial embolization, or hysterectomy.

Management due to retained products:
- Suction & curettage may be needed.

Management of Uterine inversion:
- Manual reposition of the uterus: elevate the posterior fornix is the initial management + discontinuation of uterotonic agents. Suspect if a red mass protrudes from the vagina.
- Uterine relaxing agent: Nitroglycerin, Terbutaline, Magnesium sulfate.

ECTOPIC PREGNANCY

- Implantation of the fertilized ovum outside of the uterine cavity.
- Locations **ampulla of the fallopian tube most common** (98.3%), abdomen (1.4%), ovary & cervix (0.15% each).

HIGH RISK

- **Previous ectopic strongest risk factor, history of pelvic inflammatory disease (one of the most common), IUD use,** previous abdominal or tubal surgery (due to adhesions), history of tubal ligation, endometriosis, assisted reproduction (eg, IVF).
- Intermediate: infertility, history of genital infections, multiple partners, & smoking.

CLINICAL MANIFESTATIONS

- **Classic Triad:** 1. **unilateral pelvic or lower abdominal pain** 2. **vaginal bleeding** & 3. **amenorrhea** (pregnancy). This triad also seen with threatened abortion (threatened more common than ectopic).
- Atypical: vague symptoms, menstrual irregularities.
- **Ruptured**: **severe abdominal, left shoulder pain (Kehr sign),** dizziness, nausea, & vomiting. Peritonitis (guarding, rigidity or rebound tenderness). Signs of shock (from hemorrhage): **syncope**, tachycardia, & **hypotension.**

PHYSICAL EXAMINATION

- **Adnexal mass. Cervical motion tenderness.**

DIAGNOSIS

- **Quantitative beta-hCG**: confirms pregnancy. Beta-hCG should double every 48h-72h. In ectopic, serial beta-hCG fails to double (rises <66% expected, decreases, or plateaus). If initial value <1,500, then repeat every 2-3 days.
- **Transvaginal ultrasound: absence of gestational sac with beta-hCG levels >2,000 strongly suggests ectopic** OR nonviable intrauterine pregnancy.
- Other: culdocentesis - nonclotted blood present (not done often). Laparoscopy is not used often.

MANAGEMENT OF STABLE/UNRUPTURED:

- **Methotrexate** destroys trophoblastic tissue.
  Indications for Methotrexate: hemodynamically stable patients with **early gestation (<4cm, beta-hCG <5,000, no fetal tones)** who will be compliant to follow-up & are immunocompetent. Laparoscopic salpingostomy or salpingectomy are alternatives.
- RhoGAM given to Rh-negative women.
- Laparoscopic salpingostomy or salpingectomy are alternatives.

MANAGEMENT OF UNSTABLE/RUPTURED:

- **Laparoscopic salpingostomy** often surgical procedure of choice *when possible* (may need reparative procedure to save reproductive organs) + IV fluids.
- Salpingectomy if salpingostomy cannot be performed.
- RhoGAM given to Rh-negative women.

FOLLOW UP:

- **Serial beta-hCG** to see if there is a 15% decrease in 4-7 days. Beta-hCG followed until it returns to 0.
- If Methotrexate was given and there is no significant decrease, a second dose can be given. If no response to the second dose, surgery should be performed.
- Contraception should be used for at least 2 months an ectopic pregnancy.

GESTATIONAL TROPHOBLASTIC DISEASE (MOLAR PREGNANCY)

- **Neoplasm due to abnormal placental development with trophoblastic tissue** proliferation arising from gestational tissue (not maternal in origin). 80% benign.

Complete molar pregnancy:

- **Diploid (46XX usually) –** empty (enucleated) egg with no DNA that is fertilized by 1 or 2 sperm. **All paternal chromosomes leads to the absence of fetal tissue**. Associated with higher risk of malignant development into choriocarcinoma (20%). Most common type.

Partial molar pregnancy:

- **Triploid** (69XXX or XXY) - an egg is fertilized by 2 sperm (or 1 sperm that duplicates its chromosomes). **Fetal tissue may be seen but it is always abnormal and not viable.**

RISK FACTORS

- Prior Molar pregnancy, extremes of maternal age <20y or >35y, Asian.

CLINICAL MANIFESTATIONS

- **Painless vaginal bleeding, preeclampsia before 20 weeks & hyperemesis gravidarum** (due to elevated beta-hCG levels).

PHYSICAL EXAMINATION

- **Uterine size & date discrepancies** (larger or smaller than expected).

DIAGNOSIS

- **Beta-hCG: markedly elevated with complete** (eg, >100,000 mIU/mL).
- **Pelvic ultrasound:** complete - central heterogenous mass with multiple discrete anechoic spaces **"snowstorm" or "cluster of grapes"** appearance, absence of fetal parts & heart sounds. Partial - gestational sac and fetal heart tones may be present plus abnormal tissue.

MANAGEMENT

- **Surgical uterine evacuation mainstay of treatment** as soon as possible to avoid risk of choriocarcinoma development.
- Patients are followed weekly until beta-hCG levels fall to an undetectable level. Hysterectomy also an option.
- **Obtain chest radiograph to look for METS (Choriocarcinoma).**

PRURITIC URTICARIAL PAPULES & PLAQUES OF PREGNANCY

- Common benign, self-limiting rash in pregnancy.
- Also known as Polymorphic eruption of pregnancy
- Most commonly occurs in the first pregnancy after 35 weeks or postpartum.

CLINICAL MANIFESTATIONS

- **Extremely pruritic** erythematous papules within striae that spread outward to form urticarial plaques.
- Usually spares the face, palms & soles.

MANAGEMENT

- **Topical corticosteroids** to decrease pruritus.
- Usually resolves spontaneously by 15 days postpartum.

CONTRACEPTIVE METHODS

EMERGENCY (POSTCOITAL) CONTRACEPTION

- In order of maximal to minimal efficacy: **copper IUD most effective** > Ulipristal > Levonorgestrel > Estrogen-Progestin.

LEVONORGESTREL:

- **Ideally given within 72 hours after intercourse** but effective up to 5 days (120 hours) after intercourse. Mechanism: **inhibits or delays ovulation.** Reduces the chance of pregnancy by 75% - 99%. Preferred over the Estrogen-progestin regimen. Common adverse effects are nausea & vomiting.

HIGH-DOSE ESTROGEN-PROGESTIN:

- **Ideally given within 72 hours of unprotected intercourse**.
- Mechanism: inhibits or delays ovulation. Common adverse effects are nausea & vomiting.

COPPER IUD:

- **The most effective method of emergency contraception** if inserted within 5-7 days after unprotected intercourse. Prevents up to 99% of pregnancies.

ULIPRISTAL:

- Progestin receptor modulator that delays ovulation. Must be taken within 5 days (120 hours) after intercourse. It is the most effective oral emergency contraceptive.

ESTROGEN + PROGESTERONE ORAL CONTRACEPTIVES

MECHANISM OF ACTION

- Prevents ovulation & implantation by inhibiting midcycle LH surge, thickens cervical mucosa, and thins the endometrium.
- Failure rate: average 9%. 0.3% when used correctly.
- Often started with the onset of menses or within the 5 days after the start of menses. Active pills are taken for 21 days followed by 7 days of no pills or placebos.

ADVANTAGES

- Improves dysmenorrhea, abnormal uterine bleeding, acne, & hirsutism.
- **Protects against osteoporosis, ovarian, & endometrial cancers.**
- Reduces ectopic pregnancy risk as well as decreases the incidence of ovarian cysts & benign breast disease.

DISADVANTAGES

- **Increased hypercoagulability (DVT & PE),** gallstone formation & gall stasis, increased fluid retention, increased triglycerides, cholestasis, & diabetes mellitus. Increased risk of hepatic adenoma.
- Cautious use in patients with hepatobiliary disease.

CONTRAINDICATIONS

- History of ischemic heart disease, DVT, PE or stroke, **Breast cancer**, migraine with aura.
- **Smokers should stop the use of OCPs if 35 years of age or older** (especially if smoking 15 cigarettes or more a day due to thrombogenic potential).
- *Severe* hypertension (systolic 160 mmHg or diastolic 100 mmHg).

PROGESTERONE-ONLY PILL

- **Norethindrone** "mini pill"

MECHANISM OF ACTION

- Thickens the cervical mucus, thins the endometrium, & suppresses ovulation.

INDICATIONS

- **Women in whom an estrogen-containing contraceptive is either contraindicated or causes additional health issues** (eg, Migraine with aura or women 35 years of age or older who smoke at least 15 cigarettes a day).
- Often initiated on the first day of menses. Back-up contraceptive is not necessary if POPs are started within the first 5 days of the start of menses.
- **Pills must be taken at the same time each day** to maximize efficacy.

ADVANTAGES

- **No estrogen-related adverse effects** so little effect on coagulation factors, blood pressure, glucose, and lipid levels.
- **Safe during lactation**. **Reduces the risk of Endometrial cancer**.

ADVERSE EFFECTS

- Unscheduled bleeding & changes in menses.

PROGESTERONE-ONLY CONTRACEPTIVES

NORETHINDRONE "mini pill".

INJECTABLE: **depot Medroxyprogesterone** acetate.

- 5% average failure rate. **Lasts 3 months.**
- Mechanism: suppresses pituitary FSH & LH secretion.
- Adverse effects: **may lead to calcium loss, bone weakness,** & **Osteoporosis** so not usually used more than 2 years.

PROGESTIN IMPLANTS:

- 0.05% average failure rate. **Lasts 3 years.**
- Adverse effects include headache & menstrual irregularities.

INTRAUTERINE LEVONORGESTREL:

- **Good for 5 years.** Induces inflammation, leading to a hostile environment to a fertilized ovum. Usually inserted during menses to ensure the patient is not pregnant.
- Adverse effects: uterine perforation, **increased risk of ectopic pregnancy & pelvic inflammatory disease**, cramping or bleeding with menses, and risk of spontaneous abortion if pregnancy occurs.

COPPER INTRAUTERINE DEVICE

MECHANISM OF ACTION:

- Causes inflammation that makes a hostile environment for sperm and ova.
- 0.8% average failure rate.

ADVANTAGES:

- **10 year duration of action, very effective contraceptive method**, no exogenous hormones.
- The copper IUD does not cause anovulation or amenorrhea (patients continue to have cyclic bleeding and less unscheduled bleeding compared to Levonorgestrel IUD).
- It can be used for emergency contraception and left in place for ongoing contraception.

ADVERSE EFFECTS

- **Increased incidence of Pelvic inflammatory disease.**

CLOMIPHENE CITRATE

MECHANISM OF ACTION:

- Partial estrogen receptor agonist that stimulates ovulation via the hypothalamus, leading to increased LH and FSH release.

INDICATIONS:

- **Induces ovulation to enhance fertility, especially in patients with Polycystic ovarian syndrome.**
- Infertility due to anovulation.

ADVERSE EFFECTS:

- **Hot flashes most common,** ovarian enlargement, multiple gestation pregnancy, abdominal discomfort, & visual changes.

LEUPROLIDE

- Mechanism of action: Gonadotropin releasing hormone analog (GnRH).

Indications:

- **Fertility: if given pulsatile** (the natural way the body releases GnRH).
- **Inhibition of estrogen & testosterone: if given continuously** (suppresses LH & FSH with subsequent reduction of estrogen & testosterone). Used in uterine fibroids, advanced prostate cancer (decreases testosterone), dysfunctional uterine bleeding, & premenstrual syndrome.

Adverse effects of continuous dosing:

- **Hot flashes,** depression, **osteopenia** (due to decreased estrogen). Anti-androgen adverse effects.

DANAZOL

Mechanism of action:

- **Hypoestrogenic and hyperandrogenic.**

Indications:

- Endometriosis (suppresses LH & FSH production), fibrocystic breast disease, hereditary angioedema. **Limited use due to hyperandrogenic adverse effects.**

Adverse effects:

- **Hyperandrogenic side effects** (weight gain, acne, hirsutism, virilization), & hepatic dysfunction.

BASIC PHYSIOLOGY

MENSTRUAL CYCLE OVERVIEW

Understanding the roles of the hormones in the menstrual cycle are critical to understand this chapter.

Follicular phase: during the 1st 14 days (follicular phase), the endometrium thickens under the influence of **estrogen**. In the ovaries, a dominant follicle matures, leading to ovulation.

Luteal phase: after ovulation, the ruptured follicle becomes the corpus luteum, secreting progesterone (& some estrogen). **Progesterone** enhances the lining of the uterus to prepare it for implantation. If there is no implantation, the corpus luteum degenerates, leading to a steep decrease in both estrogen & progesterone. The steep drops in both hormones leads to menstruation.

PHASE 1: FOLLICULAR (Proliferative)

Days 1-12

ESTROGEN PREDOMINATES.

- ***Pulsatile GnRH*** from the hypothalamus ⇨↑FSH & LH from the pituitary gland to stimulate the ovaries.

Ovaries:

- ↑***FSH*** causes ***follicle & egg maturation in the ovary.***
- ↑***LH stimulates*** the maturing follicle to ***produce estrogen.***

Endometrium (Uterus)

Estrogen "builds" up the endometrium (proliferative).

Estrogen causes NEGATIVE FEEDBACK in HPO system:
(Hypothalamus-Pituitary-Ovarian)

- The ↑'ing levels of estrogen inhibits hypothalamic GnRH release as well as pituitary release of LH & FSH (so no new follicles start maturing).

OVULATION: Days 12-14

- The ↑estrogen being released from the mature follicle ***switches from NEGATIVE TO POSITIVE FEEDBACK*** on GnRH, causing mutual ↑***'es in estrogen, FSH & LH.***
- The sudden ***LH surge causes ovulation*** (egg release).

PHASE 2: LUTEAL PHASE (Secretory)

Days 14 - 28

PROGESTERONE PREDOMINATES.

- The LH surge also causes the ruptured follicle to become the corpus luteum. The corpus luteum secretes ***progesterone*** & *estrogen* to maintain the endometrial lining. Estrogen & progesterone switches back to negative feedback.

If pregnancy occurs:

The blastocyst (maturing zygote) keeps the corpus luteum functional (secreting estrogen & progesterone, which keeps the endometrium from sloughing).

MENSTRUAL CYCLE

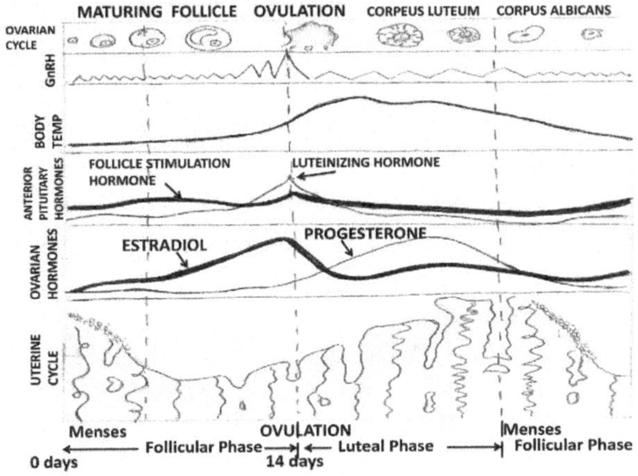

MENSTRUATION (1st days of Follicular)

If the egg is not fertilized, the corpus luteum soon deteriorates (causing a ***fall of progesterone & estrogen levels***). This has 2 effects:

- The endometrium is no longer maintained & sloughs off, leading to ***menstruation.***
- The negative feedback on GnRH subsides, causing ↑pulsatile GnRH secretion. This leads to ↑FSH & LH, which starts the follicle maturation process all over again.

GnRH pulses >1 an hour favor LH secretion. Less frequent pulses favor FSH secretion

MENSTRUAL DISORDERS

ABNORMAL UTERINE BLEEDING

- **Unexplained abnormal bleeding in a nonpregnant woman** in regards to quantity, schedule, or duration (formerly dysfunctional uterine bleeding).

- Anovulatory (90%): the ovaries produce estrogen but no ovulation = no corpus luteum formation. **Unopposed estrogen** (from no progesterone) leads to endometrial growth & unpredictable shedding.

CLINICAL MANIFESTATIONS
- Abnormal bleeding with a relatively normal physical examination.

DIAGNOSIS
- There is no specific test for DUB. Workup as indicated may include: **beta-hCG to rule out pregnancy**, hemoglobin, & hematocrit. Additional tests may be performed for particular etiologies.

- **Endometrial biopsy to rule out Endometrial carcinoma should be done in all women >35 years with obesity, hypertension or diabetes & all patients with postmenopausal bleeding**

MANAGEMENT OF ACUTE HEMORRHAGE
- IV high-dose estrogen or high-dose oral contraceptives.

CHRONIC MANAGEMENT
- **Estrogen-progestin contraceptive pills first-line.**

- Progesterone if estrogen is contraindicated.

- Levonorgestrel-releasing IUD.

- NSAIDs can be used in patients unable or unwilling to be treated with hormonal therapy.

- Surgery: if not responsive to medical treatment. **Hysterectomy is the definitive management.** **Endometrial ablation** in patients who do not want a hysterectomy.

DYSMENORRHEA

- **Painful menstruation** that affects normal activities.
- **Primary: due to increased prostaglandins** (not due to pelvic pathology). Prostaglandins cause increased uterine wall contractions. Usually starts 1-2 years after menarche onset in teenagers.
- **Secondary: due to pelvis or uterus pathology** (eg, endometriosis, PID, adenomyosis, leiomyomas).

CLINICAL MANIFESTATIONS

- **Recurrent, crampy** midline **lower abdominal or pelvic pain 1-2 days before or at the onset of menses** gradually **diminishing over 12-72 hours.**
- Pain may radiate to the lower back & thighs and may be associated with headache, nausea, or vomiting.
- Physical exam: normal if Primary dysmenorrhea.

DIAGNOSIS

- Labs & imaging not mandatory to exclude secondary but should be done if pelvic disease is suspected.

MANAGEMENT

- **Supportive therapy** includes heat compresses, vitamin B, & vitamin E started 2 days prior to and for 3 days into menses. Exercise.
- **NSAIDs or hormonal therapy first-line medical management**. NSAIDs started prior to pain onset & given for 2-3 days. Hormonal therapy: estrogen-progestin contraceptive pills or progestin only.
- **Laparoscopy: indicated if unresponsive to 3 cycles of initial therapy to rule out secondary causes** (most common causes of secondary in younger patients are PID & endometriosis).

PREMENSTRUAL SYNDROME

- **PMS:** cluster of physical, behavioral and mood changes with cyclical occurrence during the luteal phase of the menstrual cycle.
- **Premenstrual dysphoric disorder: severe PMS with functional impairment** where anger, irritability & internal tension are prominent (DSM V diagnostic criteria).

CLINICAL MANIFESTATIONS

- **Physical**: abdominal bloating & fatigue most common, breast swelling or pain, weight gain, headache, changes in bowel habits, muscle or joint pain.
- **Emotional**: **irritability most common,** tension, depression, anxiety, hostility, libido changes.
- **Behavioral**: food cravings, poor concentration, noise sensitivity, loss of motor senses.

DIAGNOSIS

- **Symptoms occurring 1-2 weeks before menses (luteal phase), relieved within 2-3 days of the onset of menses** plus at least 7 symptom-free days during the follicular phase.
- Patient should record a diary of symptoms for >2 cycles.

MANAGEMENT

- Lifestyle modifications: stress reduction & exercise most beneficial. Caffeine, alcohol, cigarette, & salt reduction. NSAIDs, vitamin B6 & E.
- **SSRIs first-line medical therapy for emotional symptoms with dysfunction** (eg, **Fluoxetine, Sertraline**, Citalopram).
- **Oral contraceptives** (especially **Drospirenone-containing** OCPs) can be used in patients who do not want to take SSRIs.
- Gonadotropin-releasing hormone (GnRH) agonist therapy with estrogen-progestin addback if no response to SSRIs or OCPs.

AMENORRHEA

PRIMARY AMENORRHEA

- Failure of menarche onset by age 15 years (in the presence of secondary sex characteristics) or age 13 years (in the absence of secondary sex characteristics).

WORKUP:

- All women with primary amenorrhea should have **hCG & FSH** testing **most importantly.**
- TSH & prolactin level also usually measured initially.
- Karyotyping done if increased FSH and little breast development (to rule out Turner's syndrome).

SECONDARY AMENORRHEA

- **Absence of menses for >3 months in a patient with previously normal menstruation** (or >6 months in a patient who was previously oligomenorrheic).

ETIOLOGIES:

- **Pregnancy is the most common cause.**
- **Hypothalamus dysfunction: functional hypothalamic amenorrhea** - puberty delay due (eg, **athletes,** illness, anorexia). **The female athlete triad: hypothalamic amenorrhea, eating disorder, & osteoporosis** (due to loss of bone protection by estrogen). FHA can cause 1ry or 2ry amenorrhea.
- **Pituitary dysfunction: Prolactinoma** or pituitary infarct (Sheehan syndrome). Associated with **decreased FSH, LH, & estrogen.**
- **Ovarian dysfunction: decreased estrogen + increased FSH & LH.** Polycystic ovarian syndrome. Premature ovarian failure: follicular failure or follicular resistance to LH or FSH. Turner syndrome. May have symptoms of estrogen deficiency (similar to menopause).
- **Uterine dysfunction: Asherman's syndrome = acquired endometrial scarring** secondary to postpartum hemorrhage, after D&C or endometrial infection. Pelvic ultrasound – absence of the normal uterine stripe. Hysteroscopy.

WORKUP

- **Beta-hCG (to rule out pregnancy) is the best initial test.**
- If hCG negative, order serum prolactin, FSH, LH, TSH, & estrogen.
- Testosterone measured if evidence of hirsutism or hyperandrogenism

	UTERUS PRESENT	**UTERUS ABSENT**
BREAST PRESENT	**Outflow obstruction:** transverse vaginal septum, imperforate hymen	• Mullerian agenesis (46 XX) • Androgen insensitivity (46 XY)
BREAST ABSENT	• **Elevated: ↑FSH, ↑LH = Ovarian causes** - Premature ovarian failure (46XX) - Gonadal dysgenesis (ex. Turner's 45XO) • **Normal/Low: ↓FSH, ↓LH** - **Hypothalamus-Pituitary Failure** - Puberty delay (eg, athletes, illness, anorexia)	Rare. Usually caused by a defect in testosterone synthesis. Presents like a phenotypic immature girl with primary amenorrhea (will often have intrabdominal testes).

LEIOMYOMA (UTERINE FIBROIDS) FIBROMYOMA

- **Benign uterine smooth muscle tumors** that derive from the muscle cells of the myometrium.
- Most common benign gynecologic tumor.
- Types: Intramural, submucosal, subserosal, parasitic.

RISK FACTORS
- Increasing age (especially >35y)
- 5 times **more common in African-Americans**
- Nulliparity, obesity, family history, & hypertension.

PATHOPHYSIOLOGY
- Growth is **estrogen dependent** – may increase in size with relation to the menstrual cycle, anovulatory states, and during pregnancy & regress after menopause.

CLINICAL MANIFESTATIONS
- **Most are asymptomatic** & found incidentally (especially if intramural).
- **Bleeding most common symptom (menorrhagia or irregular)** especially if submucosal.
- Dysmenorrhea, pelvic pressure or pain.
- May affect fertility.

PHYSICAL EXAMINATION
- Normal or may have palpable **firm, nontender, asymmetric** mobile **mass or masses in the abdomen or pelvis** on bimanual exam.

DIAGNOSIS
- **Transvaginal ultrasound: most widely used initial imaging test** for suspected fibroids: **focal heterogenic hypoechoic mass or masses with shadowing**.

MANAGEMENT
- **Observation: majority don't need treatment.** Decision to treat is determined by symptoms, size/rate of tumor growth, & the desire for fertility.
- Nonsurgical: Leuprolide is the most effective medical treatment but usually used if near menopause or to shrink fibroids prior to hysterectomy or myomectomy. Levonorgestrel-releasing IUD. NSAIDs for dysmenorrhea.

SURGICAL MANAGEMENT:
- **Hysterectomy is the definitive treatment.** Fibroids are the most common cause for hysterectomy.
- **Myomectomy:** used especially **to preserve fertility.**
- Other: uterine artery embolization (may preserve fertility if myomectomy is not an option). Endometrial ablation. Both may affect the ability to conceive.

EXAM TIP:
- Asymptomatic women: observation
- Symptomatic women who desire fertility: nonsurgical treatment or myomectomy
- Symptomatic women who do not desire fertility: nonsurgical treatment, myomectomy, myolysis, or uterine artery embolization
- Symptomatic women desiring definitive treatment: hysterectomy

MENOPAUSE

- Cessation of menses >1 year due to loss of ovarian function, leading to decreased estrogen & progesterone production.
- **Average age in the US is 50-52y.** Premature if < 40 years.

CLINICAL MANIFESTATIONS

- **Estrogen deficiency** - menstrual cycle alterations, vasomotor instability (including **hot flashes most common perimenopausal symptom**), **sleep disturbances, mood changes**, skin, nail, & hair changes, increased cardiovascular events, hyperlipidemia, osteoporosis, dyspareunia (painful intercourse), vaginal atrophy, & urinary incontinence.

PHYSICAL EXAMINATION

- Decreased bone density, dry & thin skin with decreased elasticity.
- Vaginal atrophy with thin mucosa.
- Decrease in breast size.

DIAGNOSIS

- **FSH assay most sensitive initial test (increased serum FSH** >30 IU/mL).
- **Increased LH and decreased estrogen.**
- Androstenedione levels don't change.
- Estrone is the predominant estrogen after menopause.

COMPLICATIONS

- Loss of estrogen's protective effects leads to osteoporosis, hyperlipidemia and increased cardiovascular risk.

Management of vasomotor insufficiency & hot flashes:

- Hormone replacement therapy: risks vs. benefits must be considered.
  Estrogen only (if no uterus)
  Estrogen + Progestin (if uterus still present).
- 2nd-line: SSRIs (eg, Paroxetine) or Gabapentin.

Management of vaginal atrophy: see below

VULVOVAGINAL ATROPHY

- Seen in **hypoestrogenic states** (eg, **menopause,** postpartum lactation, and postpartum women, progesterone-only or low-dose oral contraceptives).

CLINICAL MANIFESTATIONS

- **Vaginal dryness, dyspareunia**, vaginal inflammation, infection & recurrent UTIs with increased pH (loss of lactobacilli which normally converts glucose to lactic acid).

MANAGEMENT

- **Vaginal moisturizers:** improves symptoms (ex. dyspareunia, dryness) but no effect on atrophy.
- **Topical vaginal estrogens safest, most effective medical therapy** - cream, vaginal ring, vaginal troches. Adverse effects: vaginal bleeding, breast pain, nausea, thromboembolism (CVA, DVT, PE), endometrial cancer. Less risk compared to oral estrogen. Estrogen increases hepatic production of coagulation factors.
- **Ospemifene:** selective estrogen receptor modulator (SERM) that is an **estrogen agonist in the vagina & bone** and an estrogen antagonist in the breast & uterus.

HORMONAL REPLACEMENT THERAPY

- **Estrogen only (if no uterus)**
- **Estrogen + Progestin (if uterus still present).**

INDICATIONS FOR HRT:

- Healthy woman <60 years for menopause symptom relief (eg, vasomotor symptoms, mood changes, vaginal atrophy).
- Decreases Osteoporosis risk.

RISKS OF HRT:

- DVT or pulmonary embolism.
- Endometrial cancer (estrogen only).
- Breast cancer risk with estrogen-progestin therapy is controversial.

CONTRAINDICATIONS TO HORMONAL THERAPY:

- Women with increased risk of cardiovascular disease, thromboembolic disease, stroke, endometrial or breast cancer.
- History of liver disease.

TAMOXIFEN

MECHANISM OF ACTION:

- Selective estrogen receptor modulator (SERM).
- Tamoxifen is an **estrogen antagonist in the breast but an estrogen agonist in the endometrium bone,** liver, & coagulation system.

INDICATIONS:

- Adjuvant treatment in estrogen & progesterone receptor-positive **breast cancer**, **breast cancer prevention,** & **Osteoporosis prevention** in postmenopausal women.

ADVERSE EFFECTS:

- **Increased risk of Endometrial cancer, venous thromboembolism, hot flashes** (induces menopause), & ocular toxicity.

RALOXIFENE

MECHANISM OF ACTION:

- Selective estrogen receptor modulator (SERM).
- Raloxifene is an **estrogen agonist in the bone but an estrogen antagonist in the breast & endometrium.**

INDICATIONS:

- **Breast cancer prevention in high-risk women & osteoporosis prevention** in postmenopausal women.

ADVERSE EFFECTS:

- Weight gain.
- Thromboembolic events (less than Tamoxifen)
- Hot flashes (induces Menopause).

ADENOMYOSIS

- **Islands of endometrial tissue within the myometrium** (muscular layer of the uterine wall).

RISK FACTORS
- Most commonly presents later in the reproductive years (ages of 35 – 50). Endometriosis, fibroids.

CLINICAL MANIFESTATIONS
- **Menorrhagia** (progressively worsens)
- **Dysmenorrhea** & chronic pelvic pain.
- May cause infertility.

PHYSICAL EXAMINATION
- **Symmetrically (uniformly) enlarged, "globular" boggy, uterus (may be tender).**

DIAGNOSIS
- Clinical diagnosis of exclusion of 2ry amenorrhea (rule out pregnancy, endometriosis, & fibroids).
- Transvaginal ultrasound. MRI (more accurate).
- Post-total abdominal hysterectomy examination of uterus is the definitive diagnosis.

MANAGEMENT
- Conservative management: used to preserve fertility – analgesics, progestins (eg, levonorgestrel-releasing intrauterine device), aromatase inhibitors.
- **Total abdominal hysterectomy is the only effective therapy.**

ENDOMETRITIS

- **Infection of the decidua (pregnancy endometrium).**
- Usually polymicrobial (often vaginal flora, aerobic, & anaerobic bacteria).

RISK FACTORS
- Postpartum or postabortal uterine infection - **C-section biggest risk factor.**
- Prolonged rupture of membranes >24 hours, vaginal delivery, dilation & curettage (or evacuation), multiple pelvic examinations.
- Chorioamnionitis (fetal membrane infection).

DIAGNOSIS
- Mainly a clinical diagnosis - **fever** (> 38C)/100.4F)**, tachycardia, abdominal pain, & uterine tenderness 2-3 days after C-section,** postpartum, or **postabortal** (may present later).
- May have vaginal bleeding or discharge (foul-smelling lochia).

Management post C-section:
- **Clindamycin + Gentamicin first-line** (Clindamycin covers gram + & anaerobes, Gent gram -).
- May add Ampicillin for additional group B *Streptococcus* coverage.
- Ampicillin-sulbactam is an alternative.

Management after vaginal delivery or chorioamnionitis: Ampicillin + Gentamicin.

PROPHYLAXIS
- **First-generation cephalosporin** (eg, **Cefazolin**) **x 1 dose during C-section** may be given to reduce the incidence.

ENDOMETRIOSIS

- **Implantation of endometrial tissue** (stroma & gland) **outside the uterus.**

PATHOPHYSIOLOGY

- The **ectopic endometrial tissue** responds to cyclical hormonal changes.

LOCATIONS

- **Ovaries are the most common site.**
- Other sites include the posterior cul de sac, broad & uterosacral ligaments, rectosigmoid colon, bladder.

RISK FACTORS

- Prolonged estrogen exposure (eg, **nulliparity,** late first pregnancy, early menarche, short menstrual cycles), family history, heavy menstruation.
- Peak incidence 25 - 35y.

CLINICAL MANIFESTATIONS

- **Classic triad: ❶ cyclic premenstrual pelvic pain** (1-2 weeks before menstruation) **❷ dysmenorrhea** (painful menstruation) and **❸ Dyspareunia** (painful intercourse).

- May have **dyschezia** (painful defecation). **Abnormal bleeding.**
- May have back pain, pre or post menstrual spotting.
- Asymptomatic in 1/3.
- Infertility.

PHYSICAL EXAMINATION:

- Usually normal but may have a fixed tender adnexal mass, a fixed retroverted uterus or nodular thickening of the uterosacral ligament.

DIAGNOSIS:

- Clinical diagnosis.

- **Ultrasound initial imaging test of choice** to rule out other causes.

- **Laparoscopy with biopsy definitive diagnosis:**
  - Raised, patches of thickened, discolored scarred or "powder burn" appearing implants of tissue.
  - **Endometrioma** - endometriosis involving the ovaries large enough to be considered a tumor, usually filled with old blood appearing chocolate-colored "**chocolate cyst**".

MEDICAL (CONSERVATIVE) MANAGEMENT

- **Ovulation suppression - combined OCPs first-line.** NSAIDs may be given for pain. Progestins (eg Levonorgestrel-releasing IUD), Leuprolide (GnRH agonist). Danazol (an androgen not commonly used).

SURGICAL MANAGEMENT

- Conservative laparoscopy with ablation of ectopic endometrial tissue used if fertility desired (preserves uterus & ovaries).

- Total abdominal hysterectomy and bilateral salpingo-oophorectomy if no desire for fertility.

ENDOMETRIAL HYPERPLASIA

- Endometrial gland proliferation with cytologic atypia. **Precursor to Endometrial carcinoma.**
- Most common postmenopausal or increasing age in premenopausal women.

RISK FACTORS

- **Prolonged unopposed estrogen** (unopposed by progesterone) - **chronic anovulation, estrogen-only therapy,** Polycystic ovarian syndrome, obesity, perimenopause, early menarche, late menopause, Lynch syndrome, & **Tamoxifen.** Hyperplasia occurs within 3y of estrogen-only therapy.

CLINICAL MANIFESTATIONS

- **Abnormal uterine bleeding** (menorrhagia, metrorrhagia, postmenopausal bleeding).
- May be associated with a vaginal discharge.

DIAGNOSIS

- **Transvaginal ultrasound screening test – thickened endometrial stripe >4-mm.**
- **Endometrial biopsy definitive diagnosis –** indicated if >35y, increased endometrial stripe seen on TVUS, patients on unopposed estrogen therapy, Tamoxifen, persistent bleeding with thick stripe.

MANAGEMENT

- Hyperplasia **without atypia:** **Progestin** (oral or IUD). Repeat endometrial biopsy in 3-6 months.
- Hyperplasia **with atypia:** **total abdominal hysterectomy.** Progestin treatment used if not a surgical candidate or if patient wishes to preserve fertility.

ENDOMETRIAL CANCER

- **Most common gynecologic malignancy in the US** (2 times more common than Cervical cancer).
- **Adenocarcinoma most common type** (>80%). Papillary serous 10%, clear cell 5%, adenosquamous 2% and mucinous 2%.
- **Mainly affects postmenopausal women** (75%) - **50-60 year peak.** Perimenopausal 25%.
- Estrogen-dependent cancer. Associated with antecedent Endometrial hyperplasia.
- **Combination OCPs (estrogen + progesterone) are protective against both ovarian & endometrial cancers.**

RISK FACTORS

- **Increased estrogen exposure:** increased ovulatory cycles (eg, nulliparity, early menarche, late menopause), chronic anovulation, **Polycystic ovary syndrome**, obesity, estrogen-only hormonal therapy, & **Tamoxifen**. Diabetes mellitus, Lynch syndrome (HNPCC).

CLINICAL MANIFESTATIONS

- **Abnormal uterine bleeding** (eg, **postmenopausal bleeding,** pre or perimenopausal bleeding – menorrhagia or metrorrhagia).

DIAGNOSIS

- Transvaginal ultrasound – thickened endometrial stripe > 4 mm.
- Endometrial biopsy definitive diagnosis.

MANAGEMENT

- **Stage I: total abdominal hysterectomy with bilateral salpingo-oophorectomy**. May need post-op radiation therapy. Most are well differentiated (one of the most curable gynecologic cancers).
- Stage II, III: TAH-BSO + lymph node excision with or without post-op radiation therapy.
- Stage IV (advanced): systemic chemotherapy.

POST MENOPAUSAL BLEEDING

ETIOLOGIES

- **Usually benign** (eg, vaginal/endometrial atrophy, cervical polyps, submucosal fibroids).
- **10% due to Endometrial cancer**.
- ANY postmenopausal bleeding in a woman not on HRT (or on HRT with abnormal bleeding) should raise suspicion for endometrial carcinoma, hyperplasia, or Leiomyosarcoma.

DIAGNOSIS

- **Transvaginal ultrasound usually initial diagnostic test.** If endometrial stripe <4mm, repeat ultrasound in 4 months. If continued bleeding, biopsy should be performed.
- **Endometrial biopsy if stripe >4mm.**
- Hysteroscopy may be warranted if focal thickening of endometrium.

UTERINE PROLAPSE

- Uterine herniation into the vagina.

RISK FACTORS

- **Weakness of pelvic support structures: most common after childbirth** (especially traumatic), increased pelvic floor pressure: multiple vaginal births, obesity, & repeated heavy lifting.

CLINICAL MANIFESTATIONS

- Vaginal fullness, heaviness or "falling out" sensation.
- Low back pain, abdominal pain.
- Symptoms may be worse with prolonged standing and relieved with lying down.
- Urinary urgency, frequency or stress incontinence.

PHYSICAL EXAMINATION

- Bulging mass especially with increased intrabdominal pressure (eg Valsalva).
- Grades: 0 (no descent) to 4 (through the hymen).
- Grade 0: no descent
- Grade 1: uterus descent into the upper 2/3 of the vagina
- Grade 2: the cervix approaches the introitus
- Grade 3: the cervix is outside the introitus
- Grade 4: entire uterus is outside of the vagina – complete rupture
- May be accompanied by **cystocele** (posterior bladder herniating into the **anterior vagina**), **enterocele** (pouch of Douglas – small bowel herniating into the **upper vagina**) or **rectocele** (distal sigmoid colon or rectum herniating into the **posterior distal vagina**).

CONSERVATIVE MANAGEMENT

- **Kegel exercises,** behavioral modifications, weight control.
- Pessaries elevate & support the uterus.
- Estrogen treatment may improve atrophy.

SURGICAL MANAGEMENT

- Hysterectomy or uterus-sparing techniques including uterosacral or sacrospinous ligament fixation.

OVARIAN DISORDERS

PHYSIOLOGIC OVARIAN CYSTS

- Fluid-filled sac within the ovaries most commonly related to ovulation (usually unilateral).
- Common in reproductive years. **Most spontaneously resolve within a few weeks.**
- **Most are asymptomatic.** May be associated with abnormal uterine bleeding or dyspareunia.

PHYSIOLOGIC TYPES
- **Follicular cysts most common.** Occur when follicles fail to rupture & continue to grow.
- Corpus luteal cysts: fail to degenerate after ovulation.
- Theca Lutein: excess beta-hCG causes hyperplasia of theca interna cells (rare).

PHYSICAL EXAMINATION: unilateral pelvic pain or tenderness. Mobile palpable cystic adnexal mass.

DIAGNOSIS
- **Transvaginal ultrasound:** Follicular: smooth, thin-walled unilocular. Corpus luteal: complex, thicker-walled with peripheral vascularity.
  - **Low risk for malignancy: anechoic, unilocular fluid-filled cysts.**
  - High-risk for malignancy: solid, nodular, thick septations are high-risk for malignancy.
- Order beta-hCG to rule out pregnancy.
- Suspicious for malignancy: tumor markers (eg, CA-125, alpha-fetoprotein, beta-hCG).

Management if <8 cm:
- **Supportive - most cysts <8cm are functional** & **usually spontaneously resolve.** Rest, NSAIDs, **repeat ultrasound after 1-2 cycles**.
- OCPs may prevent recurrence but don't treat existing ones.

Management if >8 cm or persistent:
- Options include laparoscopy or laparotomy.

Management if postmenopausal:
- Options include laparoscopy or laparotomy if large or if tumor marker CA-125 is elevated.
- Cysts in postmenopausal women are considered to be malignant until proven otherwise.

RUPTURED PHYSIOLOGIC OVARIAN CYST

- Asymptomatic or **sudden onset of unilateral lower abdominal pain** often sharp & focal, often occurring during sexual activity or strenuous physical activity. **Abnormal uterine bleeding.**

PHYSICAL EXAMINATION
- Unilateral pelvic pain or tenderness. May have a mobile palpable cystic adnexal mass.
- May have signs of hemodynamic compromise if massive bleeding (not common).

DIAGNOSIS
- **Transvaginal ultrasound: initial test of choice - adnexal mass + pelvic fluid** in patients with symptoms consistent with rupture (fluid can be a normal finding). Beta-hCG & CBC.

MANAGEMENT
- Uncomplicated: **expectant management for most - observation, analgesics, & rest.** Uncomplicated = the absence of the following - hemodynamic instability, large volume or ongoing blood loss, fever, leukocytosis, or suspicion of malignancy.
- Stable + significant hemoperitoneum: hospitalization, close observation, & fluid replacement.
- Hemodynamically unstable or ongoing hemorrhage: laparoscopy usually preferred over laparotomy. Cystectomy is preferred over oophorectomy in premenopausal women.

OVARIAN CANCER

- 5th most common cancer in American women.
- 2nd most common gynecologic cancer with the **highest mortality of all the gynecologic cancers**.
- **>90% epithelial** (seen especially postmenopausal).

RISK FACTORS

- **Increased number of ovulatory cycles** (eg, **nulliparity,** infertility, **>50 years, early menarche, late menopause)**, family history (7% lifetime risk instead of normal 1-2%), Caucasian race.
- Genetic: **BRCA-1 or BRCA-2** (15-40%), Peutz-Jehgers, Turner's syndrome, Lynch syndrome (HNPCC).

CLINICAL MANIFESTATIONS

- **Rarely symptomatic until late in the disease course** (extensive METS).
- GI: abdominal fullness or distention, **increasing abdominal girth + weight loss**, back or abdominal pain, early satiety, constipation or bowel obstruction (intestinal compression).
- Urinary frequency. Irregular menses, menorrhagia, postmenopausal bleeding.

PHYSICAL EXAMINATION

- Palpable abdominal or ovarian mass (solid, fixed, irregular), **ascites,** pleural effusion, Sister Mary Joseph's node (METS to the umbilical lymph nodes).

DIAGNOSIS

- **Pelvic ultrasound initial test of choice**.
- Additional workup include: staging imaging (eg, CT scan of the abdomen & pelvis), baseline CA-125 levels, mammography, chest radiograph, pap smear, & colonoscopy.

MANAGEMENT

- **Stage I: surgical removal** - total abdominal hysterectomy + bilateral salpingo-oophorectomy + selective lymphadenectomy.
- Stage II – IV: **surgical removal followed by platinum-based chemotherapy** - Cisplatin or Carboplatin + Paclitaxel (Taxol).
- **Serum CA-125 levels used to monitor treatment progress.**

PROGNOSIS

- Because Ovarian cancer presents late in the disease course and is usually metastatic at presentation, it is associated with a generally poor prognosis.

BARTHOLIN CYST & ABSCESS

CLINICAL MANIFESTATIONS

- **Infected gland: pain, tenderness.** Unilateral vulvar mass, edema or inflammation. May be **fluctuant if abscess** is present. Localized pain & tenderness, dyspareunia.
- **Noninfected: nontender**, unilateral vulvar mass at Bartholin duct location.

DIAGNOSIS: CBC & culture of the drained fluid (including for STIs).

MANAGEMENT IF INFECTED

- **Incision & drainage** with or without placement of a Word catheter for continued drainage under local anesthesia. Immediate pain relief occurs upon drainage of pus. Antibiotic therapy if severe infection or patients with risk factors or for recurrent abscesses.
- Asymptomatic cyst: no intervention needed.
- Recurrent abscesses: a Word catheter can be placed after I and D to allow continued drainage. Marsupialization may be needed in patients with recurrent cysts.

BENIGN OVARIAN NEOPLASMS

- In women of reproductive age, 90% of ovarian neoplasms are benign.
- The risk of malignancy increases with age.
- Types: surface epithelial tumors, stromal tumors, and germ cell tumors.
- **Dermoid ovarian cyst (mature cystic teratoma) is the most common benign ovarian neoplasm** – may contain tissue derived from all 3 germ cell layers (eg, sebaceous fluid, hair, bone, teeth etc.). Has small malignant potential (0.2 – 2%).

CLINICAL MANIFESTATIONS
- Generally asymptomatic (usually an incidental finding).
- May lead to ovarian torsion or rarely, may rupture.

PHYSICAL EXAMINATION
- Normal or may have adnexal fullness.

DIAGNOSIS
- **Pelvic ultrasound** – cystic structure that may contain calcifications & hyperechoic nodules.

MANAGEMENT
- **Surgical removal (laparoscopic cystectomy** preferred) due to potential risk of torsion or malignant transformation.
- Salpingo-oophorectomy is another option.

OVARIAN TORSION

- Complete or partial rotation of the ovary on its ligamental supports.
- This can **compromise ovarian blood flow.** Prolonged ischemia may lead to infarction.

ETIOLOGIES
- Usually a mechanical complication in patients with functional ovarian cysts or ovarian neoplasm (especially if > 5 cm).

CLINICAL MANIFESTATIONS
- **Unilateral pelvic pain** (usually acute).
- May be associated with **nausea** & vomiting.

PHYSICAL EXAMINATION
- **Abdominal tenderness or adnexal mass.**

DIAGNOSIS
- **Ultrasound with Doppler initial test of choice – decreased ovarian blood flow.** Normal flow does not exclude torsion, so **definitive diagnosis is made during surgical exploration.** MRI

MANAGEMENT
- **Laparoscopy with detorsion** to restore blood flow.
- Ovarian cystectomy may be needed to remove the responsible cyst & preserve the ovary in premenopausal women.
- Necrotic or malignant: Salpingo-oophorectomy.

POLYCYSTIC OVARIAN SYNDROME (PCOS)

- Characterized by bilateral cystic ovaries, insulin resistance, and hyperandrogenism.
- Also known as Stein-Leventhal Syndrome.

PATHOPHYSIOLOGY
- Increased LH leads to increased testosterone production.
- Decreased FSH production leads to follicular degeneration & bilateral cystic ovaries.

CLINICAL MANIFESTATIONS
- **Menstrual dysfunction** oligomenorrhea or secondary amenorrhea.
- **Increased androgen: hirsutism** (eg, coarse hair on face, neck & abdomen, acne, & male pattern baldness).
- **Insulin resistance: type II Diabetes mellitus, obesity,** & hypertension.

PHYSICAL EXAMINATION:
- **Bilateral enlarged, smooth, mobile ovaries** on bimanual examination. Acanthosis nigricans.

DIAGNOSIS
- Diagnosis based on Rotterdam criteria (2 of 3 criteria) – ❶ lab or clinical signs (eg, hirsutism, acne, & male-pattern baldness), ❷ amenorrhea or oligomenorrhea, and ❸ cystic ovaries on ultrasound.

Labs: **increased testosterone** (eg, DHEA), **increased LH:FSH ratio ≥ 3:1**.

- Pelvic ultrasound: bilateral enlarged ovaries & multiple ovarian cysts with a **"string of pearls"** appearance.

- GnRH agonist stimulation test: rise in serum hydroxyprogesterone.

- Lipid panel, glucose tolerance test (for DM).

MANAGEMENT
- Lifestyle changes: diet, exercise, weight loss (decreases insulin resistance).

- **Combination oral contraceptives mainstay of treatment** (also reduces Endometrial hyperplasia).

- Anti-androgenic agents: **Spironolactone** (blocks testosterone receptors) may be added if symptoms persist after OCPs. Leuprolide, Finasteride are other anti-androgenics.

INFERTILITY
- **Clomiphene** selective estrogen receptor modulator that reestablishes ovulation in anovulatory women who wish to get pregnant.

- **Metformin** in patients with abnormal LH:FSH ratios **may improve menstrual frequency** by reducing insulin, leads to weight loss, and prevents Diabetes mellitus.

- Wedge resection may help to restore ovulation if Clomiphene is ineffective.

PROGNOSIS:
- Untreated PCOS is associated with increased risk of metabolic syndrome, Diabetes mellitus, cardiovascular disease, dyslipidemia, endometrial hyperplasia, and endometrial cancer.

VAGINAL CANCER

- Rare. 1% of gynecological malignancies. Peak incidence 60-65y.
- Primary tumors are rare (**Squamous cell carcinoma most common primary)**. More commonly, vaginal cancer occurs as a secondary tumor (eg, cervical, vulvar or distant source).

RISK FACTORS
- Same risk factors seen as in cervical neoplasia.
- **HPV types 16 and 18** cause approximately 70 percent of all cervical cancers worldwide and nearly 90 percent of anal cancers, oropharyngeal cancer, vulvar and vaginal cancer, and penile cancer.

CLINICAL MANIFESTATIONS
- **Abnormal vaginal bleeding most common symptom (postcoital,** intermenstrual or postmenopausal), watery vaginal discharge, dyspareunia. May be symptomatic.

DIAGNOSIS
- On visualization, the lesion may appear as a mass, plaque, or an ulcer.
- The **posterior wall of the upper one-third of the vagina is the most common site.**
- Biopsy is definitive. If a lesion is not seen, colposcopy should be performed to determine biopsy site.

MANAGEMENT
- Stage I: **surgical excision or radiation therapy for primary vaginal cancer**. Up to 15% will develop vaginal stenosis or sexual dysfunction after treatment so the use of a vaginal dilator may be needed.
- Stage II to IV: chemoradiation. Radiation alone is an alternative.

CANCER OF THE VULVA

- **Squamous cell carcinoma most common type (90%).** Malignant melanoma. Clear cell adenocarcinoma is linked to diethylstilbestrol (DES) in utero exposure.
- **Paget disease** is **vulvar intraepithelial neoplasia** that is a superficial lesion of the epithelium that has not invaded the basement membrane (pre-cancer). May progress to carcinoma-in-situ or squamous cell carcinoma.

RISK FACTORS
- **HPV types 16 and 18 cause approximately 70% of all cervical cancers worldwide and nearly 90% of anal cancers**, as well as a significant proportion of oropharyngeal cancer, **vulvar and vaginal cancer**, and penile cancer. Linked to DES exposure, smoking, immunosuppression, obesity.
- Most commonly seen in postmenopausal women.

CLINICAL MANIFESTATIONS
- Vulvar pruritus (itching), bleeding, or pain.
- The labia majora are the most common site (50%) followed by the labia minora and rarely the clitoris or Bartholin glands.

PHYSICAL EXAMINATION:
- **Red or white ulcerative or raised crusted lesion.**

DIAGNOSIS
- Biopsy – acetic acid or toluidine blue application may help aid biopsy.

Management: surgical excision, radiation therapy, chemotherapy (eg, 5-fluorouracil).

OTHER INFECTIOUS DISORDERS

PELVIC INFLAMMATORY DISEASE

- Ascending infection of the upper reproductive tract.

ETIOLOGIES

- **Usually mixed - *Chlamydia trachomatis* (most common), *Neisseria gonorrhoeae*,** *Gardnerella vaginalis, M. genitalium*, anaerobes, enteric or respiratory pathogens etc.

RISK FACTORS

- Multiple sex partners, unprotected sex, prior PID, age 15-19, nulliparous, IUD placement.

CLINICAL MANIFESTATIONS

- Pelvic or lower abdominal pain, dysuria, dyspareunia, vaginal discharge or bleeding, nausea, vomiting.
- Physical examination: **lower abdominal tenderness, fever, purulent cervical discharge. Cervical motion tenderness (chandelier sign).**

DIAGNOSIS

- Primarily clinical – ❶ abdominal tenderness + ❷ cervical motion tenderness + ❸ adnexal tenderness + plus at least 1 of the following: positive gram stain, temperature >38 C, WBC >10,000, pus on culdocentesis or laparoscopy, pelvic abnormality on bimanual exam or ultrasound, increased ESR or CRP.
- Workup includes **pregnancy test (rule out Ectopic pregnancy)** & nucleic acid amplification test (for Gonorrhea and Chlamydia).
- Laparoscopy is the most accurate test for PID (rarely performed) – may be done in uncertain cases, severe disease, or if no improvement with antibiotics

OUTPATIENT MANAGEMENT

- **Ceftriaxone** (250mg IM x 1 dose) PLUS **Doxycycline** (100mg bid x 14 days). Metronidazole 500mg bid x 14 days often added.
- Levofloxacin + Metronidazole alternative if true Penicillin allergy.

INPATIENT MANAGEMENT

- **Second generation cephalosporin** (eg, **Cefoxitin or Cefotetan**) + **IV Doxycycline.**
- Clindamycin + Gentamicin is an alternative (eg, pregnancy or true Penicillin allergy).

FITZ HUGH-CURTIS SYNDROME

- **Perihepatitis** with hepatic fibrosis, scarring & peritoneal surface of the anterior right upper quadrant **in the setting of Pelvic inflammatory disease (PID)**.
- Seen in 10% of women with PID

CLINICAL MANIFESTATIONS

- **RUQ pain** due to perihepatitis (liver capsule involvement). May radiate to the right shoulder.

PHYSICAL EXAMINATION

- Marked RUQ tenderness.

DIAGNOSIS

- **Laparoscopy - "violin-string" adhesions** on the anterior liver surface. Often have normal LFTs (or slight elevations).

BACTERIAL VAGINOSIS

- **Overgrowth of *Gardnerella vaginalis*** & anaerobes (eg, *Mobiluncus, Peptostreptococcus*) due to altered biome - **decreased *Lactobacillus acidophilus*** (*L. acidophilus* normally maintains vaginal pH).
- Although it is not a sexually transmitted infection, it is more common in sexually active women with new or multiple partners (changes the vaginal biome).

CLINICAL MANIFESTATIONS
- Vaginitis: **malodorous vaginal discharge** worse after sex, vaginal itching, burning, & dyspareunia.

DIAGNOSIS
- Amsel criteria: **copious, thin, homogenous, grayish-white vaginal discharge, vaginal pH >4.5, positive whiff-amine test – "fishy odor"** when a drop of 10% KOH is added, **clue cells** on saline wet mount (epithelial cells covered by bacteria), **few WBCs** (not inflammatory), & few lactobacilli.

MANAGEMENT
- **Metronidazole x 7 days** (gel or oral) or **Clindamycin** (oral or gel). Both are safe in pregnancy.
- **Partners do not need treatment.** Treatment for asymptomatic nonpregnant women not indicated.

PREVENTION: avoid douching & smoking.
- Pregnancy complications include Prelabor rupture of membranes, chorioamnionitis, & preterm labor.

TRICHOMONIASIS

- ***Trichomonas vaginalis*** is a flagellated protozoan that is transmitted sexually.

CLINICAL MANIFESTATIONS
- Women: **vaginitis, cystitis, or cervicitis** - copious malodorous vaginal discharge worse with menses, postcoital bleeding, dyspareunia, dysuria, & frequency.
- Men: most men are asymptomatic but may develop urethritis.

PHYSICAL EXAMINATION
- **Copious frothy yellow-green vaginal discharge,** vulvovaginal erythema.
- **Cervical petechiae (strawberry cervix).**

DIAGNOSIS
- Microscopic examination (saline wet mount) – **mobile protozoan trophozoites**, vaginal pH >4.5, increased WBCs.
- Nucleic acid amplification test (NAAT) or culture should be performed if wet mount is negative.

MANAGEMENT
- **Metronidazole 2g oral dose x 1 dose** or 500mg bid x 7 days. Tinidazole alternative. Treatment is indicated for both symptomatic & asymptomatic men & women. **Partners must be treated.**
- Follow up: because of high rate of reinfection, retesting with NAAT performed within 3 months of initial treatment.
- Reinfection: Metronidazole 500mg orally bid x 7 days (single-dose therapy should be avoided if recurrent).

COMPLICATIONS
- Increased risk of HIV transmission, complications during pregnancy.

	BACTERIAL VAGINOSIS	TRICHOMONIASIS	CANDIDA	CYTOLYTIC VAGINITIS
PATHO PHYSIOLOGY	• Decreased Lactobacilli acidophilus (normally maintains vaginal pH) ⇨ overgrowth of normal flora ex ***GARDNERELLA VAGINALIS**, anaerobes*** *(Mobiluncus, Peptostreptococcus)* • ***MC cause of vaginitis*****	• ***TRICHOMONAS VAGINALIS:*** pear shaped flagellated protozoa • Sexually transmitted	• ***Candida albicans overgrowth*** (part of the normal flora due to change in normal vaginal environment (ex . use of abx) • ↑c DM, steroid, pregnancy	• *Overgrowth of **LACTOBACILLI***
CLINICAL MANIFESTATIONS	• Vaginal odor worse after sex • ± Pruritus • >50% asymptomatic	• Vulvar pruritus, erythema, dysuria • Dyspareunia	• Vaginal & vulvar erythema, swelling, burning, pruritus • Burning when urine touches skin, Dysuria, Dyspareunia	• Vaginal or vulvar pruritus & burning • Dysuria
VAGINAL DISCHARGE	• Copious discharge • ***Thin, homogenous, watery GREY-WHITE "FISH ROTTEN"* smell***	• Copious malodorous discharge • ***FROTHY YELLOW GREEN DISCHARGE**** worse c menses • ***STRAWBERRY CERVIX*: (cervical petechiae)***	• ***THICK CURD-LIKE/COTTAGE CHEESE DISCHARGE****	Nonodorous discharge white to opaque
VAGINAL pH	***>5***	***>5***	Normal (3.8- 4.2)	Normal (3.8- 4.2)
WHIFF TEST	*Positive: **FISHY ODOR*** with **10% KOH Prep***	May be present	Negative	Copious lactobacilli Large # of epithelial cells
MICROSCOPIC	• ***CLUE CELLS:**** epithelial cells covered by bacteria. • ***Few WBC's***, few lactobacilli	• Mobile protozoa (wet mount) • WBC's	• ***HYPHAE, YEAST**** & spores on KOH prep	
MANAGEMENT	• ***METRONIDAZOLE** (Flagyl) **x 7 days*** - Safe in pregnancy - May use gel or PO • ***CLINDAMYCIN*** - May use gel or PO	• ***METRONIDAZOLE*** (Flagyl) - ***2g oral x 1 dose*** OR - 500mg bid oral x 7days - Safe in pregnancy - ***Oral preferred*** • ***TINIDAZOLE***	• ***FLUCONAZOLE*** (PO x 1 dose) • ***Intravaginal antifungals*** - Clotrimazole, Nystatin - Butoconazole - Miconazole	• ***Discontinue tampon usage*** (to decrease vaginal acidity) • ***Sodium Bicarbonate*** - Sitz bath with $NaHCO_3$ - Douche with $NaHCO_3$
PREVENTION	• ***Avoid douching*** - Douching promotes loss of Lactobacilli • ***Treating partner unnecessary*** - Unclear if sexually transmitted. - But reduced recurrence if male uses condoms	• ***Spermicidal agents:*** ex. nonoxynol 9 reduces transmission ***MUST TREAT PARTNER***	• Keep vagina dry, 100% cotton underwear, avoid tight-fitting clothes, avoid use of feminine deodorants & bubble baths	
COMPLICATIONS	Pregnancy- PROM, preterm labor, chorioamnionitis.	Perinatal complications, ↑HIV transmission		

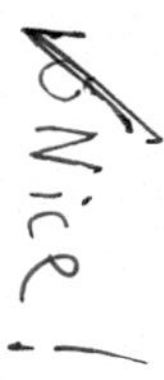

PHOTO CREDITS

Picture of Menstrual cycle
Kevin L. Young

A

I

J

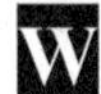

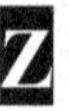

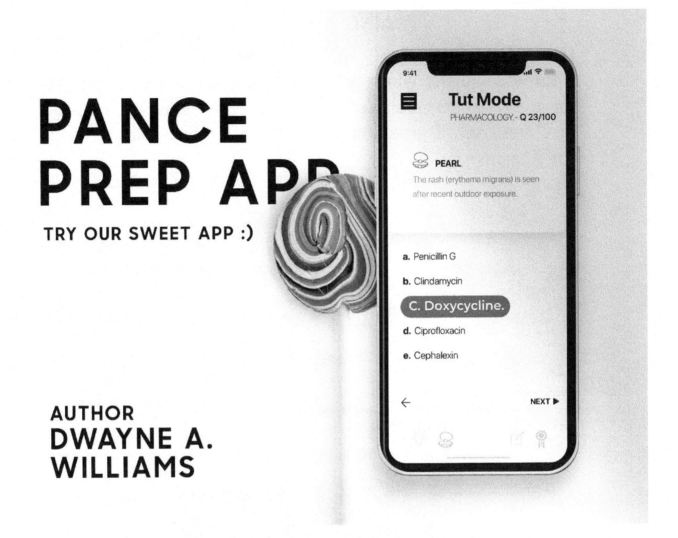

ALSO AVAILABLE

CYTOCHROME P450 INDUCERS

John was **worth**y when referred & <u>**inducted**</u> into sainthood for giving up **chronic alcohol** use & placing him**self on a real** fast, **fend**ing off **greasy carbs**, leading to **less warfare** with **theo**logians.

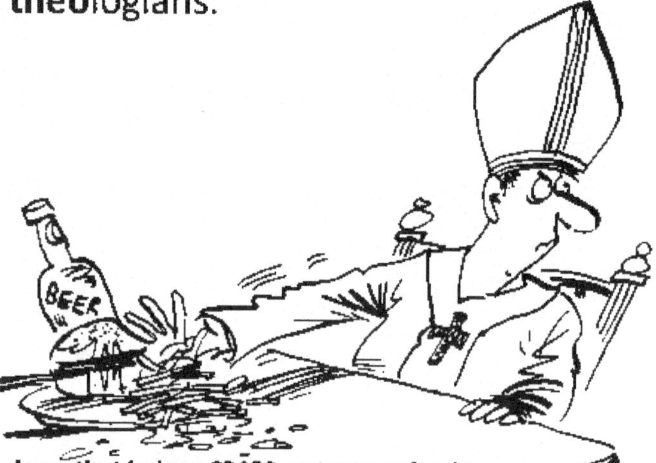

drugs that induce CP450 system can lead to decreased levels of certain drugs ex. warfarin (less warfare), theophylline (theologians) and phenytoin

<u>INDUCERS OF THE P450</u>

- **St. Johns Wort**
- **rifampin** (referred)
- **chronic alcohol use**
- **sulfonylureas** (self on a real)
- **Phenytoin**
- **Phenobarbital** (fend)
- **Griseofulvin** (greasy)
- **Carbamazepine** (carbs)

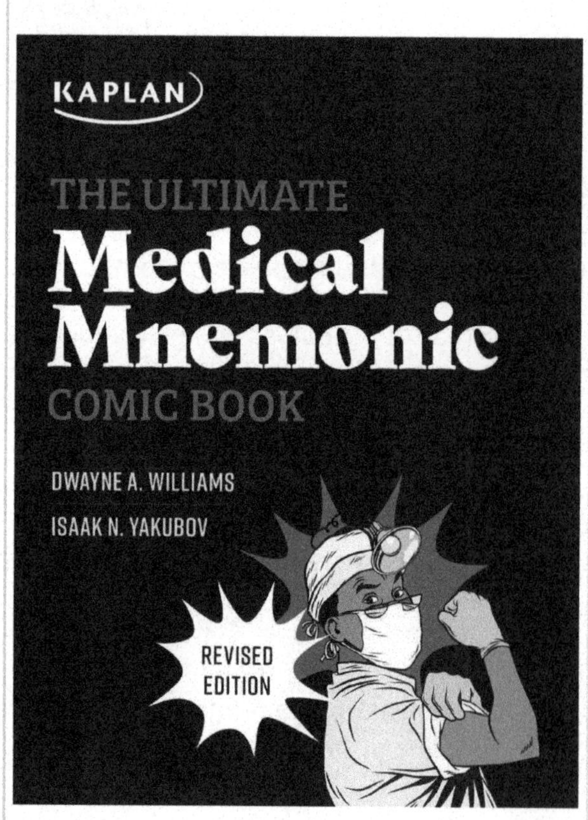

Made in USA - Kendallville, IN
1174365_9781712861165
10.19.2020 1427